Color Textbook of
Histology

Color Textbook of
Histology
Third Edition

LESLIE P. GARTNER, PhD

Professor of Anatomy
Department of Biomedical Sciences
Baltimore College of Dental Surgery
Dental School
University of Maryland
Baltimore, Maryland

JAMES L. HIATT, PhD

Professor Emeritus
Department of Biomedical Sciences
Baltimore College of Dental Surgery
Dental School
University of Maryland
Baltimore, Maryland

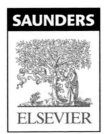

SAUNDERS

ELSEVIER

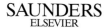

SAUNDERS
ELSEVIER

1600 John F. Kennedy Blvd.
Ste 1800
Philadelphia, PA 19103-2899

Notice

Neither the Publisher nor the Authors assume any responsibility for any loss or injury and/or damage to persons or property arising out of or related to any use of the material contained in this book. It is the responsibility of the treating practitioner, relying on independent expertise and knowledge of the patient, to determine the best treatment and method of application for the patient.

The Publisher

Library of Congress Control Number: 2006930093

Cover: *Top image* used with permission of Nature Publishing Group; from Smith CJ, Grigorieff N, Pearse BM: Clathrin coats at 21 Å resolution: A cellular assembly designed to recycle multiple membrane receptors. EMBO J 17:4943–4953, 1998. *Middle image* courtesy of Alexey Khodjakov, Wadsworth Center, Albany, New York. *Bottom image* courtesy of Drs. Gartner and Hiatt.

Acquisitions Editor: Inta Ozols
Developmental Editor: Jacquie Mahon
Publishing Services Manager: Linda Van Pelt
Project Manager: Joan Nikelsky
Design Direction: Gene Harris

Printed in China

Last digit is the print number: 9   8   7   6   5   4   3   2   1

To my wife Roseann,
my daughter Jennifer,
and my mother Mary

LPG

To my grandchildren
Nathan David,
James Mallary,
Hanna Elisabeth,
Alexandra Renate,
Eric James,
and Elise Victoria

JLH

■ ■ ■

Preface

Once again, we are gratified to release a new edition of a histology textbook that is well established not only in its original language but also in several other languages. The place of histology has changed as the biological sciences have progressed in the last half of the 20th century. It evolved from the purely descriptive science of microscopic anatomy to its current position as the linchpin between functional anatomy and molecular and cell biology.

This third edition, coming only a few short years after the second edition reached bookshelves, has been revised to reflect new information in cell and molecular biology that pertains to histology. While incorporating much new material we were mindful of the time constraints that students face due to an ever-expanding curriculum and an exponentially increasing information glut. We labored diligently to maintain readability and brevity. We revised many illustrations and added detail to figure legends.

The most visible, and we believe most valuable, addition for the student to this revision is the inclusion of a CD-ROM containing 21 brief PowerPoint presentations that give overviews of each chapter. They offer the student keys by which he or she can quickly form a basic understanding of the material.

The third edition of this textbook is bundled not only with the CD but also with access to Student Consult, a website developed by Elsevier publishing company that permits the purchaser of this book to view the entire text plus all images online. The website also provides seamless integration to related content in other Elsevier books that the reader has purchased, if that book is a title that has been selected to be a Student Consult title.

As in the first two editions, we have conveyed information as efficiently as possible. Tables and figures summarize complex topics to promote acquisition of knowledge. The text is punctuated by bulleted sections that not only organize important aspects of functional histology but also alert the reader to their significance. Important terms appear in bold type to permit rapid review as the student prepares for examinations. Clinical Correlation boxes illustrate the relevance of histology to students of the health professions. We believe that these features emphasize an important tenet of modern day histology—that structure and function are intimately related.

Although we have made every effort to present a complete and accurate account of the subject matter, we realize that there are omissions and errors in any undertaking of this magnitude. Therefore, we continue to encourage and welcome suggestions, advice, and criticism that will facilitate the improvement of this text.

Leslie P. Gartner
James L. Hiatt
lgartner@umaryland.edu

Acknowledgments

We would like to thank the following individuals for the help and support they provided in the preparation of this book. At the University of Maryland, special thanks go to Ms. Lyndsay C. Bare, a third-year dental student, for her many suggestions that helped to improve the presentation of the material.

We are truly grateful to Dr. Robert A. Bloodgood for providing us with an extensive list of suggestions for improvement. We also wish to thank Drs. Felipe A. Roberio and Joel Schechter for their helpful comments on topics related to their fields of expertise.

Histology is a visual subject; therefore, excellent graphic illustrations are imperative. For that we are indebted to Todd Smith for his careful attention to detail in revising and creating new illustrations. We also thank our many colleagues from around the world and their publishers who generously permitted us to borrow illustrative materials.

Finally, our thanks go to the project team at Elsevier for all their help, namely Inta Ozols, Jacqueline Mahon, and Joan Nikelsky.

Contents

Introduction to Histology and Basic Histological Techniques

Histology is that branch of anatomy that studies tissues of animals and plants. This textbook, however, discusses only animal, and more specifically human, tissues. In its broader aspect, the word *histology* is used as if it were a synonym for microscopic anatomy, because its subject matter encompasses not only the microscopic structure of tissues but also that of the cell, organs, and organ systems.

The body is composed of cells, intercellular matrix, and a fluid substance, extracellular fluid (tissue fluid), which bathes these components. Extracellular fluid, which is derived from plasma of blood, carries nutrients, oxygen, and signaling molecules to cells of the body. Conversely, signaling molecules, waste products, and carbon dioxide released by cells of the body reach blood and lymph vessels by way of the extracellular fluid. Extracellular fluid and much of the intercellular matrix are not visible in routine histological preparations, yet their invisible presence must be appreciated by the student of histology.

The subject of histology no longer merely deals with the structure of the body; it also concerns itself with the body's function. In fact, histology has a direct relationship to other disciplines and is essential for their understanding. This textbook, therefore, intertwines the disciplines of cell biology, biochemistry, physiology, embryology, gross anatomy, and, as appropriate, pathology. Students will recognize the importance of this subject as they refer to the text later in their careers. An excellent example of this relationship will be evident when the reader learns about the histology of the kidney and realizes it is the intricate and almost sublime structure of that organ (down to the molecular level) that is responsible for the kidney's ability to perform its function. Alterations of the kidney's structure are responsible for a great number of life-threatening conditions.

The remainder of this chapter discusses the methods used by histologists to study the microscopic anatomy of the body.

LIGHT MICROSCOPY

Tissue Preparation

Steps required in preparing tissues for light microscopy include (1) fixation, (2) dehydration and clearing, (3) embedding, (4) sectioning, and (5) mounting and staining the sections.

Various techniques have been developed to prepare tissues for study so that they closely resemble their natural, living state. The steps involved are **fixation, dehydration** and **clearing, embedding** in a suitable medium, **sectioning** into thin slices to permit viewing by transillumination, **mounting** sections onto a surface for ease of handling, and **staining** them so that the various tissue and cell components may be differentiated.

Fixation

Fixation refers to treatment of the tissue with chemical agents that not only retard the alterations of tissue subsequent to death (or after removal from the body) but also maintain its normal architecture. The most common fixative agents used in light microscopy are neutral buffered **formalin** and **Bouin's fluid.** Both of these substances cross-link proteins, thus maintaining a lifelike image of the tissue.

Dehydration and Clearing

Because a large fraction of the tissue is composed of water, a graded series of alcohol baths, beginning with 50% alcohol and progressing in graded steps to 100% alcohol, are used to remove the water *(dehydration)*. The tissue is then treated with xylene, a chemical that is miscible with melted paraffin. This process is known as *clearing*, because the tissue becomes transparent in xylene.

Embedding

In order to distinguish the overlapping cells in a tissue and the extracellular matrix from one another, the histologist must *embed* the tissues in a proper medium and then slice them into thin sections. For light microscopy, the usual embedding medium is paraffin. The tissue is placed in a suitable container of melted paraffin until it is completely **infiltrated.** Once the tissue is infiltrated with paraffin, it is placed into a small receptacle, covered with melted paraffin, and allowed to harden, forming a paraffin block containing the tissue.

Sectioning

After the blocks of tissue are trimmed of excess embedding material, they are mounted for sectioning. This task is performed using a microtome, a machine equipped with a blade and an arm that advances the tissue block in specific equal increments. For light microscopy, the thickness of each section is about 5 to 10 μm.

Sectioning also can be performed on specimens frozen either in liquid nitrogen or on the rapid-freeze bar of a cryostat. These sections are mounted by the use of a quick-freezing mounting medium and sectioned at subzero temperatures by means of a pre-cooled steel blade. The sections are placed on pre-cooled glass slides, permitted to come to room temperature, and stained with specific dyes (or treated for histochemical or immunocytochemical studies).

Mounting and Staining

Paraffin sections are mounted (placed) on glass slides and then stained by water-soluble stains that permit differentiation of the various cellular components.

The sections for conventional light microscopy, cut by stainless steel blades, are mounted on adhesive-coated glass slides. Because many tissue constituents have approximately the same optical densities, they must be stained for light microscopy, usually with water-soluble stains. Therefore, the paraffin must first be removed from the section, after which the tissue is rehydrated and stained. After staining, the section is again dehydrated so that the coverslip may be permanently affixed by the use of a suitable mounting medium. The coverslip not only protects the tissue from damage but also is necessary for viewing the section with the microscope.

Various types of stains have been developed for visualization of the many components of cells and tissues; they may be grouped into three classes:

■ Stains that differentiate between acidic and basic components of the cell
■ Specialized stains that differentiate the fibrous components of the extracellular matrix
■ Metallic salts that precipitate on tissues, forming metal deposits on them

The most commonly used stains in histology are **hematoxylin and eosin (H&E).** Hematoxylin is a base that preferentially colors the acidic components of the cell a bluish tint. Because the most acidic components are deoxyribonucleic acid (DNA) and ribonucleic acid (RNA), the nucleus and regions of the cytoplasm rich in ribosomes stain dark blue; these components are referred to as **basophilic.** Eosin is an acid that dyes the basic components of the cell a pinkish color. Because many cytoplasmic constituents have a basic pH, regions of the cytoplasm stain pink; these elements are said to be **acidophilic.** Many other stains are also used in preparation of specimens for histological study (Table 1-1).

Molecules of some stains, such as **toluidine blue,** polymerize with each other when exposed to high concentrations of polyanions in tissue. These aggregates differ in color from their individual molecules. For example, toluidine blue stains tissues blue except for those that are rich in polyanions (e.g., cartilage matrix and granules of mast cells), which stain purple. A tissue or cell component that stains purple with this stain is said to be **metachromatic,** and toluidine blue is said to exhibit **metachromasia.**

Light Microscopes

Compound microscopes are composed of a specific arrangement of lenses that permit a high magnification and good resolution of the tissues being viewed.

The present-day light microscope uses a specific arrangement of groups of lenses to magnify an image (Fig. 1-1). Because this instrument uses more than just a single lens, it is known as a **compound microscope.** The light source is an electric bulb with a tungsten filament whose light is gathered into a focused beam by the **condenser lens.**

The light beam is located below and is focused on the specimen. Light passing through the specimen

Table 1–1 Common Histological Stains and Reactions

Reagent	Result
Hematoxylin	*Blue:* nucleus; acidic regions of the cytoplasm; cartilage matrix
Eosin	*Pink:* basic regions of the cytoplasm; collagen fibers
Masson's trichrome	*Dark blue:* nuclei *Red:* muscle, keratin, cytoplasm *Light blue:* mucinogen, collagen
Orcein's elastic stain	*Brown:* elastic fibers
Weigert's elastic stain	*Blue:* elastic fibers
Silver stain	*Black:* reticular fibers
Iron hematoxylin	*Black:* striations of muscle, nuclei, erythrocytes
Periodic acid–Schiff	*Magenta:* glycogen and carbohydrate-rich molecules
Wright's and Giemsa stains (used for differential staining of blood cells)	*Pink:* erythrocytes, eosinophil granules *Blue:* cytoplasm of monocytes and lymphocytes

enters one of the objective lenses; these lenses sit on a movable turret located just above the specimen. Usually four objective lenses are available on a single turret, providing low, medium, high, and oil magnifications. Generally, in most microscopes the first three lenses magnify 4, 10, and 40 times, respectively, and are used without oil; the oil lens magnifies the image 100 times.

The image from the objective lens is gathered and further magnified by the ocular lens of the eyepiece. This lens usually magnifies the image by a factor of 10—for total magnifications of 40, 100, 400, and 1000—and focuses the resulting image on the retina of the eye.

Focusing of the image is performed by the use of knurled knobs that move the objective lenses up or down above the specimen. The coarse-focus knob moves it in larger increments than the fine-focus knob does. It is interesting that the image projected on the retina is reversed from right to left and is upside down.

The quality of an image depends not only on the capability of a lens to magnify but also on its **resolution**—the ability of the lens to show that two distinct objects are separated by a distance. The quality of a lens depends on how close its resolution approaches the theoretical limit of 0.25 μm, a restriction that is determined by the wavelength of visible light.

There are several types of light microscopes, distinguished by the type of light used as a light source and the manner in which they use the light source. However, most students of histology are required to recognize only images obtained from compound light microscopy, transmission electron microscopy, and scanning electron microscopy; therefore, the other types of light microscopes are not discussed.

Digital Imaging Techniques

Digital imaging techniques employ computer technology to capture and manipulate histologic images.

The advent of computer technology has provided a means of capturing images digitally, without the use of film. Although this method of image capturing cannot yet compete with film technology, it has several advantages that make it a valuable tool:

■ Immediate visualization of the acquired image
■ Digital modification of the image
■ Capability of enhancing the image by the use of commercially available software

In addition, because these images are stored in a digital format, hundreds of them may be archived on a single CD-ROM disk and their retrieval is almost instantaneous. Finally, their digital format permits the electronic transmission of these images by e-mail or distribution via the Internet.

Interpretation of Microscopic Sections

One of the most difficult, frustrating, and time-consuming skills needed in histology is interpreting what a two-dimensional section looks like in three dimensions. If you imagine a coiled garden hose and then take thin sections from that hose, you will see that the three-dimensional object is not necessarily discerned from any *one* of the two-dimensional sections (Fig. 1-2). However, by viewing all of the sections drawn from the coiled tube, you can mentally reconstruct the correct three-dimensional image.

Advanced Visualization Procedures
Histochemistry

Histochemistry is a method of staining tissue that provides information about the presence and location of intracellular and extracellular macromolecules.

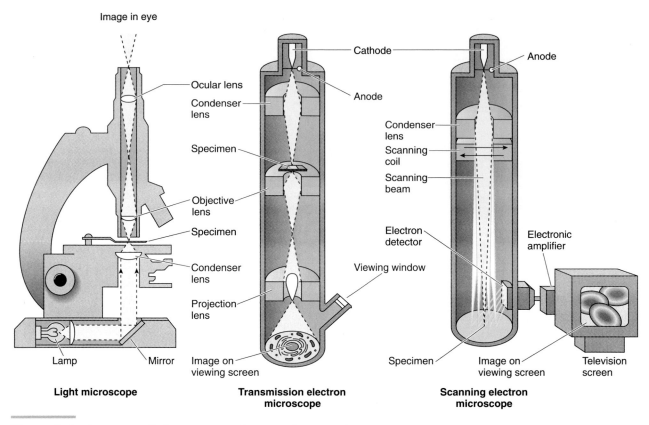

Light microscope

Image in eye
Ocular lens
Objective lens
Specimen
Condenser lens
Lamp
Mirror

Transmission electron microscope

Cathode
Anode
Condenser lens
Specimen
Objective lens
Specimen
Condenser lens
Projection lens
Viewing window
Image on viewing screen

Scanning electron microscope

Anode
Condenser lens
Scanning coil
Scanning beam
Electron detector
Electronic amplifier
Specimen
Image on viewing screen
Television screen

Figure 1–1 Comparison of light, transmission electron, and scanning electron microscopes.

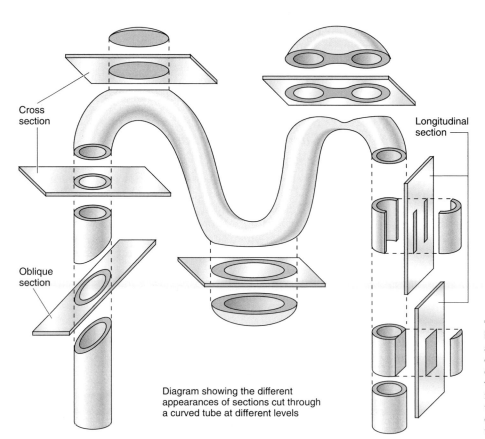

Cross section

Oblique section

Longitudinal section

Diagram showing the different appearances of sections cut through a curved tube at different levels

Figure 1–2 Histology requires a mental reconstruction of two-dimensional images into the three-dimensional solid from which they were sectioned. Here, a curved tube is sectioned in various planes to illustrate the relationship between a series of two-dimensional sections and their three-dimensional structure.

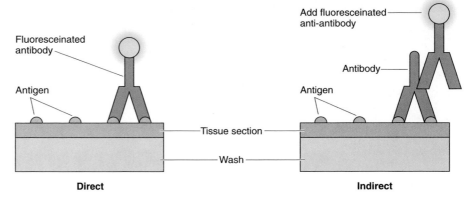

Figure 1–3 Direct and indirect methods of immunocytochemistry. *Left,* An antibody against the antigen was labeled with a fluorescent dye and viewed with a fluorescent microscope. The fluorescence occurs only over the location of the antibody. *Right,* Fluorescent-labeled antibodies are prepared against an antibody that reacts with a particular antigen. When viewed with fluorescent microscopy, the region of fluorescence represents the location of the antibody.

Specific chemical constituents of tissues and cells can be localized by the methods of histochemistry and cytochemistry. These methods capitalize on the enzyme activity, chemical reactivity, and other physicochemical phenomena associated with the constituent of interest. Reactions of interest are monitored by the formation of an insoluble precipitate that takes on a certain color. Frequently, histochemistry is performed on frozen tissues and can be applied to both light and electron microscopy.

A common histochemical reaction uses the periodic acid–Schiff (PAS) reagent, which forms a magenta precipitate with molecules rich in glycogen and carbohydrate-rich molecules. To ensure that the reaction is specific for glycogen, consecutive sections are treated with amylase. Thus, sections not treated with amylase display a magenta deposit, whereas amylase-treated sections display a lack of staining in the same region.

Although enzymes can be localized by histochemical procedures, the product of enzymatic reaction rather than the enzyme itself is visualized. The reagent is designed so that the product precipitates at the site of the reaction and is visible either as a metallic or a colored deposit.

Immunocytochemistry

> *Immunocytochemistry uses fluoresceinated antibodies and anti-antibodies to provide more precise intracellular and extracellular localization of macromolecules than is possible with histochemistry.*

Although histochemical procedures permit relatively good localization of some enzymes and macromolecules in cells and tissues, more precise localization can be achieved by the use of immunocytochemistry. This procedure requires developing an antibody against the particular macromolecule to be localized and labeling the antibody with a fluorescent dye such as fluorescein or rhodamine.

There are two methods of antibody labeling: direct and indirect. In the **direct method** (Fig. 1-3) the antibody against the macromolecule is labeled with a fluorescent dye. The antibody is then permitted to react with the macromolecule, and the resultant complex may be viewed with a fluorescent microscope (Fig. 1-4).

In the **indirect method** (see Fig. 1-3) a fluorescent-labeled antibody is prepared against the primary antibody specific for the macromolecule of interest. Once the primary antibody has reacted with the antigen, the preparation is washed to remove unbound primary antibody; the labeled antibody is then added and reacts with the original antigen-antibody complex, forming a secondary complex visible by fluorescent microscopy (Fig. 1-5). The indirect method is more sensitive than the direct method because numerous labeled anti-antibodies bind to the primary antibody, making them easier to visualize. In addition, the indirect method does not require labeling of the primary antibody, which often is available only in limited quantities.

Immunocytochemistry can be used with specimens for electron microscopy by labeling the antibody with ferritin, an electron-dense molecule, instead of with a fluorescent dye. Ferritin labeling can be applied in both the direct and indirect methods.

Autoradiography

> *Autoradiography is a method that uses the incorporation of radioactive isotopes into macromolecules, which are then visualized by the use of an overlay of film emulsion.*

Autoradiography (or radioautography) is a particularly useful method for localizing and investigating a specific temporal sequence of events. The method requires incorporation of a radioactive isotope—most commonly tritium (^{3}H)—into the compound being studied (Fig. 1-6). An example is the use of tritiated amino acid to

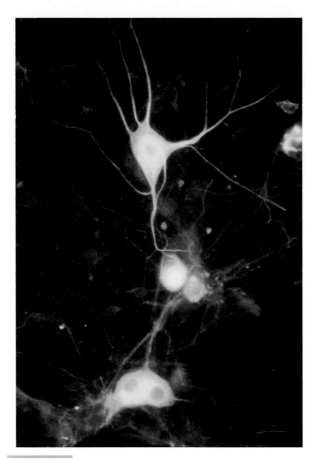

Figure 1–4 Example of direct immunocytochemistry. Cultured neurons from rat superior cervical ganglion were immunostained with fluorescent-labeled antibody specific for the insulin receptor. The bright areas correspond to sites where the antibody has bound to insulin receptors. The staining pattern indicates that receptors are located throughout the cytoplasm of the soma and processes but are missing from the nucleus. (From James S, Patel N, Thomas P, Burnstock G: Immunocytochemical localisation of insulin receptors on rat superior cervical ganglion neurons in dissociated cell culture. J Anat 182:95-100, 1993.)

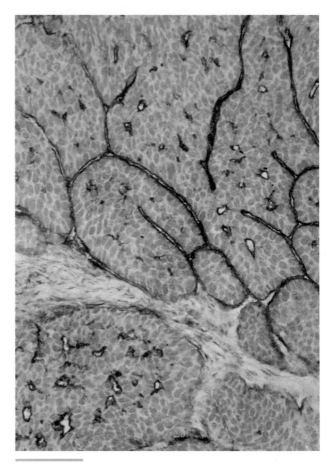

Figure 1–5 Indirect immunocytochemistry. Fluorescent antibodies were prepared against primary antibodies against type IV collagen, to demonstrate the presence of a continuous basal lamina at the interface between malignant clusters of cells and the surrounding connective tissue. (From Kopf-Maier P, Schroter-Kermani C: Distribution of type VII collagen in xenografted human carcinomas. Cell Tissue Res 272:395-405, 1993.)

track the synthesis and packaging of proteins. After the radiolabeled compound is injected into an animal, tissue specimens are taken at selected time intervals. The tissue is processed as usual and placed on a glass slide; however, instead of the tissue being sealed with a coverslip, a thin layer of photographic emulsion is placed over it. The tissue is placed in a dark box for a few days or weeks, during which time particles emitted from the radioactive isotope expose the emulsion over the cell sites where the isotope is located. The emulsion is developed and fixed by means of photographic techniques, and small silver grains are left over the exposed portions of the emulsion. The specimen then is sealed with a coverslip and viewed with a light micro-

scope. The silver grains are positioned over the regions of the specimen that incorporated the radioactive compound.

Autoradiography has been used to follow the time course of incorporation of tritiated proline into the basement membrane underlying endodermal cells of the yolk sac (see Fig. 1-6). An adaptation of the autoradiography method of electron microscopy has been used to show that the tritiated proline first appears in the cytosol of the endodermal cells, then travels to the rough endoplasmic reticulum, then to the Golgi apparatus, then into vesicles, and finally into the extracellular matrix (Fig. 1-7). In this manner, the sequence of events occurring in the synthesis of type IV collagen—the main protein in the lamina densa of the basal lamina—was visually demonstrated.

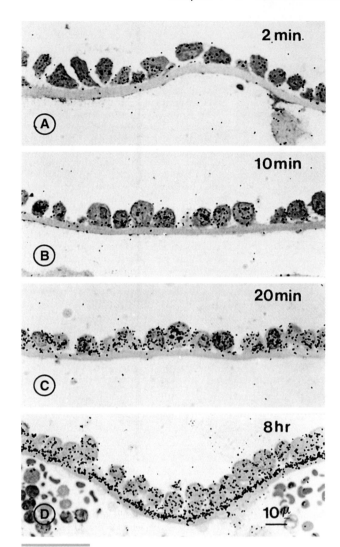

Figure 1–6 Autoradiography. Light microscopic examination of tritiated proline incorporation into the basement membrane as a function of time subsequent to tritiated proline injection (scale bar = 10 μ). In light micrographs A to C, the silver grains *(black dots)* are localized mostly in the endodermal cells; after 8 hours (light micrograph D), however, the silver grains are also localized in the basement membrane. The presence of silver grains indicates the location of tritiated proline. (From Mazariegos MR, Leblond CP, van der Rest M: Radioautographic tracing of ³H-proline in endodermal cells of the parietal yolk sac as an indicator of the biogenesis of basement membrane components. Am J Anat 179:79-93, 1987.)

CONFOCAL MICROSCOPY

Confocal microscopy relies on a laser beam for the light source and a pinhole screen to eliminate undesirable reflected light from being observed. Thus, the only light that can be observed is that which is located at the focal point of the objective lens, making the pinhole conjugate of the focal point.

In confocal microscopy, a laser beam passes through a dichroic mirror to be focused on the specimen by two motorized mirrors whose movements are computer-controlled to scan the beam along the sample. Because the sample is treated by fluorescent dyes, the impinging laser beam causes the emission of light from the dyes. The emitted light follows the same path taken by the laser beam, but in the opposite direction, and the dichroic mirror focuses this emitted light on a pinhole in a plate. A photomultiplier tube collects the emitted light passing through the pinhole while the plate containing the pinhole blocks all the extraneous light that would create a fuzzy image. It must be remembered that the light emerging from the pinhole at any particular moment in time represents a single point in the sample, and as the laser beam scans across the sample additional individual points are collected by the photomultiplier tube. All of these points gathered by the photomultiplier tube are then compiled by a computer, forming a composite image one pixel at a time (Fig. 1-8). Since the depth of field is very small (only a thin layer of the sample is observed at any one scan), the scanning may be repeated at deeper and deeper levels in the sample, allowing the compilation of a very good three-dimensional image (Fig. 1-9).

ELECTRON MICROSCOPY

The use of electrons as a light source in electron microscopy permits the achievement of much greater magnification and resolution than that realized by light microscopy.

In light microscopes, optical lenses focus visible light (a beam of photons). In electron microscopes, electromagnets serve the function of focusing a beam of electrons. Because the wavelength of an electron beam is much shorter than that of visible light, electron microscopes theoretically are capable of resolving two objects separated by 0.005 nm. In practice, however, the resolution of the **transmission electron microscope** is about 0.2 nm, which is still more than a thousand-fold greater than the resolution of the compound light microscope. The resolution of the **scanning electron microscope** is about 10 nm, considerably less than that of the transmission electron microscope. Moreover, modern electron microscopes can magnify an object as much as 150,000 times; this magnification is powerful enough to see individual macromolecules such as DNA and myosin.

Transmission Electron Microscopy

Transmission electron microscopy (TEM) uses much thinner sections compared with light microscopy and requires heavy metal precipitation techniques rather than water-soluble stains to stain tissues.

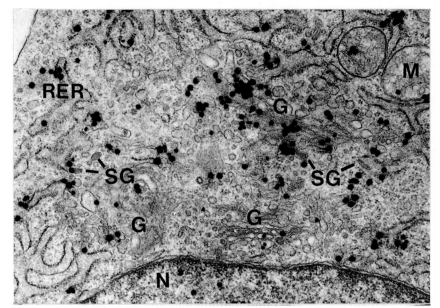

Figure 1–7 Autoradiography. In this electron micrograph of a yolk sac endodermal cell, silver grains (similar to those in Figure 1-6), representing the presence of tritiated proline, are evident overlying the rough endoplasmic reticulum (RER), Golgi apparatus (G), and secretory granules (SG). Type IV collagen, which is rich in proline, is synthesized in endodermal cells and released into the basement membrane. The tritiated proline is most concentrated in organelles involved in protein synthesis. M, mitochondria; N, nucleus. (From Mazariegos MR, Leblond CP, van der Rest M: Radioautographic tracing of ^{3}H-proline in endodermal cells of the parietal yolk sac as an indicator of the biogenesis of basement membrane components. Am J Anat 179:79-93, 1987.)

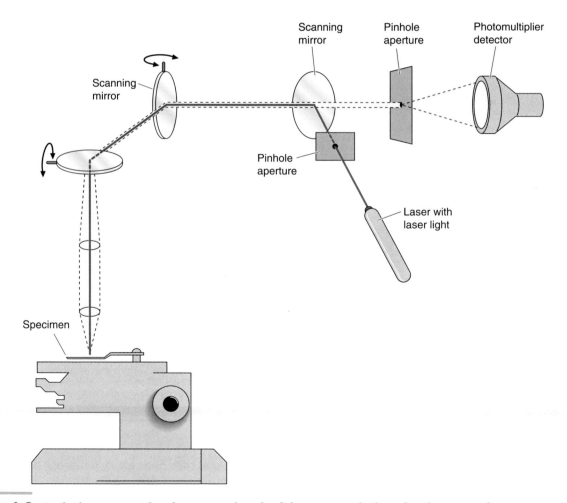

Figure 1–8 Confocal microscopy. A laser beam passes through a dichroic mirror to be focused on the specimen by two motorized mirrors whose movements are computer-controlled to scan the beam along the sample. The light emerging from the pinhole at any particular moment in time represents a single point in the sample, and as the laser beam scans across the sample additional individual points are collected by the photomultiplier tube. All the points are computer-assembled to produce the final confocal image.

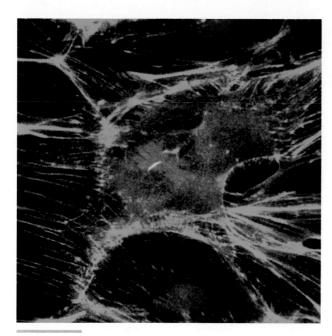

Figure 1–9 Confocal image of a metaphase Kangaroo rat cell (PtK2) stained with FITC-phalloidin for F-actin (*green*) and propidium iodide for chromosomes (*red*). (Courtesy of Dr. Matthew Schibler, University of California Brain Research Institute, Los Angeles, California.)

Preparation of tissue specimens for TEM involves the same basic steps as in light microscopy. Special fixatives have been developed for use with transmission light microscopy, because the greater resolving power of the electron microscope requires finer and more specific cross-linking of proteins. These fixatives, which include buffered solutions of **glutaraldehyde, paraformaldehyde, osmium tetroxide,** and **potassium permanganate,** not only preserve fine structural details but also act as electron-dense stains, which permit observation of the tissue with the electron beam.

Because these fixatives penetrate fresh tissues even less than fixatives for light microscopy, relatively small pieces of tissues are infiltrated in large volumes of fixatives. Tissue blocks for TEM are usually no larger than 1 mm^3. Suitable embedding media have been developed, such as epoxy resin, so that plastic-embedded tissues may be cut into extremely thin (ultra-thin) sections (25 to 100 nm) that do not absorb the beam of electrons.

Electron beams are produced in an evacuated chamber by heating a tungsten filament, the **cathode.** The electrons then are attracted to the positively charged **anode,** a donut-shaped metal plate with a central hole. With a charge differential of about 60,000 volts placed between the cathode and the anode, the electrons that pass through the hole in the anode have high kinetic energy.

The electron beam is focused on the specimen by the use of electromagnets, which are analogous to the condenser lens of a light microscope (see Fig. 1-1). Because the tissue is stained with heavy metals that precipitate preferentially on lipid membranes, the electrons lose some of their kinetic energy as they interact with the tissue. The heavier the metal encountered by an electron, the less energy the electron will retain.

The electrons leaving the specimen are subjected to the electromagnetic fields of several additional electromagnets, which focus the beam on a fluorescent plate. As the electrons hit the fluorescent plate, their kinetic energy is converted into points of light, whose intensity is a direct function of the electron's kinetic energy. You can make a permanent record of the resultant image by substituting an electron-sensitive film in place of the fluorescent plate and by producing a negative from which a black and white photomicrograph can be printed.

Freeze-Fracture Technique

The macromolecular structure of the internal aspects of membranes is revealed by the freeze-fracture technique (Fig. 1-10). Quick-frozen specimens that have been treated with cryopreservatives do not develop ice crystals during the freezing process; hence, the tissue does not suffer mechanical damage. As the frozen specimen is hit by a super-cooled razor blade, it fractures along cleavage planes, which are regions of least molecular bonding; in cells, fracture frequently occurs between the inner and outer leaflets of membranes.

The fracture face is coated at an angle by evaporated platinum and carbon, forming accumulations of platinum on one side of a projection and no accumulation on the opposite side next to the projection, thus generating a replica of the surface. The tissue is then digested away, and the replica is examined by TEM. This method allows display of the transmembrane proteins of cellular membranes.

Scanning Electron Microscopy

Scanning electron microscopy (SEM) provides a three-dimensional image of the specimen.

Unlike TEM, SEM is used to view the surface of a solid specimen. Using this technique, you can view a three-dimensional image of the object. Usually, the object to be viewed is prepared in a special manner that permits a thin layer of heavy metal, such as gold

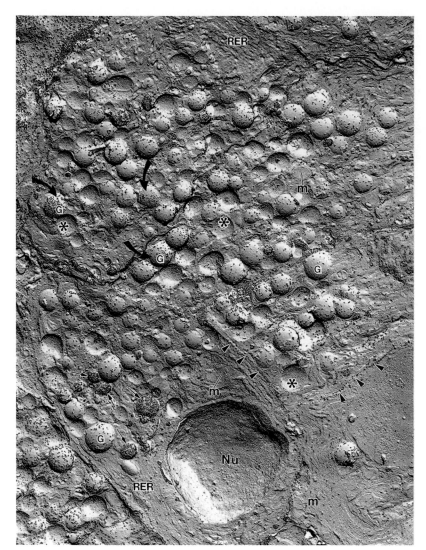

Figure 1-10 Cytochemistry and freeze-fracture. Fracture-label replica of an acinar cell of the rat pancreas. *N*-acetyl-D-galactosamine residues were localized by the use of *Helix pomatia* lectin-gold complex, which appears as black dots in the image. Arrowheads indicate cell membranes. The nucleus (Nu) appears as a depression, the rough endoplasmic reticulum (RER) as parallel lines, and secretory granules as small elevations or depressions. The elevations (G) represent the E-face half, and the depressions *(asterisks)* represent the P-face of the membrane of the secretory granule. m, mitochondria. (From Kan FWK, Bendayan M: Topographical and planar distribution of *Helix pomatia* lectin-binding glycoconjugates in secretory granules and plasma membrane of pancreatic acinar cells of the rat: Demonstration of membrane heterogeneity. Am J Anat 185:165-176, 1989.)

or palladium, to be deposited on the specimen's surface.

As a beam of electrons scans the surface of the object, some (backscatter electrons) are reflected and others (secondary electrons) are ejected from the heavy metal coat. The backscatter and secondary electrons are captured by electron detectors that are interpreted, collated, and displayed on a monitor as a three-dimensional image (see Fig. 1-1). You can make the image permanent either by photographing it or digitizing it for storage in a computer.

2

Cytoplasm

Cells are the basic functional units of complex organisms. Cells that are related or are similar to each other as well as cells that function in a particular manner or serve a common purpose are grouped together to form **tissues.** The four basic tissues (epithelium, connective tissues, muscle, and nervous tissue) that compose the body are assembled to form **organs** which, in turn, are collected into **organ systems.** The task of each organ system is specific, in that it performs a collection of associated functions, such as digestion, reproduction, and respiration.

Although the human body is composed of more than 200 different types of cells, each performing a different function, all cells possess certain unifying characteristics and thus can be described in general terms. Every cell is surrounded by a bilipid plasma membrane, possesses organelles that permit it to discharge its functions, synthesizes macromolecules for its own use or for export, produces energy, and is capable of communicating with other cells (Figs. 2-1 to 2-4).

Protoplasm, the living substance of the cell, is subdivided into two compartments: **cytoplasm,** extending from the plasma membrane to the nuclear envelope, and **karyoplasm,** the substance forming the contents of the nucleus. The cytoplasm is detailed in this chapter; the nucleus is discussed in Chapter 3.

The bulk of the cytoplasm is **water,** in which various inorganic and organic chemicals are dissolved and/or suspended. This fluid suspension is called the **cytosol.** The cytosol contains **organelles,** metabolically active structures that perform distinctive functions (Figs. 2-5 and 2-6). Additionally, the shapes of cells, their ability to move, and the intracellular pathways within cells are maintained by a system of tubules and filaments known as the **cytoskeleton.**

Finally, cells contain **inclusions,** which consist of metabolic by-products, storage forms of various nutrients, and inert crystals and pigments. The following topics discuss the structure and functions of the major constituents of the organelles, cytoskeleton, and inclusions.

ORGANELLES

Organelles are metabolically active cellular structures that execute specific functions.

Although some organelles were discovered by light microscopists, their structure and function were not elucidated until the advent of electron microscopy, separation techniques, and sensitive biochemical and histochemical procedures. As a result of the application of these methods, it is now known that the membranes of organelles are composed of a phospholipid bilayer, which not only partitions the cell into compartments but also provides large surface areas for the biochemical reactions essential for the maintenance of life.

Cell Membrane

The cell membrane forms a selectively permeable barrier between the cytoplasm and the external milieu.

Each cell is bounded by a cell membrane (also known as the **plasma membrane** or **plasmalemma**) that functions in:

- Maintaining the structural integrity of the cell
- Controlling movements of substances in and out of the cell (selective permeability)
- Regulating cell–cell interactions
- Recognizing, via receptors, antigens and foreign cells as well as altered cells
- Acting as an interface between the cytoplasm and the external milieu
- Establishing transport systems for specific molecules
- Transducing extracellular physical or chemical signals into intracellular events.

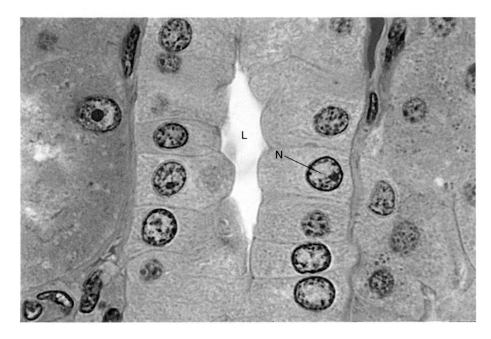

Figure 2–1 Light micrograph of typical cells from the renal cortex of a monkey (×975). Note the blue nucleus (N) and the pink cytoplasm. The boundaries of individual cells may be easily distinguished. The white area in the middle of the field is the lumen (L) of a collecting tubule.

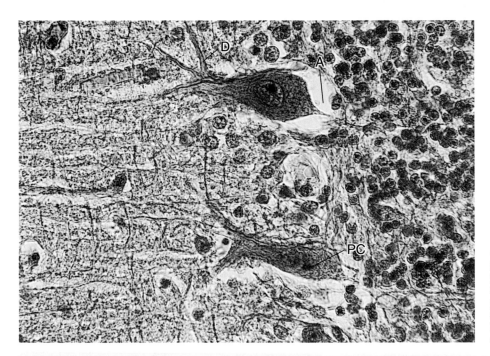

Figure 2-2 Purkinje cells (PC) from the cerebellum of a monkey (×540). Observe the long, branching processes, dendrites (D), and axon (A), of these cells. The nucleus is located in the widest portion of the cell.

Cell membranes are not visible with the light microscope. In electron micrographs, the plasmalemma is about 7.5 nm thick and appears as a trilaminar structure of two thin, dense lines with an intervening light area. Each layer is about 2.5 nm in width, and the entire structure is known as the **unit membrane** (Fig. 2-7). The inner (cytoplasmic) dense line is its **inner leaflet;** the outer dense line is its **outer leaflet.**

Molecular Composition

The plasmalemma is composed of a phospholipid bilayer and associated integral and peripheral proteins.

Each leaflet is composed of a single layer of **phospholipids** and associated **proteins,** usually in a 1:1 proportion by weight. In certain cases, such as myelin sheaths,

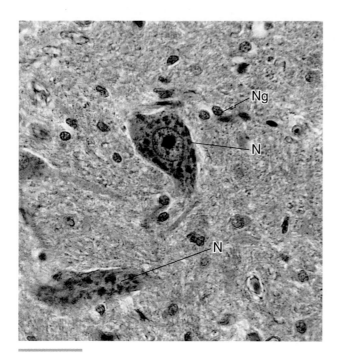

Figure 2–3 Motor neurons from the human spinal cord (×540). These nerve cells have numerous processes (axons and dendrites). The centrally placed nucleus and the single large nucleolus are clearly visible. The Nissl bodies (N; rough endoplasmic reticulum) are the most conspicuous features of the cytoplasm. Observe also the small nuclei of the neuroglia cells (Ng).

however, the lipid component outweighs the protein component by a ratio of 4 : 1. The two leaflets, composing a **lipid bilayer** in which **proteins** are suspended, constitute the basic structure of all membranes of the cell (Fig. 2-8).

Each phospholipid molecule of the lipid bilayer is composed of a **polar head,** located at the surface of the membrane, and two long **nonpolar** fatty acyl tails projecting into the center of the plasmalemma (see Fig. 2-8). The nonpolar fatty acyl tails of the two layers face each other within the membrane and form weak noncovalent bonds with each other, holding the bilayer together. Because the phospholipid molecule is composed of a **hydrophilic** head and a **hydrophobic** tail, the molecule is said to be **amphipathic.**

The polar heads are composed of **glycerol,** to which a positively charged nitrogenous group is attached by a negatively charged **phosphate group.** The two fatty acyl tails, only one of which is usually saturated, are covalently bound to glycerol. Other amphipathic molecules, such as **glycolipids** and **cholesterol,** are also present in the cell membrane. The unsaturated fatty acyl molecules increase membrane fluidity, whereas cholesterol decreases it (although cholesterol concentrations much lower than normal increase membrane fluidity).

The protein components of the plasmalemma either span the entire lipid bilayer as **integral proteins** or are attached to the cytoplasmic aspect (and at times the extracellular aspect) of the lipid bilayer as **peripheral proteins.** Because most integral proteins pass through

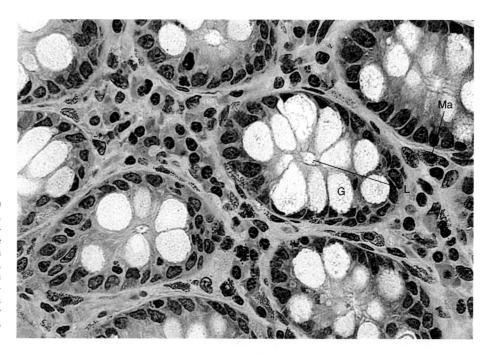

Figure 2–4 Goblet cells (G) from the monkey colon (×540). Some cells, such as goblet cells, specialize in secreting materials. These cells accumulate mucinogen, which occupies much of the cells' volume, and then release it into the lumen (L) of the intestine. During the processing of the tissue, the mucinogen is extracted, leaving behind empty spaces. Observe the presence of a mast cell (Ma).

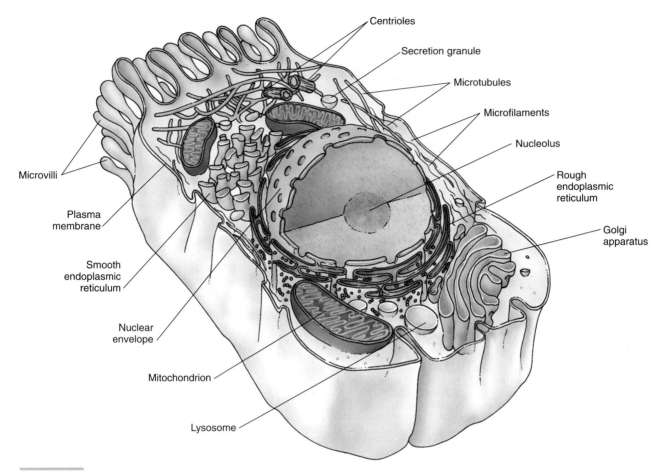

Figure 2–5 Three-dimensional illustration of an idealized cell, as visualized by transmission electron microscopy. Various organelles and cytoskeletal elements are displayed.

the thickness of the membrane, they are also referred to as **transmembrane proteins.** Those regions of transmembrane proteins that project into the cytoplasm or the extracellular space are composed of hydrophilic amino acids, whereas the intramembrane region consists of hydrophobic amino acids. Transmembrane proteins frequently form ion channels and carrier proteins that facilitate the passage of specific ions and molecules across the cell membrane.

Many of these transmembrane proteins are quite long and are folded so that they make several passes through the membrane and thus are known as **multipass proteins.** The cytoplasmic and extracytoplasmic aspects of these proteins commonly possess receptor sites that are specific for particular **signaling molecules.** Once these molecules are recognized at these receptor sites, the integral proteins can alter their conformation and can perform a specific function.

Because the same integral membrane proteins have the ability to float like icebergs in the sea of phospho-

lipids, this model is referred to as the **fluid mosaic model** of membrane structure. However, the integral proteins frequently possess only limited mobility, especially in polarized cells, in which particular regions of the cell serve specialized functions.

Peripheral proteins do not usually form covalent bonds with either the integral proteins or the phospholipid components of the cell membrane. Although they are usually located on the cytoplasmic aspect of the cell membrane, they may also be on the extracellular surface. These proteins may form bonds either with the phospholipid molecules or with the transmembrane proteins. Frequently, they are associated with the secondary messenger system of the cell (see below) or with the cytoskeletal apparatus.

Using freeze-fracture techniques, you can cleave the plasma membrane into its two leaflets in order to view the hydrophobic surfaces (Figs. 2-9 and 2-10). The outer surface of the inner leaflet is referred to as the **P-face** (closer to the *p*rotoplasm); the inner surface of

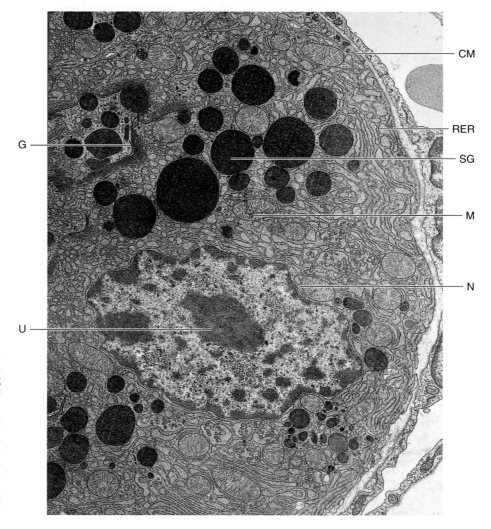

CM

RER

SG

M

N

G

U

Figure 2–6 Electron micrograph of an acinar cell from the urethral gland of a mouse illustrating the appearance of some organelles (×11,327). CM, cell membrane; G, Golgi apparatus; M, mitochondria; N, nucleus; RER, rough endoplasmic reticulum; SG, secretory granules; U, nucleolus. (From Parr MB, Ren HP, Kepple L, et al: Ultrastructure and morphometry of the urethral glands in normal, castrated, and testosterone-treated castrated mice. Anat Rec 236:449-458, 1993.)

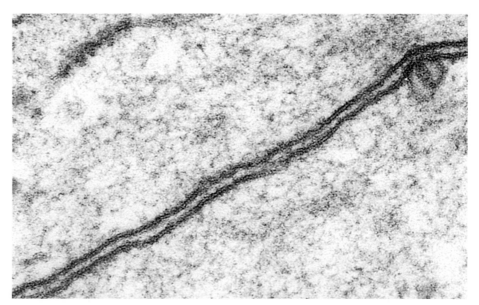

Figure 2–7 Electron micrograph showing a junction between two cells that demonstrates the trilaminar structures of the two cell membranes (×240,000). (From Leeson TS, Leeson CR, Papparo AA: Text/Atlas of Histology. Philadelphia, WB Saunders, 1988.)

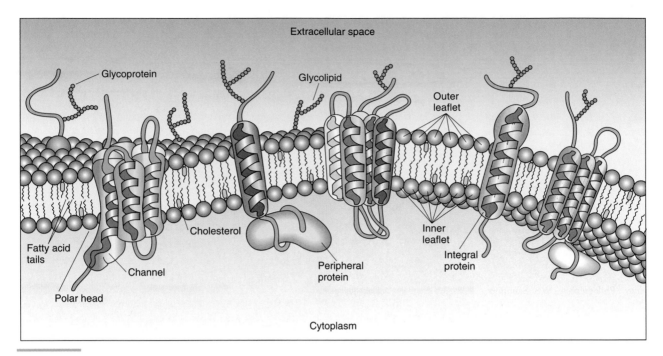

Figure 2–8 A fluid mosaic model of the cell membrane.

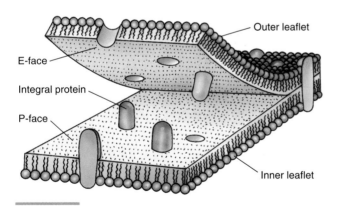

Figure 2–9 The E-face and the P-face of the cell membrane.

the outer leaflet is known as the **E-face** (closer to the *e*xtracellular space). Electron micrographs of freeze-fractured plasma membranes show that the integral proteins, visualized by shadowing replica, are more numerous on the P-face than on the E-face (see Fig. 2-10).

Glycocalyx

Glycocalyx, composed usually of carbohydrate chains, coats the cell surface.

A fuzzy coat, referred to as the **cell coat,** or glycocalyx, is often evident in electron micrographs of the cell membrane. This coat is usually composed of carbohydrate chains that are covalently attached to transmembrane proteins and/or phospholipid molecules of the outer leaflet (see Fig. 2-8). Additionally, some of the extracellular matrix molecules, adsorbed to the cell surface, also contribute to its formation. Its intensity and thickness vary, but it may be as thick as 50 nm on some epithelial sheaths, such as those lining regions of the digestive system.

Because of its numerous negatively charged sulfate and carboxyl groups, the glycocalyx stains intensely with lectins as well as with dyes such as ruthenium red and Alcian blue, permitting its visualization with light microscopy. The most important function of the glycocalyx is protection of the cell from interaction with inappropriate proteins, from chemical injury, and from physical injury. Other cell coat functions include cell–cell recognition and adhesion, as occurs between endothelial cells and neutrophils, in blood clotting, and in inflammatory responses.

Membrane Transport Proteins

Membrane transport proteins are of two types, channel proteins and carrier proteins; they facilitate the movement of aqueous molecules and ions across the plasmalemma.

Although the hydrophobic components of the plasma membrane limit the movement of polar molecules

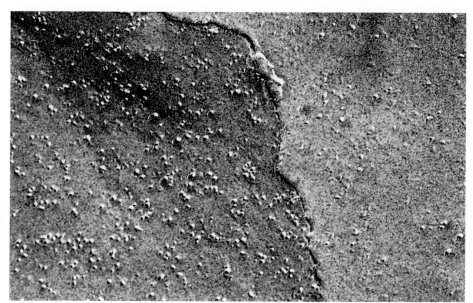

Figure 2–10 Freeze-fracture replica of a cell membrane (×168,000). The E-face (*right*) is closer to the extracellular space, and the P-face (*left*) is closer to the protoplasm. Note that the integral proteins are more numerous on the P-face than on the E-face side. (From Leeson TS, Leeson CR, Papparo AA: Text/Atlas of Histology. Philadelphia, WB Saunders, 1988.)

across it, the presence and activities of specialized transmembrane proteins facilitate the transfer of these hydrophilic molecules across this barrier. These transmembrane proteins and protein complexes form **channel proteins** and **carrier proteins,** which are specifically concerned with the transfer of ions and small molecules across the plasma membrane.

A few nonpolar molecules (e.g., benzene, oxygen, nitrogen) and uncharged polar molecules (e.g., water, glycerol) can move across the cell membrane by **simple diffusion** down their concentration gradients. Even when driven by a concentration gradient, however, movement of most ions and small molecules across a membrane requires the aid of membrane transport proteins, either channel proteins or carrier proteins. This process is known as **facilitated diffusion.** Because both types of diffusion occur without any input of energy other than that inherent in the concentration gradient, they represent **passive transport** (Fig. 2-11). By expending energy, cells can transport ions and small molecules against their concentration gradients. Only carrier proteins can mediate such energy-requiring **active transport.** The several channel proteins involved in facilitated diffusion are discussed first, and the more versatile carrier proteins are considered afterward.

Channel Proteins

Channel proteins may be gated or ungated; they are incapable of transporting substances against a concentration gradient.

Channel proteins participate in the formation of hydrophilic pores, called **ion channels,** across the plas-

malemma. In order to form hydrophilic channels, the proteins are folded so that the hydrophobic amino acids are positioned peripherally, interacting with the fatty acyl tails of the phospholipid molecules of the lipid bilayer, whereas the hydrophilic amino acids face inward, forming a polar inner lining for the channel.

There are more than 100 different types of ion channels; some of these are specific for one particular ion but others permit the passage of several different ions and small water-soluble molecules. Although these ions and small molecules follow chemical or electrochemical concentration gradients for the direction of their passage, cells have the capability of preventing these substances from entering these hydrophilic tunnels by means of controllable **gates** that block their opening. Most channels are **gated channels;** only a few are **ungated.** Gated channels are classified according to the control mechanism required to open the gate.

VOLTAGE-GATED CHANNELS

These channels go from the closed to the open position, permitting the passage of ions from one side of the membrane to the other. The most common example is depolarization in the transmission of nerve impulses. In some channels, such as Na^+ channels, the open position is unstable and the channel goes from an open to an **inactive position,** in which the passage of the ion is blocked and for a short time (a few milliseconds) the gate cannot be opened again. This is the **refractory period** (see Chapter 9 on the nervous tissue). The velocity of response to depolarization may also vary, and some of those channels are referred to as **velocity-dependent.**

A Passive Transport

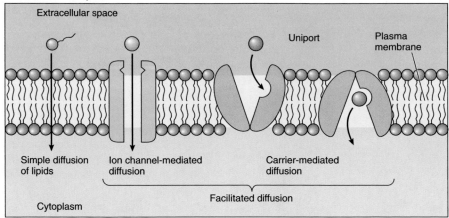

B Active Transport

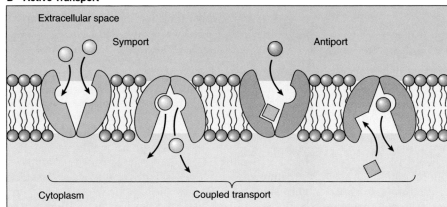

Figure 2–11 Types of transport. **A,** Passive transport: facilitated diffusion, which includes ion channel-mediated diffusion and carrier-mediated diffusion. **B,** Active transport: coupled transport.

LIGAND-GATED CHANNELS

Channels that require the binding of a **ligand** (signaling molecule) to the channel protein to open their gate are known as ligand-gated channels. Unlike voltage-gated channels, these channels remain open until the ligand dissociates from the channel protein; they are referred to as **ion channel–linked receptors.** Some of the ligands controlling these gates are neurotransmitters, whereas others are nucleotides.

Neurotransmitter-gated channels are usually located on the postsynaptic membrane. The neurotransmitter binds to a specific site on the protein, altering its molecular conformation, and thus opening the channel or gate and permitting the influx of a specific ion into the cell. Some neurotransmitters are **excitatory,** whereas others are **inhibitory.** Excitatory neurotransmitters (e.g., acetylcholine) facilitate depolarization; inhibitory neurotransmitters facilitate hyperpolarization of the membrane.

In **nucleotide-gated channels,** the signal molecule is a nucleotide (e.g., **cyclic adenosine monophosphate [cAMP]** in olfactory receptors and **cyclic**

guanosine monophosphate [cGMP] in rods of the retina) that binds to a site on the protein and, by altering the conformation of the protein complex, permits the flow of a particular ion through the ion channel.

MECHANICALLY-GATED CHANNELS

In these channels, an actual physical manipulation is required to open the gate. An example of this mechanism is found in the hair cells of the inner ear. These cells, located on the basilar membrane, possess **stereocilia** that are embedded in a matrix known as the **tectorial membrane.** Movement of the basilar membrane causes a shift in the positions of the hair cells, resulting in the bending of the stereocilia. This physical distortion opens the mechanically-gated channels of the stereocilia located in the inner ear, permitting the entry of cations into the cell, depolarizing it. This event generates impulses that the brain interprets as sound.

G-PROTEIN–GATED ION CHANNELS

Certain gated ion channels (e.g., muscarinic acetylcholine receptors of cardiac muscle cells) require the interaction between a receptor molecule and a G-protein complex (discussed later) with the resultant activation of the G protein. The activated G protein then interacts with the channel protein, modulating the ability of the channel to open or close.

UNGATED CHANNELS

One of the most common forms of an ungated channel is the **potassium (K$^+$) leak channel,** which permits the movement of K$^+$ across it and is instrumental in the creation of an **electrical potential (voltage) difference** between the two sides of the cell membrane. Because this channel is ungated, the transit of K$^+$ ions is not under the cell's control; rather, the direction of ion movement reflects its concentration on the two sides of the membrane.

AQUAPORINS

Currently, twelve different types of aquaporins have been identified. They are a family of multipass proteins that form channels designed for the passage of water from one side of the cell membrane to the other. Some of these channels are pure water transporters (e.g., AqpZ) whereas others transport glycerol (GlpF). These aquaporins discriminate in the transport of the two molecules by restricting the pore sizes in such a fashion that glycerol is too large to pass through pores of the AqpZ channel. An interesting property of aquaporins is that they are completely impermeable to protons, so that streams of protons cannot traverse the channel even though they readily pass through water molecules via the process of donor-acceptor configurations. Aquaporins interfere with this donor-acceptor model by forcing the water molecules to flip-flop halfway along the channel, so that water molecules enter the channel face up (hydrogen side up and oxygen side down) and leave the channel face down (oxygen side up and hydrogen side down). Properly functioning aquaporins in the kidney may transport as much as 20 L of water per hour, whereas improperly functioning aquaporins may result in diseases such as diabetes insipidus and congenital cataracts of the eye.

Carrier Proteins

Carrier proteins can utilize ATP-driven transport mechanisms to ferry specific substances across the plasmalemma against a concentration gradient.

Carrier proteins are **multipass** membrane transport proteins that possess binding sites for specific ions or molecules on both sides of the lipid bilayer. When a solute binds to the binding site, the carrier protein undergoes *reversible* conformational changes; as the molecule is released on the other side of the mem-brane, the carrier protein returns to its previous conformation.

As stated previously, transport by carrier proteins may be **passive**—along an electrochemical concentration gradient—or **active**—against a gradient. Transport may be **uniport**—a single molecule moving in one direction—or **coupled**—two different molecules moving in the same **(symport)** or opposite **(antiport)** directions (see Fig. 2-11). Coupled transporters convey the solutes either simultaneously or sequentially.

PRIMARY ACTIVE TRANSPORT BY THE NA$^+$-K$^+$ PUMP

Normally, the concentration of Na$^+$ is much greater outside the cell than inside, and the concentration of K$^+$ is much greater inside the cell than outside. The cell maintains this concentration differential by expending **adenosine triphosphate (ATP)** to drive a coupled antiport carrier protein known as the Na$^+$-K$^+$ pump. This pump transports K$^+$ ions into and Na$^+$ ions out of the cell, each against a steep concentration gradient. Because this concentration differential is essential for the survival and normal functioning of practically every animal cell, the plasma membrane of all animal cells possesses a large number of these pumps.

The Na$^+$-K$^+$ pump possesses two binding sites for K$^+$ on its extracellular aspect and three binding sites for Na$^+$ on its cytoplasmic aspect; thus, for every two K$^+$ ions conveyed into the cell, three Na$^+$ ions are transported out of the cell.

Na$^+$,K$^+$-ATPase has been shown to be associated with the Na$^+$-K$^+$ pump. When three Na$^+$ ions bind on the cytosolic aspect of the pump, ATP is hydrolyzed to **adenosine diphosphate (ADP)** and the released phosphate ion is used to phosphorylate the ATPase, resulting in alteration of the conformation of the pump, with the consequent transfer of Na$^+$ ions out of the cell. Binding of two K$^+$ ions on the external aspect of the pump causes dephosphorylation of the ATPase with an ensuing return of the carrier protein to its previous conformation, resulting in the transfer of the K$^+$ ions into the cell.

The constant operation of this pump reduces the intracellular ion concentration, resulting in decreased intracellular osmotic pressure. If the osmotic pressure within the cell were not reduced by the Na$^+$-K$^+$ pump, water would enter the cell in large quantities, causing the cell to swell and eventually to succumb to osmotic lysis (i.e., burst). Hence it is through the operation of this pump that the cell is able to regulate its osmolarity and, consequently, its volume. Additionally, this pump assists the K$^+$ leak channels in the maintenance of the cell membrane potential.

Because the binding sites on the external aspect of the pump bind not only K$^+$ but also the glycoside **ouabain,** this glycoside inhibits the Na$^+$-K$^+$ pump.

SECONDARY ACTIVE TRANSPORT BY COUPLED CARRIER PROTEINS

The ATP-driven transport of Na$^+$ out of the cell establishes a low intracellular concentration of that ion. The energy reservoir inherent in the sodium ion gradient can be utilized by carrier proteins to transport ions or other molecules against a concentration gradient. Frequently, this mode of active transport is referred to as secondary active transport, distinct from the primary active transport, which utilizes the energy released from the hydrolysis of ATP.

The carrier proteins that participate in secondary active transport are either symports or antiports. As a Na$^+$ ion binds to the extracellular aspect of the carrier protein, another ion or small molecule (e.g., **glucose**) also binds to a region on the same aspect of the carrier protein, inducing in it a conformational alteration. The change in conformation results in the transfer and subsequent release of both molecules on the other side of the membrane.

Cell Signaling

Cell signaling is the communication that occurs when signaling cells release signaling molecules that bind to cell surface receptors of target cells.

When cells communicate with each other, the one that sends the signal is called the **signaling cell;** the cell receiving the signal is called the **target cell.** Transmission of the information may occur either by the secretion or presentation of **signaling molecules,** which contact **receptors** on the target cell membrane (or intracellularly either in the cytosol or in the nucleus), or by the formation of intercellular pores known as **gap junctions,** which permit the movement of ions and small molecules (e.g., cAMP) between the two cells. (Gap junctions are discussed in Chapter 5.)

The signaling molecule, or **ligand,** may be either secreted and released by the signaling cell or may remain bound to its surface and be presented by the signaling cell to the target cell. A cell-surface receptor usually is a transmembrane protein, whereas an intracellular receptor is a protein that resides in the cytosol or in the nucleus of the target cell. Ligands that bind to cell-surface receptors usually are **polar** molecules; those that bind to intracellular receptors are **hydrophobic** and thus can diffuse through the cell membrane.

In the most selective signaling process, **synaptic signaling,** the signaling molecule, a neurotransmitter, is released so close to the target cell that only a single cell is affected by the ligand. A more generalized but still local form of signaling, **paracrine signaling,** occurs when the signaling molecule is released into the intercellular environment and affects cells in its immediate vicinity. Occasionally, the signaling cell is also the target cell, resulting in a specialized type of paracrine signaling known as **autocrine signaling.** The most widespread form of signaling is **endocrine signaling;** in this case, the signaling molecule enters the bloodstream to be ferried to target cells situated at a distance from the signaling cell.

Signaling Molecules

Signaling molecules bind to extracellular or intracellular receptors to elicit a specific cellular response.

Most signaling molecules are hydrophilic (e.g., **acetylcholine**) and cannot penetrate the cell membrane. Therefore, they require receptors on the cell surface. Other signaling molecules are either hydrophobic, such as **steroid hormones**, or are small nonpolar molecules, such as **nitric oxide (NO),** which have the ability to diffuse through the lipid bilayer. These ligands require the presence of an intracellular receptor. Hydrophilic ligands have a very short life span (a few milliseconds to minutes at most), whereas steroid hormones last for extended time periods (several hours to days).

Signaling molecules often act in concert, in that several different ligands are required before a specific cellular response is elicited. Moreover, the same ligand or combination of ligands may elicit different responses from different cells. For instance, acetylcholine causes skeletal muscle cells to contract, cardiac muscle cells to relax, endothelial cells of blood vessels to release nitric oxide, and parenchymal cells of some glands to release the contents of their secretory granules.

Binding of signaling molecules to their receptors activates an intracellular **second messenger system,** initiating a cascade of reactions that result in the required response. A hormone, for example, binds to its receptors on the cell membrane of its target cell. The receptor alters its conformation, with the resultant activation of **adenylate cyclase,** a transmembrane protein, whose cytoplasmic region catalyzes the transformation of **ATP** to **cAMP,** one of the most common second messengers.

cAMP activates a cascade of enzymes within the cell, thus multiplying the effects of a very few molecules of hormones on the cell surface. The specific intracellular event depends on the enzymes located within the cell; thus, cAMP activates one set of enzymes within an endothelial cell and another set of enzymes within a follicular cell of the thyroid gland. Therefore, the same molecule can have a different effect in different cells. The system is known as a second messenger system because the hormone is the first messenger that activates the formation of cAMP, the second messenger. Other second messengers include calcium (Ca^{2+}), cGMP, inositol triphosphate (IP$_3$), and diacylglycerol.

Steroid hormones (e.g., cortisol) can also diffuse through the cell membrane. Once in the cytosol, they bind to **steroid hormone receptors** (members of the **intracellular receptor family**), and the ligand-receptor complex activates gene expression, or **transcription** (the formation of **messenger ribonucleic acid [mRNA]**). Transcription may be induced directly, resulting in a fast **primary response**, or indirectly, bringing about a slower, **secondary response.** In the secondary response, the mRNA codes for the protein that is necessary to activate the expression of additional genes.

Cell-Surface Receptors

Cell-surface receptors are of three types: ion channel-linked, enzyme-linked, and G-protein–linked.

Most cell-surface receptors are integral **glycoproteins** that function in recognizing signaling molecules and in **transducing** the signal into an intracellular action. The three main classes of receptor molecules are ion channel-linked receptors (see earlier), enzyme-linked receptors, and G-protein–linked receptors.

ENZYME-LINKED RECEPTORS

These receptors are transmembrane proteins whose extracellular regions act as receptors for specific ligands. When a signaling molecule binds to the receptor site, the receptor's intracellular domain becomes activated so that it now possesses enzymatic capabilities. These enzymes then either induce the formation of second messengers, such as cGMP, or permit the assembly of intracellular signaling molecules that relay the signal intracellularly. This signal then elicits the required response by activating additional enzyme systems or by stimulating gene regulatory proteins to initiate the transcription of specific genes.

G-PROTEIN–LINKED RECEPTORS

These receptors are multipass proteins whose extracellular domains act as receptor sites for ligands. Their intracellular regions have two separate sites, one that binds to G proteins and another that becomes phosphorylated during the process of receptor desensitization.

Most cells possess two types of GTPases (monomeric and trimeric), each of which has the capability of binding **guanosine triphosphate (GTP)** and **guanosine diphosphate (GDP).** Trimeric GTPases, or **G proteins,** are composed of a large α subunit and two small β and γ subunits, and can associate with G-protein–linked receptors. There are several types of G proteins, including:

■ Stimulatory (G_s)
■ Inhibitory (G_i)
■ Pertussis toxin–sensitive (G_o)

■ Pertussis toxin–insensitive (G_{Bq})
■ Transducin (G_t)

G proteins act by linking receptors with enzymes that modulate the levels of the intracellular signaling molecules (second messengers) cAMP or Ca^{2+}.

Signaling via G_s and G_i Proteins

G_s proteins (Fig. 2-12) are usually present in the **inactive** state, in which a GDP molecule is bound to the a subunit. When a ligand binds to the G-protein–linked receptor, it alters the receptor's conformation, permitting it to bind to the a subunit of the G_s protein, which in turn exchanges its GDP for GTP. The binding of GTP causes the a subunit to dissociate not only from the receptor but also from the other two subunits and to bind with **adenylate cyclase,** a transmembrane protein. This binding activates adenylate cyclase to form

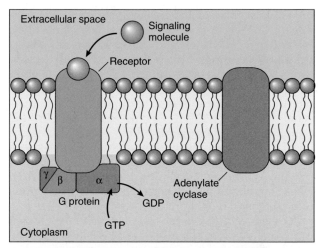

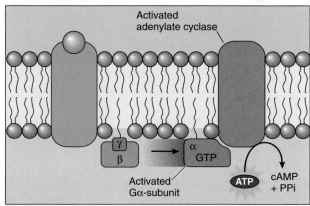

Figure 2–12 G-protein–linked receptor. When the signaling molecule contacts its receptor, the a subunit dissociates from the G protein and contacts and activates adenylate cyclase, which converts adenosine triphosphate (ATP) to cyclic adenosine monophosphate (cAMP). GDP, guanosine disphosphate; GTP, guanosine triphosphate; PPi, pyrophosphate.

many molecules of cAMP from ATP molecules. As the activation of adenylate cyclase is occurring, the ligand uncouples from the G-protein–linked receptor, returning the receptor to its original conformation without affecting the activity of the a subunit. Within a few seconds, the a subunit hydrolyzes its GTP to GDP, detaches from adenylate cyclase (thus deactivating it), and reassociates the β and γ subunits.

G_i behaves similarly to G_s, but instead of activating adenylate cyclase, it inhibits it, so that cAMP is not being produced. The lack of cAMP prevents the phosphorylation, and thus activation, of enzymes that would elicit a particular response. Hence, a particular ligand binding to a particular receptor may activate or inactivate the cell, depending on the type of G protein that couples it to adenylate cyclase.

Cyclic Adenosine Monophosphate As a Second Messenger

cAMP is an intracellular signaling molecule that activates cAMP-dependent protein kinase (**A-kinase**) by binding to it. The activated A-kinase dissociates into its **regulatory component** and two **active catalytic subunits.** The active catalytic subunits phosphorylate other enzymes in the cytosol, thus initiating a cascade of phosphorylations and resulting in a specific response. Elevated levels of cAMP in some cells result in the transcription of those genes whose regulatory regions possess **cAMP response elements (CREs).** A-kinase phosphorylates, and thus activates, a gene regulatory protein known as **CRE-binding protein (CREB)** whose binding to the CRE stimulates the transcription of those genes.

As long as cAMP is present at a high enough concentration, a particular response is elicited from the target cell. In order to prevent responses of unduly long duration, cAMP is quickly degraded by **cAMP phosphodiesterases** to 5′-AMP, which is unable to activate A-kinase. Moreover, the enzymes phosphorylated during the cascade of phosphorylations become deactivated by becoming dephosphorylated by another series of enzymes (**serine/threonine phosphoprotein phosphatases**).

Signaling via G_o Protein

When a ligand becomes bound to G_o-protein–linked receptor, the receptor alters its conformation and binds with G_o. This trimeric protein dissociates, and its subunit activates **phospholipase C,** the enzyme responsible for cleaving the membrane phospholipid phosphatidylinositol bisphosphate (PIP_2) into **IP_3** and **diacylglycerol.** IP_3 leaves the membrane and diffuses to the endoplasmic reticulum, where it causes the release of Ca^{2+}—another second messenger—into the cytosol. Diacylglycerol remains attached to the inner leaflet of the plasma membrane and, with the assistance of Ca^{2+}, activates the enzyme protein kinase C (**C-kinase**). C-kinase, in turn, initiates a phosphorylation cascade, whose end result is the activation of gene regulatory proteins that initiate transcription of specific genes.

IP_3 is rapidly inactivated by being dephosphorylated, and diacylglycerol is catabolized within a few seconds after its formation. These actions ensure that responses to a ligand are of limited duration.

Note that because cytosolic Ca^{2+} acts as an important second messenger, its cytosolic concentration must be carefully controlled by the cell. These control mechanisms include the sequestering of Ca^{2+} by the endoplasmic reticulum, specific Ca^{2+}-binding molecules in the cytosol and mitochondria, and the active transport of this ion out of the cell.

When IP_3 causes elevated cytosolic Ca^{2+} levels, the excess ions bind to **calmodulin,** a protein found in high concentration in most animal cells. The Ca^{2+}-calmodulin complex activates a group of enzymes known as **Ca^{2+}-calmodulin–dependent protein kinases (CaM-kinases).** CaM-kinases have numerous regulatory functions in the cell, such as initiation of glycogenolysis, synthesis of catecholamines, and contraction of smooth muscle.

Protein Synthetic and Packaging Machinery of the Cell

The primary components of the protein synthetic machinery of the cell are ribosomes (and polyribosomes), rough endoplasmic reticulum, and the Golgi apparatus.

Ribosomes

Ribosomes are small particles, approximately 12 nm wide and 25 nm long, composed of proteins and **ribosomal RNA (rRNA).** They function as a surface for the synthesis of proteins. Each ribosome is composed of a **large subunit** and a **small subunit,** both of which are manufactured or assembled in the nucleolus and released as separate entities into the cytosol. The small subunit has a sedimentation value of 40S and is composed of 33 proteins and an 18S rRNA. The sedimentation value of the large subunit is 60S, and it consists of 49 s and 3 rRNAs. The sedimentation values of the RNAs are 5S, 5.8S, and 28S.

The small subunit has a site for binding mRNA, a **P-site** for binding peptidyl **transfer ribonucleic acid (tRNA),** an **A-site** for binding aminoacyl tRNA, and an **E-site** where the tRNA that gave up its amino acid exits the ribosome. Some of the rRNAs of the large subunit are referred to as **ribozymes** since they have enzymatic activity and catalyze peptide bond formation. The small and large subunits are present in the cytosol individually and do not form a ribosome until protein synthesis begins.

Endoplasmic Reticulum

Endoplasmic reticulum (ER) is the largest membranous system of the cell, comprising approximately half of the total membrane volume. It is a system of interconnected tubules and vesicles whose lumen is referred to as the **cistern.** ER has two components: **smooth endoplasmic reticulum (SER)** and **rough endoplasmic reticulum (RER).** Although only the RER participates in protein synthesis, the SER is also discussed at this point, but only as an aside, and the reader should keep in mind that distinction.

Smooth Endoplasmic Reticulum

A system of anastomosing tubules and occasional flattened membrane-bound vesicles constitute SER (Fig. 2-13). The lumen of SER is assumed to be continuous with that of the rough endoplasmic reticulum. Except for cells active in synthesis of steroids, cholesterol, and triglycerides, and cells that function in detoxification of toxic materials (e.g., alcohol and barbiturates), most cells do not possess an abundance of SER. SER has become specialized in some cells (e.g., skeletal muscle cells), where it is known as **sarcoplasmic reticulum.** Here, it functions in sequestering calcium ions from the cytosol, assisting in the control of muscle contraction.

Rough Endoplasmic Reticulum

Cells that function in the synthesis of proteins that are to be exported are richly endowed with RER (see Fig. 2-6). The membranes of this organelle are somewhat different from those of its smooth counterpart, because it possesses integral proteins that function in recognizing and binding ribosomes to its cytosolic surface and

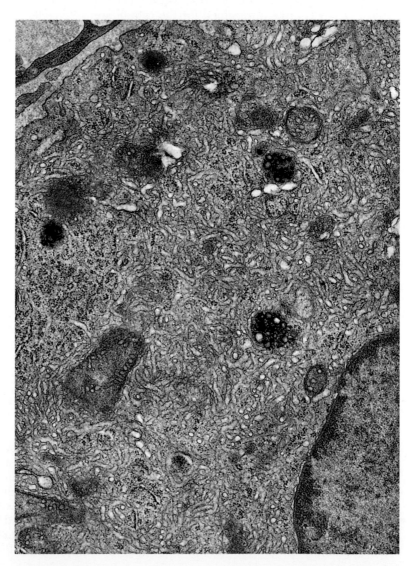

Figure 2–13 Electron micrograph of the smooth endoplasmic reticulum of the human suprarenal cortex. (From Leeson TS, Leeson CR, Papparo AA: Text/Atlas of Histology, Philadelphia, WB Saunders, 1988.)

also maintains the flattened morphology of the RER. For the purposes of this textbook, the integral proteins of interest are (1) **signal recognition particle receptor (docking protein),** (2) **ribosome receptor protein** (ribophorin I and ribophorin II), and (3) **pore protein.** Their functions are discussed later.

RER participates in the synthesis of all proteins that are to be packaged or delivered to the plasma membrane. It also performs post-translational modifications of these proteins, including sulfation, folding, and glycosylation. Additionally, lipids and integral proteins of all membranes of the cell are manufactured by the RER. The cisterna of RER is continuous with the perinuclear cistern, the space between the inner and outer nuclear membranes.

Polyribosomes

Proteins to be packaged are synthesized on the RER surface, whereas proteins destined for the cytosol are manufactured within the cytosol. The information for the primary structure of a protein (sequence of amino acids) is housed in the **deoxyribonucleic acid (DNA)** of the nucleus. This information is **transcribed** into a strand of mRNA, which leaves the nucleus and enters the cytoplasm. The sequence of **codons** of the mRNA thus represents the chain of amino acids, in which each codon is composed of three consecutive nucleotides. Because any three consecutive nucleotides constitute a codon, it is essential that the protein synthetic machinery recognizes the beginning and the end of the message; otherwise, an incorrect protein will be manufactured.

The three types of RNA play distinctive roles in protein synthesis. **mRNA** carries the coded instructions specifying the sequence of amino acids. **tRNA** forms covalent bonds with amino acids, forming **aminoacyl tRNA.** These enzyme-catalyzed reactions are specific; that is, each tRNA reacts with its own corresponding amino acid. Each tRNA also contains the **anticodon** that recognizes the codon in mRNA corresponding to the amino acid it carries. Finally, several **rRNAs** associate with a large number of proteins to form the small and large ribosomal subunits.

Protein Synthesis (Translation)

> *Protein synthesis (translation) occurs on ribosomes in the cytosol or on the surface of the rough endoplasmic reticulum.*

The requirements for protein synthesis are:

- An mRNA strand
- **tRNAs,** each of which carries an amino acid and possesses the anticodon that recognizes the codon of the mRNA coding for that particular amino acid
- Small and large ribosomal subunits

It is interesting that the approximate time of synthesis of a protein composed of 400 amino acids is about 20 seconds. Because a single strand of mRNA may have as many as 15 ribosomes translating it simultaneously, a large number of protein molecules may be synthesized in a short period of time. This conglomeration of an mRNA-ribosome complex, which usually has a spiral or long hairpin form, is referred to as a **polyribosome,** or **polysome** (Fig. 2-14).

Synthesis of Cytosolic Proteins

The general process of protein synthesis in the cytosol is outlined in Figure 2-15.

STEP 1

- The process begins when the P-site of the small ribosomal subunit is occupied by an **initiator tRNA** whose anticodon recognizes the triplet **codon AUG,** coding for the amino acid **methionine.**
- An **mRNA** binds to the small subunit.
- The small subunit assists the anticodon of the tRNA molecule to recognize the **start codon AUG** on the mRNA molecule. This step acts as a registration step so that the next three nucleotides of the mRNA molecule may be recognized as the next codon.

STEP 2

The large ribosomal subunit binds to the small subunit and the ribosome moves along the mRNA chain, in a 5′ to 3′ direction, until the next codon lines up with the A-site of the small subunit.

STEP 3

An acylated tRNA (tRNA bearing an amino acid) compares its anticodon with the codon of the mRNA; if they match, the tRNA binds to the A-site.

STEP 4

- The amino acids at the A-site and the P-site form a peptide bond.
- The tRNA on the P-site yields its amino acid to the tRNA at the A-site, which now has two amino acids attached to it. These reactions are catalyzed by the rRNA-based enzyme of the large subunit known as **peptidyl transferase.**

STEP 5

The deaminated tRNA leaves the P-site and binds to the E-site; the tRNA with its two amino acids attached moves from the A-site to the P-site. Concurrently, the ribosome moves along the mRNA chain until the next codon lines up with the A-site of the small ribosomal subunit and the tRNA from the E-site is ejected. The energy required by this step is derived from the hydrolysis of GTP.

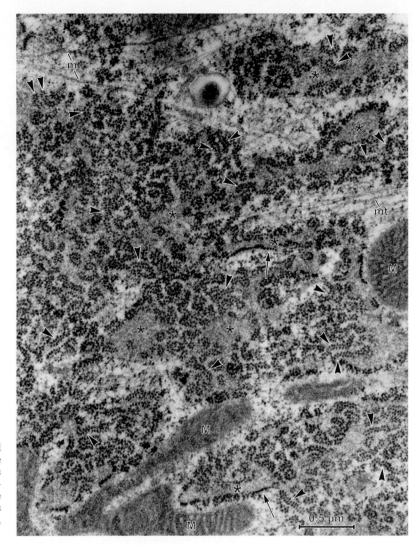

Figure 2–14 Electron micrograph of bound polysome. Arrowheads indicate rough endoplasmic reticulum; arrows indicate ribosomes; asterisks indicate cisternae; M, mitochondrion; mt, microtubule. (From Christensen AK, Bourne CM: Shape of large bound polysomes in cultured fibroblasts and thyroid epithelial cells. Anat Rec 255: 116-129, 1999.)

STEP 6

- Steps 3 through 5 are repeated, elongating the polypeptide chain until the stop codon is reached.
- There are three stop codons **(UAG, UAA, and UGA),** each one of which may halt translation.

STEP 7

- When the A-site of the small ribosomal subunit reaches a stop codon, a **release factor** binds to the A-site.
- This factor is responsible for releasing the newly formed polypeptide chain from the tRNA of the P-site into the cytosol.

STEP 8

The tRNA moves from the P-site to the E-site, the release factor is released from the A-site, and the small and large ribosomal subunits leave the mRNA.

Synthesis of Proteins on the Rough Endoplasmic Reticulum

Proteins that need to be packaged either for delivery to the outside of the cell or merely isolated from the cytosol must be identified and be delivered **cotranslationally** (during the process of synthesis) into the RER cistern. The mode of identification resides in a small segment of the mRNA, located immediately following the start codon, which codes for a sequence of amino acids known as the **signal peptide.**

Employing the sequence just outlined for the synthesis of protein in the cytosol, the mRNA begins to be translated, forming the signal peptide (Fig. 2-16). This peptide is recognized by a protein-RNA complex located in the cytosol, the **signal recognition particle (SRP).** The SRP attaches to the signal peptide and by occupying the P-site on the small subunit of the

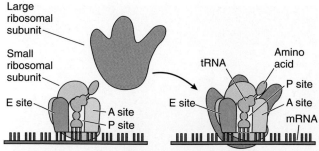
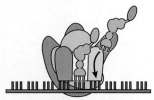
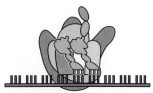

Initiation begins when the small ribosomal subunit binds with messenger RNA (mRNA). The initiator transfer RNA (tRNA) binds with its associated amino acid, methionine, to the P site.

The large subunit joins the initial complex. The empty A site is now ready to receive an aminoacyl-tRNA.

A second aminoacyl-tRNA, bearing an amino acid, binds to the empty A site.

A peptide bond is formed between the two amino acids. This bond formation brings the acceptor end of the A site tRNA into the P site as it picks up the peptidyl chain.

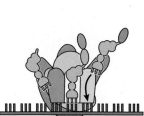
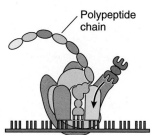
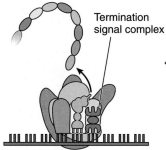
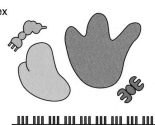

The P site tRNA moves to the E site and the A site tRNA, with the attached peptidyl chain, moves to the vacated P site. As a new aminoacyl-tRNA bearing an amino acid occupies the A site, the spent tRNA on the E site drops off the ribosome. A peptide bond is formed, and the ribosome moves down the mRNA. The cycle of adding to the forming protein chain continues.

Polypeptide synthesis continues until the ribosome encounters a "stop" or "nonsense codon" which signals the end of the polypeptide chain.

The terminal signal complex, a release factor which promotes polypeptide release, docks at the A site. The polypeptide chain is released.

Once protein synthesis is completed, the two ribosomal subunits dissociate from the mRNA, and return to the cytosol.

Figure 2–15 Protein synthesis in the cytosol.

ribosome halts translation; it then directs the polysome to migrate to the RER.

The SRP receptor protein (docking protein) in the RER membrane contacts the SRP, and the ribosome receptor protein contacts the large subunit of the ribosome, attaching the polysome to the cytosolic surface of the RER. The following events then occur almost simultaneously:

1 The pore proteins assemble, forming a **pore** through the lipid bilayer of the RER.
2 The signal peptide contacts the pore protein and begins to be translocated (amino terminus first) into the cistern of the RER.
3 The SRP is dislodged, reenters the cytosol, and frees the P-site on the small ribosomal subunit. The ribosome remains on the RER surface.

4 As translation resumes, the nascent protein continues to be channeled into the cistern of the RER.
5 An enzyme attached to the cisternal aspect of the RER membrane, known as **signal peptidase,** cleaves the signal peptide from the forming protein. The signal peptide becomes degraded into its amino acid components.
6 As detailed previously, when the stop codon is reached, protein synthesis is completed, and the small and large ribosomal subunits dissociate and reenter the cytosol to join the pool of ribosomal subunits.
7 The newly formed proteins are folded, glycosylated, and undergo additional post-translational modifications within the RER cisternae.
8 The modified proteins leave the cistern via small **transport vesicles** (without a clathrin coat) at regions of the RER devoid of ribosomes.

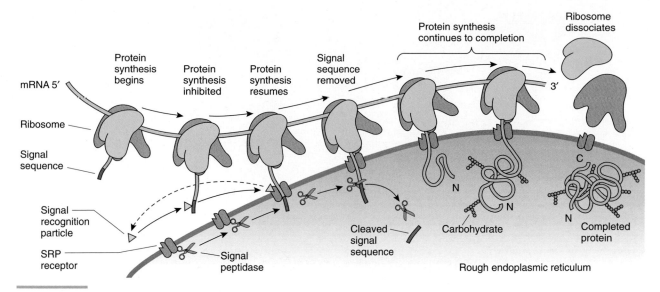

Figure 2–16 Protein synthesis on the rough endoplasmic reticulum. C, carboxyl terminus; mRNA, messenger RNA; N, amino terminus; SRP, signal recognition particle.

Golgi Apparatus

The Golgi apparatus functions in the synthesis of carbohydrates and in the modification and sorting of proteins manufactured on the RER.

Proteins manufactured and packaged in the RER follow a **default pathway** to the Golgi apparatus for post-translational modification and packaging. Proteins destined to remain in the RER or to go to a compartment other than the Golgi apparatus possess a signal that will divert them from the default pathway.

The Golgi apparatus is composed of one or more series of flattened, slightly curved membrane-bounded **cisternae,** the **Golgi stack,** which resemble a stack of pita breads that do not quite contact each other (Figs. 2-17 to 2-19). The periphery of each cisterna is dilated and is rimmed with vesicles that are in the process of either fusing with or budding off that particular compartment.

Each Golgi stack has three levels of cisternae:

- The *cis*-face (or *cis* Golgi network)
- The medial face (intermediate face)
- The *trans*-face

The *cis*-face is closest to the RER. It is convex in shape and is considered to be the entry face, because newly formed proteins from the RER enter the *cis*-face before they are permitted to enter the other cisternae of the Golgi apparatus. The *trans*-face is concave in shape and is considered to be the exit face, because the modified protein is ready to be packaged and to be sent to its destination from here.

There are two additional compartments of interest, one associated with the *cis*-face and the other with the *trans*-face. Located between the RER and the *cis*-face of the Golgi apparatus is an intermediate compartment of vesicles, or **endoplasmic reticulum/Golgi intermediate compartment (ERGIC)** and the *trans* **Golgi network (TGN),** located at the distal side of the Golgi apparatus. The ERGIC, also known as the tubulovesicular complexes, is a collection of vesicles and tubules formed from the fusion of **transfer vesicles** derived from the final cisterna of the RER, known as **transitional endoplasmic reticulum (TER).** These transfer vesicles bud off the TER and contain nascent proteins synthesized on the surface and modified within the cisternae of the RER.

Vesicles derived from the ERGIC make their way to and fuse with the periphery of the *cis*-face of the Golgi apparatus, thus delivering the protein to this compartment for further modification. The modified proteins are transferred from the *cis* to the medial and finally to the *trans* cisternae via vesicles that bud off and fuse with the rims of the particular compartment (Fig. 2-20). As the proteins pass through the Golgi apparatus, they are modified within the Golgi stack. Proteins that form the cores of glycoprotein molecules become heavily glycosylated, whereas other proteins acquire or lose sugar moieties.

Mannose phosphorylation occurs within the *cis*-face cisterna, whereas the removal of mannose from certain proteins takes place within the *cis* and medial compartments of the Golgi stack. *N*-acetylglucosamine is added to the protein within the medial cisternae. Addition of sialic acid (*N*-acetylneuraminic acid) and galactose, as

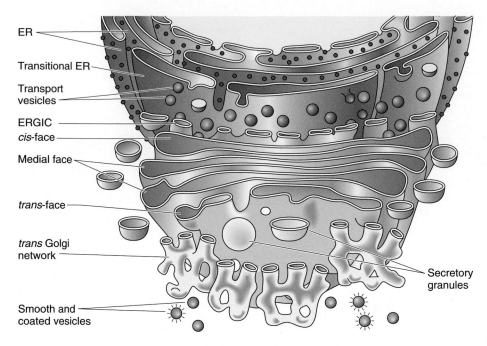

ER
Transitional ER
Transport vesicles
ERGIC
cis-face
Medial face
trans-face
trans Golgi network
Smooth and coated vesicles
Secretory granules

Figure 2–17 Rough endoplasmic reticulum (ER) and the Golgi apparatus. Transfer vesicles contain newly synthesized protein and are ferried to the endoplasmic reticulum/Golgi intermediate compartment (ERGIC) and from there to the Golgi apparatus. The protein is modified in the various faces of the Golgi complex and enters the *trans* Golgi network for packaging.

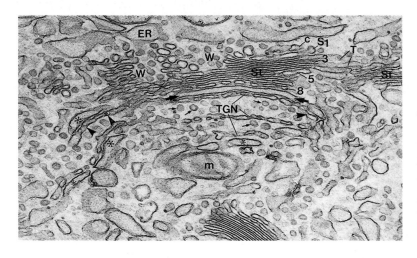

Figure 2–18 Electron micrograph of the Golgi apparatus of the rat epididymis. ER, endoplasmic reticulum; m, mitochondrion; TGN, *trans* Golgi network. Numbers represent the saccules of the Golgi apparatus. (From Hermo L, Green H, Clermont Y: Golgi apparatus of epithelial principal cells of the ependymal initial segment of the rat: Structure, relationship with endoplasmic reticulum, and role in the formation of secretory vesicles. Anat Rec 229:159-176, 1991.)

well as phosphorylation and sulfation of amino acids, occurs in the *trans*-face.

Golgi- and Rough Endoplasmic Endothelium–Associated Vesicles

Vesicles associated with the RER and Golgi apparatus possess a protein coat as well as surface markers.

Vesicles that transport proteins **(cargo)** between organelles and regions of organelles, must have a way of budding off the organelle and must be labeled as to their destination. The process of budding is facilitated by the assembly of a proteinaceous coat on the cytosolic

aspect of the organelle. Three types of coat proteins (COPs), or **coatamers,** are known to elicit the formation of cargo-bearing vesicles: **coatomer I (COP I), coatomer II (COP II),** and **clathrin**. At the site of future vesicle formation, these proteins coalesce, attach to the membrane, draw out the vesicle, and coat its cytosolic surface. Thus, there are COP I–coated, COP II–coated, and clathrin-coated vesicles.

Transport vesicles leaving the transitional ER are always COP II–coated until they reach the ERGIC, where they shed their COP II coat, which is recycled. Vesicles that arise from the ERGIC to carry recently delivered cargo to the *cis*-face require the assistance of COP I, as do all other vesicles that proceed through the medial to the

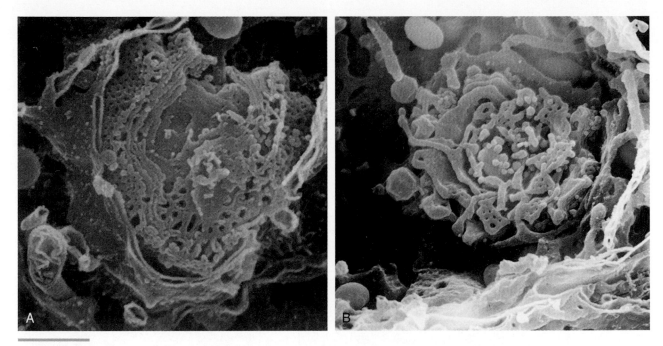

Figure 2–19 **A,** Face view of the *cis* Golgi network in a step 6 spermatid. The *cis*-most saccule is a regular network of anastomotic membranous tubules, capped by the endoplasmic reticulum. Some of the medial saccules with fewer but larger and more irregular pores are visible under the *cis* Golgi saccule. **B,** Face view of another *cis* Golgi network in a step 6 spermatid. Note the fenestration at the edges of the irregular *trans* Golgi saccules. (From Ho HC, Tang CY, Suarez SS: Three-dimensional structure of the Golgi apparatus in mouse spermatids: A scanning electron microscopic study. Anat Rec 256:189-194, 1999.)

trans-face and the *trans* Golgi network. Most of the vesicles that arise from the *trans* Golgi network, however, require the presence of clathrin for their formation.

The transport mechanism has a quality control aspect, in that if RER (or transitional ER) resident proteins are packaged in vesicles and these "stowaway" molecules reach the ERGIC, they are returned to the RER in COP I–coated vesicles. This is referred to as **retrograde transport,** in contrast to **anterograde transport** of cargo, described earlier.

Because these vesicles are formed at a particular site in the cell and must reach their destination, an additional set of information should be considered; namely, how the vesicles are transported to their destination. Although these are interesting concepts to contemplate, the complexity of the mechanism precludes a complete discussion here; instead, a cursory overview is presented. (For more information, consult a textbook on cell biology.)

As the cargo-containing vesicles form, they possess not only a coatomer or clathrin coat but also other surface markers and receptors. Some of these receptors interact with microtubules and the motor protein complexes that are responsible for vesicle movement. As discussed later (see *Cytoskeleton*), microtubules are long, straight, rigid, tubule-like structures that originate in the **microtubule organizing center (MTOC)** and

extend to the cell periphery. The major MTOC of the cell is known as the centrosome and it houses a pair of centrioles embedded in a matrix of proteins rich in γ-tubulin ring complexes.

The MTOC is located in the vicinity of the Golgi complex, and these ends of the microtubules, each emanating from a γ-tubulin ring complex, are referred to as the **minus end;** the other end of each microtubule, near the periphery of the cell, is the **plus end.** The molecular motor that drives vesicles to the minus end (toward the MTOC) is dynein and its accessory protein complex. The molecular motor that drives vesicles toward the positive end (away from the MTOC) is kinesin and its associated protein complex. Thus, vesicles derived from the ER as well as from the ERGIC are driven toward the MTOC and are driven by dynein, whereas vesicles that leave the Golgi complex in a retrograde direction to the ERGIC or to the RER are driven by kinesin.

Sorting in the *Trans* Golgi Network

The trans *Golgi network is responsible for the sorting of proteins to their respective pathways so that they reach the plasma membrane, secretory granules, or lysosomes.*

Cargo that leaves the TGN is enclosed in vesicles that may do one of the following (see Fig. 2-20):

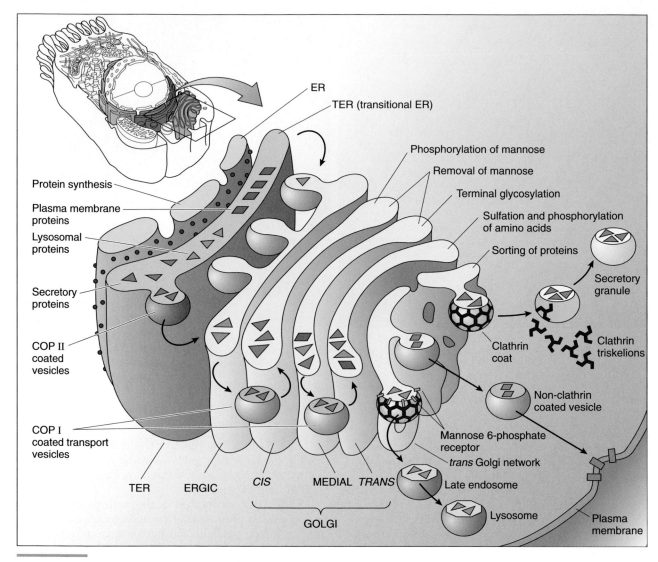

Figure 2–20 The Golgi apparatus and packaging in the *trans* Golgi network. ER, endoplasmic reticulum; ERGIC, endoplasmic reticulum/Golgi intermediate compartment; COP, coat protein (coatomer).

- Insert into the cell membrane as membrane proteins and lipids
- Fuse with the cell membrane such that the protein they carry is *immediately* released into the extracellular space
- Congregate in the cytoplasm near the apical cell membrane as **secretory granules (vesicles),** and, upon a given signal, fuse with the cell membrane for *eventual* release of the protein outside the cell
- Fuse with **late endosomes** (see later), releasing their content into that organelle, which then becomes a lysosome

The first three processes are known as **exocytosis,** because material leaves the cytoplasm proper. Neither immediate release into the extracellular space nor insertion into the cell membrane requires a particular regulatory process; thus, both processes are said to follow the **constitutive secretory pathway (default pathway).** In contrast, the pathways to lysosomes and to secretory vesicles are known as the **regulated secretory pathway.**

TRANSPORT OF LYSOSOMAL PROTEINS

The sorting process begins with the phosphorylation of mannose residues of the lysosomal proteins (lysosomal hydrolases) in the *cis* cisterna of the Golgi stack. When these proteins reach the *trans* Golgi network, their mannose-6-phosphate (M6P) is recognized as a signal,

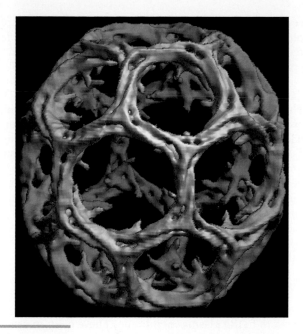

Figure 2–21 A map of clathrin coat at 21 Å resolution. To allow a clear view of the path of the triskelion legs, the amino-terminal domain and most of the linker have been removed from this map. (From Smith CJ, Grigorieff N, Pearse BM: Clathrin coats at 21 Å resolution: A cellular assembly designed to recycle multiple membrane receptors. EMBO J 17:4943-4953, 1998.)

and they become bound to mannose-6-phosphate receptors, transmembrane proteins of the TGN membrane.

A small pit is formed with the assistance of **clathrin triskelions,** protein complexes composed of three heavy and three light chains forming a structure with three arms that radiate from a central point (Fig. 2-21; also see Fig. 2-20). The triskelions self-assemble, coating the cytoplasmic aspect of the TGN rich in M6P receptors to which M6P is bound. As the pit deepens, it pinches off the TGN and forms a **clathrin-coated vesicle.** The clathrin coat is also referred to as the **clathrin basket.**

The clathrin-coated vesicle quickly loses its clathrin coat, which, unlike the formation of the clathrin basket, is an energy-requiring process. The uncoated vesicle reaches, fuses with, and releases its contents into the late endosome (endosomes are discussed later).

Because clathrin coats are utilized for many other types of vesicles, an intermediary protein, **adaptin,** is interposed between the cytoplasmic aspect of the receptor molecule and the clathrin. Many different types of adaptins exist. Each has a binding site for a particular receptor as well as a binding site for clathrin.

TRANSPORT OF REGULATED SECRETORY PROTEINS

Proteins that are to be released into the extracellular space in a discontinuous manner also require the for-

mation of clathrin-coated vesicles. The signal for their formation is not known; however, the mechanism is believed to be similar to that for lysosomal proteins.

Unlike vesicles that ferry lysosomal enzymes, secretory granules are quite large and carry many more proteins than there are receptors on the vesicle surface. Additionally, the contents of the secretory granules become condensed with time as a result of the loss of fluid from the secretory granules (see Figs. 2-6 and 2-20). During this process of increasing concentration, these vesicles are frequently referred to as **condensing vesicles.** Moreover, secretory granules of polarized cells remain localized in a particular region of the cell. They remain as clusters of secretory granules that, in reaction to a particular signal (e.g., neurotransmitter or hormone), fuse with the cell membrane to release their contents into the intercellular space.

TRANSPORT ALONG THE CONSTITUTIVE PATHWAY

All vesicles that participate in nonselective transport, such as those passing between the RER and the *cis* Golgi network or among the cisternae of the Golgi stack or utilizing the constitutive pathway between the TGN and the plasma membrane, also require a coated vesicle (see Fig. 2-20). However, the coating is composed of a seven-unit protein (**coatomer)** complex instead of clathrin. Each protein of the coatomer complex is referred to as a **coat protein (COP) subunit,** whose assembly, unlike that of clathrin, is energy-requiring and remains with the vesicle until it reaches its intended target. As indicated previously, there are two types of coatomers, **COP I** and **COP II.**

Vesicles derived from the TGN are driven along microtubule tracts by the use of kinesin and its associated protein complex. However, these vesicles also use an alternative, and perhaps their primary, pathway of actin filaments. The motor that drives these vesicles is myosin II; it is believed that myosin II is brought to the *trans* Golgi network subsequent to, or in conjunction with, the recruitment of the clathrin triskelions to the site of vesicle formation.

Alternative Concept of the Golgi Apparatus

An alternative concept of the Golgi apparatus suggests the occurrence of cisternal maturation instead of anterograde vesicle transport.

The two predominant theories of **anterograde vesicle transport** (already described) and **cisternal maturation** are mutually incompatible, and ample evidence exists to support both theories. The theory of cisternal maturation suggests that instead of the cargo being ferried through the various regions of the Golgi apparatus, it remains stationary and the various enzyme systems of the Golgi are transported in a retrograde fashion in the correct sequence and at the designated time, so that a given sedentary cisterna matures into the subsequent cisternae.

At first glance, the cisternal maturation theory may appear to be dubious; however, it may be illustrated by a commonly observed phenomenon. If one is sitting in a stationary train and watches another stationary train on the neighboring railroad track when one of the trains begins to move, it is difficult initially to determine which train is moving, and without external visual aids we cannot make a reasonable determination. The current state of research cannot determine which of the two theories is correct, but most histology and cell biology textbooks favor the anterograde vesicle transport theory.

Endocytosis, Endosomes, and Lysosomes

Endocytosis, endosomes, and lysosomes are involved in the ingestion, sequestering, and degradation of substances internalized from the extracellular space.

The process whereby a cell ingests macromolecules, particulate matter, and other substances from the extracellular space is referred to as **endocytosis.** The endocytosed material is engulfed in a vesicle appropriate for its volume. If the vesicle is large (>250 nm in diameter), the method is called **phagocytosis** (cell eating) and the vesicle is a **phagosome.** If the vesicle is small (<150 nm in diameter), the type of endocytosis is called **pinocytosis** (cell drinking) and the vesicle is a **pinocytotic vesicle.**

Endocytotic Mechanisms

Endocytosis is divided into two categories: phagocytosis and pinocytosis.

Phagocytosis

The process of engulfing larger particulate matter, such as microorganisms, cell fragments, and cells (e.g., defunct red blood cells), is usually performed by specialized cells known as **phagocytes.** The most common phagocytes are the white blood cells, the **neutrophils,** and the **monocytes.** When monocytes leave the bloodstream and enter the connective tissue domain to perform their task of phagocytosis, they become known as **macrophages.**

Phagocytes can internalize particulate matter because they possess receptors that recognize certain surface features of the material to be engulfed. Two of the better understood of these surface features come from the study of immunology and are the **constant regions (Fc regions)** of antibodies and a blood-borne series of proteins known as **complement.** Because the variable region of the antibody binds to the surface of a microorganism, the Fc region projects away from its surface.

Macrophages and neutrophils possess Fc receptors that bind the Fc regions of the antibody upon contact. This relationship acts as a signal for the cell to extend pseudopods, surround the microorganism, and internalize the microorganism by forming a **phagosome.** Complement on the surface of the microorganism probably assists phagocytosis in a similar manner, because macrophages also possess complement receptors on their surface. Interaction between complement and its receptor presumably activates the cell to form pseudopods and engulf the offending microorganism.

Pinocytosis

Because most cells export substances into the intercellular space, they continually add the membranes of vesicles that transport those substances from the *trans* Golgi network to the plasma membrane. These cells, in order to maintain their shape and size, must continually remove the excess membrane and return it for recycling. This cycle of membrane shuffling during exocytosis and endocytosis is known as **membrane trafficking,** the movement of membranes to and from various compartments of the cell. In most cells, pinocytosis is the most active transporting process and contributes most to the recapturing of membranes (Fig. 2-22).

RECEPTOR-MEDIATED ENDOCYTOSIS

Many cells specialize in the pinocytosis of several types of macromolecules. The most efficient form of capturing these substances depends on the presence of receptor proteins (**cargo receptors**) in the cell membrane. Cargo receptors are transmembrane proteins that become associated with the particular macromolecule (**ligand**) extracellularly and with a **clathrin coat** intracellularly (see Fig. 2-20).

The assembly of clathrin triskelions beneath the cargo receptors pulls on the plasma membrane, forming a clathrin-coated pit (Figs. 2-23 and 2-24), which eventually becomes a **pinocytotic vesicle,** enclosing the ligand as a droplet of fluid about to drip from a surface. To release this pinocytotic vesicle, several molecules of **dynamin,** a GTPase, surround the constricted neck of the vesicle, pinch its neck closed, and the pinocytotic vesicle is released from its membrane origin into the cytoplasm. This method of endocytosis permits the cell to increase the concentration of the ligand (e.g., low-density lipoprotein) within the pinocytotic vesicle.

A typical pinocytotic vesicle may have as many as 1000 cargo receptors of several types, for they may bind different macromolecules. Each cargo receptor is

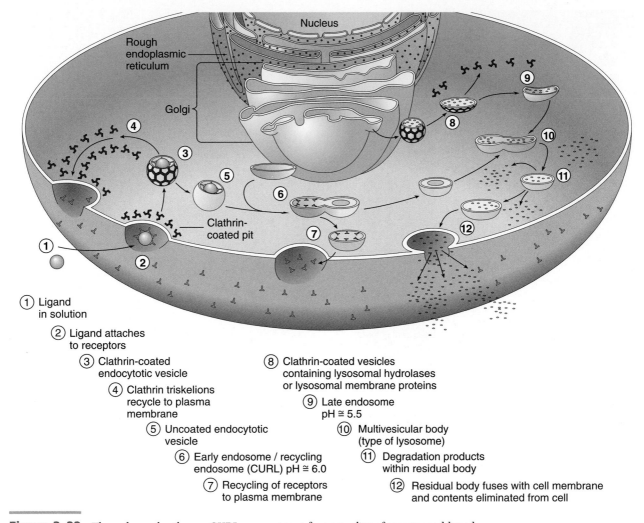

1. Ligand in solution
2. Ligand attaches to receptors
3. Clathrin-coated endocytotic vesicle
4. Clathrin triskelions recycle to plasma membrane
5. Uncoated endocytotic vesicle
6. Early endosome / recycling endosome (CURL) pH ≅ 6.0
7. Recycling of receptors to plasma membrane
8. Clathrin-coated vesicles containing lysosomal hydrolases or lysosomal membrane proteins
9. Late endosome pH ≅ 5.5
10. Multivesicular body (type of lysosome)
11. Degradation products within residual body
12. Residual body fuses with cell membrane and contents eliminated from cell

Figure 2–22 The endosomal pathways. CURL, *c*ompartment for *u*ncoupling of *r*eceptor and *l*igand.

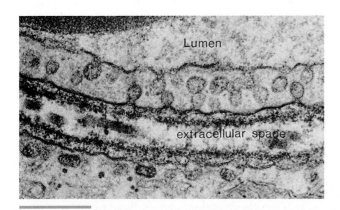

Figure 2–23 Electron micrograph of endocytosis in a capillary. (From Hopkins CR: Structure and Function of Cells. Philadelphia, WB Saunders, 1978.)

linked to its own adaptin, the protein with a binding site for the cytoplasmic aspect of the receptor, as well as a binding site for the clathrin triskelion.

Endosomes

Endosomes are divided into two compartments: early endosomes, near the periphery of the cell, and late endosomes, situated deeper within the cytoplasm.

Shortly after their formation, pinocytotic vesicles lose their clathrin coats (which return to the pool of clathrin triskelions in the cytosol) and fuse with **early endosomes** (Fig. 2-25; also see Fig. 2-22), a system of vesicles and tubules located near the plasma membrane. If the entire contents of the pinocytotic vesicle require degradation, the material from the early endosome is transferred to a **late endosome.** This similar set of

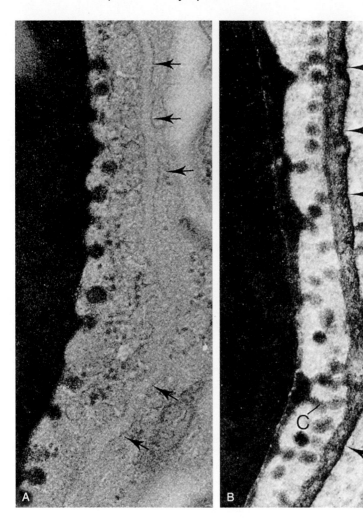

Figure 2–24 Electron micrographs of transport of microperoxidase, a trace molecule, across the endothelial cell of a capillary (×35,840). **A,** The lumen of the capillary is filled with the tracer; note its uptake of pinocytotic vesicles on the luminal aspect. Arrows indicate the extracellular space. **B,** One minute later, the tracer has been conveyed across the endothelial cell and exocytosed on the connective tissue side into the extracellular space (*arrows*). Note the region of fused vesicles (C), forming a temporary channel between the lumen of the capillary and the extracellular space. (From Hopkins CR: Structure and Function of Cells. Philadelphia, WB Saunders, 1978.)

tubules and vesicles, located deeper in the cytoplasm near the Golgi apparatus, helps to prepare its contents for eventual destruction by lysosomes.

Early and late endosomes, collectively, constitute the **endosomal compartment.** The membranes of all endosomes contain ATP-linked H^+ pumps that acidify the interior of the endosomes by actively pumping H^+ ions into the interior of the endosome so that the early endosome has a pH of 6.0 and the late endosome a pH of 5.5.

Material entering the early endosome may be retrieved from that compartment and returned to its earlier location, as occurs with cargo receptors that need to be recycled. When the pinocytotic vesicle fuses with the early endosome, the acidic environment causes an uncoupling of the ligand from its receptor molecule. The ligand remains within the lumen of the early endosome, whereas the receptor molecules (e.g., low-density lipoprotein receptors) are returned to the plasma membrane where they originated, or to the plasma membrane of another region of the cell, a process known as

transcytosis. Some authors refer to this type of early endosome as a **CURL** (*c*ompartment for *u*ncoupling of *r*eceptor and *l*igand) or, more recently, as a **recycling endosome** (see Figs. 2-22 and 2-25).

Within 10 to 15 minutes of entering the early endosome, the ligand either is transferred to a late endosome (as in the case of low-density lipoprotein) or is packaged to be returned to the cell membrane, where it is released (e.g., transferrin) into the extracellular space. Occasionally, both the receptor and the ligand (e.g., epidermal growth factor and its receptor) are transferred to the late endosome, and then to a lysosome, for eventual degradation.

The transport between early and late endosomes has not been elucidated. Some authors suggest that early endosomes migrate along microtubule pathways into a deeper location within the cell and become late endosomes. Others postulate that early and late endosomes are two separate compartments and that specific **endosomal carrier vesicles** ferry material from early to late

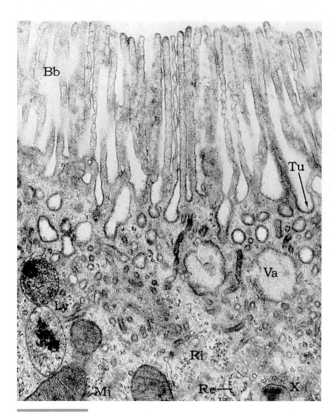

Figure 2–25 Endocytotic vesicles (Tu) of the proximal tubule cell of the kidney cortex (×25,000). Note the presence of microvilli (Bb), lysosomes (Ly), mitochondria (Mi), rough endoplasmic reticulum (Re), free ribosomes (Ri), and, possibly, early endosomes (Va). (From Rhodin JAG: An Atlas of Ultrastructure. Philadelphia, WB Saunders, 1963.)

endosomes. These are believed to be large vesicles containing numerous small vesicles that have been noted as **multivesicular bodies** in electron micrographs. Both theories recognize the presence of a system of microtubules along which either the early endosome or the endosomal carrier vesicle negotiates its way to the late endosome.

Lysosomes

Lysosomes have an acidic pH and contain hydrolytic enzymes.

The contents of late endosomes are delivered for enzymatic digestion into the lumina of specialized organelles known as lysosomes (Fig. 2-26; also see Fig. 2-25). Each lysosome is round to polymorphous in shape. Its average diameter is 0.3 to 0.8 μm, and it contains at least 40 different types of **acid hydrolases,** such as sulfatases, proteases, nucleases, lipases, and glycosidases, among others. Because all of these enzymes require an acid environment for optimal function, lysosomal membranes possess proton pumps that actively transport H^+ ions into the lysosome, maintaining its lumen at a pH of 5.0 (see Fig. 2-22).

Lysosomes aid in digesting not only macromolecules, phagocytosed microorganisms, cellular debris, and cells but also excess or senescent organelles, such as mitochondria and RER. The various enzymes digest the engulfed material into small, soluble end products that are transported by carrier proteins in the lysosomal membrane from the lysosomes into the cytosol and are either reused by the cell or exported from the cell into the extracellular space.

Formation of Lysosomes

Lysosomes receive their hydrolytic enzymes as well as their membranes from the *trans* Golgi network (TGN); however, they arrive in different vesicles. Although both types of vesicles possess a clathrin coat as they pinch off the TGN, the clathrin coat is lost shortly after formation. The uncoated vesicles then fuse with late endosomes.

Vesicles ferrying lysosomal enzymes possess **mannose-6-phosphate receptors,** to which these enzymes are bound. In the acidic environment of the late endosome, the lysosomal enzymes dissociate from their receptors, their mannose residue becomes dephosphorylated, and the receptors are recycled by being returned to the TGN. It should be understood that the dephosphorylated lysosomal hydrolases can no longer bind to the mannose-6-phosphate receptors and therefore stay in the late endosome (see Figs. 2-20 and 2-22).

When late endosomes possess both enzymatic and membrane components, some authors hypothesize that the late endosome fuses with a lysosome. However, others suggest that it matures to become a lysosome.

Transport of Substances into Lysosomes

Substances destined for degradation within lysosomes reach these organelles in one of three ways: through phagosomes, pinocytotic vesicles, or autophagosomes (see Fig. 2-22).

Phagocytosed material, contained within **phagosomes,** moves toward the interior of the cell. The phagosome joins either a lysosome or a late endosome. The hydrolytic enzymes digest most of the contents of the phagosome, especially the protein and carbohydrate components. Lipids, however, are more resistant to complete digestion, and they remain enclosed within the spent lysosome, now referred to as a **residual body.**

Senescent organelles such as mitochondria and organelles no longer required by the cell, or the RER of a quiescent fibroblast, need to be degraded. The organelles in question become surrounded by elements of the endoplasmic reticulum and are enclosed in vesicles called **autophagosomes.** These structures fuse

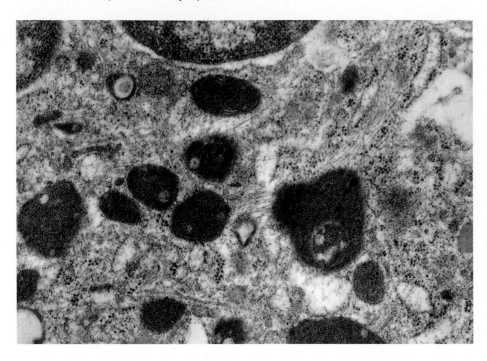

Figure 2–26 Lysosomes of rat cultured alveolar macrophages (×45,000). (From Sakai M, Araki N, Ogawa K: Lysosomal movements during heterophagy and autophagy: With special reference to nematolysosome and wrapping lysosome. J Electron Microsc Tech 12:101-131, 1989.)

either with late endosomes or with lysosomes and share the same subsequent fate as the phagosome.

CLINICAL CORRELATIONS

Certain individuals with hereditary enzyme deficiencies are incapable of completely degrading various macromolecules into soluble by-products. A **lysosomal storage disorder** generally results. As the insoluble intermediaries of these substances become amassed within the lysosomes of their cells, the size of these lysosomes increases sufficiently to interfere with the abilities of these cells to perform their function (Table 2-1).

Probably the most commonly known of these conditions is **Tay-Sachs disease,** occurring mostly in children of Northeast European Jewish ancestry and in certain individuals of Cajun ancestry in Louisiana. These children display a deficiency in the enzyme hexosaminidase and cannot catabolize GM_2 gangliosides. Although most cells in these children accumulate GM_2 ganglioside in the lysosomes, it is the neurons in their central and peripheral nervous systems that are the most problematic. Lysosomes of these cells become so engorged that they interfere with neuronal function, causing the children to become vegetative within the first year or two and to die by the third year of life.

Peroxisomes

Peroxisomes are self-replicating organelles that contain oxidative enzymes.

Peroxisomes (microbodies) are small (0.2 to 1.0 μm in diameter), spherical to ovoid membrane-bound organelles that contain more than 40 oxidative enzymes, especially **urate oxidase, catalase,** and **D-amino acid oxidase** (Fig. 2-27). They are present in almost all animal cells and function in the catabolism of long-chained fatty acids (**beta oxidation**), forming **acetyl coenzyme A (CoA)** as well as **hydrogen peroxide (H_2O_2)** by combining hydrogen from the fatty acid with molecular oxygen. Acetyl CoA is used by the cell for its own metabolic needs or is exported into the intercellular space to be used by neighboring cells. Hydrogen peroxide detoxifies various noxious agents (e.g., ethanol) and kills microorganisms. Excess hydrogen peroxide is degraded into water and molecular oxygen by the enzyme **catalase.**

Proteins destined for peroxisomes are not manufactured on the RER but in the cytosol and are transported into the peroxisomes by two specific peroxisome targeting signals that direct the protein from the cytosol to the peroxisome, where they recognize membrane-bound import receptors unique to the targeting signal. However, some peroxisomal membrane proteins may be manufactured on and targeted to the peroxisomes via the RER. Similar to mitochondria, peroxisomes increase in size and undergo fission to form new peroxisomes; however, they possess no genetic material of their own.

TABLE 2–1 Major Lysosomal Storage Diseases

Type	Specific Disease	Enzyme Deficiency	Metabolite Buildup
Glycogenosis	Pompe's disease (glycogen storage disease, type II)	Lysosomal glucosidase	Glycogen
Sphingolipidosis	GM_1 gangliosidoses	GM_1 ganglioside beta-galactosidase	GM_1 ganglioside; oligosaccharides containing galactose
	GM_2 gangliosidoses		
	Tay-Sachs disease	Hexosaminidase A	GM_2 ganglioside
	Gaucher's disease	Glucocerebrosidase	Glucocerebroside
	Niemann-Pick disease	Sphingomyelinase	Sphingomyelin
Mucopolysaccharidosis (MPS)			
MPS I	Hurler's syndrome	α-L-Iduronidase	Heparan sulfate, dermatan sulfate
MPS II	Hunter's syndrome	L-Iduronosulfate sulfatase	Heparan sulfate, dermatan sulfate
Glycoproteinosis		Enzymes that degrade polysaccharide side chains of glycoproteins	Several, depending on enzyme

Modified from Kumar V, Cotran RS, Robbins SL: Basic Pathology, 5th ed. Philadelphia, WB Saunders, 1992.

Proteasomes

Proteasomes are small organelles composed of protein complexes that are responsible for proteolysis of malformed and ubiquitin-tagged proteins.

The protein population of a cell is in a constant flux as a result of the continuous synthesis, export, and degradation of these macromolecules. Frequently, proteins, such as those that act in metabolic regulation, have to be degraded to ensure that the metabolic response to a single stimulus is not prolonged. Additionally, proteins that have been denatured, damaged, or malformed have to be eliminated; moreover, antigenic proteins that have been endocytosed by antigen-presenting cells (APCs) have to be cleaved into small polypeptide fragments **(epitopes)** so that they can be presented to T lymphocytes for recognition and the mounting of an immune response.

The process of cytosolic proteolysis is carefully controlled by the cell, and it requires that the protein be recognized as a potential candidate for degradation. This recognition involves **ubiquination,** a process whereby several ubiquitin molecules (a 76-amino acid long polypeptide chain) are attached to a lysine residue of the candidate protein to form a **polyubiquinated protein.** Once a protein has been thus tagged, it is degraded by **proteasomes,** multisubunit protein complexes that have a molecular weight in excess of 2 million daltons. During proteolysis, the ubiquitin molecules are released and reenter the cytosolic pool. The mechanism of ubiquitination requires:

- The cooperation of a series of enzymes, including **ubiquitin-activating enzyme**
- A family of **ubiquitin-conjugating enzymes**
- A number of **ubiquitin ligases** each of which recognizes one or more substrate proteins

Ubiquitination, the release of ubiquitin from the candidate protein, and the mechanism of protein degradation by the proteasome are all energy-requiring processes. An average cell may have as many as 30,000 proteasomes

Mitochondria

Mitochondria possess their own DNA and perform oxidative phosphorylation and lipid synthesis.

Mitochondria are flexible, rod-shaped organelles, about 0.5 to 1 μm in girth and sometimes as much as 7 μm in length. Most animal cells possess a large number of mitochondria (as many as 2000 in each liver cell) because, via **oxidative phosphorylation,** they produce ATP, a stable storage form of energy that can be used by the cell for its various energy-requiring activities.

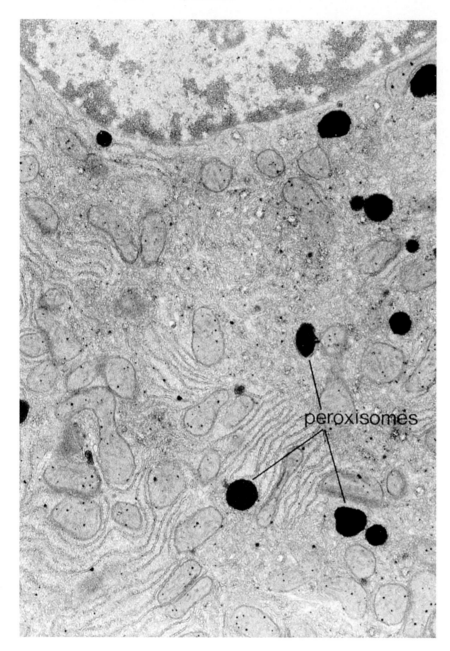

Figure 2-27 Peroxisomes in hepatocytes (×10,700). The cells were treated with 3′,3′-diaminobenzidine and osmium tetroxide, yielding a black reaction product caused by the enzyme catalase located within peroxisomes. (From Hopkins CR: Structure and Function of Cells. Philadelphia, WB Saunders, 1978.)

Each mitochondrion possesses a smooth **outer membrane** and a folded **inner membrane** (Fig. 2-28; also see Fig. 2-6). The folds of the inner membrane, known as **cristae,** greatly increase the surface area of the membrane. The number of cristae possessed by a mitochondrion is related directly to the energy requirement of the cell; thus, a cardiac muscle cell mitochondrion has more cristae than an osteocyte mitochondrion has. The narrow space (10 to 20 nm in width) between the inner and outer membranes is called the **intermembrane space,** whereas the large space enclosed by the inner membrane is termed the

matrix space (intercristal space). The contents of the two spaces differ somewhat and are discussed later.

Outer Mitochondrial Membrane and Intermembrane Space

The outer mitochondrial membrane possesses a large number of **porins,** multipass transmembrane proteins. Each porin forms a large aqueous channel through which water-soluble molecules, as large as 10 kD, may pass. Because this membrane is relatively permeable to

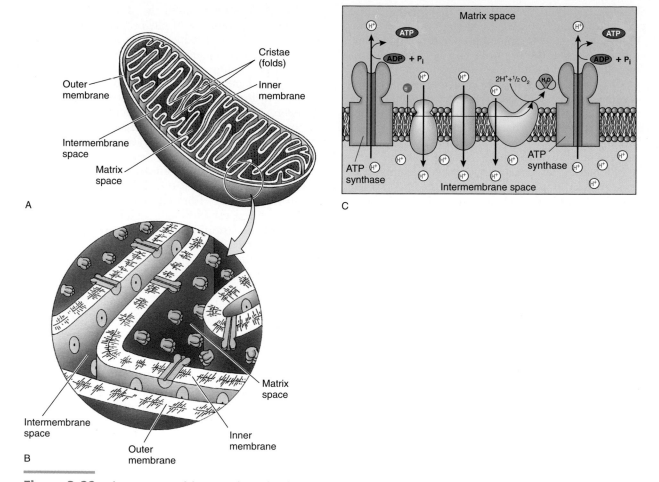

Figure 2–28 The structure and function of mitochondria. **A,** Mitochondrion sectioned longitudinally to demonstrate its outer and folded inner membranes. **B,** Enlarged region of the mitochondrion, displaying the inner membrane subunits and ATP synthase. **C,** Two ATP synthase complexes and three of the five members of the electron transport chain that also function to pump hydrogen (H^+) from the matrix into the intermembrane space. ADP, adenosine diphosphate; ATP, adenosine triphosphate; P_i, inorganic phosphate.

small molecules, including proteins, the contents of the **intermembrane space** resemble the cytosol. Additional proteins located in the outer membrane are responsible for the formation of mitochondrial lipids.

Inner Mitochondrial Membrane

The inner mitochondrial membrane is folded into cristae to provide a larger surface area for ATP synthase and the respiratory chain.

The inner mitochondrial membrane, which encloses the matrix space, is folded to form cristae. This membrane is richly endowed with **cardiolipin,** a phospholipid that possesses four, rather than the usual two, fatty acyl chains. The presence of this phospholipid in high concentration makes the inner membrane nearly impermeable to ions, electrons, and protons.

In certain regions, the outer and inner mitochondrial membranes contact each other; these **contact sites** act as pathways for proteins and small molecules to enter and leave the matrix space. The contact sites are composed of carrier proteins for the transport and regulatory proteins for the recognition of markers denoting the transportability of the specific macromolecules. These same contact sites are also used for the transport of proteins into the intermembrane space, provided that the proteins bear markers specific for entry into that space.

Additional sites are also available for the transport of macromolecules that are destined for the outer or inner mitochondrial membrane or for the matrix. At these sites, the two membranes do not contact one another, but both inner and outer membranes possess receptor molecules that recognize not only the macromolecule that is being transported but also cytosolic carrier molecules (and chaperones) responsible for the delivery of that particular macromolecule.

Viewed in negatively stained preparations, the inner membrane displays the presence of a large number of lollipop-like inner membrane subunits, protein complexes known as **ATP synthase,** which are responsible for the generation of ATP from ADP and inorganic phosphate. The globular head of the subunit, about 10 nm in diameter, is attached to a narrow, flattened, cylinder-like stalk, 4 nm wide and 5 nm long, projecting from the inner membrane into the matrix space (see Fig. 2-28).

Additionally, a large number of protein complexes, the **respiratory chains,** are present in the inner membrane. Each respiratory chain is composed of three respiratory enzyme complexes: (1) **NADH dehydrogenase complex,** (2) **cytochrome b-c₁ complex,** and (3) **cytochrome oxidase complex.** These complexes form an **electron transport chain** that is responsible for the passage of electrons along this chain and, more important, that function as proton pumps that transport H^+ from the matrix into the intermembrane space, establishing an **electrochemical gradient** that provides energy for the ATP-generating action of ATP synthase.

Matrix

The matrix space is filled with a dense fluid composed of at least 50% protein, which accounts for its viscosity. Much of the protein component of the matrix is enzymes responsible for the stepwise degradation of fatty acids and pyruvate to the metabolic intermediate **acetyl CoA** and the subsequent oxidation of this intermediate in the **tricarboxylic acid (Krebs) cycle.** Mitochondrial ribosomes, tRNA, mRNA, and dense spherical **matrix granules** (30 to 50 nm in diameter) are also present in the matrix.

The function of matrix granules is not understood. They are composed of phospholipoprotein, although in some cells, especially cells of bone and cartilage, they may also bind magnesium and calcium. Moreover, in injured cells whose cytosolic Ca^{2+} levels are dangerously high, matrix granules may sequester calcium to protect the cell from calcium toxicity.

The matrix also contains the double-stranded mitochondrial **circular deoxyribonucleic acid (cDNA)** and the enzymes necessary for the expression of the mitochondrial genome. cDNA contains information for the formation of only 13 mitochondrial proteins, 16S and 12S rRNA, and genes for 22 tRNAs. Therefore, most of the codes necessary for the formation and functioning of mitochondria are located in the genome of the nucleus.

Oxidative Phosphorylation

Oxidative phosphorylation is the process responsible for the formation of ATP.

Acetyl CoA, formed through the β-oxidation of fatty acids and the degradation of glucose, is oxidized in the citric acid cycle to produce, in addition to carbon dioxide (CO_2), large quantities of the reduced cofactors nicotinamide adenine dinucleotide (NADH) and flavin adenine dinucleotide ($FADH_2$). Each of these cofactors releases a hydride ion (H^+) which is stripped of its two high-energy electrons and becomes a proton (H^+). The electrons are transferred to the electron transport chain and during mitochondrial respiration reduce oxygen (O_2) to form water (H_2O).

According to the **chemiosmotic theory,** the energy released by the sequential transfer of the electrons is used to transport H^+ from the matrix into the intermembrane space, establishing a high proton concentration in that space exerting a **proton motive force** (see Fig. 2-28). Only through ATP synthase may these protons leave the intermembrane space and reenter the matrix. As the protons pass down this electrochemical gradient, the energy differential in the proton motive force is transformed into the stable high-energy bond of ATP by the globular head of the inner membrane subunit, which catalyzes the formation of ATP from ADP + P_i, where P_i is inorganic phosphate. The newly formed ATP either is utilized by the mitochondrion or is transported, through an ADP-ATP antiport system, into the cytosol. During the entire process of glycolysis, tricarboxylic acid cycle, and electron transport, each glucose molecule yields 36 molecules of ATP.

In some cells, such as the brown fat cells of hibernating animals, oxidation is uncoupled from phosphorylation, resulting in the formation of heat instead of ATP. This uncoupling is dependent on the presence of proton shunts, known as **thermogenins,** that resemble ATP synthase but that cannot generate ATP. As the protons pass through thermogenins to reenter the matrix, the energy of the proton motive force is transformed into heat. It is this heat that awakens the animal from its state of hibernation.

Origin and Replication of Mitochondria

Because of the presence of the mitochondrial genetic apparatus, it is believed that mitochondria were free-living organisms that either invaded or were phagocytosed by anaerobic eukaryotic cells, developing a **symbiotic relationship.** The mitochondrion-like organism received protection and nutrients from its host and provided its host with the capability of reducing its O_2 content and simultaneously supplying it with a stable form of chemical energy.

Mitochondria are self-replicating, in that they are generated from preexisting mitochondria. These organelles enlarge in size, replicate their DNA, and undergo fission. The division usually occurs through the intracristal space of one of the centrally located cristae. The outer mitochondrial membrane of the opposing halves extends through that intracristal space; the halves meet and fuse with each other, thus dividing the mitochondrion into two nearly equal halves. The two new mitochondria move away from each other. The average life span of a mitochondrion is about 10 days.

Annulate Lamella

Annulate lamellae are parallel aggregates of membranes that enclose cistern-like spaces, thus resembling multiple copies, usually six to ten, of nuclear envelopes. They possess nuclear pore complex-like regions (**annuli**) that are in register with those of neighboring membranes. The cisternae of these organelles are relatively evenly spaced, separated by about 80 to 100 nm, and are continuous with the cisternae of the RER.

These organelles are normally present only in cells that have high mitotic indices, such as oocytes, tumor cells, and embryonic cells. Because of their resemblance to the nuclear envelope, some authors suggest that they act as reserves for the nuclear envelope in these rapidly dividing cells. However, immunocytochemical studies of annulate lamellae do not lend support to that supposition, and neither their function nor their significance is understood.

INCLUSIONS

Inclusions are considered to be nonliving components of the cell that do not possess metabolic activity and are not bounded by membranes. The most common inclusions are glycogen, lipid droplets, pigments, and crystals.

Glycogen

Glycogen is the storage form of glucose.

Glycogen is the most common storage form of glucose in animals and is especially abundant in cells of muscle and liver. It appears in electron micrographs as clusters, or **rosettes,** of β particles (and larger α particles in the liver) that resemble ribosomes, located in the vicinity of the SER. On demand, enzymes responsible for glycogenolysis degrade glycogen into individual molecules of glucose.

CLINICAL CORRELATIONS

Some individuals suffer from **glycogen storage disorders** as a result of their inability to degrade glycogen, resulting in excess accumulation of this substance in the cells. There are three classifications of this disease: (1) hepatic, (2) myopathic, and (3) miscellaneous. The lack or malfunction of one of the enzymes responsible for the degradation is responsible for these disorders (Table 2-2).

Lipids

Lipids are storage forms of triglycerides.

Lipids, triglycerides in storage form, not only are stored in specialized cells (**adipocytes**) but also are located as individual droplets in various cell types, especially **hepatocytes.** Most solvents used in histological preparations extract triglycerides from cells, leaving empty spaces indicative of the locations of lipids. However, with the use of osmium and glutaraldehyde, the lipids (and cholesterol) may be fixed in position as gray-to-black intracellular droplets. Lipids are very efficient forms of energy reserves; twice as many ATPs are derived from 1 g of fat as from 1 g of glycogen.

TABLE 2–2   Major Subgroups of Glycogen Storage Disorders

Type (Specific Disease)	Deficient Enzyme	Tissue Changes	Clinical Signs
Hepatic Hepatorenal (von Gierke's disease)	Glucose-6-phosphatase	Intracellular accumulation of glycogen in hepatocytes and cortical tubules of kidneys	Enlarged liver and kidneys; hypoglycemia with subsequent convulsions; gout; bleeding; 50% mortality rate
Myopathic (McArdle's syndrome)	Muscle phosphorylase	Glycogen accumulation in skeletal muscle cells	Cramps following vigorous exercise; adult onset
Miscellaneous (Pompe's disease)	Lysosomal acid maltase	Glycogen accumulation Enlarged lysosomes in hepatocytes	Massively enlarged heart; cardiac and respiratory failure within 2 years of onset; adults have milder form involving only skeletal muscle

Pigments

The most common pigment in the body, besides **hemoglobin** of red blood cells, is **melanin,** manufactured by melanocytes of the skin and hair, pigment cells of the retina, and specialized nerve cells in the substantia nigra of the brain. These pigments have protective functions in skin and aid in the sense of sight in the retina, but their role in hair and neurons is not understood. Additionally, in long-lived cells, such as neurons of the central nervous system and cardiac muscle cells, a yellow-to-brown pigment, **lipofuscin,** has been demonstrated. Unlike other inclusions, lipofuscin pigments are membrane-bound and are believed to represent the indigestible remnants of lysosomal activity. They are formed from fusion of several **residual bodies.**

Crystals

Crystals are not commonly found in cells, with the exception of Sertoli cells **(crystals of Charcot-Böttcher),** interstitial cells **(crystals of Reinke)** of the testes, and occasionally in macrophages (Fig. 2-29). It is believed that these structures are crystalline forms of certain proteins.

CYTOSKELETON

The cytoskeleton has three major components: thin filaments, intermediate filaments, and microtubules.

The cytoplasm of animal cells contains a cytoskeleton, an intricate three-dimensional meshwork of protein filaments that are responsible for the maintenance of cellular morphology. Additionally, the cytoskeleton is an active participant in cellular motion, whether of organelles or vesicles within the cytoplasm, regions of the cell, or the entire cell. The cytoskeleton has three components: thin filaments (microfilaments), intermediate filaments, and microtubules.

Thin Filaments

Thin filaments are actin filaments that interact with myosin to bring about intracellular or cellular movement.

Thin filaments (microfilaments) are composed of two chains of globular subunits **(G-actin)** coiled around each other to form a filamentous protein, **F-actin** (Figs. 2-30 and 2-31). Actin constitutes about 15% of the total protein content of non-muscle cells. Only about half of their total actin is in the filamentous form, because the monomeric G-actin form is bound by small proteins, such as **profilin** and **thymosin,** which prevent their polymerization. Actin molecules, present in the cells of many different vertebrate and invertebrate species, are very similar to each other in their amino acid sequence, attesting to their highly conserved nature.

Thin filaments are 6-nm thick and possess a faster-growing **plus end** and a slower-growing **minus end.** When the actin filament reaches its desired length,

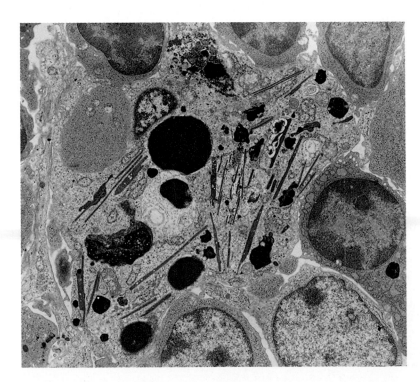

Figure 2–29 Electron micrograph of crystalloid inclusions in a macrophage (×5100). (From Yamazaki K: Isolated cilia and crystalloid inclusions in murine bone marrow stromal cells. Blood Cells 13:407-416, 1988.)

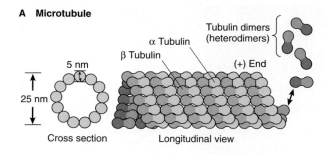

A **Microtubule**

5 nm

25 nm

Cross section

Longitudinal view

β Tubulin

α Tubulin

Tubulin dimers (heterodimers)

(+) End

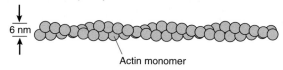

B **Thin filaments (actin)**

6 nm

Actin monomer

C **Intermediate filaments**

8–10 nm

Fibrous subunit

D **Centriole**

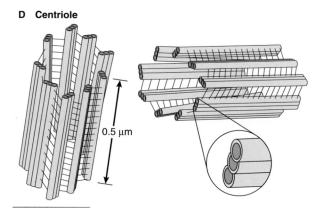

0.5 μm

Figure 2–30 Elements of the cytoskeleton and centriole. **A,** Microtubule; **B,** thin filaments (actin); **C,** intermediate filaments; **D,** centriole.

members of a family of small proteins, **capping proteins,** attach to the plus end, terminating the lengthening of the filament. The process of shortening of actin filaments is regulated in the presence of ATP, ADP, and Ca^{2+} by capping proteins, such as gelsolin, which prevent polymerization of the filament. The cell membrane phospholipid **polyphosphoinositide** has the

opposite effect: it removes the gelsolin cap, permitting elongation of the actin filament.

Depending on their isoelectric point, there are three classes of actin: **α-actin** of muscle, and **β-actin** and **γ-actin** of non-muscle cells. Although actin participates in the formation of various cellular extensions as well as in assembling structures responsible for motility, its basic composition is unaltered. It is capable of fulfilling its many roles via its association with different actin-binding proteins. The most commonly known of these proteins is **myosin,** but numerous other proteins, such as α-actinin, spectrin, fimbrin, filamin, gelsolin, and talin, also bind to actin to perform essential cellular functions (Table 2-3).

Actin filaments form bundles of varied lengths, depending on the function that they perform in non-muscle cells. These bundles form three types of associations:

■ Contractile bundles
■ Gel-like networks
■ Parallel bundles

Contractile bundles, such as those responsible for the formation of cleavage furrows (contractile rings) during mitotic division, are usually associated with myosin. Their actin filaments are arranged loosely, parallel to each other, with the plus and minus ends alternating in direction. These assemblies are responsible for movement not only of organelles and vesicles within the cell but also for cellular activities, such as exocytosis and endocytosis, as well as the extension of filopodia and cell migration.

The myosin associated with these contractile bundles may be one of several types: **myosin-I** through **myosin-IX.** Myosin-II forms **thick filaments** (15 nm in diameter) and moves actin filaments, especially in muscle cells. Myosin-V can bind not only to actin filaments but also to other cytoplasmic components, such as vesicles, moving them along an actin filament from one position in the cell to another, whereas myosin-I has been implicated in the formation and retraction of actin-directed protrusions of the cell cortex, such as in the formation of pseudopods.

Gel-like networks provide the structural foundation of much of the cell cortex. Their stiffness is due to the protein filamin, which assists in the establishment of a loosely organized network of actin filaments resulting in localized high viscosity. During the formation of filopodia, the gel is liquefied by proteins such as **gelsolin,** which, in the presence of ATP and high Ca^{2+}, cleaves the actin filaments and, by forming a cap over their plus end, prevents them from lengthening.

The proteins **fimbrin** and **villin** are responsible for forming actin filaments into closely packed **parallel bundles** that form the core of microspikes and microvilli, respectively. These bundles of actin filaments are

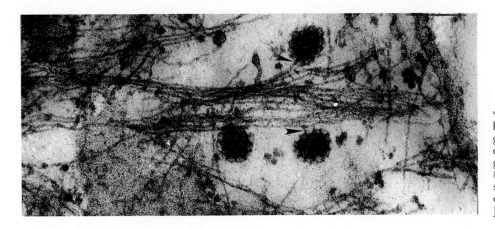

Figure 2–31 Electron micrograph of clathrin-coated vesicles contacting filaments *(arrowheads)* in granulosa cells of the rat ovary (×35,000). (From Batten BE, Anderson E: The distribution of actin in cultured ovarian granulosa cells. Am J Anat 167:395-404, 1983.)

TABLE 2–3 Actin-Binding Proteins

Protein	Molecular Mass of Each Subunit (Da)	Number of Subunits	Function
α-Actinin	100,000	2	Bundling actin filaments for contractile bundles
Fimbrin	68,000	1	Bundling actin filaments for parallel bundles
Filamin	270,000	2	Cross-link actin filaments into gel-like network
Myosin-II	260,000	2	Contraction by sliding actin filaments
Myosin-V	150,000	1	Movement of vesicles and organelles along actin filaments
Spectrin α β	265,000 260,000	2 2	Forms supporting network for plasma membrane of red blood cell
Gelsolin	90,000	1	Cleaves and caps actin filaments
Thymosin	5000	1	Binds to G-actin subunits, maintaining them in monomeric form

anchored in the **terminal web,** a region of the cell cortex composed of a network of intermediate filaments and the protein **spectrin.** Spectrin molecules are flexible, rod-like tetramers that assist the cell in maintaining the structural integrity of the cortex.

Actin is also important in the establishment and maintenance of **focal contacts** of the cell with extracellular matrix (Fig. 2-32). At focal contacts, the **integrin** (a transmembrane protein) of the cell membrane binds to structural glycoproteins, such as **fibronectin,** of the extracellular matrix, permitting the cell to maintain its attachment. Simultaneously, the intracellular region of the integrin contacts the cytoskeleton via intermediary proteins that attach it to actin filaments. The mode of attachment involves integrin binding to **talin,** which contacts both **vinculin** and the actin fila-

ment. Vinculin binds to α-actinin, the actin-binding protein that assembles actin into contractile bundles. These contractile bundles, referred to as **stress fibers** in fibroblasts maintained in tissue culture, resemble myofibrils of striated muscle. Stress fibers may extend between two focal points or a focal point and intermediate filaments and assist the cell in exerting a tensile force on the extracellular matrix (as in the wound contraction function of fibroblasts).

Intermediate Filaments

Intermediate filaments and their associated proteins assist in the establishment and maintenance of the three-dimensional framework of the cell.

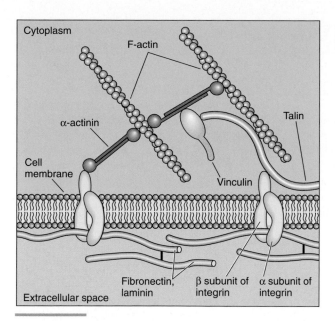

Cytoplasm
F-actin
α-actinin
Talin
Cell membrane
Vinculin
Fibronectin, laminin
β subunit of integrin
α subunit of integrin
Extracellular space

Figure 2–32 The cytoskeleton. Fibronectin and laminin receptor regions of integrin molecules bind to fibronectin and laminin, respectively, in the extracellular space. Intracellular talin-binding or α-actinin–binding regions of integrin molecules bind to talin or α-actinin, respectively. Thus, integrin molecules bridge the cytoskeleton to an extracellular support framework.

Electron micrographs display a category of filaments in the cytoskeleton whose diameter of 8 to 10 nm places them between thick and thin filaments and they are consequently named intermediate filaments (see Fig. 2-30). These filaments and their associated proteins accomplish the following:

■ Provide structural support for the cell
■ Form a deformable three-dimensional structural framework for the cell
■ Anchor the nucleus in place
■ Provide an adaptable connection between the cell membrane and the cytoskeleton
■ Furnish a structural framework for the maintenance of the nuclear envelope as well as its reorganization subsequent to mitosis

When microbeads bound to integrin molecules of the cell membrane are micromanipulated, as when one pulls on them, the tensile forces produce distortion of the cytoskeleton, with resultant deformation of the nucleus and rearrangement of the nucleoli. Thus, it appears that the cytoskeleton, and specifically the intermediate filaments, react to forces generated in the extracellular matrix, and by forcing modulations in the shape and location of cellular constituents, they protect the structural and functional integrity of the cell from external stresses and strains.

Biochemical investigations have determined that there are several categories of intermediate filaments that share

the same morphological and structural characteristics. These rope-like intermediate filaments are constructed of tetramers of rod-like proteins that are tightly bundled into long helical arrays. The individual subunit of each tetramer differs considerably for each type of intermediate filament. The categories of intermediate filaments include keratins, desmin, vimentin, glial fibrillary acidic protein, neurofilaments, and nuclear lamins (Table 2-4).

Several intermediate filament-binding proteins have been discovered. As they bind to intermediate filaments, they link them into a three-dimensional network that facilitates the formation of the cytoskeleton. Four of the best known of these proteins have the following characteristics:

1 **Filaggrin** binds keratin filaments into bundles.
2 **Synamin** and **plectin** bind desmin and vimentin, respectively, into three-dimensional intracellular meshworks.
3 **Plakins** assist the maintenance of contact between the keratin intermediate filaments and hemidesmosomes of epithelial cells as well as actin filaments with neurofilaments of sensory neurons.

CLINICAL CORRELATIONS

Immunocytochemical methods, utilizing specific immunofluorescent antibodies, are employed to distinguish intermediate filament types in tumors of unknown origin. Knowledge of the source of these tumors assists not only in their diagnosis but also in devising effective treatment plans.

Microtubules

Microtubules are long, straight, rigid tubular-appearing structures that act as intracellular pathways.

The **centrosome** is the region of the cell in the vicinity of the nucleus that houses the centrioles (see later), as well as several hundred ring-shaped **γ-tubulin ring complex** molecules. These γ-tubulin molecules act as nucleation sites for **microtubules,** which are long, straight, rigid, hollow-like cylindrical structures 25 nm in outer diameter, with a luminal diameter of 15 nm (Fig. 2-33; also see Fig. 2-30). Therefore, the centrosome is considered to be the **MTOC** of the cell.

Microtubules are polarized, having a rapidly growing plus end as well as a minus end, which must be stabilized or it will depolymerize, thus shortening the microtubule. The minus end is stabilized by being embedded in a γ-tubulin molecule. Microtubules are dynamic structures that frequently change their length by undergoing growth spurts and then becoming shorter; both

TABLE 2–4 Predominant Types of Intermediate Filaments

Filament	Polypeptide Component Size (Da)	Cell Type	Function
Keratins (30 variations) Type I (acidic) Type II (neutral/basic)	40,000-70,000 40,000-70,000	Epithelial cells Cells of hair and nails	Support cell assemblies and provide tensile strength to cytoskeleton
Tonofilaments	40,000-70,000	Epithelial cells, especially stratified squamous keratinized	Assist in formation of desmosomes and hemidesmosomes
Desmin	53,000	All types of muscle cells	Links myofibrils in striated muscle (around Z disks); attaches to cytoplasmic densities in smooth muscle
Vimentin	54,000	Cells of embryo as well as cells of mesenchymal origin: fibroblasts, leukocytes, endothelial cells	Surrounds nuclear envelope; is associated with cytoplasmic aspect of nuclear pore complex
Glial fibrillary acidic protein (GFAP)	50,000	Astrocytes, Schwann cells, oligodendroglia	Supports glial cell structure
Neurofilaments L: low molecular weight (NF-L) M: medium molecular weight (NF-M) H: high molecular weight (NF-H)	68,000 160,000 210,000	Neurons	Form cytoskeleton of axons and dendrites; assist in the formation of the gel state of the cytoplasm; cross-linking responsible for great tensile strength
Nuclear lamins A, B, and C	65,000-75,000	Lining of nuclear envelopes of all cells	Control and assembly of the nuclear envelope; organization of perinuclear chromatin

processes occur at the plus ends, so that the average half-life of a microtubule is only about 10 minutes. The main functions of microtubules are to:

■ Provide rigidity and maintain cell shape
■ Regulate intracellular movement of organelles and vesicles
■ Establish intracellular compartments
■ Provide the capability of ciliary (and flagellar) motion

Each microtubule consists of 13 parallel **protofilaments** composed of heterodimers of the globular polypeptide α- and β-tubulin subunits, each consisting of about 450 amino acids and each having a molecular mass of about 50,000 daltons (see Fig. 2-30). Polymer-ization of the heterodimers requires the presence of magnesium (Mg^{2+}) and GTP. During cell division, rapid polymerization of existing as well as new microtubules is responsible for the formation of the spindle apparatus.

CLINICAL CORRELATIONS

The polymerization process is disrupted by antimitotic drugs, such as colchicine, that block the mitotic event by binding to the tubulin molecules, preventing their assembly into the protofilament.

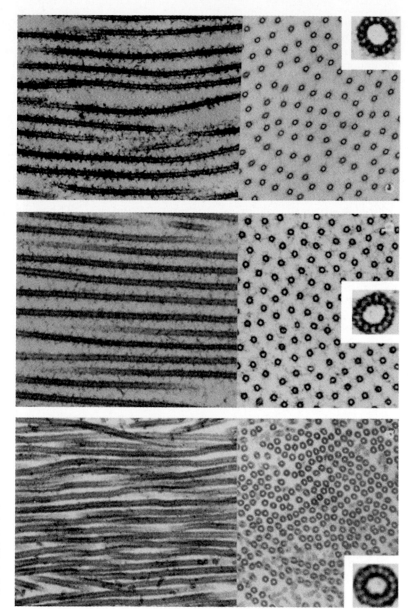

Figure 2–33 Electron micrograph of microtubules assembled with and without microtubule-associated proteins (MAPs) (×65,790). *Top,* Microtubules assembled from unfractionated MAPs. *Center,* Microtubules assembled in the presence of MAP₂ subfraction only. *Bottom,* Microtubules assembled without MAPs. (From Leeson TS, Leeson CR, and Papparo AA: Text/Atlas of Histology. Philadelphia, WB Saunders, 1988.)

Microtubule-Associated Proteins

Microtubule-associated proteins are motor proteins that assist in the translocation of organelles and vesicles inside the cell.

In addition to tubulin heterodimers, microtubules also possess microtubule-associated proteins (MAPs) bound to their periphery at 32-nm intervals. There are various types of MAPs, ranging in molecular weight from about 50,000 to more than 300,000 daltons. Their primary functions are to prevent depolymerization of microtubules and to assist in the intracellular movement of organelles and vesicles.

Movement along a microtubule occurs in both directions and is toward both the plus end and the minus end. The two major families of microtubule motor proteins, the MAPs **dynein** and **kinesin,** bind to the microtubule as well as to vesicles (and organelles). It is believed that different members of each motor protein family transport their cargo at disparate, meticulously controlled rates and that different organelles have their own particular motor protein. In the presence of ATP, dynein moves the vesicle toward the minus end of the microtubule. Kinesin effects vesicular (and organelle) transport in the opposite direction, toward the plus end, but the mechanism of ATP utilization by these MAPs is not understood. Additionally, dynein and kinesin participate in the organization of the minus and plus ends, respectively.

Centrioles

Centrioles are small, cylindrical structures composed of nine microtubule triplets; they constitute the core of the microtubule organizing center, or the centrosome.

Centrioles are small, cylindrical structures, 0.2 μm in diameter and 0.5 μm in length (see Fig. 2-30). Usually, they are paired structures, arranged perpendicular to each other, and are located in the microtubule organizing center, the centrosome, in the vicinity of the Golgi apparatus. The centrosome assists in the formation and organization of microtubules as well as in its self-duplication before cell division.

Centrioles are composed of a specific arrangement of nine triplets of microtubules arranged around a central axis. Each microtubule triplet consists of one complete and two incomplete microtubules fused to each other, so that the incomplete ones share three protofilaments. The complete microtubule "A" is posi-tioned closest to the center of the cylinder; "C" is the farthest away. Adjacent triplets are connected to each other by a fibrous substance of unknown composition, extending from microtubule A to microtubule C. Each triplet is arranged so that it forms an oblique angle with the adjacent triplet and a straight angle with the fifth triplet.

During the S phase of the cell cycle, each centriole of the pair replicates, forming a procentriole in some unknown manner, at 90 degrees to itself. This procentriole initially possesses no microtubules, but tubulin molecules begin to polymerize closest to the parent centriole, with the plus end growing away from the parent. The actual replication of the centriole requires the presence of γ-tubulin rings, structures that do not become part of but serve to direct the elongation of the forming microtubules by occupying the forming plus and minus ends. It is believed that the γ-tubulin rings and pericentrin serve as beams that support the developing centriole. Additionally, δ-tubulins, related to the α- and β-tubulin superfamily, are also required to form the triplet structure of the microtubule arrays.

Centrioles function in the formation of the centrosome, and during mitotic activity they are responsible for the formation of the spindle apparatus. Additionally, centrioles are the basal bodies that guide the formation of cilia and flagella.

Nucleus

3

The nucleus is the largest organelle of the cell (Fig. 3-1). It contains nearly all of the **deoxyribonucleic acid (DNA)** possessed by the cell as well as the mechanisms for **ribonucleic acid (RNA)** synthesis, and its resident nucleolus is the location for the assembly of ribosomal subunits. The nucleus, bounded by two lipid membranes, houses three major components:

- **Chromatin,** the genetic material of the cell
- The **nucleolus,** the center for ribosomal RNA (rRNA) synthesis
- **Nucleoplasm,** containing macromolecules and nuclear particles involved in the maintenance of the cell.

The nucleus is usually spherical and is centrally located in the cell; however, in some cells it may be spindle-shaped to oblong-shaped, twisted, lobulated, or even disk-shaped. Although usually each cell has a single nucleus, some cells (such as osteoclasts) possess several nuclei, whereas mature red blood cells have extruded nuclei. The size, shape, and form of the nucleus are generally constant for a particular cell type, a fact useful in clinical diagnoses of the degree of malignancy of certain cancerous cells.

NUCLEAR ENVELOPE

The nuclear envelope is composed of two parallel unit membranes that fuse with each other at certain regions to form perforations known as nuclear pores.

The nucleus is surrounded by the nuclear envelope, composed of two parallel unit membranes: the **inner** and **outer nuclear membranes,** separated from each other by a 10- to 30-nm space called the **perinuclear cisterna** (Figs. 3-2 and 3-3). The nuclear envelope is perforated at various intervals by **nuclear pores** (discussed later) that permit communication between the cytoplasm and the nucleus. At these pores, the inner

and outer nuclear membranes are continuous with one another. The nuclear envelope helps to control movement of macromolecules between the nucleus and the cytoplasm and assists in organizing the chromatin.

Inner Nuclear Membrane

The inner nuclear membrane is about 6-nm thick and faces the nuclear contents. It is in close contact with the **nuclear lamina,** an interwoven meshwork of intermediate filaments, 80- to 100-nm thick, composed of **lamins A, B,** and **C** and located at the periphery of the nucleoplasm. The nuclear lamina help in organizing and providing support to the lipid bilayer membrane and the perinuclear chromatin, as well as play a role in the assembly of vesicles to re-form the nuclear envelope subsequent to cell division. Certain integral proteins of the inner nuclear membrane act either directly or via other nuclear matrix proteins as contact sites for nuclear RNAs and chromosomes.

Outer Nuclear Membrane

The outer nuclear membrane is also about 6-nm thick, faces the cytoplasm, and is continuous with the rough endoplasmic reticulum (RER). It is considered by some authors as a specialized region of the RER (see Figs. 3-2 and 3-3). Its cytoplasmic surface is surrounded by a thin, loose meshwork of the intermediate filaments, termed **vimentin.** Its cytoplasmic surface usually possesses ribosomes actively synthesizing transmembrane proteins that are destined for the outer or inner nuclear membranes.

Nuclear Pores

Nuclear pores are interruptions in the nuclear envelope, where the inner and outer nuclear membranes fuse with each other, establishing sites where communication may occur between the nucleus and the cytoplasm.

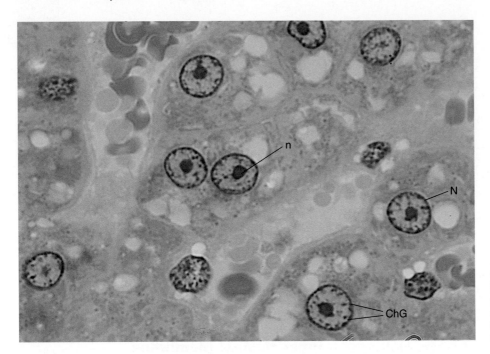

Figure 3–1 Cell nuclei. Light micrograph (×1323). Typical cells, each containing a spherical nucleus (N). Observe the chromatin granules (ChG) and the nucleolus (n).

At certain locations on the surface of the nuclear envelope, the outer and inner nuclear membranes are continuous with each other, creating openings known as nuclear pores, which permit communication between the nuclear compartment and the cytoplasm (Fig. 3-4). The number of nuclear pores ranges from a few dozen to several thousand, correlated directly with the metabolic activity of the cell.

High-resolution electron microscopy has revealed that the nuclear pore is surrounded by **nonmembranous structures** (glycoproteins) embedded in its rim. These structures and the pore are called the **nuclear pore complex,** which selectively guards passage through the pore (Fig. 3-5). Evidence suggests that each of the nuclear pore complexes is in communication with the others via the nuclear lamina and certain pore-connecting fibers.

Nuclear Pore Complex

The nuclear pore complex is composed of the nuclear pore and its associated glycoproteins.

The nuclear pore complex is about 100 to 125 nm in diameter and spans the two nuclear membranes. It is composed of three ring-like arrays of proteins stacked on top of the other, each ring displaying eight-fold symmetry and interconnected by a series of spokes arranged in a vertical fashion. In addition, the nuclear pore complex has cytoplasmic fibers, a transporter, and a nuclear basket (Fig. 3-6).

Associated Glycoproteins

The **cytoplasmic ring,** composed of eight subunits, is located on the rim of the cytoplasmic aspect of the nuclear pore. Each subunit possesses a cytoplasmic filament, believed to be a Ran-binding protein (a family of guanosine triphosphate [GTP]-binding proteins), that extends into the cytoplasm. It has been suggested that these fibers may mediate import into the nucleus through the nuclear pore complex by moving substrates along their length toward the center of the pore.

The **luminal spoke ring (middle ring)** is composed of a set of eight transmembrane proteins that project into the lumen of the nuclear pore as well as into the perinuclear cistern. These spoke-like proteins appear to anchor the glycoprotein components of the nuclear pore complex into the rim of the nuclear pore.

The center of the middle ring is occupied by an oblong-shaped structure known as the **transporter,** which is coupled to the spoke-like proteins of the luminal ring. Note that the presence of the transporter (central plug) is not universally accepted because some investigators consider it to be the material being transported into or out of the nucleus; thus it is not presented within the model in Figure 3-6. The central lumen of the middle ring is believed to be a gated channel that restricts passive diffusion between the cytoplasm and the nucleoplasm. It is associated with additional protein complexes that facilitate the regulated transport of materials across the nuclear pore complex.

A **nuclear ring (nucleoplasmic ring),** analogous to the cytoplasmic ring, is located on the rim of the nucleo-

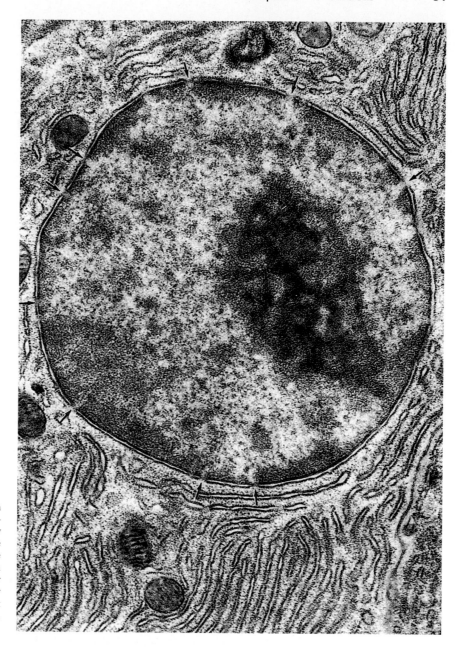

Figure 3–2 Cell nucleus. Electron micrograph (×16,762). Observe the electron-dense nucleolus, the peripherally located dense heterochromatin, and the light euchromatin. The nuclear envelope surrounding the nucleus is composed of an inner nuclear membrane and an outer nuclear membrane that is interrupted by the nuclear pores *(arrows)*. (From Fawcett DW: The Cell. Philadelphia, WB Saunders, 1981.)

plasmic aspect of the nuclear pore and assists in the export of several types of RNA. A filamentous, flexible, basket-like structure, the **nuclear basket,** appears to be suspended from the nucleoplasmic ring and protruding into the nucleoplasm. The nuclear basket becomes deformed during the process of nuclear export. Attached to the distal aspect of the nuclear basket is the **distal ring.**

Nuclear Pore Function

The nuclear pore functions in bidirectional nucleocytoplasmic transport.

Although the nuclear pore is relatively large, it is nearly filled with the structures constituting the nuclear pore complex. Because of the structural conformation of those subunits, several 9- to 11-nm wide channels are available for simple diffusion of ions and small molecules. However, macromolecules and particles larger than 11 nm cannot reach or leave the nuclear compartment via simple diffusion; instead, they are selectively transported via a **receptor-mediated transport** process. Signal sequences of molecules to be transported through the nuclear pores must be recognized by one of the many receptor sites of the nuclear pore

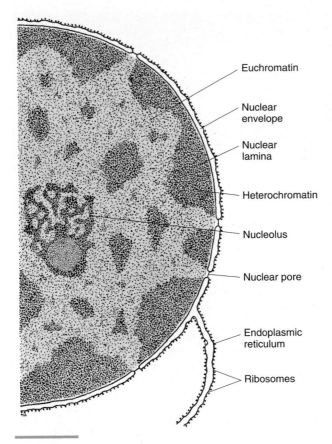

Euchromatin

Nuclear
envelope

Nuclear
lamina

Heterochromatin

Nucleolus

Nuclear pore

Endoplasmic
reticulum

Ribosomes

Figure 3–3 Nucleus. The outer nuclear membrane is studded with ribosomes on its cytoplasmic surface, and it is continuous with the rough endoplasmic reticulum. The space between the inner and outer nuclear membranes is the perinuclear cistern. Observe that the two membranes are united at the nuclear pores.

complex. Transport across the nuclear pore complex is frequently an energy-requiring process.

The bidirectional traffic between the nucleus and the cytoplasm is mediated by a group of target proteins containing **nuclear localization signals (NLSs),** known as importins, and **nuclear export signals (NESs),** known as **exportins** (also known as karyopherins, PTACs, transportins, and Ran-binding proteins). **Exportins** transport macromolecules (e.g., RNA) from the nucleus into the cytoplasm, whereas **importins** transport cargo (e.g., protein subunits of ribosomes) from the cytoplasm into the nucleus. Exportin and importin transport is regulated by a family of GTP-binding proteins known as **Ran** (Fig. 3-7). These specialized proteins along with other **nucleoporins** located along receptor sites in the nuclear pore complex facilitate the signal-mediated import and export processes.

Some protein trafficking is more like shuttling, because some proteins pass back and forth between the cytoplasm and the nucleus in a continuous fashion.

Recently it has been reported that certain other transport mechanisms literally shuttle in both directions. These transport signals are called **nucleocytoplasmic shuttling (NS)** signals. Proteins that carry this signal interact with mRNA.

CHROMATIN

Chromatin is a complex of DNA and proteins and represents the relaxed, uncoiled chromosomes of the interphase nucleus.

DNA, the cell's genetic material, resides in the nucleus in the form of **chromosomes,** which are clearly visible during cell division. In the interval between cell divisions, the chromosomes are unwound in the form of chromatin (see Figs. 3-2 and 3-3). Depending on its transcriptional activity, chromatin may be condensed as heterochromatin or extended as euchromatin.

Heterochromatin, a condensed inactive form of chromatin, stains deeply with Feulgen stains, which make it visible with the light microscope. It is located mostly at the periphery of the nucleus. The remainder of the chromatin, scattered throughout the nucleus and not visible with the light microscope, is **euchromatin.** This is the active form of chromatin in which the genetic material of the DNA molecules is being transcribed into RNA.

When euchromatin is examined with electron microscopy, it is seen to be composed of a thread-like material 30-nm thick. More careful evaluation indicates that these threads may be unwound, resulting in an 11-nm wide structure resembling "beads on a string." The beads are termed **nucleosomes,** and the string, which is the **DNA molecule,** appears as a thin filament 2 nm in diameter (Fig. 3-8).

Each nucleosome is composed of an octomer of proteins, duplicates of each of four types of **histones (H_2 A, H_2 B, H_3, and H_4).** The nucleosome is also wrapped with two complete turns (~150 nucleotide pairs) of the DNA molecule that continues as **linker DNA** extending to the next "bead." The spacing between each nucleosome is about 200 base pairs. This configuration of the nucleosome with its coils of DNA represents the simplest arrangement of chromatin packaging in the nucleus. Because only a small amount of the chromatin in the cell is in this configuration, it is thought to represent regions where the DNA is being transcribed.

During the cell cycle, **chromatin assembly factor 1 (CAF-1)** expedites the rapid assembly of the nucleosomes of the newly synthesized DNA into chromatin so that it cannot become a template. Therefore, the nucleosome/histone assembly not only provides a structural framework for the chromatin but also imparts control mechanisms important in DNA repair, replication, and transcription.

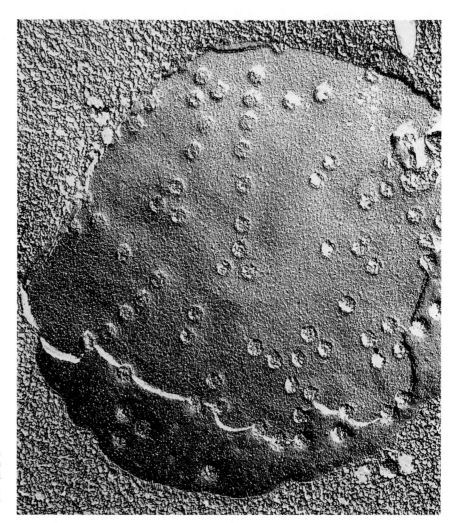

Figure 3–4 Nuclear pores. Electron micrograph (×47,778). Many nuclear pores may be observed in this freeze-fractured preparation of a nucleus. (From Leeson TS, Leeson CR, Paparo AA: Text/Atlas of Histology. Philadelphia, WB Saunders, 1988.)

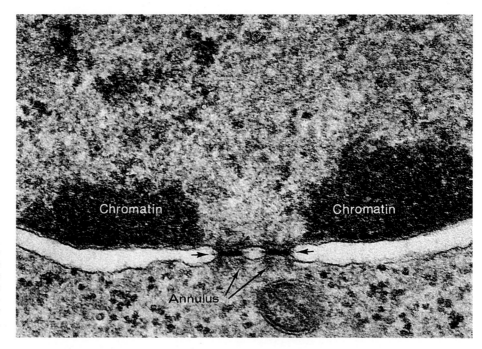

Figure 3–5 Nuclear pore. Electron micrograph (×24,828). Note the heterochromatin adjacent to the inner nuclear membrane and that the inner and outer nuclear membranes are continuous at the nuclear pore. (From Fawcett DW: The Cell. Philadelphia, WB Saunders, 1981.)

NUCLEAR PORE COMPLEX

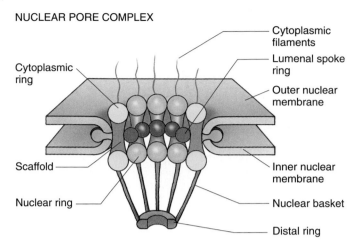

Figure 3–6 Nuclear pore complex. This illustration of the current understanding of the structure of the nuclear pore complex demonstrates that it is made up of several combinations of eight units each. Note that the model does not include a transporter (see text). (Based on Alberts B, Bray D, Lewis J, et al: Molecular Biology of the Cell, 3rd ed. New York, Garland Publishing, 1994; and on Beck M, Förster F, Ecke M, et al: Nuclear pore complex structure and dynamics revealed by cryoelectron tomography. Science 306:1387-1390, 2004.)

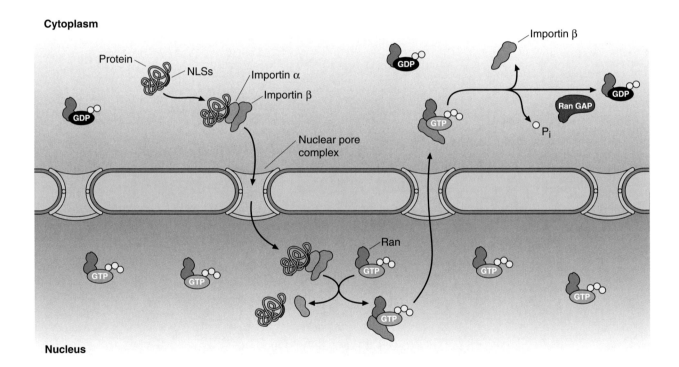

Figure 3-7 Role of Ran in nuclear import. Ran/guanosine diphosphate (GDP) is present in high concentration in the cytoplasm whereas Ran/guanosine triphosphate (GTP) is present in high concentration in the nucleus. Proteins to be imported into the nucleus form complexes with nuclear localization signals (NLSs) importin α and importin β. Upon import through the nuclear pore complex, Ran/GTP binds to importin β, thus releasing importin α and the imported protein. To complete the cycle, the Ran/GTP/importin β complex exits the nucleus to enter the cytoplasm via the nuclear pore complex. Here the Ran/GTPase-activating protein (RanGAP) hydrolyzes GTP, forming Ran/GDP, thus releasing importin β back into the cytoplasm.

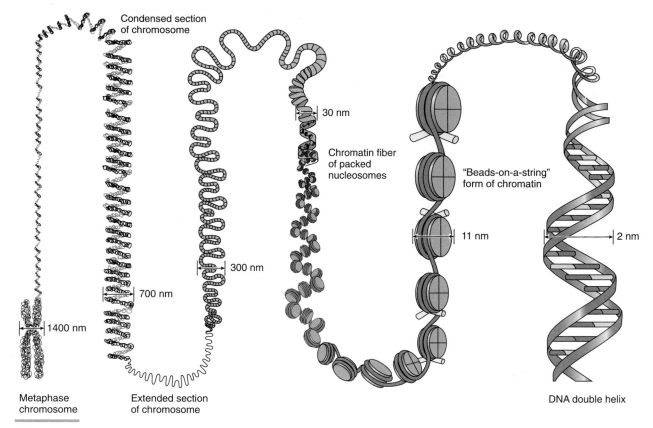

Condensed section
of chromosome

30 nm

Chromatin fiber
of packed
nucleosomes

"Beads-on-a-string"
form of chromatin

11 nm

2 nm

300 nm

700 nm

1400 nm

Metaphase
chromosome

Extended section
of chromosome

DNA double helix

Figure 3–8 Chromatin packaging. Note the complex packaging of chromatin to form a chromosome.

Electron microscopic studies of the nuclear contents following more careful manipulation has revealed chromatin fibers exhibiting 30-nm diameters. Packaging of chromatin into 30-nm threads is believed to occur by helical coiling of consecutive nucleosomes at six nucleosomes per turn of the coil and cooperatively bound there with **histone H₁** (see Fig. 3-8). Nonhistone proteins are also associated with the chromatin, but their function is not clear.

Chromosomes

Chromosomes are chromatin fibers that become so condensed and tightly coiled during mitosis and meiosis that they are visible with the light microscope.

As the cell leaves the interphase stage and prepares to undergo mitotic or meiotic activity, the chromatin fibers are extensively condensed to form **chromosomes,** visible with light microscopy. Tighter condensing of the chromatin material is accomplished by looping the coiled 30-nm fibers into 300-nm-diameter loops, held together by specific protein/DNA-bound complexes located at their bases. Further coiling of the 300-nm loops into tightly woven 700-nm helical loops forms the

maximally condensed chromosomes observed in the metaphase stage of mitosis or meiosis (see Fig. 3-8).

The number of chromosomes in somatic cells is specific for the species and is called the **genome,** the total genetic makeup. In humans, the genome consists of 46 chromosomes, representing 23 homologous pairs of chromosomes. One member of each of the chromosome pairs is derived from the maternal parent; the other comes from the paternal parent. Of the 23 pairs, 22 are called **autosomes;** the remaining pair, which determines gender, are the **sex chromosomes.** The sex chromosomes of the female are two X chromosomes (**XX**); those of the male are the X and Y chromosomes (**XY**) (Fig. 3-9).

Sex Chromatin

Only one of the two X chromosomes in female somatic cells is transcriptionally active. The inactive X chromosome, randomly determined early in development, remains inactive throughout the life of that individual.

Microscopic study of interphase nuclei of cells from females displays a very tightly coiled clump of chromatin, the **sex chromatin (Barr body),** the inactive counterpart of the two X chromosomes. Epithelial cells obtained from the lining of the cheek and neutrophils

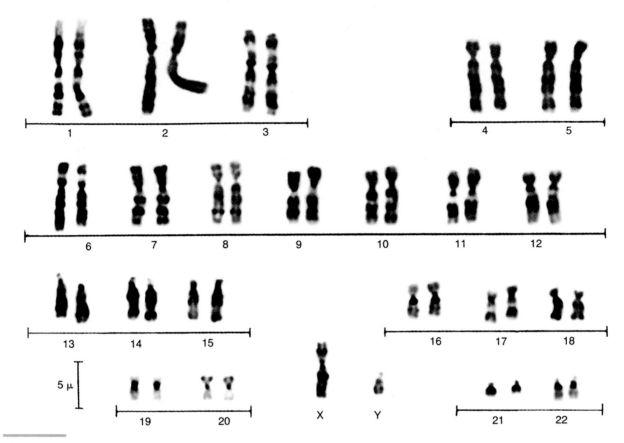

Figure 3–9 Human karyotype. A normal human karyotype illustrating banding. (From Bibbo M: Comprehensive Cytopathology. Philadelphia, WB Saunders, 1991.)

obtained from blood smears are especially useful for studying sex chromatin. The sex chromatin is observed at the edge of the nuclear envelope in smears of the oral epithelial cells and as a small drumstick-like evagination of the nuclei of the neutrophils. A number of cells must be examined to observe sex chromatin because the X chromosome must be in the proper orientation to be displayed for observation.

Ploidy

Cells containing the full complement of chromosomes (46) are said to be **diploid (2n).** Germ cells (mature ova or spermatozoa) are said to be **haploid (ln);** that is, only one member of each of the homologous pairs of chromosomes is present. Upon fertilization, the chromosomal number is restored to the diploid (2n) amount as the nuclei of the two germ cells unite.

Certain alkaloids, such as colchicine, a plant derivative, arrest a dividing cell in the metaphase stage of mitosis when the chromosomes are maximally condensed, thus permitting the pairing and numbering of the chromosomes via a conventional system of **karyotyping,** an analysis of chromosome number (see Fig. 3-9).

CLINICAL CORRELATIONS

One item that may be observed from the karyotype is **aneuploidy,** an abnormal chromosome number. People with **Down syndrome,** for example, have an extra chromosome 21 (**trisomy 21);** they exhibit mental retardation, stubby hands, and many congenital malformations, especially of the heart, among other manifestations.

Certain syndromes are associated with abnormalities in the number of sex chromosomes. **Klinefelter syndrome** results when an individual possesses three sex chromosomes (**XXY).** These persons exhibit the male phenotype, but they do not develop secondary sexual characteristics and are usually sterile. **Turner syndrome** is another example of aneuploidy called **monosomy** of the sex chromosomes. The karyotype exhibits only one sex chromosome (**XO).** These individuals are females whose ovaries never develop and who have undeveloped breasts, a small uterus, and mental retardation.

Giemsa reagent stains the adenine-thymine–rich regions of chromosomes, producing a pattern of **G bands** that is unique for each chromosome pair and is characteristic for each species. Careful analysis of the G bands can help reveal deletions of certain portions of the chromosome, nondisjunctions, translocations, and so on, that may assist in the diagnosis of certain genetic disorders or diseases resulting from chromosomal anomalies.

Deoxyribonucleic Acid

DNA, the genetic material of the cell, is located in the nucleus, where it acts as a template for RNA transcription.

Nearly all of the DNA, a double-stranded polynucleotide chain wound into a double helix, is housed in the nucleus of the cell. Each nucleotide is composed of a nitrogenous base, a deoxyribose sugar, and a phosphate molecule. Further, the nucleotides are linked to one another by phosphodiester bonds formed between the sugar molecules.

There are two types of bases: **purines** (adenine and guanine) and **pyrimidines** (cytosine and thymine). A double helix is established by the formation of hydrogen bonds between complementary bases on each strand of the DNA molecule. These bonds are formed between adenine (A) and thymine (T) and between guanine (G) and cytosine (C).

Genes

The biological information that is passed from one cell generation to the next—the units of heredity—are located at specific regions on the DNA molecule called **genes.** Each gene represents a specific segment of the DNA molecule that codes for the synthesis of a particular protein. The sequential arrangement of bases constituting the gene represents the sequence of amino acids of the protein. The genetic code is designed in such a manner that a triplet of consecutive bases, a **codon,** denotes a particular amino acid. Each amino acid is represented by a different codon.

Prior to beginning the Human Genome Project, it was believed that the 3 billion nucleotide bases in the human genome represented about 100,000 genes. Preliminary analysis at the conclusion of the Project indicated that the number of genes was far less than expected. Currently the data indicate that the human genome contains about 25,000 genes, all of which have been sequenced and mapped. Findings from this and other studies have already increased our understanding of some genetic disorders as well as indicated better treatment modalities for several diseases, with the promise of many other discoveries and applications in the years to come.

Ribonucleic Acid

RNA is similar to DNA except that it is single-stranded, one of its bases is uracil instead of thymine, and its sugar is ribose instead of deoxyribose.

Like DNA, RNA is composed of a linear sequence of nucleotides, but RNA is single-stranded and the sugar in RNA is ribose, not deoxyribose. One of the bases, thymine, is replaced by uracil (U), which, similar to thymine, is complementary to adenine.

The DNA in the nucleus serves as a template for synthesis of a complementary strand of RNA, a process called **transcription** (Fig. 3-10). Synthesis of the three types of RNA is catalyzed by three different **RNA polymerases:**

■ **Messenger RNA (mRNA)** by RNA polymerase II
■ **Transfer RNA (tRNA)** by RNA polymerase III
■ **Ribosomal RNA (rRNA)** by RNA polymerase I

The mechanism of transcription is generally the same for all three types of RNA.

Messenger RNA

Messenger RNA carries the genetic code from the nucleus to the cytoplasm to act as a template for protein synthesis.

mRNA serves as an intermediary for carrying the genetic information encoded in DNA that specifies the primary sequence of proteins from the nucleus to the protein-synthesizing machinery in the cytoplasm (see Fig. 3-10). Each mRNA is a complementary copy of the region of the DNA molecule that constitutes one gene. An mRNA molecule thus consists of a series of codons corresponding to particular amino acids. It also contains a **start codon** (AUG), which is necessary for initiating protein synthesis, and one or more **stop codons** (UAA, UAG, or UGA), which act to terminate protein synthesis. Once formed in the nucleus, mRNA is transported to the cytoplasm, where it is translated into protein (see Chapter 2).

TRANSCRIPTION

Transcription of DNA into mRNA begins with attachment of RNA polymerase II to a **core promoter,** a specific DNA sequence located adjacent to a gene. In the presence of a series of cofactors, RNA polymerase II initiates transcription by unwinding the double helix of the DNA two turns, thus exposing the nucleotides and, therefore, the codons on the DNA strand. The enzyme uses one of the exposed DNA strands as a template on which to assemble and polymerize complementary bases of the RNA molecule.

TRANSCRIPTION

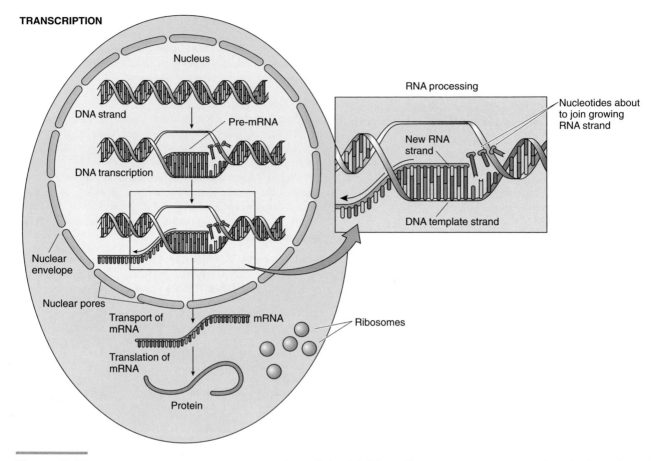

Figure 3–10 DNA transcription into messenger RNA (mRNA). (Modified from Alberts B, Bray D, Lewis J, et al: Molecular Biology of the Cell, 3rd ed. New York, Garland Publishing, 1994.)

The process is repeated as a new region of the DNA double helix is unwound and more nucleotides are polymerized into the growing mRNA chain. As the enzyme moves along the DNA molecule, the polymerized mRNA chain is separated from the template DNA strand, permitting the two DNA strands to re-form into the double helix configuration (see Fig. 3-10).

Transcription begins at a DNA triplet corresponding to the start codon AUG and is concluded when the RNA polymerase II recognizes a **chain-terminator** site complementary to the stop codons UAA, UAG, or UGA. When the enzyme reaches the chain terminator, it is released from the DNA molecule, permitting it to repeat the process of transcription. Simultaneously, the newly formed RNA strand (primary transcript) is released from the DNA molecule, leaving it free in the nucleoplasm.

The primary transcript is a long, single-stranded RNA molecule, called **precursor messenger RNA (pre-mRNA).** It contains both coding segments **(exons)** and noncoding segments **(introns).** The introns must be removed and the exons have to be spliced together. For that to occur, pre-mRNA and nuclear processing proteins form complexes of **heterogenous nuclear ribonucleoprotein particles (hnRNPs)** that begin **RNA splicing,** thus reducing the length of the pre-mRNA molecule. Additional processing involves **spliceosomes,** complexes of five **small nuclear ribonucleoprotein particles (snRNPs)** and a large number of **non-snRNP splicing factors** that assist in the splicing mechanism to produce **messenger ribonucleoprotein (mRNP).** Finally, the nuclear processing proteins are removed from the complex, leaving mRNA ready to be transported out of the nucleus via the nuclear pore complexes (see Fig. 3-10).

Because there is an abundance of DNA within the euykaryotic genome, much of it was believed to be evolutionary remnants without coding function. During transcription, DNA unwinds and codes for strands of RNA comprising *exons* (coding segments) and *introns* (noncoding segments). Later in this process, the exons are spliced together to form continual sequences of mRNA for translation to a protein in the cytoplasm. The introns removed from the primary RNA transcript were thought to have no function, even though their RNA represents about 95% more RNA than the protein-coding genes.

Recent evidence suggests that although these intronic RNA segments do not encode protein, they perform regulatory functions that are in parallel with regulatory proteins. Their role may relate to differentiation, development, gene expression, and evolution. If proved correct, this could have a profound impact on understanding certain disease processes and their treatment. For example, it is known that noncoding RNAs are linked to several cancers, autism, and schizophrenia.

This description of mRNA synthesis is only a brief overview and omits many details. Readers desiring more information should consult texts in molecular and cellular biology.

Transfer RNA

Transfer RNA ferries activated amino acids to the ribosome/mRNA complex, resulting in the formation of the protein.

tRNA is a small RNA molecule produced from DNA by RNA polymerase III. It is about 80 nucleotides in length and is folded upon itself to resemble a cloverleaf with base pairing between some of the nucleotides.

Two regions of the tRNA are of special significance. One of these, the **anticodon,** recognizes the codon of the mRNA; the other is the amino acid-bearing region, which resides at the 3' end of the molecule. tRNA is aminoacylated not only in the cytoplasm but also in the nucleus. This is believed to be a "proofreading" step that facilitates functional readiness in the cytoplasm. tRNA then transfers activated amino acids to the ribosome-mRNA complex, where they are incorporated into the polypeptide chain forming the protein (see Chapter 2).

Ribosomal RNA

Ribosomal RNA forms associations with proteins and enzymes in the nucleus to form ribosomes.

rRNA is synthesized in the fibrillar (pars fibrosa) region of the nucleolus by RNA polymerase I (Fig. 3-11). The primary transcript is called **45S rRNA (pre-rRNA),** a huge molecule of about 13,000 nucleotides. A 5S rRNA molecule, synthesized in the nucleus, and ribosomal proteins, synthesized in the cytoplasm, are transported into the nucleolus. Here they associate with the 45S rRNA molecule, forming a very large **ribonucleoprotein particle (RNP).** This RNP is processed by several resident molecules into precursors of the large and small ribosomal subunits in the pars granulosa region of the nucleolus. Thereafter, assembled small ribosomal subunits, made up of 18S rRNAs and other ribosomal proteins, make their way from the nucleolus to the cytoplasm by transport via the nuclear pore complexes. The

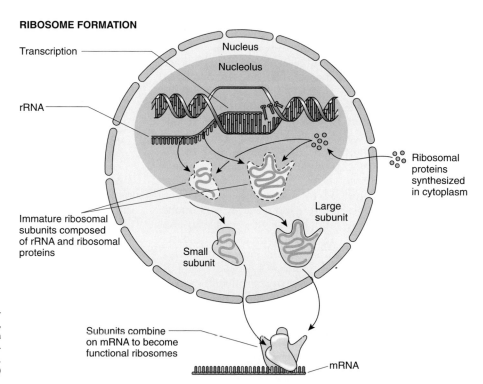

RIBOSOME FORMATION

Transcription

Nucleus

Nucleolus

rRNA

Ribosomal proteins synthesized in cytoplasm

Immature ribosomal subunits composed of rRNA and ribosomal proteins

Large subunit

Small subunit

Subunits combine on mRNA to become functional ribosomes

mRNA

Figure 3–11 Ribosome formation. mRNA, messenger RNA; rRNA, ribosomal RNA. (Modified from Alberts B, Bray D, Lewis J, et al: Molecular Biology of the Cell, 3rd ed. New York, Garland Publishing, 1994.)

remaining 28S, 5.8S, and 5S rRNAs are assembled into large ribosomal subunits and are transported out of the nucleus to the cytoplasm by way of the nuclear pore complexes.

Nucleoplasm

The nucleoplasm consists of interchromatin and perichromatin granules, RNPs, and the nuclear matrix.

Interchromatin granules (IGs), which are 20 to 25 nm in diameter, contain RNPs and several enzymes, including adenosine triphosphatase (ATPase), guanosine triphosphatase (GTPase), β-glycerophosphatase, and nicotinamide adenine dinucleotide (NAD) pyrophosphatase. They are located in clusters scattered throughout the nucleus among the chromatin material and appear to be connected to each other by thin fibrils. Their function is unclear.

Perichromatin granules are 30 to 50 nm in diameter and are located at the margins of the heterochromatin. These electron-dense particles are surrounded by a 25-nm wide halo of a less dense region. They are composed of densely packed fibrils of 4.7S low molecular weight RNA complexed to two peptides, resembling hnRNPs.

snRNPs participate in splicing, cleaving, and transporting hnRNPs. Although most snRNPs are located in the nucleus, some are limited to nucleoli. Several minor subgroups of these particles have been discovered recently, but their function has yet to be elucidated.

Nuclear Matrix

The nuclear matrix is defined both in structural and biochemical terms. It appears that differences reported in its components may be due to the extraction methods employed in studying its contents. Biochemically, the matrix contains about 10% of the total protein, 30% of the RNA, 1% to 3% of the total DNA, and 2% to 5% of the total nuclear phosphate. The structural components include the nuclear pore–nuclear lamina complex, residual nucleoli, residual RNP networks, and fibrillar elements. Recent studies have revealed that the nucleus possesses a nucleoplasmic reticulum that is continuous with the endoplasmic reticulum of the cytoplasm and the nuclear envelope. This reticulum houses nuclear calcium that functions within the nucleus. Further, this reticulum possesses receptors for inositol 1,4,5-trisphosphate that ultimately regulate calcium signals within certain compartments of the nucleus—namely, regions dedicated to protein transport, transcription of certain genes, and possibly others.

Functionally, the nuclear matrix is associated with DNA replication sites, rRNA and mRNA transcription and processing, steroid receptor binding, heat shock proteins, carcinogen binding, DNA viruses, and viral proteins. This list is not inclusive and does not address the functional natures of each of these associations because they are still unclear. It has been suggested, however, that the nucleus may contain many interactive subcompartments that function spatially and temporally in a tightly coordinated fashion to facilitate gene expression.

Nucleolus

The nucleolus is the deeply staining non–membrane-bounded structure within the nucleus that is involved in rRNA synthesis and in the assembly of small and large ribosomal subunits

The nucleolus, a dense nonmembranous structure located in the nucleus, is observed only during interphase because it dissipates during cell division. It stains basophilic with hematoxylin and eosin, being rich in rRNA and protein. The nucleolus contains only small amounts of DNA, which is also inactive and thus does not stain with Feulgen stains. Usually, there are no more that two or three nucleoli per cell; however, their number, size, and shape generally are species-specific and relate to the synthetic activity of the cell. In cells that are actively synthesizing protein, the nucleolus may occupy up to 25% of the nuclear volume. Densely staining regions are the **nucleolus-associated chromatin,** which is being transcribed into rRNA (see Figs. 3-2 and 3-3).

Four distinct areas of the nucleolus have been described:

- **A pale-staining fibrillar center,** containing inactive DNA (not being transcribed)
- **Pars fibrosa,** containing nucleolar RNAs being transcribed
- **Pars granulosa,** in which maturing ribosomal subunits are assembled
- **Nucleolar matrix,** a network of fibers active in nucleolar organization

Also located in the pale-staining regions are the tips of chromosomes 13, 14, 15, 21, and 22 (in humans), containing the **nucleolar-organizing regions,** where gene loci that encode rRNA are located.

The cell's ribosomal subunits are organized and assembled within the nucleolus, except those located in the mitochondria. However, recent evidence shows that the nucleolus performs additional functions. These include regulating some of the events in the cell cycle such as cytokinesis; inactivating mitotic cyclin-dependent kinases by sequestering cell cycle regulatory proteins; modifying small RNAs that moderate and modify pre-rRNA; assembling RNP; engaging in nuclear export; and playing a role in aging.

CLINICAL CORRELATIONS

Some suggest that the rDNA in the nucleolus may become unstable, thereby accelerating the aging process. In malignant cells, the nucleolus may become hypertrophic. Furthermore, it is known that in tumor cells the nucleolar-organizing regions become larger and more numerous, thus indicating a poorer clinical prognosis.

THE CELL CYCLE

The cell cycle is a series of events within the cell that prepare the cell for dividing into two daughter cells.

The cell cycle is divided into two major events: **interphase**, a long period of time during which the cell increases its size and content and replicates its genetic material (Fig. 3-12), and **mitosis**, a shorter period of time during which the cell divides its nucleus and cytoplasm,

CELL CYCLE

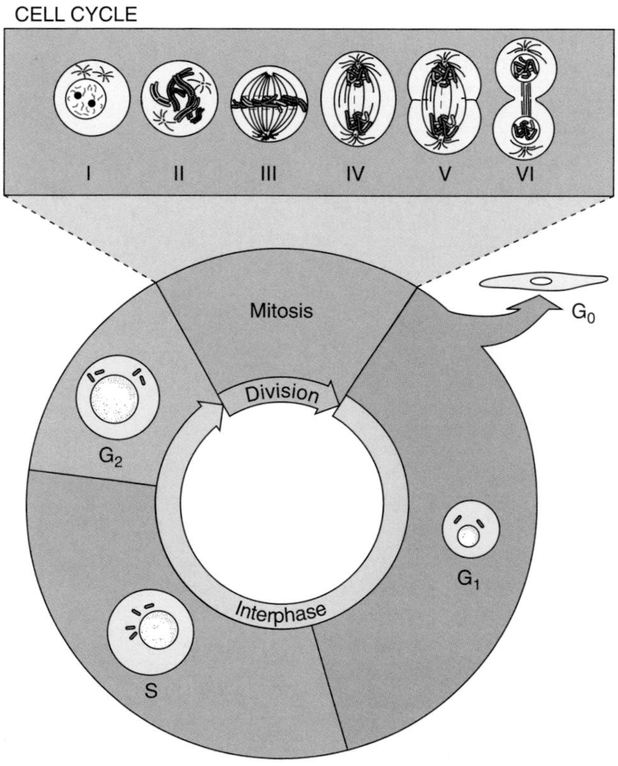

Figure 3–12 The cell cycle in actively dividing cells. Nondividing cells, such as neurons, leave the cycle to enter the G_0 phase (resting stage). Other cells, such as lymphocytes, may return to the cell cycle.

giving rise to two daughter cells. The cell cycle may be thought of as beginning at the conclusion of the telophase stage in mitosis, after which the cell enters interphase.

Cells that become highly differentiated after the last mitotic event may cease to undergo mitosis either permanently (e.g., neurons, muscle cells) or temporarily (e.g., peripheral lymphocytes) and return to the cell cycle at a later time. Cells that have left the cell cycle are said to be in a resting stage, the G_0 **(outside) phase,** or the **stable phase.**

Interphase

Interphase is subdivided into three phases:

- G_1 **(gap) phase,** when the synthesis of macromolecules essential for DNA duplication begins
- **S (synthetic) phase,** when the DNA is duplicated
- G_2 **phase,** when the cell undergoes preparations for mitosis

Gap 1

The G_1 phase (gap 1 phase) is a period of cell growth, RNA synthesis, and other events in preparation for the next mitosis.

Daughter cells formed during mitosis enter the G_1 **phase.** During this phase, the cells synthesize RNA, regulatory proteins essential to DNA replication, and enzymes necessary to carry out these synthetic activities. Thus, the cell volume, reduced by dividing the cell in half during mitosis, is restored to normal. Additionally, the nucleoli are reestablished during the G_1 phase. It is during this time that the centrioles begin to duplicate themselves, a process that is completed by the G_2 **phase.**

The triggers inducing the cell to enter the cell cycle may be (1) a mechanical force (e.g., stretching of smooth muscle), (2) injury to the tissue (e.g., ischemia), and (3) cell death. All of these incidents cause the release of ligands by signaling cells in the involved tissue. Frequently these ligands are growth factors that indirectly induce the expression of **proto-oncogenes,** genes that are responsible for controlling the proliferative pathways of the cell.

Obviously the expression of proto-oncogenes must be very strictly regulated to prevent unwanted and uncontrolled cell proliferation. Mutations in proto-oncogenes that enable the cell to escape control and divide in an unrestrained fashion are responsible for many cancers. Such mutated proto-oncogenes are known as **oncogenes.**

Ligands designed to induce proliferation bind to cell surface receptor proteins of the target cell and activate one of the **signal transduction pathways** described in Chapter 2. Hence, extracellular signals that are perceived at the cell surface are transmuted into intracellular events, most of which involve the sequential activation of a cascade of cytoplasmic **protein kinases.** These kinases activate a series of intranuclear **transcription factors** that regulate the expression of proto-oncogenes, resulting in cell division.

The capability of the cell to begin and advance through the cell cycle is governed by the presence and interactions of a group of related proteins known as **cyclins,** with specific **cyclin-dependent kinases (CDKs).** Thus:

- *Cyclin D*, synthesized during **early G₁ phase,** binds to CDK4 as well as to CDK6. Additionally, in the **late G₁ phase** cyclin E is synthesized and binds to CDK2. These three complexes, through other intermediaries, permit the cell to enter and progress through the **S phase.**
- *Cyclin A* binds to CDK2 and CDK1 and these complexes permit the cell to leave the S phase and enter the G₂ phase and induce the formation of cyclin B.
- *Cyclin B* binds to CDK1, and this complex allows the cell to leave the G₂ phase and enter the **M phase.**

Once the cyclins have performed their specific functions, they enter the ubiquitin-proteasome pathway, where they are degraded into their component molecules. The cell also employs quality control mechanisms, known as **checkpoints,** to safeguard against early transition between the phases. These checkpoints ensure the meticulous completion of essential events, such as adequate cell growth, correct DNA synthesis, and proper chromosome segregation, before permitting the cell to leave its current phase of the cell cycle. The cell accomplishes such delays in the progression through the cell cycle by activating inhibitory pathways and/or by suppressing activating pathways.

The actual control mechanisms are considerably more involved and complicated than the steps just described. For example, it appears that the nucleolus plays a regulatory role in the cell cycle by sequestering certain proteins, thus inhibiting their function. The complete sequence of steps is beyond the scope of this textbook. (For more details, see relevant textbooks of cell biology as well as current literature on the cell cycle.)

S Phase

DNA synthesis occurs during the S phase.

During the S phase, the synthetic phase of the cell cycle, the genome is duplicated. All of the requisite nucleoproteins, including the histones, are imported and incorporated into the DNA molecule, forming the chromatin material. The cell now contains twice the normal complement of its DNA. The amount of DNA present in autosomal and germ cells also varies. Autosomal cells contain the diploid (2n) amount of DNA before the synthetic (S) phase of the cell cycle when the diploid (2n) amount of DNA is doubled (4n) in preparation for cell

division. In contrast, germ cells produced by meiosis possess the haploid (1n) number of chromosomes and also the haploid (1n) amount of DNA.

G₂ Phase

The gap 2 phase (G₂ phase) is the period between the end of DNA synthesis and the beginning of mitosis.

During the G₂ phase, the RNA and proteins essential to cell division are synthesized, the energy for mitosis is stored, tubulin is synthesized for assembly into microtubules required for mitosis, DNA replication is analyzed for possible errors, and any of these errors is corrected.

Mitosis

Mitosis is the process of cell division that results in the formation of two identical daughter cells.

Mitosis (M) occurs at the conclusion of the G₂ phase and thus completes the cell cycle. Mitosis is the process whereby the cytoplasm and the nucleus of the cell are divided equally into two identical daughter cells (Figs. 3-13 to 3-15). First, the nuclear material is divided in a process called **karyokinesis,** followed by division of the cytoplasm, called **cytokinesis.** The process of mitosis is divided into five distinct stages: **prophase, prometaphase, metaphase, anaphase,** and **telophase** (Fig. 3-16).

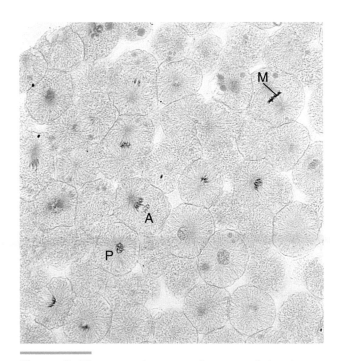

Figure 3–13 Stages of mitosis. Light micrograph (×270). Note the various stages: A, anaphase; M, metaphase; P, prophase.

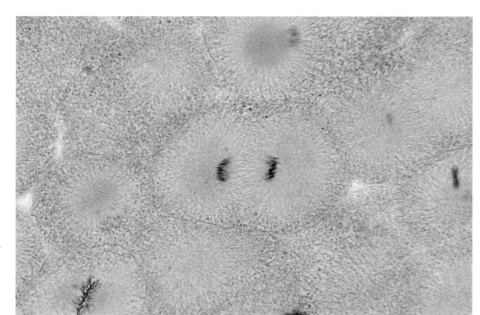

Figure 3–14 Anaphase stage of mitosis. Light micrograph (×540). Sister chromatids have separated from the metaphase plate and are now migrating away from each other to opposite poles.

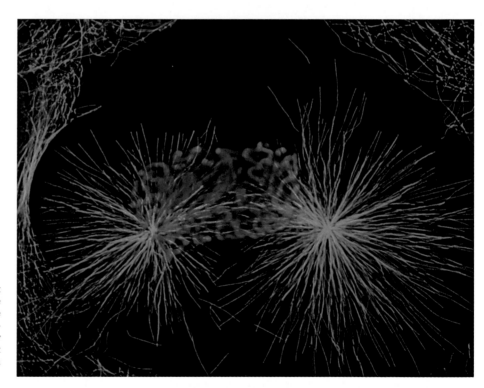

Figure 3–15 Immunoflorescent image of a cell in the prometaphase stage of mitosis. Note the spindle microtubules *(green)* and the chromosomes *(blue)*. (Courtesy of Alexey Khodjakov, PhD, Research Scientist and Associate Professor, Wadsworth Center, Albany, New York.)

Prophase

During prophase, the chromosomes condense and the nucleolus disappears.

At the beginning of prophase, the chromosomes are condensing, and thus becoming visible microscopically.

Each chromosome consists of two parallel **sister chromatids,** joined together at one point along their length, the **centromere.** As chromosomes condense, the nucleolus disappears. The **centrosome** also divides into two regions, each half containing a pair of **centrioles** and a **microtubule-organizing center (MTOC),** which migrate away from each other to opposite poles of the cell.

MITOSIS

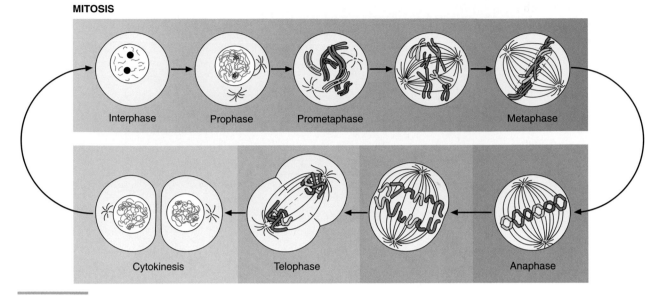

Figure 3–16 Stages of mitosis in a cell containing a diploid (2n) number of 6 chromosomes.

From each MTOC, **astral rays** and **spindle fibers** develop, giving rise to the **mitotic spindle apparatus.** It is thought that the astral rays (microtubules that radiate out from the pole of the spindle) may assist in orienting the MTOC at the pole of the cell. Those microtubules that attach to the centromere region of the chromosome are the **spindle fibers,** which assist in directing the chromosome migration to the pole. In the absence of centrioles, the microtubule-nucleating material is dispersed within the cytoplasm with the result that astral rays and spindle fibers do not form properly, and mitosis does not proceed in the appropriate manner.

At the centromere region of each chromatid, a new MTOC, the **kinetochore,** develops. Spindle fibers bind to the kinetochore in preparation for chromatid migration to effect karyokinesis.

Prometaphase

Prometaphase begins when the nuclear envelope disappears.

Prometaphase begins as the nuclear lamins are phosphorylated, resulting in the breakdown and disappearance of the nuclear envelope. During this phase, the chromosomes are arranged randomly throughout the cytoplasm. Microtubules that become attached to the kinetochores are known as **mitotic spindle microtubules,** whereas microtubules that do not become incorporated into the spindle apparatus are called **polar microtubules.** Some believe that the polar microtubules are responsible for maintaining the spacing between the two poles during the mitotic event. The mitotic spindle microtubules assist in

migration of the chromosomes so that they become oriented into an alignment with the mitotic spindle.

Metaphase

Metaphase begins as the newly duplicated chromosomes align themselves on the equator of the mitotic spindle.

During metaphase, the chromosomes become maximally condensed and are lined up at the equator of the mitotic spindle (**metaphase plate** configuration). Each chromatid parallels the equator, and spindle microtubules are attached to its kinetochore, radiating to the spindle pole. Sister chromatids must be maintained in close proximity as the chromosome condenses and aligns on the metaphase mitotic spindle. During anaphase, cohesion proteins located between the chromatids disappear.

Anaphase

During anaphase, the sister chromatids separate and begin to migrate to opposite poles of the cell, and a cleavage furrow begins to develop.

Anaphase begins when sister chromatids, located at the equator of the metaphase plate, pull apart and begin their migration toward the opposite poles of the mitotic spindle. The spindle/kinetochore attachment site leads the way, with the arms of the chromatids simply trailing, contributing nothing to the migration or its pathway.

It has been postulated that the observed movement of the chromatids toward the pole in anaphase may be the result of shortening of the microtubules via depolymerization at the kinetochore end. This, coupled with the recent discovery of dynein associated with the kinetochore, may be analogous to vesicle transport along microtubules. In **late anaphase,** a cleavage furrow begins to form at the plasmalemma, indicating the region where the cell will be divided during cytokinesis.

Telophase

Telophase, the terminal phase of mitosis, is characterized by cytokinesis, reconstitution of the nucleus and nuclear envelope, disappearance of the mitotic spindle, and unwinding of the chromosomes into chromatin.

At telophase, each set of chromosomes has reached its respective pole, the nuclear lamins are dephosphory-

lated and the nuclear envelope is reconstituted. The chromosomes uncoil and become organized into heterochromatin and euchromatin of the interphase cell. The nucleolus is developed from the **nuclear-organizing regions** on each of five pairs of chromosomes.

Cytokinesis is the division of the cytoplasm into two equal parts during mitosis. The cleavage furrow continues to deepen until only the **midbody,** a small bridge of cytoplasm, and remaining polar microtubules connect the two daughter cells (Fig. 3-17). The polar microtubules are surrounded by a **contractile ring,** which lies just inside the plasma membrane. The contractile ring is composed of **actin** and **myosin filaments** attached to the plasma membrane. Constriction of the ring is followed by depolymerization of the remaining spindle microtubules separating the two daughter cells. During separation of the daughter

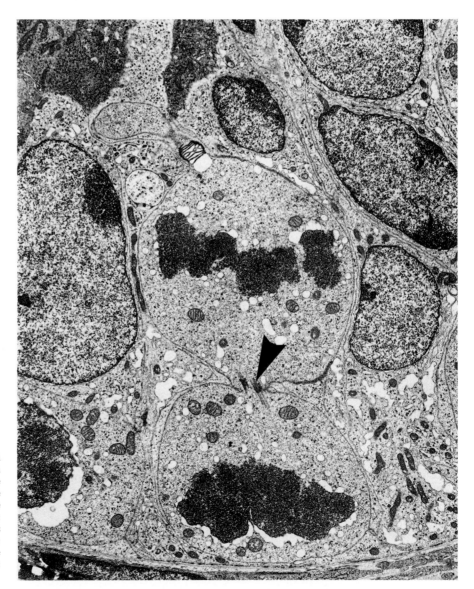

Figure 3–17 Cytokinesis. Electron micrograph (×8092). A spermatogonium in late telophase demonstrating the forming midbody *(arrowhead).* The chromosomes in the daughter nuclei are beginning to uncoil. (From Miething A: Intercellular bridges between germ cells in the immature golden hamster testis: Evidence for clonal and nonclonal mode of proliferation. Cell Tissue Res 262: 559-567, 1990.)

cells and shortly thereafter, the elements of the contractile ring and the remaining microtubules of the mitotic apparatus are disassembled, concluding cytokinesis.

Each daughter cell resulting from mitosis is identical in every respect, including the entire genome, and each daughter cell possesses a diploid (2n) number of chromosomes.

CLINICAL CORRELATIONS

A more complete understanding of mitosis and the cell cycle has greatly aided cancer chemotherapy, making it possible to use drugs at the time when the cells are in a particular stage of the cell cycle. For example, **vincristine** and similar drugs disrupt the mitotic spindle, arresting the cell in mitosis. **Colchicine,** another plant alkaloid that produces the same effect, has been used extensively in studies of individual chromosomes and karyotyping. **Methotrexate,** which inhibits purine synthesis, and **5-fluorouracil,** which inhibits pyrimidine synthesis, both halt the cell cycle in the S phase, preventing cell division; both are common chemotherapy agents.

Oncogenes are mutated forms of normal genes called proto-oncogenes, which code for proteins that control cell division. Oncogenes may result from a viral infection or random genetic accidents. When present in a cell, oncogenes dominate genes over the normal proto-oncogene alleles, causing unregulated cell division and proliferation. Examples of cancer cells arising from oncogenes include **bladder cancer** and **acute myelogenous leukemia.**

Meiosis

Whereas mitosis is cell division of somatic cells into two identical daughter cells, meiosis is a special type of cell division resulting in the formation of gametes (spermatozoa or ova) whose chromosome number has been reduced from the diploid (2n) to the haploid (1n) number.

Meiosis begins at the conclusion of interphase in the cell cycle. It produces the germ cells—the ova and the spermatozoa. This process has two crucial results:

1 Reduction in the number of chromosomes from the **diploid (2n)** to the **haploid (1n)** number, ensuring that each gamete carries the haploid amount of DNA and the haploid number of chromosomes.
2 Recombination of genes, ensuring genetic variability and diversity of the gene pool.

Meiosis is divided into two separate events:

Meiosis I, or reductional division (first event). Homologous pairs of chromosomes line up, members of each pair separate and go to opposite poles, and the cell divides; thus, each daughter cell receives half the number of chromosomes (haploid number).

Meiosis II, or equatorial division (second event). The two **chromatids** of each chromosome are separated, as in mitosis, followed by migration of the chromatids to opposite poles and the formation of two daughter cells. These two events produce four cells (gametes), each with the haploid number of chromosomes and haploid DNA content.

Meiosis I

Meiosis I (reductional division) separates the homologous pairs of chromosomes, thus reducing the number from diploid (2n) to haploid (1n).

MEIOSIS I

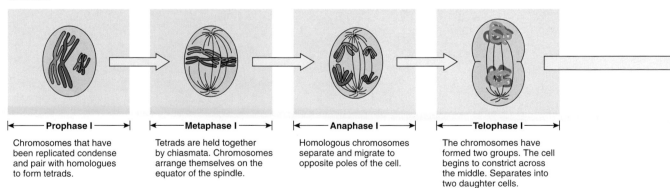

|← Prophase I →| |← Metaphase I →| |← Anaphase I →| |← Telophase I →|

Chromosomes that have been replicated condense and pair with homologues to form tetrads.

Tetrads are held together by chiasmata. Chromosomes arrange themselves on the equator of the spindle.

Homologous chromosomes separate and migrate to opposite poles of the cell.

The chromosomes have formed two groups. The cell begins to constrict across the middle. Separates into two daughter cells.

Figure 3–18 Stages of meiosis in an idealized cell containing a diploid (2n) number of 4 chromosomes.

In gametogenesis, when the germ cells are in the **S phase** of the cell cycle preceding meiosis, the amount of DNA is doubled to **4n** but the chromosome number remains at **2n** (46 chromosomes). Meiosis I proceeds as outlined in Figure 3-18.

Prophase I

> *Prophase I, the commencement of meiosis, begins after the DNA has been doubled to 4n in the S phase.*

Prophase of meiosis I lasts a long time and is subdivided into the following five phases:

1 *Leptotene.* Individual chromosomes, composed of two chromatids joined at the centromere, begin to condense, forming long strands in the nucleus.
2 *Zygotene.* Homologous pairs of chromosomes approximate each other, lining up in register (gene locus to gene locus), and make synapses via the **synaptonemal complex,** forming a tetrad.
3 *Pachytene.* Chromosomes continue to condense, becoming thicker and shorter; **chiasmata** (crossing over sites) are formed as random exchange of genetic material occurs between homologous chromosomes.
4 *Diplotene.* Chromosomes continue to condense and then begin to separate, revealing chiasmata.
5 *Diakinesis.* Chromosomes condense maximally and the nucleolus disappears, as does the nuclear envelope, freeing the chromosomes into the cytoplasm.

Metaphase I

> *Metaphase I is characterized by homologous pairs of chromosomes, each composed of two chromatids, lining up on the equatorial plate of the meiotic spindle.*

During **metaphase I,** homologous chromosomes align as pairs on the equatorial plate of the spindle apparatus in random order, ensuring a subsequent reshuffling of the maternal and paternal chromosomes. Spindle fibers become attached to the kinetochores of the chromosomes.

Anaphase I

> *Anaphase I is evident when the homologous pairs of chromosomes begin to pull apart, commencing their migrations to opposite poles of the cell.*

In **anaphase I,** homologous chromosomes migrate away from each other, going to opposite poles. Each chromosome still consists of two chromatids.

Telophase I

> *During Telophase I, the migrating chromosomes, each consisting of two chromatids, reach opposite poles.*

Telophase I is similar to telophase of mitosis. The chromosomes reach the opposing poles, nuclei are re-formed and cytokinesis occurs, giving rise to two daughter cells. Each cell possesses 23 chromosomes, the haploid (**1n**) number, but because each chromosome is composed of two chromatids, the DNA content is still diploid. Each of the two newly formed daughter cells enters meiosis II.

MEIOSIS II

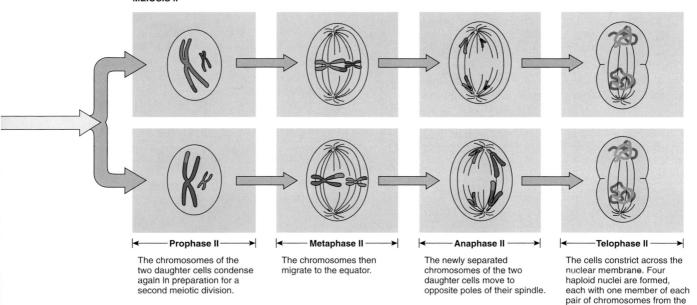

|←——— **Prophase II** ———→| |←——— **Metaphase II** ———→| |←——— **Anaphase II** ———→| |←——— **Telophase II** ———→|

The chromosomes of the two daughter cells condense again in preparation for a second meiotic division.

The chromosomes then migrate to the equator.

The newly separated chromosomes of the two daughter cells move to opposite poles of their spindle.

The cells constrict across the nuclear membrane. Four haploid nuclei are formed, each with one member of each pair of chromosomes from the original nucleus.

Meiosis II

Meiosis II (equatorial division) occurs without DNA synthesis and proceeds rapidly through four phases and cytokinesis to form four daughter cells each with the haploid chromosome number.

The equatorial division is not preceded by an S phase. It is very similar to mitosis and is subdivided into **prophase II, metaphase II, anaphase II, telophase II,** and **cytokinesis** (see Fig. 3-18). The chromosomes line up on the equator, the kinetochores attach to spindle fibers, followed by the chromatids migrating to opposite poles, and cytokinesis divides each of the two cells, resulting in a total of four daughter cells from the original diploid germ cell. Each of the four cells contains a haploid amount of DNA and a haploid chromosome number.

Unlike the daughter cells resulting from mitosis, each of which contains the diploid number of chromosomes and is an identical copy of the other, the four cells resulting from meiosis contain the haploid number of chromosomes and are genetically distinct because of reshuffling of the chromosomes and crossing over. Thus, every gamete contains its own unique genetic complement.

CLINICAL CORRELATIONS

Abnormalities in chromosome numbers may occur during meiosis. During meiosis I, when homologous pairs normally separate, **nondisjunction** may occur; thus, one daughter cell will have both rather than one chromosome of the homologous pair, resulting in 24 chromosomes, whereas the other daughter cell will have only 22 chromosomes. At fertilization with a normal gamete (containing 23 chromosomes), the resultant zygote will have either 47 chromosomes (**trisomy**) or 45 chromosomes (**monosomy**). Nondisjunction occurs more frequently with certain chromosomes (i.e., trisomy of chromosomes 8, 9, 13, 18, 21) that produce unique characteristics (e.g., the characteristics of Down syndrome [trisomy 21]).

APOPTOSIS

Cells die as a result of various factors, including (1) acute injury, (2) accidents, (3) lack of a vascular supply, (4) destruction by pathogens or the immune system, and (5) genetic programming. During embryogenesis, many cells, such as those that would give rise to a tail in the human embryo, are driven into the genetically determined process of dying. This process continues on throughout adult life to establish a balance between cell proliferation and cell death. For example, in the adult human billions of cells die each hour within the bone marrow and digestive tract to balance cell proliferation in these tissues. Cell death by this means is called **programmed cell death (apoptosis).** In contrast to apoptosis, during necrosis the cell dies because of attack or injury that causes the cell to rupture, thereby exposing its contents to neighboring cells and thus initiating an inflammatory response. Because apoptosis has formidable consequences for the cell involved as well as for the organism, it must be carefully regulated, controlled, and monitored.

The process of apoptosis is regulated by a number of highly conserved genes that code for a family of enzymes known as **caspases,** which degrade regulatory and structural proteins in the nucleus and in the cytoplasm. Activation of caspases is induced when certain cytokines, such as **tumor necrosis factor (TNF),** released by signaling cells, binds to the TNF receptor of the target cell. These TNF receptors are transmembrane proteins whose cytoplasmic aspect binds to adapter molecules to which caspases are bound. Once TNF binds to the extracellular moiety of its receptor, the signal is transduced and caspase becomes activated. The activated caspase is released and, in turn, triggers a cascade of caspases that results in the degradation of chromosomes, nuclear lamins, and cytoskeletal proteins. Finally, the entire cell becomes fragmented. The cell fragments are then phagocytosed by macrophages. However, these macrophages do not release cytokines that would initiate an inflammatory response.

4

Extracellular Matrix

Cells of multicellular organisms congregate to form structural and functional associations, known as **tissues**. Each of the four basic tissues of the body—epithelium, connective tissue, muscle, and nervous tissue—possesses specific, defined characteristics, which are detailed in subsequent chapters. However, all tissues are composed of **cells** and an **extracellular matrix (ECM)**, a complex of nonliving macromolecules manufactured by the cells and exported by them into the extracellular space.

Some tissues, such as epithelium, form sheets of cells with only a scant amount of ECM. At the opposite extreme is connective tissue, composed mostly of ECM with a limited number of cells scattered throughout the matrix. Cells maintain their associations with the ECM by forming specialized junctions that hold them to the surrounding macromolecules. This chapter explores the nature of the ECM not only as it relates to the tissues that house it but also as it relates to the cells contained within it. Although it was initially believed that the ECM merely forms the skeletal elements of the tissue in which it resides, it is now known that it may also:

- Modify the morphology and functions of cells
- Modulate the survival of cells
- Influence the development of cells
- Regulate the migration of cells
- Direct mitotic activity of cells
- Form junctional associations with cells

The ECM of the connective tissue proper, the most common connective tissue of the body, is composed of a hydrated gel-like **ground substance** with **fibers** embedded in it. Ground substance resists forces of compression, and fibers withstand tensile forces. The water of hydration permits the rapid exchange of nutrients and waste products carried by the extracellular fluid as it percolates through the ground substance (Fig. 4-1).

GROUND SUBSTANCE

Ground substance is an amorphous gel-like material composed of glycosaminoglycans, proteoglycans, and glycoproteins.

The three families of macromolecules that compose ground substance form various interactions with each other, with fibers, and with the cells of connective tissue and epithelium (Fig. 4-2).

Glycosaminoglycans

Glycosaminoglycans (GAGs) are negatively charged, long, rod-like chains of repeating disaccharides that have the capability of binding large quantities of water.

GAGs are long, inflexible, unbranched polysaccharides composed of chains of repeating disaccharide units. One of the two repeating disaccharides is always an **amino sugar** (*N*-acetylglucosamine or *N*-acetylgalactosamine); the other typically is a **uronic acid** (iduronic or glucuronic) (Table 4-1). Because the amino sugar is usually sulfated and because these sugars also have carboxyl groups projecting from them, they are negatively charged and thus attract cations such as sodium (Na^+). A high sodium concentration in the ground substance attracts extracellular fluid, which (by hydrating the intercellular matrix) assists in the resistance to forces of compression. As these molecules come into close proximity to each other, their negative charges repel one another, which causes them to have a slippery texture, as evidenced by the slickness of mucus, vitreous humor of the eye, and synovial fluid.

All but one of the major GAGs of the ECM matrix are sulfated, each consisting of fewer than 300 repeating disaccharide units (see Table 4-1). The sulfated

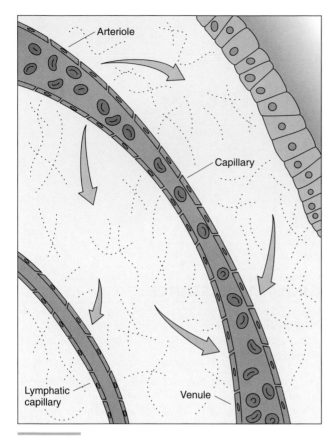

Figure 4–1 Tissue fluid flow. Fluid from the higher pressure arterial ends of the capillary bed enters the connective tissue spaces and becomes known as extracellular fluid, which percolates through the ground substance. Some, but not all, of the extracellular fluid then reenters the blood circulatory system at the lower-pressure venous end of the capillary bed and the venules. The extracellular fluid that did not reenter the blood vascular system will enter the even lower-pressure lymphatic system which will eventually deliver it to the blood vascular system.

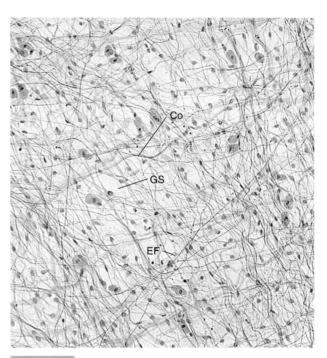

Figure 4–2 Light micrograph (×132) of areolar connective tissue, displaying cells, collagen fibers (Co), elastic fibers (EF), and ground substance (GS). Observe that in this very loose type of connective tissue the fibers, although interwoven, present a relatively haphazard arrangement, thus permitting stretching of the tissue in any direction. The cells of areolar connective tissue are principally of three types: fibroblast, macrophages, and mast cells. The extensive extracellular spaces are occupied by ground substance composed mainly of glycosaminoglycans and proteoglycans, a large component of which is aggrecan aggregate, a highly hydrated macromolecule.

GAGs include keratan sulfate, heparan sulfate, heparin, chondroitin 4-sulfate, chondroitin 6-sulfate, and dermatan sulfate. These GAGs are usually linked covalently to protein molecules to form proteoglycans. The only nonsulfated GAG is **hyaluronic acid (hyaluronan),** which may have as many as 10,000 repeating disaccharide units. It is a very large macromolecule that does not form covalent links to protein molecules (although proteoglycans do become attached to it via link proteins).

Note that all GAGs are synthesized within the Golgi apparatus by resident enzymes—except hyaluronic acid, which is synthesized as a free linear polymer at the cytoplasmic face of the plasma membrane by hyaluronan synthases. These enzymes are integral membrane proteins that not only catalyze the polymerization but also facilitate the transfer of the newly formed macro-

molecule into the ECM. It has been suggested that this macromolecule also has intracellular functions. Some of the newly released hyaluronic acid is endocytosed by some cells, especially during the cell cycle, where it has a role in maintaining space and modulating microtubular activities during the metaphase and anaphase stages of mitosis, thus facilitating chromosomal movements. Additional intracellular roles may involve modulation of intracellular trafficking and influencing intracytoplasmic-specific and intranuclear-specific kinases.

Proteoglycans

Proteoglycans constitute a family of macromolecules; each is composed of a protein core to which glycosaminoglycans are covalently bonded.

When sulfated GAGs form covalent bonds with a protein core, they form a family of macromolecules known as proteoglycans, many of which occupy huge domains. These large structures look like a bottle brush,

TABLE 4–1 Types of Glycosaminoglycans (GAGs)

Type	Molecular Mass (Da)	Repeating Disaccharides	Covalent Linkage To Protein	Location In Body
Hyaluronic acid	10^7-10^8	D-Glucuronic acid-beta-1,3-N-acetyl-D-glucosamine	No	Most connective tissue, synovial fluid, cartilage, dermis
Keratan sulfate I and II	10,000-30,000	Galactose-beta-1,4-N-acetyl-D-glucosamine-6-SO_4	Yes	Cornea (keratan sulfate I), Cartilage (keratan sulfate II)
Heparan sulfate	15,000-20,000	D-Glucuronic acid-beta-1,3-N-acetyl galactosamine L-Iduronic acid-2 or -SO_4-beta-1,3-N-acetyl-D-galactosamine	Yes	Blood vessels, lung, basal lamina
Heparin (90%) (10%)	15,000-20,000	L-Iduronic acid-beta-1,4-sulfo-D-glucosamine-6-SO_4 D-Glucuronic acid-beta-1,4-N-acetylglucosamine-6-SO_4	No	Mast cell granule, liver, lung, skin
Chondroitin 4-sulfate	10,000-30,000	D-Glucuronic acid-beta-1,3-N-acetylgalactosamine-6-SO_4	Yes	Cartilage, bone, cornea, blood vessels
Chondroitin 6-sulfate	10,000-30,000	D-Glucuronic acid-beta-1,3-N-acetylgalactosamine-6-SO_4	Yes	Cartilage, Wharton's jelly, blood vessels
Dermatan sulfate	10,000-30,000	L-Iduronic acid-alpha-1,3-N-acetylglucosamine-4-SO_4	Yes	Heart valves, skin, blood vessels

with the protein core resembling the wire stem and the various sulfated GAGs projecting from its surface in three-dimensional space, as do the bristles of the brush (Fig. 4-3).

Proteoglycans are of various sizes, ranging from about 50,000 Da (decorin and betaglycan) to as many as 3 million Da (aggrecan). The protein cores of proteoglycans are manufactured on the rough endoplasmic reticulum (RER); they are then transported to the Golgi apparatus, where resident enzymes covalently bind tetrasaccharides to its serine side chains; the GAG is then assembled by the addition of sugars one at a time. Sulfation, catalyzed by sulfotransferases, and epimerization (rearrangement of various groups around the carbon atoms of the sugar units) also occur in the Golgi apparatus.

Many proteoglycans, especially **aggrecan,** a macromolecule found in cartilage and connective tissue proper, attach to hyaluronic acid (see Fig. 4-3). The mode of attachment involves a noncovalent ionic interaction between the sugar groups of the hyaluronic acid and the core protein of the proteoglycan molecule. The connection is reinforced by small **link proteins** that form bonds with both the core protein of aggrecan as well as with the sugar groups of hyaluronic acid. Because hyaluronic acid may be as much as 20 μm in length, the result of this association is an aggrecan composite that occupies a very large volume and may have a molecular mass as large as several hundred million Da. This immense molecule is responsible for the gel state of the ECM and acts as a barrier to fast diffusion of aqueous deposits, as when one observes the slow disappearance of an aqueous bubble after its subdermal injection.

CLINICAL CORRELATIONS

Many pathogenic bacteria, such as *Staphylococcus aureus,* secrete **hyaluronidase,** an enzyme that cleaves hyaluronic acid into numerous small fragments, thus converting the gel state of the ECM to a sol state. The consequence of this reaction is to permit the rapid spread of the bacteria through the connective tissue spaces.

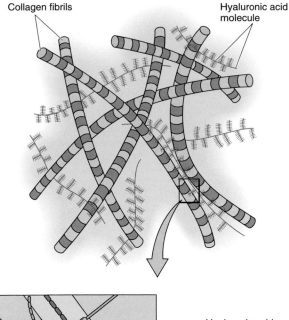

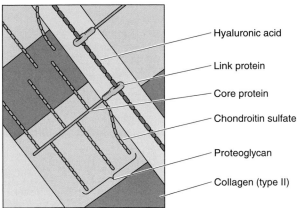

Hyaluronic acid

Link protein

Core protein

Chondroitin sulfate

Proteoglycan

Collagen (type II)

Figure 4–3 The association of aggrecan molecules with collagen fibers. *Inset* displays a higher magnification of the aggrecan molecule, indicating the core protein of the proteoglycan molecule to which the glycosaminoglycans are attached. The core protein is attached to the hyaluronic acid by link proteins. (Adapted from Fawcett DW: Bloom and Fawcett's A Textbook of Histology, 11th ed. Philadelphia, WB Saunders, 1986.)

Functions of Proteoglycans

Proteoglycans have numerous functions. By occupying a large volume, they resist compression and retard the rapid movement of microorganisms and metastatic cells; however, in the same fashion, they facilitate normal cellular locomotion by permitting migrating cells to move into the space that these hydrated macromolecules occupied. In addition, in association with the basal lamina, they form molecular filters of varying pore sizes and charge distributions that selectively screen and retard macromolecules as they pass through them.

Proteoglycans also possess binding sites for certain signaling molecules, such as transforming growth factor-β. By binding these signaling molecules, proteoglycans can either impede their function by preventing the molecules from reaching their destinations, or enhance their function by concentrating them in a specific location. Some proteoglycans, such as decorins, are required for the formation of collagen fibers; mutated mice that cannot produce decorins or that produce defective decorins, possess skin with reduced tensile strength.

Some proteoglycans, such as **syndecans,** instead of being released into the ECM, remain attached to the cell membrane. The core proteins of syndecans act as transmembrane proteins and are attached to the actin filaments of the cytoskeleton. Their extracellular moieties bind to components of the ECM, thus permitting the cell to become attached to macromolecular components of the matrix. In addition, syndecans of fibroblasts function as co-receptors because they bind fibroblast growth factor and present it to cell membrane fibroblast growth factor receptors in their vicinity.

Glycoproteins

Cell adhesive glycoproteins have binding sites for several components of the ECM as well as for integrin molecules of the cell membrane that facilitate the attachment of cells to the ECM.

The ability of cells to adhere to components of the ECM is mediated to a great extent by cell adhesive glycoproteins. These large macromolecules have several domains, at least one of which usually binds to cell surface proteins called **integrins,** one to collagen fibers, and one to proteoglycans. In this manner, adhesive glycoproteins fasten the various components of tissues to each other. The major types of adhesive glycoproteins are fibronectin, laminin, entactin, tenascin, chondronectin, and osteonectin.

Fibronectin is a large dimer composed of two similar polypeptide subunits, each about 220,000 Da, attached to one another at their carboxyl ends by disulfide bonds. Each arm of this V-shaped macromolecule has binding sites for various extracellular components (e.g., collagen, heparin, heparan sulfate, and hyaluronic acid) and for integrins of the cell membrane. The region of the fibronectin that is specific for adhering to the cell membrane has the three-residue sequence arginine, glycine, and aspartate, referred to as the **RGD sequence.** This sequence of amino acids is characteristic of the integrin binding site in many adhesive glycoproteins. Fibronectin is produced mainly by connective tissue cells known as **fibroblasts.** The actin components of the cytoskeleton of these cells and their associated myosin counterparts interact, placing tension on their plasmalemma. The integrin molecules relay the tensile forces to the newly exocytosed fibronectin molecules, stretching them just enough to expose hidden binding sites that permit fibronectins to bind to each other, thus forming the fibronectin matrix.

Fibronectin is also present in blood as **plasma fibronectin,** where it facilitates wound healing, phagocytosis, and coagulation. Fibronectin may be temporarily attached to the plasma membrane as **cell-surface fibronectin.** Fibronectin marks migratory pathways for embryonic cells so that the migrating cells of the developing organism can reach their destination.

Laminin is a very large glycoprotein (950,000 Da), composed of three large polypeptide chains, A, B_1, and B_2. The B chains wrap around the A chain, forming a cross-like pattern of one long and three short chains. The three chains are held in position by disulfide bonds. The location of laminin is almost strictly limited to the basal lamina; therefore, this glycoprotein has binding sites for heparan sulfate, type IV collagen, entactin, and the cell membrane.

The sulfated glycoprotein **entactin** (also known as **nidogen**) binds to the laminin molecule where the three short arms of that molecule meet each other. Entactin also binds to type IV collagen, thus facilitating the binding of laminin to the collagen meshwork.

Tenascin is a large glycoprotein composed of six polypeptide chains held together by disulfide bonds. This macromolecule, which resembles a bug whose six legs project radially from a central body, has binding sites for the transmembrane proteoglycan syndecans and for fibronectin. Tenascin's distribution is usually limited to embryonic tissue, where it marks migratory pathways for specific cells.

Chondronectin and **osteonectin** are similar to fibronectin. The former has binding sites for type II collagen, chondroitin sulfates, hyaluronic acid, and integrins of chondroblasts and chondrocytes. Osteonectin possesses domains for type I collagen, proteoglycans, and integrins of osteoblasts and osteocytes. In addition, it may facilitate the binding of calcium hydroxyapatite crystals to type I collagen in bone.

FIBERS

Collagen and elastic fibers, the two major fibrous proteins of connective tissue, have distinctive biochemical and mechanical properties as a consequence of their structural characteristics.

The fibers of the ECM provide tensile strength and elasticity to this substance. Classical histologists have described three types of fibers on the basis of their morphology and reactivity with histological stains: **collagen, reticular,** and **elastic** (see Fig. 4-2). Although it is now known that reticular fibers are in fact a type of collagen fiber, many histologists retain the term *reticular fibers* not only for historical reasons but also for con-

venience when describing organs that possess large quantities of this particular collagen type.

Collagen Fibers: Structure and Function

Collagen fibers are composed of tropocollagen subunits whose α-chain amino acid sequences permit the classification of collagen into at least 20 different fiber types. There are three categories of collagen: fibril-forming, fibril-associated, and network-forming; there are also collagen-like proteins that form an additional category.

The capability of the ECM to withstand compressive forces is due to the presence of the hydrated matrix formed by GAGs and proteoglycans. Tensile forces are resisted by fibers of the tough, firm, inelastic protein collagen. This family of proteins is very abundant, constituting about 20% to 25% of all the proteins in the body. Collagens are classified into three categories, fibril-forming, fibril-associated, and network-forming collagens. An additional category, collagen-like proteins, is also recognized.

Fibril-forming collagen, as its classification implies, forms flexible fibers (Fig. 4-4) whose tensile strength is greater than that of stainless steel of comparable diameter. Large collections of collagen fibers appear glistening white in live tissue; therefore, collagen fiber bundles are also referred to as *white fibers.* Collagen fibers of connective tissue are usually less than 10 μm in diameter and are colorless when unstained. Stained with hematoxylin and eosin, they appear as long, wavy, pink fiber bundles.

Electron micrographs of collagen fibers stained with heavy metals display cross-banding at regular intervals of 67 nm, a characteristic property of these fibers. These fibers are formed from parallel aggregates of thinner fibrils 10 to 300 nm in diameter and many micrometers in length (Fig. 4-5). The fibrils themselves are fashioned from a highly regular assembly of even smaller subunits, **tropocollagen (collagen) molecules,** each about 280 nm long and 1.5 nm in diameter. Individual tropocollagen molecules are composed of three polypeptide chains, called **α-chains,** wrapped around each other in a triple helical configuration.

Each α-chain possesses about 1000 amino acid residues. Every third amino acid is glycine, and most of the remaining amino acids are composed of proline, hydroxyproline, and hydroxylysine. It is believed that glycine, because of its small size, permits the close association of the three α-chains; the hydrogen bonds of hydroxyproline hold the three α-chains together; and hydroxylysine permits the formation of fibrils by binding the tropocollagen molecules to each other.

Although at least 20 different types of collagen are known, depending on the amino acid sequence of their α-chains, only 10 of them are of interest in this

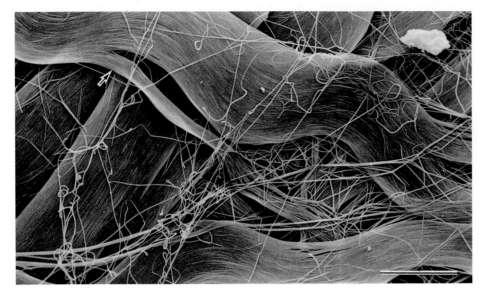

Figure 4–4 Scanning electron micrograph of collagen fiber bundles from the epineurium of the rat sciatic nerve (×2034). Note that the thick fiber bundles are interwoven and that they are arranged in an almost haphazard manner. Also, fiber bundles split *(arrow)* into thinner bundles (or thinner bundles coalesce to form larger bundles). Moreover, each of the thick fiber bundles is composed of numerous fine fibrils that run a parallel course in each bundle. (From Ushiki T, Ide C: Three-dimensional organization of the collagen fibrils in the rat sciatic nerve as revealed by transmission and scanning electron microscopy. Cell Tissue Res 260:175-184, 1990.)

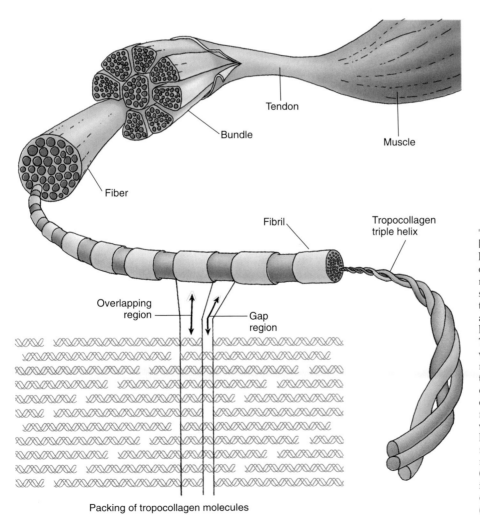

Figure 4–5 Components of a collagen fiber. The ordered arrangement of the tropocollagen molecules gives rise to gap and overlap regions, responsible for the 67-nm cross-banding of type I collagen. The *gap region* is the area between the head of one tropocollagen molecule and the tail of the next. The *overlapping region* is the area where the tail of one tropocollagen molecule overlaps the tail of another in the row above or below. In three dimensions, the overlap region coincides with numerous other overlap regions, and the gap regions coincide with numerous other gap regions. The heavy metals that are used in electron microscopy precipitate into the gap regions and make them visible as the 67-nm cross-banding. Type I collagen is composed of two identical a1(I) chains *(blue)* and one a2(I) chain *(pink)*.

textbook. Each α-chain is coded by a separate messenger ribonucleic acid (mRNA). These different collagen types are located in specific regions of the body, where they serve various functions (Table 4-2; Fig. 4-6).

CLINICAL CORRELATIONS

At the end of surgery, the cut surfaces of skin are carefully sutured; usually, a week later the sutures are removed. The tensile strength of the dermis at that point is only about 10% that of normal skin. Within the next 4 weeks, the tensile strength increases to about 80% of normal, but in many cases it never reaches 100%. The initial weakness is attributed to the formation of type III collagen during early wound healing, whereas the later improvement in tensile strength is due to scar maturation, when type III collagen is replaced by type I collagen.

Some individuals, especially blacks, are predisposed to an excessive accumulation of collagen during wound healing. In these patients, the scar forms an elevated growth known as a **keloid.**

Collagen Synthesis

The synthesis of collagen occurs on the rough endoplasmic reticulum as individual preprocollagen chains (α-chains).

The synthesis of collagen occurs on the RER as individual **preprocollagen** chains (Fig. 4-7), which are α-chains possessing additional amino acid sequences, known as **propeptides,** at both the amino and carboxyl ends. As a preprocollagen molecule is being synthesized, it enters the cisterna of the RER, where it is modified. First, the signal sequence directing the molecule to the RER is removed; then some of the proline and lysine residues are hydroxylated (by the enzymes peptidyl proline hydroxylase and peptidyl lysine hydroxylase) in a process known as post-translational modification to form hydroxyproline and hydroxylysine, respectively. Subsequently, selected hydroxylysines are glycosylated by the addition of glucose and galactose.

Three preprocollagen molecules align with each other and assemble to form a tight helical configuration known as a **procollagen molecule.** It is believed that the precision of their alignment is accomplished by the propeptides. Because these propeptides do not wrap around each other, the procollagen molecule resembles a tightly wound rope with frayed ends. The propeptides apparently have the additional function of keeping the procollagen molecules soluble, thus preventing their spontaneous aggregation into collagen fibers within the cell.

The procollagen molecules leave the RER via transfer vesicles that transport them to the Golgi apparatus, where they are further modified by the addition of oligosaccharides. The modified procollagen molecules are packaged in the *trans* Golgi network and are immediately ferried out of the cell.

As procollagen enters the extracellular environment, proteolytic enzymes, called **procollagen peptidases,** cleave the propeptides (removing a portion of the frayed ends) from both the amino and carboxyl ends (see Fig. 4-7). The newly formed molecule is shorter (280 nm in length) and is known as a **tropocollagen (collagen) molecule.** Tropocollagen molecules spontaneously self-assemble (see Fig. 4-7), in a specific head-to-tail

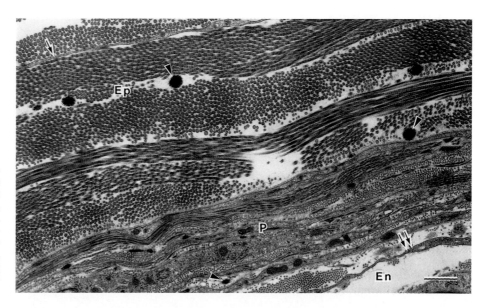

Figure 4–6 Electron micrograph (×22,463) of collagen fibers from the perineurium of the rat sciatic nerve. Ep, epineurium; En, endoneurium; P, perineurium. (From Ushiki T, Ide C: Three-dimensional organization of the collagen fibrils in the rat sciatic nerve, as revealed by transmission and scanning electron microscopy. Cell Tissue Res 260:175-184, 1990.)

TABLE 4–2 Major Types and Characteristics of Collagen

Molecular Type	Molecular Formula	Synthesizing Cells	Function	Location in Body
I (fibril-forming); most common of all collagens	$[\alpha(I)]_2\alpha 2(I)$	Fibroblasts, osteoblasts, odontoblasts, cementoblasts	Resists tension	Dermis, tendon, ligaments, capsules of organs, bone, dentin, cementum
II (fibril-forming)	$[\alpha 1(II)]_3$	Chondroblasts	Resists pressure	Hyaline cartilage, elastic cartilage
III (fibril-forming); also known as reticular fibers. Highly glycosylated	$[\alpha 1(III)]_3$	Fibroblasts, reticular cells, smooth muscle cells, hepatocytes	Forms structural framework of spleen, liver, lymph nodes, smooth muscle, adipose tissue	Lymphatic system, spleen, liver, cardiovascular system, lung, skin
IV (network-forming); do not display 67-nm periodicity and α-chains retain propeptides	$[\alpha 1(IV)]_2\alpha 2(IV)$	Epithelial cells, muscle cells, Schwann cells	Forms meshwork of the lamina densa of the basal lamina to provide support and filtration	Basal lamina
V (fibril-forming)	$[\alpha 1(V)]_2\alpha 2(V)$	Fibroblasts, mesenchymal cells	Associated with type I collagen, also with placental ground substance	Dermis, tendon, ligaments, capsules of organs, bone, cementum, placenta
VII (network-forming); form dimers that assemble into anchoring fibrils	$[\alpha 1(VII)]_3$	Epidermal cells	Forms anchoring fibrils that fasten lamina densa to underlying lamina reticularis	Junction of epidermis and dermis
IX (fibril-associated); decorate the surface of type II collagen fibers	$[\alpha 1(IX)\alpha 2(IX)\alpha 3(IX)]$	Epithelial cells	Associates with type II collagen fibers	Cartilage
XII (fibril-associated); decorate the surface of type I collagen fibers	$[\alpha 1(XII)]_3$	Fibroblasts	Associates with type I collagen fibers	Tendons, ligaments, and aponeuroses
XVII (collagen-like protein); a transmembrane protein, formerly known as bullous pemphigoid antigen	$[\alpha 1(XVII)]_3$	Epithelial cells	?	Hemidesmosomes
XVIII (collagen-like protein); cleavage of its C-terminal forms endostatin and angiogenesis inhibitor	$[\alpha 1(XVIII)]_3$	Endothelial cells	?	Basal lamina of endothelial cells

direction, into a regularly staggered array, fashioning fibrils that display a 67-nm wide banding representative of collagen types I, II, III, and V (see Fig. 4-5). The formation and maintenance of the fibrillar structure are augmented by covalent bonds formed between lysine and hydroxylysine residues of neighboring tropocollagen molecules.

As the tropocollagen molecules self-assemble in a three-dimensional array, the spaces between the heads and tails of successive molecules in a single row line up as repeating **gap regions** (every 67 nm), not in adjoining but in neighboring rows (see Figs. 4-5 and 4-7). Similarly, the overlaps of heads and tails in neighboring rows

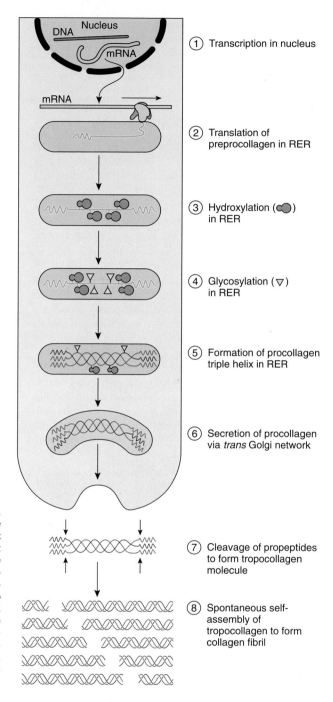

1. Transcription in nucleus

2. Translation of preprocollagen in RER

3. Hydroxylation (◐) in RER

4. Glycosylation (▽) in RER

5. Formation of procollagen triple helix in RER

6. Secretion of procollagen via *trans* Golgi network

7. Cleavage of propeptides to form tropocollagen molecule

8. Spontaneous self-assembly of tropocollagen to form collagen fibril

Figure 4–7 Sequence of events in the synthesis of type I collagen. Messenger RNA (mRNA) leaves the nucleus and attracts small and large subunits of ribosomes. As translation begins, the polysome complex translocates to the rough endoplasmic reticulum (RER), and the nascent alpha chains enter the lumen of the RER. Within the lumen, some proline and lysine residues of the α-chains are hydroxylated, and the preprocollagen molecule is glycosylated. Three α-chains form a helical configuration—the procollagen triple helix. The procollagen is transferred to the Golgi complex where further modification occurs. At the *trans* Golgi network the procollagen is packaged in clathrin-coated vesicles, and the procollagen is exocytosed. As the procollagen leaves the cell, a membrane-bound enzyme called procollagen peptidase cleaves the propeptides from both the carboxyl- and the amino-end of procollagen, transforming it into tropocollagen. These newly formed macromolecules self-assemble into collagen fibrils.

are in register with one another as the **overlap regions.** Heavy metal stains used in electron microscopy preferentially deposit in the gap regions. Consequently, viewed in the electron microscope, collagen displays alternating dark and light bands; the dark bands represent the gap regions filled with heavy metal, and the light bands represent overlap regions, where the heavy metal cannot be deposited (see Fig. 4-6).

The alignment of the collagen fibrils and fiber bundles is determined by the cells that synthesize them. The procollagen is released into folds and furrows of the plasmalemma, which act as molds that arrange the forming fibrils in the proper direction. The fibril orientation is further enhanced as the cells tug on the fibrils and physically drag them to fit the required pattern.

Fibrillar structure is absent in **type IV** and **type VII collagen** because the propeptides are not removed from the procollagen molecule. Its procollagen molecules assemble into dimers, which then form a felt-like meshwork.

CLINICAL CORRELATIONS

Hydroxylation of proline residues requires the presence of vitamin C. In individuals who suffer from a deficiency of this vitamin, the α-chains of the tropocollagen molecules are unable to form stable helices, and the tropocollagen molecules are incapable of aggregating into fibrils. This condition, known as **scurvy,** first affects connective tissues with a high turnover of collagen, such as the periodontal ligament and gingiva (Fig. 4-8). Because these two structures are responsible for maintaining teeth in their sockets, the symptoms of scurvy include bleeding gums and loose teeth. If the vitamin C deficiency is prolonged, other sites are also affected. These symptoms may be alleviated by eating foods rich in vitamin C.

Deficiency of the enzyme **lysyl hydroxylase,** a genetic disorder known as **Ehlers-Danlos syndrome,** results in abnormal cross-links among tropocollagen molecules. Individuals afflicted with this anomalous condition possess abnormal collagen fibers that result in hypermobile joints and hyperextensive skin. In many instances, the skin of affected patients is readily traumatized and the patient is subject to dislocation of the affected joints.

Elastic Fibers

Elastic fibers, unlike collagen, are highly accommodating and may be stretched one and a half times their resting length without breaking. When the force is released, elastic fibers return to their resting length.

The elasticity of connective tissue is due, in great part, to the presence of elastic fibers in the ECM (Figs. 4-9 and 4-10; also see Fig. 4-2). These fibers are usually slender, long, and branching in loose connective tissue, but they may form coarser bundles in ligaments and fenestrated sheets. Such bundles are found in the ligamentum flava of the vertebral column, and concentric sheets occur in the walls of larger blood vessels. In fact, elastic fibers constitute about 50% of the aorta by dry weight.

Elastic fibers are manufactured by fibroblasts of connective tissue as well as by smooth muscle cells of blood vessels. They are composed of **elastin,** a protein that is rich in glycine, lysine, alanine, valine, and proline but that has no hydroxylysine. Elastin chains are held together in such a fashion that four lysine molecules, each belonging to a different elastin chain, form covalent bonds with each other to form **desmosine cross-links.** These desmosine residues are highly deformable and they impart a high degree of elasticity to elastic fibers to such an extent that these fibers may be stretched to about 150% of their resting lengths before breaking. After being stretched, elastic fibers return to their resting length.

The core of elastic fibers is composed of elastin and is surrounded by a sheath of **microfibrils;** each microfibril is about 10 nm in diameter and is composed of the glycoprotein **fibrillin** (Fig. 4-11). During the for-

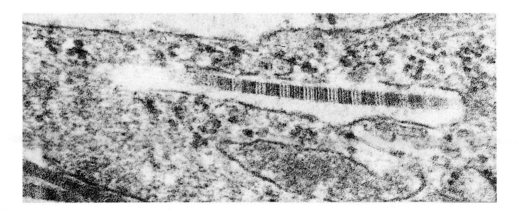

Figure 4–8 Degradation of type I collagen by fibroblasts. Collagen turnover is relatively slow in some regions of the body (e.g., in bone, where it may be stable for as long as 10 years), whereas in other regions, such as the gingiva and the periodontal ligament, the half-life of collagen may be weeks or months. Fibroblasts of the gingiva and periodontal ligament are responsible not only for the synthesis but also for the resorption of collagen. (From Ten Cate AR: Oral Histology: Development, Structure, and Function, 4th ed. St. Louis, Mosby–Year Book, 1994.)

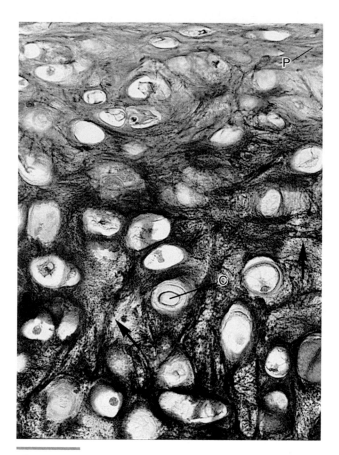

Figure 4–9 Light micrograph of elastic cartilage (×270). Note the presence of elastic fibers (*arrows*) in the matrix. The large chondrocytes of elastic cartilage occupy spaces known as lacunae in the proteoglycan-rich matrix. The large bundles of elastic fibers are clearly evident, and they appear to be arranged in a haphazard fashion. Observe that the thicker elastic fibers are composed of fine fibrils. C, chondrocyte; P, perichondrium.

mation of elastic fibers, the microfibrils are elaborated first, and the elastin is then deposited in the space surrounded by the microfibrils (Fig. 4-12).

CLINICAL CORRELATIONS

The integrity of elastic fibers depends on the presence of microfibrils. Patients with **Marfan syndrome** have a defect in the gene on chromosome 15 that codes for fibrillin; therefore, their elastic fibers do not develop normally. People who are severely affected with this condition are predisposed to fatal rupture of the aorta.

BASEMENT MEMBRANE

The basement membrane seen with light microscopy is shown by electron microscopy to be composed of the basal lamina and lamina reticularis.

The interface between epithelium and connective tissue is occupied by a narrow, acellular region—the basement membrane—which is well stained by the PAS reaction and by other histological stains that detect GAGs. A structure similar to the basement membrane, the **external lamina,** surrounds smooth and skeletal muscle cells, adipocytes, and Schwann cells. Electron microscopy shows that the basement membrane has two constituents: the **basal lamina,** elaborated by epithelial cells, and the **lamina reticularis,** manufactured by cells of the connective tissue (Fig. 4-13). The epithelial sheath is bound to the underlying connective tissue by these resilient acellular interfaces, the basal lamina and lamina reticularis.

Basal Lamina

The basal lamina manufactured by the epithelium is composed of the lamina lucida and the lamina densa.

Electron micrographs of the basal lamina display its two regions: the lamina lucida, a 50-nm-thick electron-lucent region just beneath the epithelium, and the lamina densa, a 50-nm-thick electron-dense region (Figs. 4-13 to 4-15). The **lamina lucida** consists mainly of the extracellular glycoproteins laminin and entactin, as well as of **integrins** and **dystroglycans,** transmembrane laminin receptors (both discussed later), that project from the epithelial cell membrane into the basal lamina. In rapidly frozen tissues, the lamina lucida is frequently absent, suggesting that it may be an artifact of fixation and that the lamina densa may be closer to the integrins and dystroglycans of the basal cell membrane than previously believed.

The **lamina densa** comprises a meshwork of type IV collagen, which is coated on both the lamina lucida and lamina reticularis sides by the proteoglycan **perlacan.** The **heparan sulfate** side chains projecting from the protein core of perlacan form a polyanion. The lamina reticularis aspect of the lamina densa also possesses **fibronectin.**

Laminin has domains that bind to type IV collagen, heparan sulfate, and the integrins and dystroglycans of the epithelial basal cell membrane, thus anchoring the epithelial cell to the basal lamina. The basal lamina appears to be well anchored to the reticular lamina by several substances, including fibronectin, anchoring fibrils (type VII collagen), and microfibrils (fibrillin), all elaborated by fibroblasts of connective tissue (Fig. 4-16).

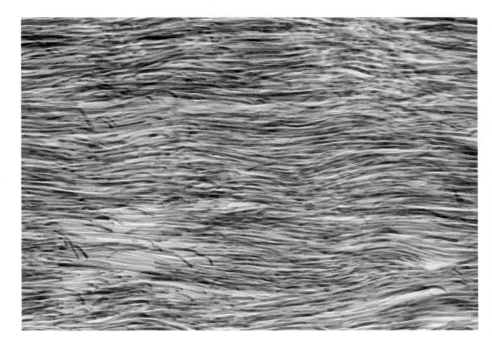

Figure 4–10 Light micrograph of dense, regular elastic connective tissue (x270). Note that the elastic fibers are short and are arranged almost parallel with each other and that their ends are somewhat curled. Unlike collagen fibers of dense regular connective tissue, where the collagen fibrils and fibers closely parallel each other, these elastic fibers appear to be somewhat misaligned.

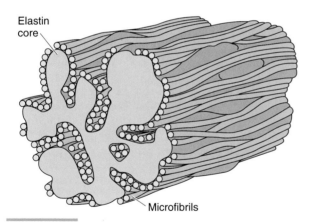

Elastin core

Microfibrils

Figure 4–11 An elastic fiber, showing microfibrils surrounding the amorphous elastin.

The basal lamina functions both as a molecular filter and as a flexible, firm support for the overlying epithelium. The filtering aspect is due not only to the type IV collagen, whose interwoven meshwork forms a physical filter of specific pore size, but also to the negative charges of its heparan sulfate constituent, which preferentially restricts the passage of negatively charged molecules. Additional functions of the basal lamina include facilitating mitotic activity and cell differentiation, modulating cellular metabolism, assisting in the establishment of cell polarity, playing a role in the modification of the arrangement of the integral proteins localized in the basal cell membrane, and acting as a path for cellular migration, as in re-epithelialization during wound repair or in the reestablishment of myoneural junctions during regeneration of motor nerves.

Lamina Reticularis

The lamina reticularis is derived from the connective tissue component and is responsible for affixing the lamina densa to the underlying connective tissue.

The **lamina reticularis** (see Figs. 4-13, 4-14, and 4-16), a region of varying thickness, is manufactured by fibroblasts and is composed of type I and type III collagen. It is the interface between the basal lamina and the underlying connective tissue, and its thickness varies with the amount of frictional force on the overlying epithelium. Thus, it is quite thick in skin and very thin beneath the epithelial lining of the alveolus of the lung.

Type I and type III collagen fibers of the connective tissue loop into the lamina reticularis, where they interact with and are bound to the microfibrils and anchoring fibrils of the lamina reticularis. Moreover, the basic groups of the collagen fibers form bonds with the acidic groups of the GAGs of the lamina densa. In addition, collagen-binding domains and GAG domains of fibronectin further assist in anchoring the basal lamina to the lamina reticularis.

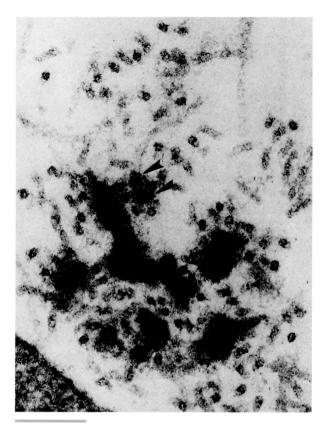

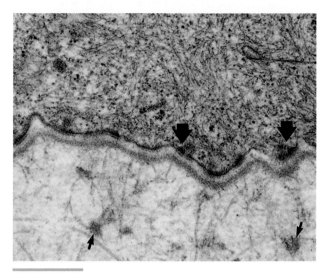

Figure 4-13 Electron micrograph of the basal lamina of the human cornea (×50,000). Note the hemidesmosomes *(large arrows)* and the anchoring plaques among the anchoring fibrils *(small arrows).* Observe that the basal cell membrane is clearly visible and that the plaques of the hemidesmosomes are attached to the cytoplasmic surface of the basal plasmalemma. The dense, amorphous-appearing line that follows the contour of the basal plasma membrane is the lamina densa, and the clear area between it and the basal cell membrane is the lamina lucida. (From Albert D, Jakobiec FA: Principles and Practice of Ophthalmology: Basic Sciences. Philadelphia, WB Saunders, 1994.)

Figure 4–12 Electron micrograph of elastic fiber development. Note the presence of microfibrils surrounding the amorphous matrix of elastin as if a small space were to be delineated by slats of a picket fence *(arrowheads).* These fibrillin-containing microfibrils are elaborated and released first, and then the manufacturing cell—a fibroblast of connective tissue proper or a smooth muscle cell of a blood vessel—releases elastin into the space enclosed by the microfibrils. (From Fukuda Y, Ferrans VJ, Crystal RG: Development of elastic fibers of nuchal ligament, aorta, and lung of fetal and postnatal sheep: An ultrastructural and electron microscopic immunohistochemical study. Am J Anat 170:597-629, 1984.)

INTEGRINS AND DYSTROGLYCANS

Integrins and dystroglycans are transmembrane glycoproteins that act as laminin receptors as well as organizers of basal lamina assembly.

Integrins are transmembrane proteins that are similar to cell membrane receptors in that they form bonds with ligands. However, unlike those of receptors, their cytoplasmic regions are linked to the cytoskeleton, and their ligands are not signaling molecules but structural members of the ECM such as collagen, laminin, and fibronectin. Moreover, the association between an integrin and its ligand is much weaker than that between a receptor and its ligand. Integrins are much more numerous than receptors, thus compensating for the bond weakness and also permitting the migration of cells along a surface of the ECM.

Integrins are heterodimers (~250,000 Da) composed of α and β glycoprotein chains whose carboxyl ends are linked to talin and α-actinin of the cytoskeleton. Their amino ends possess binding sites for macromolecules of the ECM (see Chapter 2, Fig. 2-32). Because integrins link the cytoskeleton to the ECM, they are also called **transmembrane linkers.** The α-chain of the integrin molecule binds Ca^{2+} or Mg^{2+}, divalent cations necessary for the maintenance of proper binding with the ligand.

Many integrins differ in their ligand specificity, cellular distribution, and function. Some are commonly referred to as *receptors* for their ligands (e.g., laminin receptor, fibronectin receptor). Cells can modulate the affinity of their receptor for its ligand by regulating the availability of divalent cations, modifying the conformation of the integrin, or otherwise altering the integrin's affinity for the ligand. In this manner, cells are not locked into a particular position once their integrins bind to the macromolecules of the ECM but can release their integrin-ligand bonds and move away from that particular location.

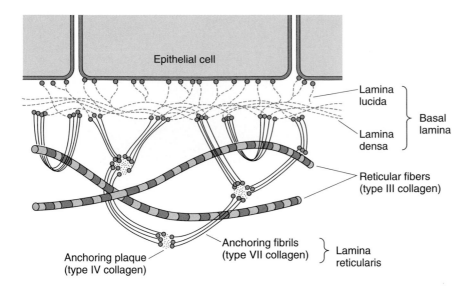

Figure 4–14 Basal lamina and lamina reticularis. (Adapted from Fawcett DW: Bloom and Fawcett's A Textbook of Histology, 12th ed. New York, Chapman and Hall, 1994.)

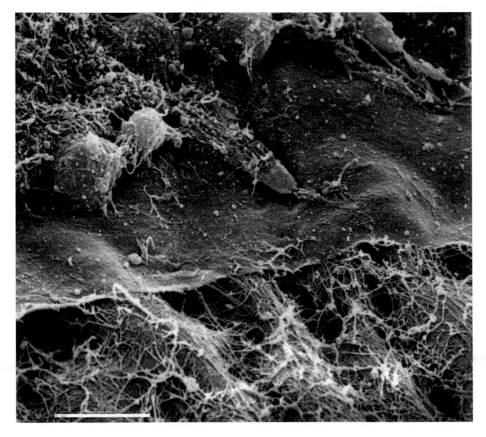

Figure 4–15 This scanning electron micrograph is of a 6-day chick embryo cornea from which a portion of the epithelium has been removed, exposing epithelial cells on the underlying basement membrane. The membrane itself has been partially removed, revealing the underlying primary corneal stroma composed of orthogonally arrayed collagen fibrils. The *white bar* at the lower left is the 10-μm mark. (© Robert L. Trelstad.)

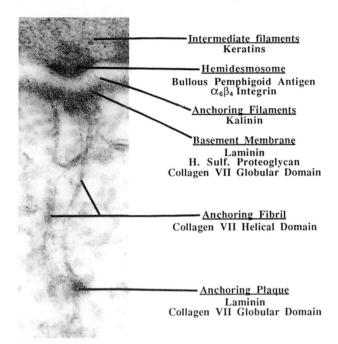

Intermediate filaments
Keratins

Hemidesmosome
Bullous Pemphigoid Antigen
$\alpha_6\beta_4$ Integrin

Anchoring Filaments
Kalinin

Basement Membrane
Laminin
H. Sulf. Proteoglycan
Collagen VII Globular Domain

Anchoring Fibril
Collagen VII Helical Domain

Anchoring Plaque
Laminin
Collagen VII Globular Domain

Figure 4–16 Electron micrograph of the basal lamina of the corneal epithelium (×165,000). H. Sulf., Heparan sulfate-rich. (From Albert D, Jakobiec FA: Principles and Practice of Ophthalmology: Basic Sciences. Philadelphia, WB Saunders, 1994.)

In addition to their roles in adhesion, integrins function in transducing biochemical signals into intracellular events by activating second messenger system cascades. The versatility of integrins in biochemical transduction is evidenced by their ability to stimulate diverse signaling pathways, including mitogen-activated protein kinase, protein kinase C, and phosphoinositide pathways that lead to activation of the cell cycle, cell differentiation, cytoskeletal reorganization, regulation of gene expression, and even programmed cell death via apoptosis. Frequently, integrins have to be activated by focal adhesion kinase, a protein tyrosine kinase; otherwise, they cannot initiate their signaling functions.

Dystroglycans are glycoproteins that are also composed of two subunits, a transmembrane β-dystroglycan and an extracellular α-dystroglycan. The α-dystroglycan binds to the laminin of the basal lamina but at different sites than does the integrin molecule. The intracellular moiety of the β-dystroglycan binds to the actin-binding protein **dystrophin,** which, in turn, binds to α-actinin of the cytoskeleton.

Dystroglycans and integrins have significant roles in the assembly of basal laminae because embryos lacking either or both of these glycoproteins are unable to form normal basal laminae.

CLINICAL CORRELATIONS

Individuals with the autosomal recessive disorder **leukocyte adhesion deficiency** are incapable of synthesizing the β-chain of the white blood cell integrins. Their leukocytes are incapable of adhering to the endothelial cells of blood vessels and thus cannot migrate to sites of inflammation. Patients with this disease have difficulty in fighting bacterial infections.

Epithelium and Glands

5

The approximately 200 distinctly different types of cells composing the human body are arranged and cooperatively organized into four basic **tissues.** Groups of these tissues are assembled in various organizational and functional arrangements into **organs,** which carry out functions of the body. The four basic tissue types are **epithelium, connective tissue, muscle,** and **nervous tissue.** This and the next four chapters discuss each of these tissues and the cells that constitute them.

EPITHELIAL TISSUE

Epithelial tissue is present in two forms: (1) as sheets of contiguous cells (epithelia) that cover the body on its external surface and line the body on its internal surface, and (2) as glands, which originate from invaginated epithelial cells.

Epithelia are derived from all three embryonic germ layers, although most of the epithelia are derived from ectoderm and endoderm. The **ectoderm** gives rise to the oral and nasal mucosae, cornea, epidermis of the skin, and glands of the skin and the mammary glands. The liver, the pancreas, and the lining of the respiratory and gastrointestinal tract are derived from the **endoderm.** The uriniferous tubules of the kidney, the lining of the male and female reproductive systems, the endothelial lining of the circulatory system, and the mesothelium of the body cavities develop from the **mesodermal** germ layer.

Epithelial tissues have numerous functions:

- **Protection** of underlying tissues of the body from abrasion and injury
- **Transcellular transport** of molecules across epithelial layers
- **Secretion** of mucus, hormones, enzymes, and so forth, from various glands
- **Absorption** of material from a lumen (e.g., intestinal tract or certain kidney tubules)

- **Control of movement** of materials between body compartments via **selective permeability** of intercellular junctions between epithelial cells
- **Detection of sensations** via taste buds, retina of the eye, and specialized hair cells in the ear.

Epithelium

Tightly bound contiguous cells forming sheets covering or lining the body are known as an epithelium.

The sheets of contiguous cells in the epithelium are tightly bound together by junctional complexes. Epithelia display little intercellular space and little extracellular matrix. They are separated from the underlying connective tissue by an extracellular matrix, the **basal lamina** (discussed in Chapter 4), synthesized by the epithelial cells. Because epithelium is avascular, the adjacent supporting connective tissue through its capillary beds supplies nourishment and oxygen via diffusion through the basal lamina.

Classification of Epithelial Membranes

Cell arrangement and morphology are the bases of classification of epithelium.

Epithelial membranes are classified according to the number of cell layers between the basal lamina and the free surface and by the morphology of the epithelial cells (Table 5-1). If the membrane is composed of a single layer of cells, it is called **simple epithelium;** if it is composed of more than one cell layer, it is called **stratified epithelium** (Fig. 5-1). The morphology of the cells may be squamous (flat), cuboidal, or columnar when viewed in sections taken perpendicular to the basement membrane. Stratified epithelia are classified by the morphology of the cells in their superficial layer

TABLE 5–1 Classification of Epithelia

Type	Shape of Surface Cells	Sample Locations	Functions
Simple Squamous	Flattened	*Lining:* pulmonary alveoli, loop of Henle, parietal layer of Bowman capsule, inner and middle ears, blood and lymphatic vessels, pleural and peritoneal cavities	Limiting membrane, fluid transport, gaseous exchange, lubrication, reducing friction (thus aiding movement of viscera), lining membrane
Cuboidal	Cuboidal	Ducts of many glands, covering of ovary, form kidney tubules	Secretion, absorption, protection
Columnar	Columnar	*Lining:* oviducts, ductuli efferentes of testis, uterus, small bronchi, much of digestive tract, gallbladder, large ducts of some glands	Transportation, absorption, secretion, protection
Pseudostratified	All cells rest on basal lamina but not all reach epithelial surface; surface cells are columnar	*Lining:* most of trachea, primary bronchi, epididymis and ductus deferens, auditory tube, part of tympanic cavity, nasal cavity, lacrimal sac, male urethra, large excretory ducts	Secretion, absorption lubrication, protection, transportation
Stratified Squamous, nonkeratinized	Flattened (with nuclei)	*Lining:* mouth, epiglottis, esophagus, vocal folds, vagina	Protection, secretion
Squamous, keratinized	Flattened (without nuclei)	Epidermis of skin	Protection
Cuboidal	Cuboidal	*Lining:* ducts of sweat glands	Absorption, secretion
Columnar	Columnar	Conjunctiva of eye, some large excretory ducts, portions of male urethra	Secretion, absorption, protection
Transitional	Dome-shaped (relaxed), flattened (distended)	*Lining:* urinary tract from renal calyces to urethra	Protection, distensible

only. In addition to these two major classes of epithelia, which are further identified by cellular morphology, there are two other distinct types: pseudostratified and transitional (see Fig. 5-1).

Simple Squamous Epithelium

Simple squamous epithelium is formed of a single layer of flat cells.

Simple squamous epithelium is composed of a single layer of tightly packed, thin, or low-profile polygonal cells. When viewed from the surface, the epithelial sheet looks much like a tile floor with a centrally placed, bulging nucleus in each cell (Fig. 5-2A). Viewed in

section, however, only some cells display nuclei, because the plane of section frequently does not encounter the nucleus. Simple squamous epithelia line pulmonary alveoli, compose the loop of Henle and the parietal layer of Bowman's capsule in the kidney, and form the endothelial lining of blood and lymph vessels as well as the mesothelium of the pleural and peritoneal cavities.

Simple Cuboidal Epithelium

Simple cuboidal epithelium is composed of a single layer of cells shaped like truncated hexagonal solids.

A single layer of polygon-shaped cells constitutes simple cuboidal epithelium (see Fig. 5-2A). When viewed in a

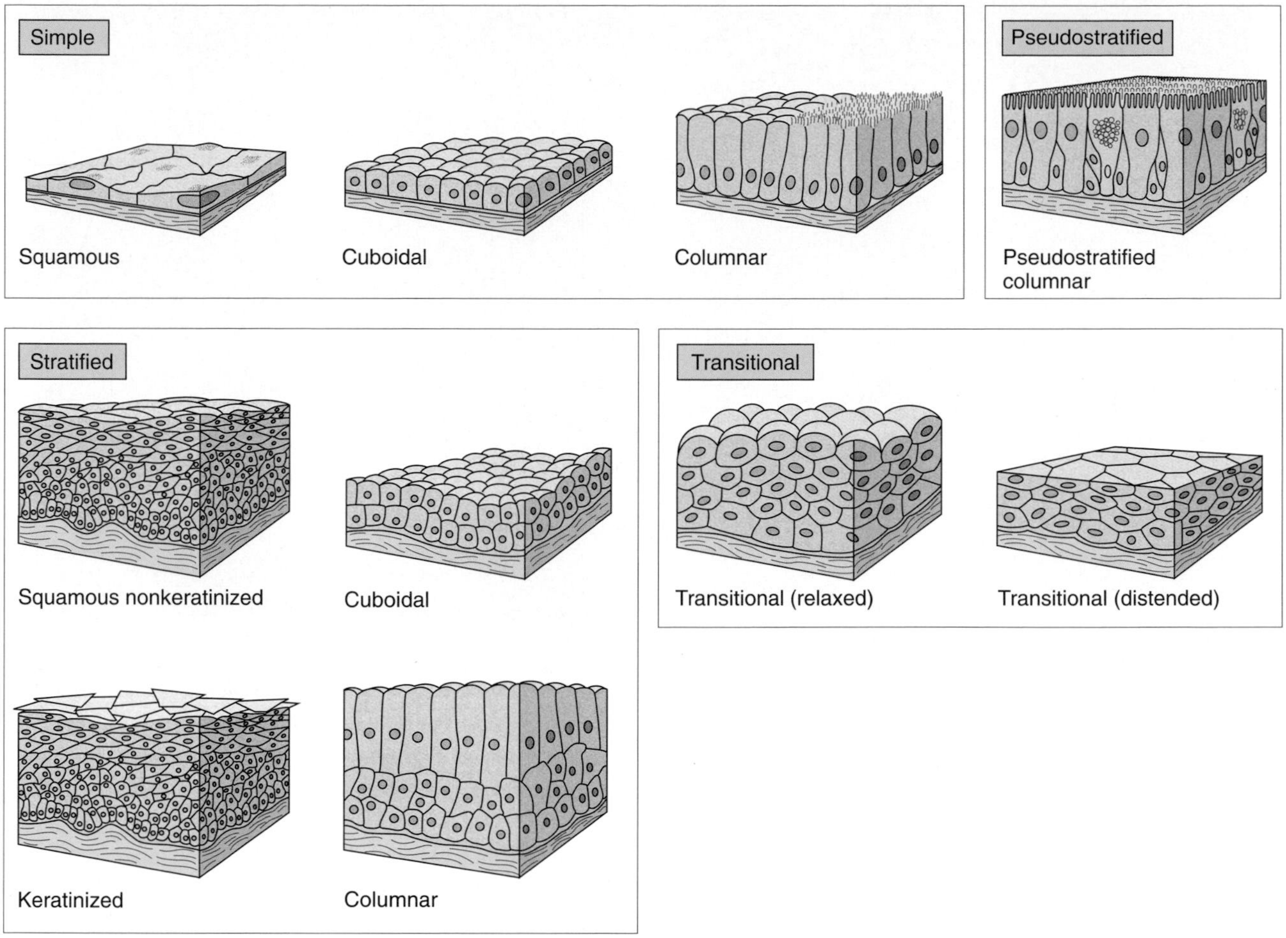

Figure 5–1 Types of epithelia.

section cut perpendicular to the surface, the cells present a square profile with a centrally placed round nucleus. Simple cuboidal epithelia make up the ducts of many glands of the body, form the covering of the ovary, and compose some kidney tubules.

Simple Columnar Epithelium

Simple columnar epithelium is composed of a single layer of tall cells shaped like hexagonal solids.

The cells of simple columnar epithelium appear much like those of simple cuboidal epithelium in a surface view; when viewed in longitudinal section, however, they are tall, rectangular cells whose ovoid nuclei are usually located at the same level in the basal half of the cell (Fig. 5-2B). Simple columnar epithelium is found in the lining of much of the digestive tract, gallbladder, and large ducts of glands. Simple columnar epithelium may exhibit a striated border, or **microvilli** (narrow, finger-like cytoplasmic processes), projecting from the apical surface of the cells. The simple columnar epithelium that lines the uterus, oviducts, ductuli efferentes, and small bronchi is ciliated. In these organs, **cilia** (hair-like structures) project from the apical surface of the columnar cells into the lumen.

Stratified Squamous Epithelium

Stratified squamous (nonkeratinized) epithelium comprises several layers of cells; the surface-most layer possesses nuclei. Stratified squamous (keratinized) epithelium is distinct in that the layers of cells composing the free surface are dead, non-nucleated, and filled with keratin.

NONKERATINIZED

Stratified squamous (nonkeratinized) epithelium is thick; because it is composed of several layers of cells, only the deepest layer is in contact with the basal lamina (Fig. 5-3A). The most basal (deepest) cells of this

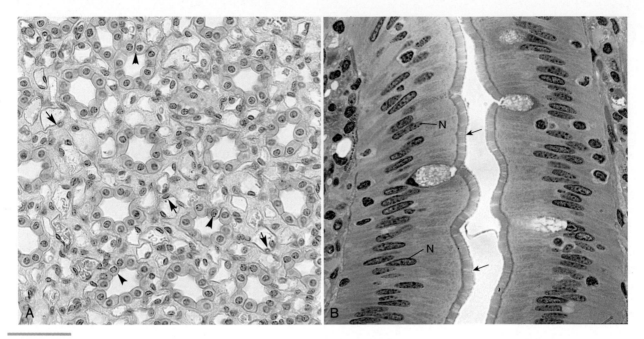

Figure 5–2 Light micrographs of simple epithelia. **A,** Simple squamous epithelium *(arrows)* (×270). Note the morphology of the cells and their nuclei. Also present is simple cuboidal epithelium *(arrowheads)*. Note the round, centrally placed nuclei. **B,** Simple columnar epithelium (×540). Observe the oblong nuclei (N) and the striated border *(arrows)*.

epithelium are cuboidal in shape; those located in the middle of the epithelium are polymorphous; and the cells composing the free surface of the epithelium are flattened (squamous)—hence the name *stratified squamous*. Because the surface cells are nucleated, this epithelium is called nonkeratinized. It is usually wet and is found lining the mouth, oral pharynx, esophagus, true vocal folds, and vagina.

KERATINIZED

Stratified squamous keratinized epithelium is similar to stratified squamous nonkeratinized epithelium, except that the superficial layers of the epithelium are composed of dead cells whose nuclei and cytoplasm have been replaced with keratin (Fig. 5-3B). This epithelium constitutes the epidermis of skin, a tough layer that resists friction and is impermeable to water.

Stratified Cuboidal Epithelium

Stratified cuboidal epithelium, which contains only two layers of cuboidal cells, lines the ducts of the sweat glands (Fig. 5-3C).

Stratified Columnar Epithelium

Stratified columnar epithelium comprises more than one layer of cells. The superficial layer is columnar in shape.

Stratified columnar epithelium is composed of a low polyhedral to cuboidal deeper layer in contact with the basal lamina and a superficial layer of columnar cells. This epithelium is found only in a few places in the body—namely, the conjunctiva of the eye, certain large excretory ducts, and regions of the male urethra.

Transitional Epithelium

Transitional epithelium consists of several layers of cells. The surface layer is large and dome-shaped.

Transitional epithelium received its name because it was erroneously believed to be in transition between stratified columnar and stratified squamous epithelia. This epithelium is now known to be a distinct type located exclusively in the urinary system, where it lines the urinary tract from the renal calyces to the urethra.

Transitional epithelium is composed of many layers of cells; those located basally are either low columnar or cuboidal cells. Polyhedral cells compose several layers above the basal cells. The most superficial cells of the empty bladder are large, are occasionally binucleated, and exhibit rounded dome-shaped tops that bulge into the lumen (Fig. 5-3D). These dome-shaped cells become flattened and the epithelium becomes thinner when the bladder is distended.

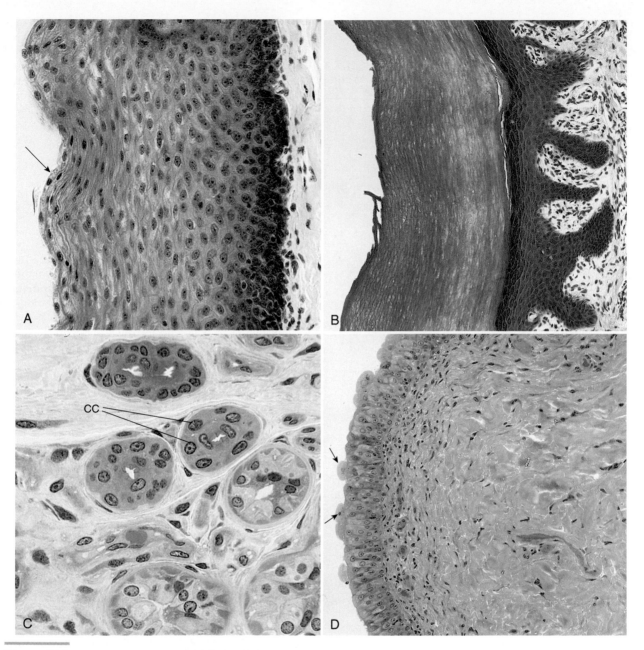

Figure 5–3 Light micrographs of stratified epithelia. **A,** Stratified squamous nonkeratinized epithelium (×509). Observe the many layers of cells and flattened (squamous) nucleated cells in the top layer (*arrow*). **B,** Stratified squamous keratinized epithelium (×125). **C,** Stratified cuboidal epithelium of the duct of a sweat gland (CC) (×509). **D,** Transitional epithelium (×125). Observe that the surface cells facing the lumen of the bladder are dome-shaped (*arrows*), which characterizes transitional epithelium.

Pseudostratified Columnar Epithelium

Pseudostratified columnar epithelium only appears stratified; all cells are in contact with the basal lamina.

As the name implies, pseudostratified columnar epithelium appears to be stratified but it is actually composed of a single layer of cells. All of the cells in pseudostratified columnar epithelium are in contact with the basal lamina, but only some cells reach the surface of the epithelium (Fig. 5-4). Cells not extending to the surface usually have a broad base and become narrow at their apical end. Taller cells reach the surface and possess a narrow base in contact with the basal lamina and a

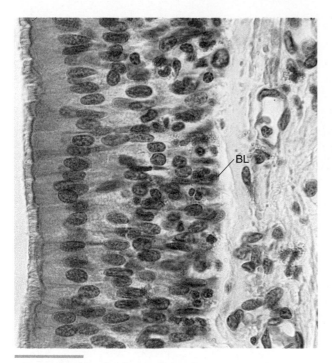

Figure 5-4 Light micrograph of pseudostratified columnar epithelia (×540). This type of epithelium appears to be stratified; however, all of the epithelial cells in this figure stand on the basal lamina (BL).

broadened apical surface. Because the cells of this epithelium are of different heights, their nuclei are located at different levels, giving the impression of a stratified epithelium even though it is composed of a single layer of cells. Pseudostratified columnar epithelium is found in the male urethra, epididymis, and larger excretory ducts of glands.

The most widespread type of pseudostratified columnar epithelium is **ciliated,** having cilia on the apical surface of the cells that reach the epithelial surface. Pseudostratified ciliated columnar epithelium is found lining most of the trachea and primary bronchi, the auditory tube, part of the tympanic cavity, the nasal cavity, and the lacrimal sac.

Polarity and Cell-Surface Specializations

Epithelial cell polarity and cell-surface specializations are related to cellular morphology and function.

Most epithelial cells have distinct morphological, biochemical, and functional domains and thus commonly display a polarity that may be related to one or all of these differences. Such polarized cells, for instance, possess an apical domain that faces a lumen and a basolateral domain whose basal component is in contact

with the basal lamina. Because these regions are distinct functionally, each may have surface modifications and specializations related to that function. For example, the apical surfaces of many epithelial cells possess microvilli or cilia, whereas their basolateral regions may exhibit many types of junctional specializations and intercellular interdigitations. The apical and basolateral domains are separated from each other by tight junctions that encircle the apical aspect of the cell.

Apical Domain

The apical domain represents the free surface of the epithelial cells.

The apical domain, the region of the epithelial cell facing the lumen, is rich in ion channels, carrier proteins, H^+-ATPase (adenosine triphosphatase), glycoproteins, and hydrolytic enzymes, as well as **aquaporins,** channel-forming proteins that function in regulation of water balance. It also is the site where regulated secretory products are delivered for release. Several surface modifications are necessary for the apical domain of an epithelium to carry out its many functions. These include microvilli with associated glycocalyx and, in some cases, stereocilia, cilia, and **flagella.** Note that the only cells in the human body that possess flagella are the spermatozoa. The structure of flagella is discussed in Chapter 21, which covers the male reproductive system.

MICROVILLI

Microvilli are small finger-like cytoplasmic projections emanating from the free surface of the cell into the lumen.

When observed by electron microscopy, absorptive columnar (and cuboidal) epithelial cells exhibit closely packed microvilli, which are cylindrical, membrane-bound projections of the cytoplasm emanating from the apical (luminal) surface of these cells (Fig. 5-5). Microvilli represent the **striated border** of the intestinal absorptive cells and the **brush border** of the kidney proximal tubule cells observed by light microscopy.

In less active cells, microvilli may be sparse and short; in intestinal epithelia, whose major function is transport and absorption, they are crowded and 1 to 2 μm in length, thus greatly increasing the surface area of the cells. Each microvillus contains a core of 25 to 30 **actin filaments,** cross-linked by **villin,** attached to an amorphous region at its tip and extending into the cytoplasm, where the actin filaments are embedded in the terminal web. The **terminal web** is a complex of actin and spectrin molecules as well as intermediate filaments located at the cortex of the epithelial cells (Figs. 5-6 to 5-8). At regular intervals, **myosin-I** and **calmodulin**

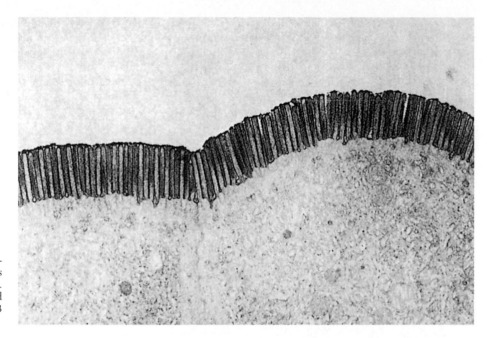

Figure 5–5 Electron micrograph of microvilli of epithelial cells from the small intestine (×2800). (From Hopkins CR: Structure and Function of Cells. Philadelphia, WB Saunders, 1978.)

connect the actin filaments to the plasma membrane of the microvillus, giving it support. Epithelia not functioning in absorption or transport may exhibit microvilli without cores of actin filaments.

Light microscopy of epithelia stained for carbohydrates reveals the glycocalyx, evident in electron micrographs as an amorphous, fuzzy coating over the luminal surface of the microvilli. The **glycocalyx** represents carbohydrate residues attached to the transmembrane proteins of the plasmalemma. These glycoproteins function in protection and cell recognition (see Chapter 2).

Stereocilia (not be confused with cilia) are long microvilli found only in the epididymis and on the sensory hair cells of the cochlea (inner ear). It is believed that these nonmotile structures are unusually rigid because of their core of actin filaments. In the epididymis, they probably function in increasing the surface area; in the hair cells of the ear, they function in signal generation.

CILIA

Cilia are long, motile, hair-like structures emanating from the apical cell surface. Their core is composed of a complex arrangement of microtubules known as the axoneme.

Cilia are motile, hair-like projections (diameter, 0.2 μm; length, 7 to 10 μm) that emanate from the surface of certain epithelial cells. In the ciliated epithelia of the respiratory system (e.g., trachea and bronchi) and in the oviduct, there may be hundreds of cilia in orderly arrays on the luminal surface of the cells. Other epithelial cells, such as the hair cells of the vestibular apparatus in the inner ear, possess only a single cilium, which functions in a sensory mechanism.

Cilia are specialized to function in propelling mucus and other substances over the surface of the epithelium via rapid rhythmic oscillations. Cilia of the respiratory tree, for example, move mucus and debris toward the oropharynx, where it may be swallowed or expectorated. Cilia of the oviduct move the fertilized ovum toward the uterus.

Electron microscopy reveals that cilia possess a specific internal structure that is consistently conserved throughout the plant and animal kingdoms (Figs. 5-9 and 5-10). The core of the cilium contains a complex of uniformly arranged microtubules called the **axoneme.** The axoneme is composed of a constant number of longitudinal microtubules arranged in a consistent 9 + 2 organization (Fig. 5-10B). Two centrally placed microtubules **(singlets)** are evenly surrounded by nine **doublets** of microtubules. The two microtubules located in the center of the core are separated from each other, each displaying a circular profile in cross section, composed of 13 protofilaments. Each of the nine doublets is composed of two subunits. In cross section, **subunit A** is a microtubule composed of 13 protofilaments, exhibiting a circular profile. **Subunit B** possesses 10 protofilaments, exhibits an incomplete circular profile in cross section, and shares three protofilaments of subunit A.

Several elastic protein complexes are associated with the axoneme. **Radial spokes** project from subunit A of each doublet inward toward the **central sheath** surrounding the two singlets. Neighboring doublets are connected by **nexin,** another elastic protein, extending

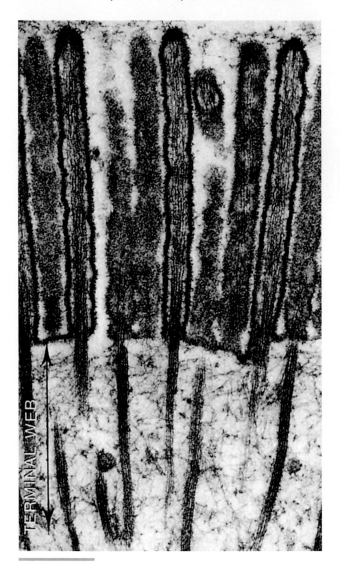

Figure 5–6 High-magnification electron micrograph of microvilli (×60,800). (From Hopkins CR: Structure and Function of Cells. Philadelphia, WB Saunders, 1978.)

from subunit A of one doublet to subunit B of the adjacent doublet (see Fig. 5-9).

The microtubule-associated protein **dynein,** also active in flagella, which has ATPase activity, radiates from subunit A of one doublet toward subunit B of the neighboring doublet. These dynein arms are arranged at 24-nm intervals along the length of subunit A. Dynein ATPase, by hydrolyzing ATP, provides the energy for the ciliary bending. Movement of the cilia is initiated by the dynein arms transiently attaching to specific sites on the protofilaments of the adjacent doublets, sliding them toward the tip of the cilium. However, nexin, an elastic protein extending between adjacent doublets, restrains this action to some degree, thus translating the

sliding movement into a bending motion. As the cilium bends, an energy-requiring process, the elastic protein complex is stretched. When the dynein arms release their hold on the B subunit, the elastic protein complex returns to its original length, snapping the cilium back to its straight position (which does not require energy), effecting movement of material at the tip of the cilium.

CLINICAL CORRELATIONS

Kartagener's syndrome results from hereditary defects in the ciliary dynein that would normally provide the energy for ciliary bending. Thus, ciliated cells without functional dynein are prohibited from functioning. Persons having this syndrome are susceptible to lung infections since their ciliated respiratory cells fail to clear the tract of debris and bacteria. Additionally, males with this syndrome are sterile since their sperm are immotile.

The 9 + 2 microtubule arrangement within the axoneme continues throughout most of the length of the cilium except at its base, where it is attached to the basal body (see Fig. 5-9). The morphology of the **basal body** is similar to that of a centriole, in that it is composed of nine triplets and no singlets.

Basal bodies develop from **procentriole organizers.** As tubulin dimers are added, the procentriole lengthens to form the nine triplet microtubules characteristic of the basal body. After formation, the basal body migrates to the apical plasmalemma and gives rise to a cilium. Nine doublet microtubules develop from the nine triplets of the basal body, and a single pair of microtubules form to give the cilium its characteristic 9 + 2 microtubule arrangement.

Basolateral Domain

The basolateral domain includes the basal and lateral aspects of the cell membrane.

The basolateral domain may be subdivided into two regions: the lateral plasma membrane and the basal plasma membrane. Each region possesses its own junctional specializations and receptors for hormones and neurotransmitters. In addition, these regions are rich in Na^+,K^+-ATPase and ion channels and are sites for constitutive secretion.

LATERAL MEMBRANE SPECIALIZATIONS

Lateral membrane specializations reveal the presence of junctional complexes.

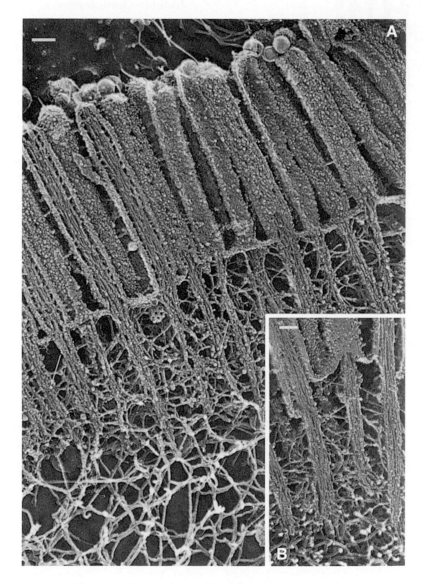

Figure 5–7   Electron micrograph of the terminal web and microvillus. Observe that the actin filaments of the microvilli are attached to the terminal web. **A**, ×83,060; **B** *(inset),* ×66,400. (From Hirokana N, Tilney LG, Fujiwara K, Heuser JE: Organization of actin, myosin, and intermediate filaments in the brush border of intestinal epithelial cells. J Cell Biol 94:425-443, 1982.)

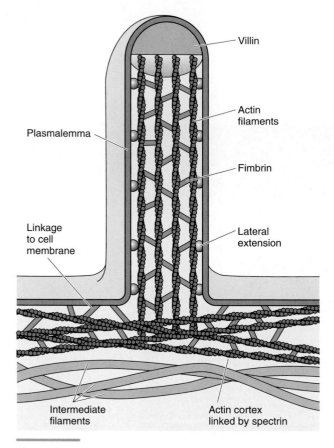

Figure 5–8 The structure of a microvillus.

Light microscopy reveals zones, called **terminal bars,** where epithelial cells are in contact and, presumably, attached to each other. Especially notable in the apical region of the simple columnar epithelium lining the gut, terminal bars were once thought to be composed of an amorphous intercellular cement substance. Horizontal sections through the terminal bars showed that they were continuous around the entire circumference of each cell, indicating that these cells were attached to every adjacent cell. Electron microscopy has revealed that terminal bars are in fact composed of intricate **junctional complexes.** These complexes, which hold contiguous epithelial cells together, may be classified into three types (Fig. 5-11):

- **Occluding junctions** function in joining cells to form an impermeable barrier, preventing material from taking an intercellular route in passing across the epithelial sheath.
- **Anchoring junctions** function in maintaining cell-to-cell or cell-to-basal lamina adherence.
- **Communicating junctions** function in permitting movement of ions or signaling molecules between

cells, thus coupling adjacent cells both electrically and metabolically.

The three components of the junctional complex are the zonulae occludentes, zonulae adherentes, and desmosomes (maculae adherentes).

Zonulae Occludentes

Zonulae occludentes prevent movement of membrane proteins and function to prevent intercellular movement of water-soluble molecules.

Also known as tight junctions, zonulae occludentes are located between adjacent plasma membranes and are the most apically located junction between the cells of the epithelia (see Fig. 5-11). They form a "belt-like" junction that encircles the entire circumference of the cell. In electron micrographs, the adjoining cell membranes approximate each other; their outer leaflets fuse, then diverge, and then fuse again several times within a distance of 0.1 to 0.3 μm (Fig. 5-12). At the fusion sites, transmembrane junctional proteins called **claudins** and **occludins** bind to each other, thus forming a seal occluding the intercellular space. Freeze-fracture analysis of cell membranes at the zonulae occludentes displays a "quilted" appearance of anastomosing strands, known as **tight junction strands,** on the P-face and a corresponding network of grooves on the E-face (Fig. 5-13).

Although both occludin and claudins participate in the formation of the tight junction, it appears that claudins have a more active role because these are the proteins that are probably responsible for the obliteration of the intercellular space by forming the tight junction strands described earlier. Not only are claudins calcium-independent, they do not form strong cell adhesions. As a result, their contact must be reinforced by **cadherins** as well as by cytoplasmic zonula occludens proteins such as ZO1, ZO2, and ZO3.

Tight junctions function in two ways: (1) they prevent the movement of membrane proteins from the apical domain to the basolateral domain; (2) they fuse plasma membranes of adjacent cells to prohibit water-soluble molecules from passing between cells. Depending on the numbers and patterns of the strands in the zonula, some tight junctions are said to be "tight," whereas others are "leaky." These terms reflect the efficiency of the cells in maintaining the integrity of the epithelial barrier between two adjacent body compartments.

Zonulae Adherentes

Zonulae adherentes are belt-like junctions that assist adjoining cells to adhere to one another.

Zonulae adherentes of the junctional complex are located just basal to the zonulae occludentes and also

Text continued on p. 99

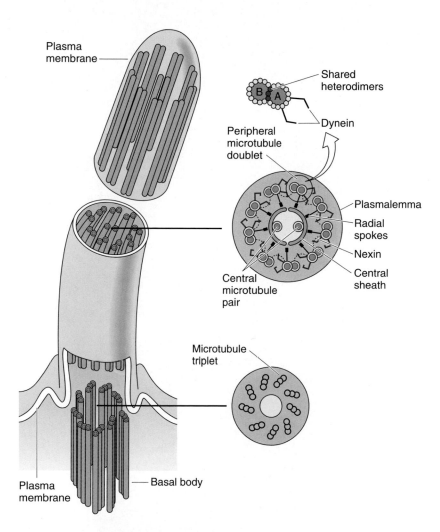

Figure 5–9 The microtubular arrangement of the axoneme in the cilium.

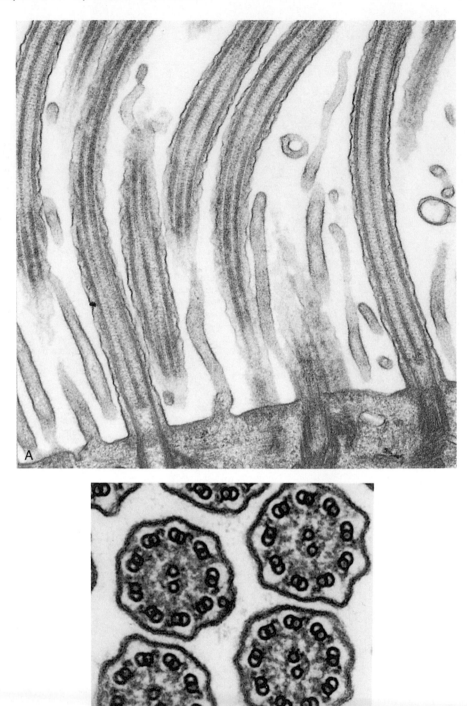

Figure 5–10 Electron micrographs of cilia. **A,** Longitudinal section of cilia (×36,000). **B,** Cross sectional view demonstrating microtubular arrangement in cilia (×88,000). (From Leeson TS, Leeson CR, Paparo AA: Text/Atlas of Histology. Philadelphia, WB Saunders, 1988.)

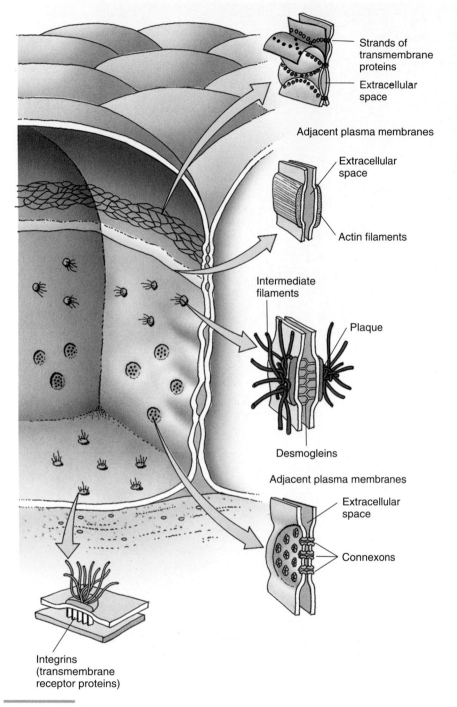

Figure 5–11 Junctional complexes, gap junctions, and hemidesmosomes.

Strands of transmembrane proteins

Extracellular space

Adjacent plasma membranes

Extracellular space

Actin filaments

Intermediate filaments

Plaque

Desmogleins

Adjacent plasma membranes

Extracellular space

Connexons

Integrins (transmembrane receptor proteins)

Zonulae occludentes
Extend along entire circumference of the cell. Prevent material from taking paracellular route in passing from the lumen into the connective tissues.

Zonulae adherentes
Basal to zonulae occludentes. E-cadherins bind to each other in the intercellular space and to actin filaments, intracellularly.

Maculae adherentes
E-cadherins are associated with the plaque; intermediate filaments form hairpin loops.

Gap junctions
Communicating junctions for small molecules and ions to pass between cells. Couple adjacent cells metabolically and electrically.

Hemidesmosomes
Attach epithelial cells to underlying basal lamina.

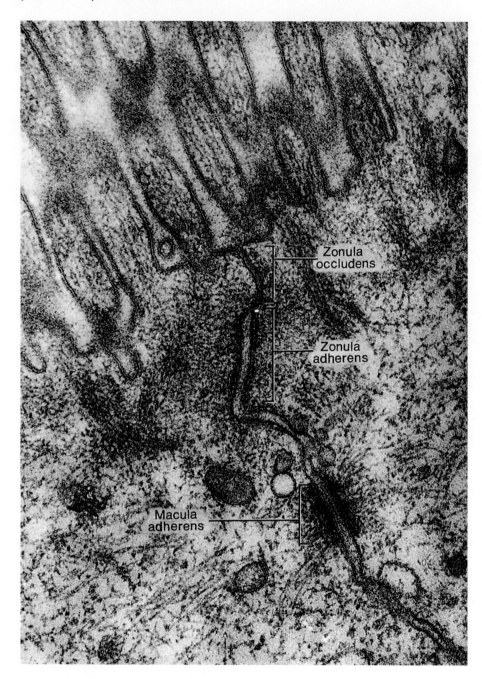

Figure 5–12 Electron micrograph of the junctional complex. (From Fawcett DW: The Cell, 2nd ed. Philadelphia, WB Saunders, 1981.)

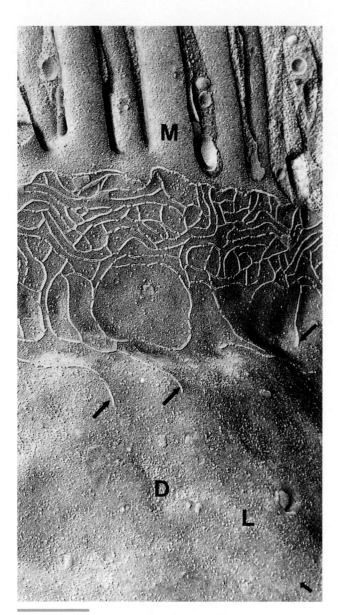

Figure 5–13 Freeze-fracture replica displaying the tight junction (zonula occludens) in guinea pig small intestine (×60,000). The P-face of the microvillar membrane (M) possesses fewer intramembrane particles than the P-face of the lateral cell membrane (L). Note the free terminal ridge-shaped protrusions (*arrows*) and desmosome (D). (From Trier JS, Allan CH, Marcial MA, Madara JL: Structural features of the apical and tubulovesicular membranes of rodent small intestinal tuft cells. Anat Rec 219:69-77, 1987.)

encircle the cell (see Fig. 5-11). The intercellular space of 15 to 20 nm between the outer leaflets of the two adjacent cell membranes is occupied by the extracellular moieties of **cadherins** (see Fig. 5-12). These Ca^{2+}-dependent integral proteins of the cell membrane are **transmembrane linker proteins.** Their intracytoplas-

mic aspect binds to a specialized region of the cell web, specifically a bundle of actin filaments that run parallel to and along the cytoplasmic aspect of the cell membrane. The actin filaments are attached to each other and to the cell membrane by the anchor proteins **catenin, vinculin,** and **α-actinin** (see Chapter 2). The extracellular region of the cadherins of one cell forms bonds with those of the adjoining cell participating in the formation of the zonula adherens. Thus, this junction not only joins the cell membranes to each other but also links the cytoskeleton of the two cells via the transmembrane linker proteins.

Fascia adherens is similar to zonula adherens but does not go around the entire circumference of the cell. Instead of being belt-like, it is "ribbon-like." Cardiac muscle cells, for example, are attached to each other at their longitudinal terminals via the fascia adherens.

Desmosomes (Maculae Adherentes)

Desmosomes are weld-like junctions along the lateral cell membranes that help to resist shearing forces.

Desmosomes are the last of the three components of the junctional complex. These "spot weld"-like junctions also appear to be randomly distributed along the lateral cell membranes of simple epithelia and throughout the cell membranes of stratified squamous epithelia, especially in the epidermis.

Disk-shaped **attachment plaques** (~400 × 250 × 10 nm) are located opposite each other on the cytoplasmic aspects of the plasma membranes of adjacent epithelial cells (Fig. 5-14; also see Fig. 5-11). Each plaque is composed of a series of attachment proteins, the best characterized of which are **desmoplakins** and **pakoglobins.**

Intermediate filaments (see Chapter 2) of cytokeratin are observed to insert into the plaque, where they make a hairpin turn, then extend back out into the cytoplasm. These filaments are thought to be responsible for dispersing the shearing forces on the cell.

In the region of the opposing attachment plaques, the intercellular space is up to 30 nm in width and contains filamentous materials with a thin, dense, vertical line located in the middle of the intercellular space. High-resolution electron microscopy reveals that the filamentous material is **desmoglein** and **desmocollin,** extracellular components of the Ca^{2+}-dependent transmembrane linker proteins of the cadherin family. In the presence of Ca^{2+}, they bond with transmembrane linker proteins from the adjoining cell. In the presence of a calcium-chelating agent, the desmosomes break into two halves and the cells separate. Thus, two cells are required for the formation of a desmosome. The cytoplasmic aspects of the transmembrane linker proteins bind to the desmoplakins and pakoglobins constituting the plaque.

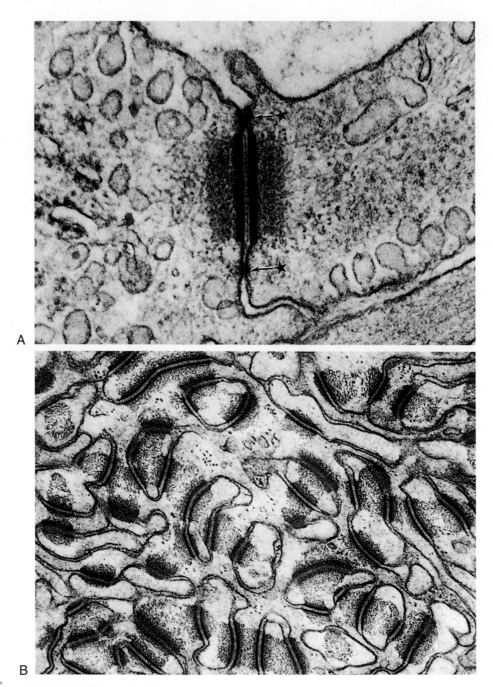

Figure 5–14 Electron micrographs of a desmosome. Observe the dense accumulation of intracellular intermediate filaments inserting into the plaque of each cell *(asterisk).* (From Fawcett DW: The Cell, 2nd ed. Philadelphia, WB Saunders, 1981.)

CLINICAL CORRELATIONS

Some people produce autoantibodies against desmosomal proteins, especially those in the skin, resulting in a skin disease called **pemphigus vulgaris.** Binding of the autoantibodies to desmosomal proteins disrupts cell adhesion, leading to widespread blistering and consequent loss of extracellular fluids; if untreated, this condition leads to death. Treatment with systemic steroids and immunosuppressive agents usually controls the condition.

Gap Junctions

Gap junctions, also called nexus or communicating junctions, are regions of intercellular communication.

Gap junctions are widespread in epithelial tissues throughout the body as well as in cardiac muscle cells, smooth muscle cells, and neurons, but not in skeletal muscle cells. They differ from the occluding and anchoring junctions in that they mediate intercellular communication by permitting the passage of various small molecules between adjacent cells. The intercellular cleft at the gap junction is narrow and constant, about 2 to 4 nm.

Gap junctions are built by six closely packed transmembrane channel-forming proteins **(connexins)** that assemble to form channel-structures called **connexons,** aqueous pores through the plasma membrane that juts out about 1.5 nm into the intercellular space (see Fig. 5-11). Presently it is believed that there may be more than 20 different connexins which can assemble into many different arrays of connexons that may be related to their specific function. Each gap junction may be formed by clusters of a few to many thousands of connexons. When a connexon of one plasma membrane is in register with its counterpart of the adjacent plasma membrane, the two connexons fuse, forming a functional intercellular hydrophilic communication channel (Fig. 5-15). With a diameter of 1.5 to 2.0 nm, the hydrophilic channel permits the passage of ions, amino acids, vitamins, cyclic adenosine monophosphate (cAMP), certain hormones, and molecules smaller than 1 kDa in size.

Gap junctions are regulated, and may be opened or closed rapidly. Although the opening and closing mechanism is not fully understood, it has been shown

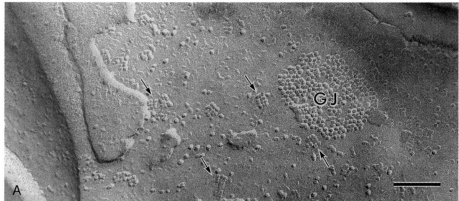

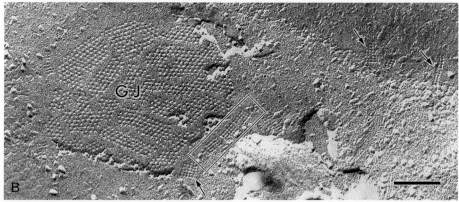

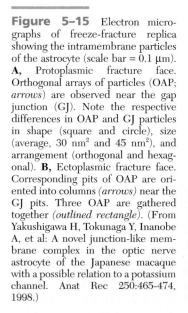

Figure 5–15 Electron micrographs of freeze-fracture replica showing the intramembrane particles of the astrocyte (scale bar = 0.1 μm). **A,** Protoplasmic fracture face. Orthogonal arrays of particles (OAP; *arrows*) are observed near the gap junction (GJ). Note the respective differences in OAP and GJ particles in shape (square and circle), size (average, 30 nm² and 45 nm²), and arrangement (orthogonal and hexagonal). **B,** Ectoplasmic fracture face. Corresponding pits of OAP are oriented into columns (*arrows*) near the GJ pits. Three OAP are gathered together (*outlined rectangle*). (From Yakushigawa H, Tokunaga Y, Inanobe A, et al: A novel junction-like membrane complex in the optic nerve astrocyte of the Japanese macaque with a possible relation to a potassium channel. Anat Rec 250:465-474, 1998.)

experimentally that a decrease in cytosolic pH or an increase in cytosolic Ca^{2+} concentrations closes gap junctions. Conversely, high pH or low Ca^{2+} concentrations opens the channels. In addition, gap junctions exhibit different properties with diverse channel permeabilities in different cells.

Gap junctions exhibit many diverse functions within the body, including cellular sharing of molecules for coordinating physiological continuity within a particular tissue. For example, when glucose is needed in the bloodstream, the nervous system stimulates liver cells (hepatocytes) to initiate glycogen breakdown. Because not all hepatocytes are individually stimulated, the signal is dispersed to other hepatocytes via gap junctions, thus coupling the hepatocytes. Gap junctions also function in electrical coupling of cells (i.e., in heart muscle and in smooth muscle cells of the gut during peristalsis), thus coordinating the activities of these cells. Gap junctions also are important during embryogenesis in coupling the cells of the developing embryo electrically and in distributing informational molecules throughout the migrating cell masses, thus keeping them coordinated in the proper development pathway.

CLINICAL CORRELATIONS

Mutations in connexin genes have been linked to a genetically based **nonsyndromic deafness** and to **erythrokeratodermia variabilis,** a skin disorder. In addition, dysfunctional migration of neural crest cells during development have been linked to mutations in the connexin genes, resulting in defects in the formation of the pulmonary vessels of the heart.

BASAL SURFACE SPECIALIZATIONS

Basal surface specializations include the basal lamina, plasma membrane enfoldings, and hemidesmosomes.

Three important features mark the basal surface of epithelia: the basal lamina, plasma membrane enfoldings, and hemidesmosomes, which anchor the basal plasma membrane to the basal lamina. The basal lamina is an extracellular supporting structure secreted by an epithelium and is located at the boundary between the epithelium and the underlying connective tissue. The structure and appearance of the basal lamina are discussed in Chapter 4.

Plasma Membrane Enfoldings

Enfoldings of the basal plasma membrane increase the surface area available for transport.

The basal surface of some epithelia, especially those involved in ion transport, possesses multiple finger-like enfoldings of the basal plasma membranes that increase the surface area of the plasmalemma and partition the mitochondria-rich basal cytoplasm. The mitochondria provide the energy required for active transport of ions in establishing osmotic gradients to ensure the movement of water across the epithelium, such as those of the kidney tubules. The compactness of the enfolded plasma membranes coupled with the arrangement of the mitochondria within the enfoldings gives a striated appearance when viewed with the light microscope; this is the origin of the term **striated ducts** describing certain ducts of the pancreas and salivary glands.

Hemidesmosomes

Hemidesmosomes attach the basal cell membrane to the underlying basal lamina.

Hemidesmosomes resemble half desmosomes and serve to attach the basal cell membrane to the basal lamina (Fig. 5-16; also see Fig. 5-11). **Attachment plaques,** composed of desmoplakins, plectin, and other associated proteins, are present on the cytoplasmic aspect of the plasma membrane. **Keratin tonofilaments** insert into these plaques, unlike those in the desmosome, where the filaments enter the plaque and then make a sharp turn to exit it. The cytoplasmic aspects of **transmembrane linker proteins** are attached to the plaque, whereas their extracellular moieties bind to **laminin** and **type IV collagen** of the basal lamina. The transmembrane linker proteins of hemidesmosomes are **integrins,** a family of extracellular matrix receptors, whereas those of desmosomes belong to the cadherin family of cell-to-cell adhesion proteins.

Renewal of Epithelial Cells

Cells making up the epithelial tissues generally exhibit a high turnover rate, which is related to their location and function. The time frame for cell renewal remains constant for a particular epithelium.

Cells of the epidermis, for example, are constantly being renewed at the basal layer by cell division. From here the cells begin their migration from the germinal layer to the surface, being keratinized on their route until they reach the surface, die, and are sloughed—the total event taking approximately 28 days. Other epithelial cells are renewed in less time.

Cells lining the small intestine are replaced every 4 to 6 days by regenerative cells in the base of the crypts. The new cells then migrate to the tips of the villi, die, and are sloughed. Still other epithelia, for example, are renewed periodically until adulthood is reached; subsequently, the cell population remains for life. Even then, however, when a large number of cells are lost because

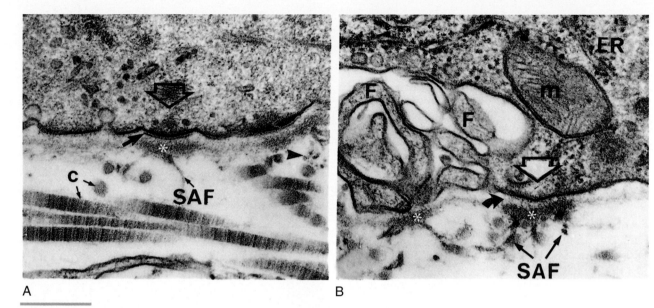

A   B

Figure 5–16   Electron micrographs of hemidesmosomes illustrating the relationship of striated anchoring fibers (SAFs), composed of type VII collagen, with the lamina densa and type III collagen of the lamina reticularis. c, Collagen fibers; ER, endoplasmic reticulum; F, cell extensions. *Wide arrows* indicate the cytoplasmic aspect of hemidesmosomes; *asterisk* indicates SAF plaque. (From Clermont Y, Xia L, Turner JD, Hermo L: Striated anchoring fibrils-anchoring plaque complexes and their relation to hemidesmosomes of myoepithelial and secretory cells in mammary glands of lactating rats. Anat Rec 237:318-325, 1993.)

of injury or acute toxic destruction, cell proliferation is triggered and the cell population is restored.

CLINICAL CORRELATIONS

Each epithelium within the body has its own unique characteristics, location, cell morphology, and so on, all of which are related to function. In certain pathological conditions, the cell population of an epithelium may undergo **metaplasia,** transforming it into another epithelial type.

Pseudostratified ciliated columnar epithelium of the bronchi of heavy smokers may undergo **squamous metaplasia,** transforming it into stratified squamous epithelium. This change impairs function, but the process may be reversed when the pathological insult is removed.

Tumors that arise from epithelial cells may be benign (nonmalignant) or malignant. Malignant tumors arising from epithelia are called **carcinomas;** those arising from glandular epithelial cells are called **adenocarcinomas.** It is interesting to note that cancers in adults are most often adenocarcinomas and after age 45 about 90% are of epithelial cell origin. However, in children under 10 years of age, epithelium-derived cancers are the least prevalent type of cancer.

GLANDS

Glands originate from epithelial cells that leave the surface where they developed and penetrate into the underlying connective tissue, manufacturing a basal lamina around themselves. The secretory units, along with their ducts, are the **parenchyma** of the gland, whereas the **stroma** of the gland represents the elements of the connective tissue that invade and support the parenchyma.

Glandular epithelia manufacture their product intracellularly by synthesis of macromolecules that are usually packaged and stored in vesicles called **secretory granules.** The secretory product may be a polypeptide hormone (e.g., from the pituitary gland); a waxy substance (e.g., from the ceruminous glands of the ear canal); a mucinogen (e.g., from the goblet cells); or milk, a combination of protein, lipid, and carbohydrates (e.g., from the mammary glands). Other glands (such as sweat glands) secrete little besides the exudate they receive from the bloodstream. In addition, striated ducts (e.g., those of the major salivary glands) act as ion pumps that modify the substances produced by their secretory units.

Glands are classified into two major groups on the basis of the method of distribution of their secretory products:

■ **Exocrine glands** secrete their products via ducts onto the external or internal epithelial surface from which they originated.

■ **Endocrine glands** are **ductless,** having lost their connections to the originating epithelium, and thus secrete their products into the blood or lymphatic vessels for distribution.

Many cell types secrete signaling molecules called **cytokines,** which perform the function of cell-to-cell communication. Cytokines are released by **signaling cells** and act on **target cells,** which possess receptors for the specific signaling molecule. (Hormone signaling is discussed in detail in Chapter 2.)

Depending on the distance the cytokine must travel to reach its target cell, its effect may be one of the following:

■ **Autocrine:** The signaling cell is its own target; thus the cell stimulates itself.
■ **Paracrine:** The target cell is located in the vicinity of the signaling cell; thus, the cytokine does not have to enter the vascular system for distribution to its target.
■ **Endocrine:** The target cell and signaling cell are far from each other; thus, the cytokine has to be transported either by the blood or by the lymph vascular system.

Glands that secrete their products via a **constitutive secretory pathway** do so continuously, releasing their secretory products immediately without storage and without requiring a prompt by signaling molecules. Glands that exhibit a **regulated secretory pathway** concentrate and store their secretory products until the proper signaling molecule for its release is received (see Chapter 2; Figs. 2-20 and 2-22).

Exocrine Glands

Exocrine glands secrete their products via a duct to the surface of their epithelial origin.

Exocrine glands are classified according to the nature of their secretion, their mode of secretion, and the number of cells (unicellular or multicellular). Many exocrine glands in the digestive, respiratory, and urogenital systems secrete substances that are described as mucous, serous, or mixed (both) types.

Mucous glands secrete **mucinogens,** large glycosylated proteins that, upon hydration, swell to become a thick, viscous, gel-like protective lubricant known as **mucin,** a major component of **mucus.** Examples of mucous glands include goblet cells and the minor salivary glands of the tongue and palate.

Serous glands (Fig. 5-17), such as the pancreas, secrete an enzyme-rich watery fluid.

Mixed glands contain acini (secretory units) that produce mucous secretions as well as acini that produce serous secretions; in addition, some of the mucous acini possess **serous demilunes,** a group of cells that secrete

a serous fluid. The sublingual and submandibular glands are examples of mixed glands (Fig. 5-18).

Cells of exocrine glands exhibit three different mechanisms for releasing their secretory products: (1) holocrine, (2) merocrine, and (3) apocrine (Fig. 5-19). The release of the secretory product of **merocrine glands** (e.g., parotid gland) occurs via exocytosis; as a

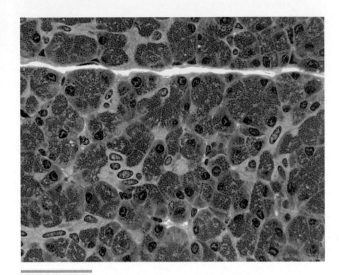

Figure 5–17 Serous gland. Light micrograph of a plastic-embedded monkey pancreas (×540).

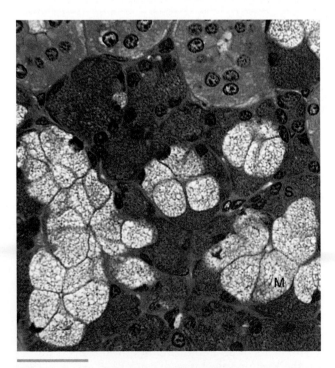

Figure 5–18 Light micrograph of the monkey submandibular gland (×540). M, mucous acini; S, serous demilunes.

A   B   C

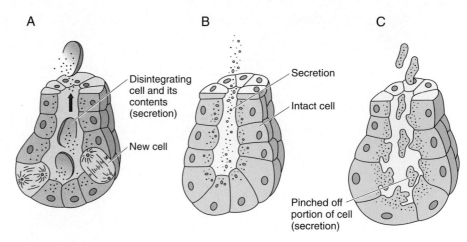

Figure 5–19 Modes of secretion: **A,** holocrine; **B,** merocrine; **C,** apocrine.

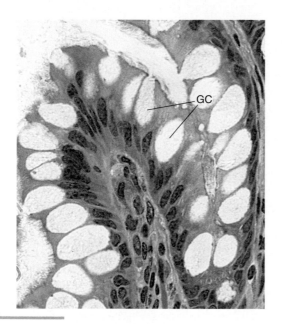

Figure 5–20 Light micrograph of goblet cells (GC) in the epithelial lining of monkey ileum (×540).

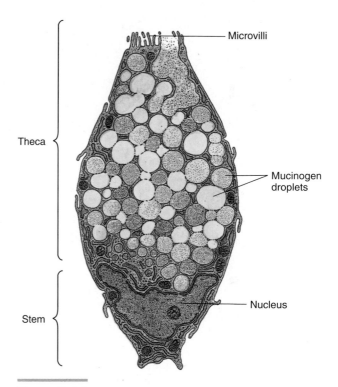

Figure 5–21 Ultrastructure of a goblet cell illustrating the tightly packed secretory granules of the theca. (From Lentz TL: Cell Fine Structure: An Atlas of Drawings of Whole-Cell Structure. Philadelphia, WB Saunders, 1971.)

result, neither cell membrane nor cytoplasm becomes a part of the secretion. Although many investigators question the existence of the apocrine mode of secretion, historically it was believed that in **apocrine glands** (e.g., lactating mammary gland), a small portion of the apical cytoplasm is released along with the secretory product. In **holocrine glands** (e.g., sebaceous gland), as a secretory cell matures, it dies and becomes the secretory product.

Unicellular Exocrine Glands

Unicellular exocrine glands are the simplest form of exocrine gland.

Unicellular exocrine glands, represented by isolated secretory cells in an epithelium, are the simplest form of exocrine gland. A primary example is the **goblet cell,** which is dispersed individually in the epithelia lining the digestive tract and portions of the respiratory tract (Figs. 5-20 and 5-21). The secretions released by these mucous glands protect the linings of these tracts.

Goblet cells derive their name from their shape, that of a goblet (Fig. 5-22). Their thin basal region sits on

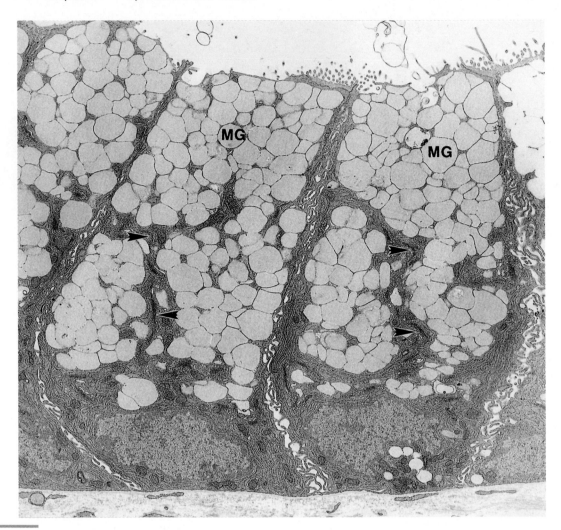

Figure 5–22 Electron micrograph of goblet cells from the colon of a rabbit (×9114). Note the presence of several Golgi complexes (*arrowheads*) and the numerous, compactly packed mucinogen granules (MG) that occupy much of the apical portion of the cells. (From Radwan KA, Oliver MG, Specian RD: Cytoarchitectural reorganization of rabbit colonic goblet cells during baseline secretion. Am J Anat 198:365-376, 1990.)

the basal lamina, whereas their expanded apical portion, the **theca,** faces the lumen of the digestive tube or respiratory tract. The theca is filled with membrane-bound secretory droplets, which displace the cytoplasm to the cell's periphery and the nucleus toward its base. The process of mucinogen release is regulated and stimulated by chemical irritation and parasympathetic innervation, resulting in exocytosis of the entire secretory contents of the cell, thus lubricating and protecting the epithelial sheet.

Multicellular Exocrine Glands

Multicellular exocrine glands exist as organized clusters of secretory units.

Multicellular exocrine glands consist of clusters of secretory cells arranged in varying degrees of organization. These secretory cells do not act alone and independently but instead function as secretory organs. Multicellular glands may have a simple structure, exemplified by the glandular epithelium of the uterus and gastric mucosa, or a complex structure, composed of various types of secretory units and organized in a compound branching fashion.

Because of their structural arrangement, multicellular glands are subclassified according to the organization of their secretory and duct components as well as according to the shape of their secretory units (Fig. 5-23).

Multicellular glands are classified as **simple** if their ducts do not branch and **compound** if their ducts

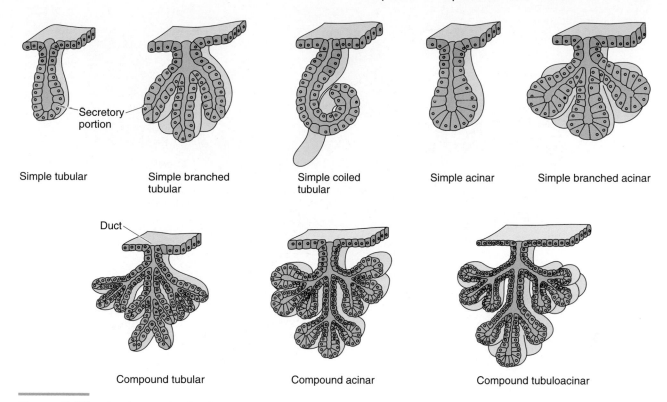

Simple tubular

Simple branched tubular

Simple coiled tubular

Simple acinar

Simple branched acinar

Compound tubular

Compound acinar

Compound tubuloacinar

Figure 5–23 Classification of multicellular exocrine glands. *Green* represents the secretory portion of the gland; *lavender* represents the duct portion.

branch. They are further categorized according to the morphology of their secretory units as **tubular, acinar** (also referred to as **alveolar,** resembling a grape), or **tubuloalveolar.**

Larger multicellular glands are surrounded by a collagenous connective tissue **capsule,** which sends **septae** (strands of connective tissue) into the gland, subdividing it into smaller compartments known as **lobes** and **lobules** (Fig. 5-24). Vascular elements, nerves, and ducts utilize the connective tissue septa to enter and exit the gland. In addition, the connective tissue elements provide structural support for the gland.

Acini of many multicellular exocrine glands such as sweat glands and major salivary glands possess **myoepithelial cells** that share the basal lamina of the acinar cells. Although myoepithelial cells are of epithelial origin, they have some characteristics of smooth muscle cells, particularly contractility. These cells exhibit small nuclei and sparse fibrillar cytoplasm radiating out from the cell body, wrapping around the acini and some of the small ducts (Fig. 5-25; also see Fig. 5-24). Their contractions assist in expressing secretions from the acini and from some small ducts.

Endocrine Glands

Endocrine glands are ductless, and thus their secretory products are released directly into the bloodstream or the lymphatic system.

Endocrine glands release their secretions (hormones) into blood or lymphatic vessels for distribution to target organs. The major endocrine glands of the body include the suprarenal (adrenal), pituitary, thyroid, parathyroid, and pineal glands and the ovaries, placenta, and testes.

The islets of Langerhans and the interstitial cells of Leydig are unusual because they are composed of clusters of cells ensconced within the connective tissue stroma of other organs (the pancreas and the testes, respectively). Hormones secreted by endocrine glands include peptides, proteins, modified amino acids, steroids, and glycoproteins. Because of their complexity and important role in regulating bodily processes, the endocrine glands are discusses in detail in Chapter 13.

The secretory cells of endocrine glands are organized either in cords of cells or in a follicular arrangement. In the **cord** type, the most common arrangement, cells

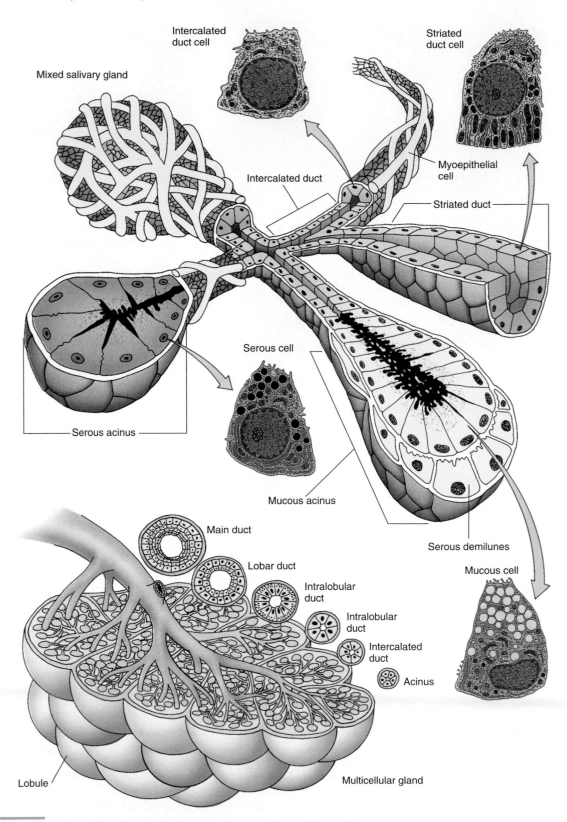

Figure 5–24 Salivary gland: its organization, secretory units, and system of ducts.

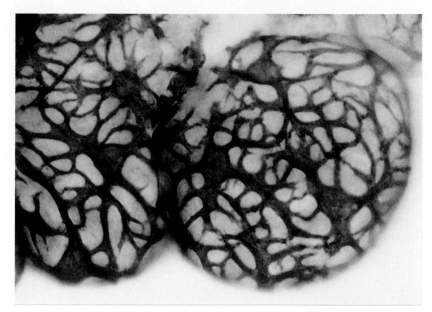

Figure 5–25 Light micrograph of myoepithelial cells immunostained for actin (×640). Myoepithelial cells surround the acini. (From Satoh Y, Habara Y, Kanno T, Ono K: Carbamylcholine-induced morphological changes and spatial dynamics of [Ca²⁺]c in harderian glands of guinea pigs: Calcium-dependent lipid secretion and contraction of myoepithelial cells. Cell Tiss Res 274:1-14, 1993.)

form anastomosing cords around capillaries or blood sinusoids. The hormone to be secreted is stored intracellularly and is released upon the arrival of the proper signaling molecule or neural impulse. Examples of the cord type of endocrine gland are the suprarenal gland, anterior lobe of the pituitary gland, and parathyroid gland.

In the **follicle** type of endocrine gland, secretory cells (**follicular cells**) form follicles that surround a cavity that receives and stores the secreted hormone. When a release signal is received, the stored hormone is resorbed by the follicular cells and released into the connective tissue to enter the blood capillaries. An example of a follicle type of endocrine gland is the thyroid gland.

Some glands of the body are mixed; for example, the parenchyma contains both exocrine and endocrine secretory units. In these mixed glands (e.g., pancreas, ovary, and testes), the exocrine portion of the gland secretes its product into a duct, whereas the endocrine portion of the gland secretes its product into the bloodstream.

Diffuse Neuroendocrine System

The diffuse neuroendocrine system produces paracrine and endocrine hormones.

Widespread throughout the digestive tract and in the respiratory system are endocrine cells interspersed among other secretory cells. These cells, members of the diffuse neuroendocrine system (DNES), manu-

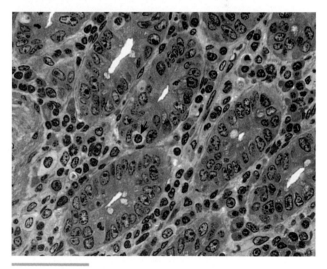

Figure 5–26 Light micrograph of diffuse neuroendocrine system (DNES) cell (×540). Note the pale-staining DNES cells (APD) located in the mucosa of the ileum (*arrow*).

facture various paracrine and endocrine hormones (Fig. 5-26). Because these cells are capable of taking up precursors of amines and decarboxylating amino acids, they were also called **APUD** (*a*mine *p*recursor *u*ptake and *d*ecarboxylation) **cells.** At one time some of these cells were called **argentaffin** and **argyophil cells** because of the way they stained with silver salts. This entire cell group is now called the **DNES,** which is described in greater detail in Chapter 17.

Connective Tissue

6

Connective tissue, as the name implies, forms a continuum with epithelial tissue, muscle, and nervous tissue as well as with other components of connective tissues to maintain a functionally integrated body. Most connective tissues originate from **mesoderm,** the middle germ layer of the embryonic tissue. From this layer, the multipotential cells of the embryo, the **mesenchyme,** develop, although in certain areas of the head and neck, mesenchyme also develops from neural crest cells of the developing embryo. Mesenchymal cells migrate throughout the body, giving rise to the connective tissues and their cells, including those of bone, cartilage, tendons, capsules, blood and hemopoietic cells, and lymphoid cells (Fig. 6-1).

Mature connective tissue is classified as **connective tissue proper,** the major subject of this chapter, or **specialized connective tissue** (i.e., cartilage, bone, and blood), detailed in Chapters 7 and 10.

Connective tissue is composed of cells and extracellular matrix consisting of ground substance and fibers (Figs. 6-2 and 6-3). The cells are the most important components in some connective tissues, whereas fibers are the most important component in other connective tissue types. For example, fibroblasts are the most important cell component of loose connective tissue because these cells manufacture and maintain the fibers and ground substance composing the extracellular matrix. In contrast, fibers are the most important component of tendons and ligaments. In still other connective tissues, the ground substance is most important component because it is the site where certain specialized connective tissue cells carry out their functions. Thus, all three components are critical to the role of connective tissue function in the body.

FUNCTIONS OF CONNECTIVE TISSUE

Although many functions are attributed to connective tissue, its primary functions include:

- Providing structural **support**
- Serving as a **medium for exchange**
- Aiding in the **defense** and **protection** of the body
- Forming a site for **storage of fat**

Bones, cartilage, and the ligaments holding the bones together, as well as the tendons attaching muscles to bone, act as **support.** Similarly, the connective tissue that forms the capsules encasing organs and the stroma forming the structural framework within organs has support functions. Connective tissue also functions as a **medium for exchange** of metabolic waste, nutrients, and oxygen between the blood and many of the cells of the body.

The functions of **defense** and **protection** are carried out by (1) the body's phagocytic cells, which engulf and destroy cellular debris, foreign particles, and microorganisms; (2) the body's immunocompetent cells, which produce antibodies against antigens; and (3) certain cells that produce pharmacological substances that help in controlling inflammation. Connective tissues also help protect the body by forming a physical barrier to invasion by and dissemination of microorganisms.

EXTRACELLULAR MATRIX

The extracellular matrix, composed of ground substance and fibers, resists compressive and stretching forces. The components of the extracellular matrix are described in Chapter 4, and their salient features are reviewed briefly here.

Ground Substance

Ground substance is a hydrated, amorphous material that is composed of **glycosaminoglycans,** long unbranched polymers of repeating disaccharides; **proteoglycans,** protein cores to which various glycosaminoglycans are covalently linked; and **adhesive glycoproteins,** large macromolecules responsible for fastening the various components of the extracellular

111

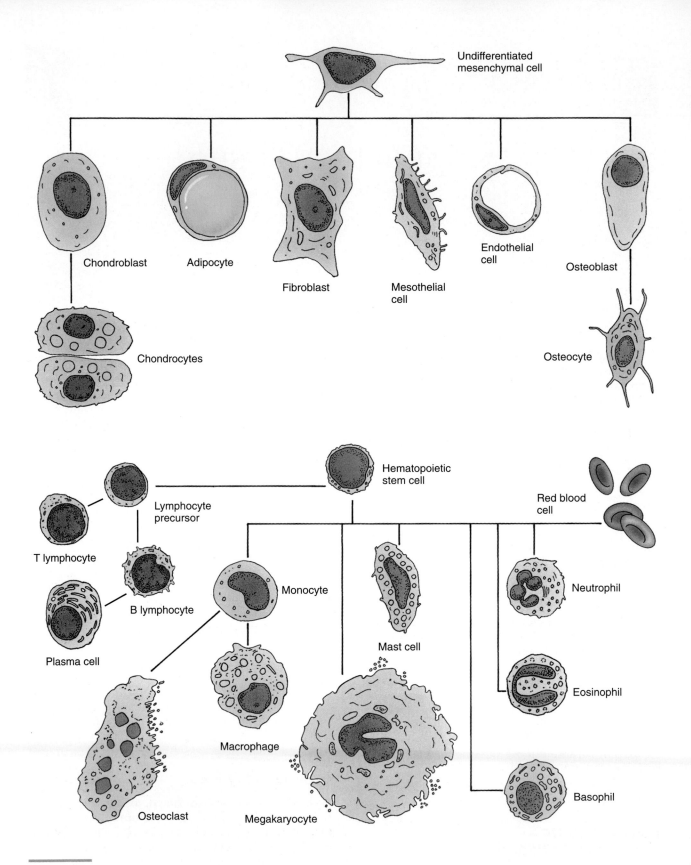

Figure 6–1 Origins of connective tissue cells (not drawn to scale).

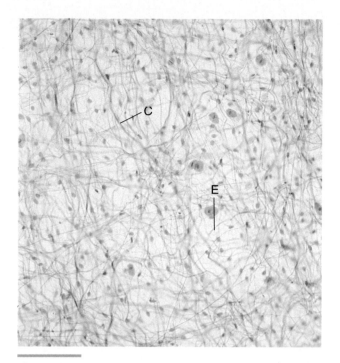

Figure 6–2 Light micrograph of loose (areolar) connective tissue displaying collagen (C) and elastic (E) fibers and some of the cell types common to loose connective tissue (×132).

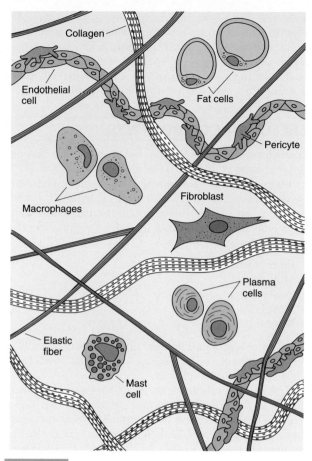

Figure 6–3 Cell types and fiber types in loose connective tissue (not drawn to scale).

matrix to one another and to integrins and dystroglycans of the cell membrane (see Chapter 4 and Fig. 4-3).

Glycosaminoglycans are of two major types: sulfated, including keratan sulfate, heparan sulfate, heparin, chondroitin sulfates, and dermatan sulfate; and nonsulfated, including hyaluronic acid.

Proteoglycans are covalently linked to hyaluronic acid, forming huge macromolecules called **aggrecan aggregates,** which are responsible for the gel state of the extracellular matrix.

Adhesive glycoproteins are of various types. Some are localized preferentially to the basal lamina, such as **laminin,** or to cartilage and bone, such as **chondronectin** and **osteonectin,** respectively. Still others are generally dispersed throughout the extracellular matrix, such as **fibronectin.**

Fibers

Fibers of the extracellular matrix are collagen (and reticular) and elastic fibers. **Collagen** fibers are inelastic and possess great tensile strength. Each fiber is composed of fine subunits, the **tropocollagen** molecule, composed of three α-chains wrapped around one another in a helical configuration. About 20 different types of collagen fibers are known, which vary in the amino acid sequences of their α-chains. The most common amino acids of collagen are **glycine, proline,** **hydroxyproline,** and **hydroxylysine.** The six major collagen types (see Table 4-2) are:

- **Type I:** in connective tissue proper, bone, dentin, and cementum
- **Type II:** in hyaline and elastic cartilages
- **Type III:** reticular fibers
- **Type IV:** lamina densa of the basal lamina
- **Type V:** in the placenta; associated with type I collagen
- **Type VII:** attaching the basal lamina to the lamina reticularis

Most of the fiber types display a 67-nm periodicity in electron micrographs, which is due to the deposition of heavy metals in the **gap regions** of the fiber (see Fig. 4-5). **Type IV collagen** is not assembled into fibers and thus does not possess a periodicity.

Elastic fibers are composed of elastin and microfibrils. These fibers are highly elastic and may be stretched to 150% of their resting length without breaking. Their elasticity is due to the protein elastin, and their stability is due to the presence of microfibrils. **Elastin** is an amorphous material whose main amino acid components are **glycine** and **proline.** Additionally, elastin is rich in lysine, the amino acid responsible for the formation of the highly deformable **desmosine residues** that impart a high degree of elasticity to these fibers.

CELLULAR COMPONENTS

The cells in connective tissues are grouped into two categories: fixed cells and transient cells (see Fig. 6-1).

Fixed cells are a resident population of cells that have developed and remain in place within the connective tissue, where they perform their functions. The fixed cells are a stable and long-lived population that includes:

- Fibroblasts
- Adipose cells
- Pericytes
- Mast cells
- Macrophages

Additionally, some authors consider certain cells of the macrophages (e.g., Kupffer cells of the liver) to be fixed connective tissue cells.

Transient cells (free or wandering cells) originate mainly in the bone marrow and circulate in the bloodstream. Upon receiving the proper stimulus or signal, these cells leave the bloodstream and migrate into the connective tissue to perform their specific functions. Because most of these motile cells are usually short-lived, they must be replaced continually from a large population of stem cells. Transient cells include:

- Plasma cells
- Lymphocytes
- Neutrophils
- Eosinophils
- Basophils
- Monocytes
- Macrophages

Fixed Connective Tissue Cells

The four connective tissue cell types that are clearly fixed are described here. Macrophages, which exhibit some fixed and some transient properties, are discussed later under "Macrophages."

Fibroblasts

Fibroblasts, the most abundant cell type in the connective tissue, are responsible for the synthesis of almost all of the extracellular matrix.

Fibroblasts, the most abundant and most widely distributed resident cells of connective tissue, are derived from undifferentiated mesenchymal cells and synthesize the extracellular matrix of connective tissue (see Fig. 6-1). Fibroblasts are the least specialized of the cells making up connective tissue and may even be represented by several different functioning populations within certain areas of the body. Because mature and immature fibroblasts may exist side by side, the immature cells, difficult to distinguish from mysenchymal cells, may—depending upon the signal proteins present—differentiate into other cell members of connective tissue (i.e., fat cells, osteoblasts, chondroblasts and myofibroblasts).

Fibroblasts may occur in either an active state or a quiescent state. Some histologists differentiate between them, calling the quiescent cells **fibrocytes;** however, because the two states are transitory, the term fibroblast is used in this text.

Active fibroblasts often reside in close association with collagen bundles, where they lie parallel to the long axis of the fiber (Fig. 6-4). Such fibroblasts are elongated, fusiform cells possessing pale-staining cytoplasm, which is often difficult to distinguish from collagen when stained with hematoxylin and eosin (H&E) (see Fig. 6-18). The most obvious portion of the cell is the darker-stained, large, granular, ovoid nucleus containing a well-defined nucleolus. Electron microscopy reveals a prominent Golgi apparatus and abundant rough endoplasmic reticulum (RER) in the fibroblast, especially when the cell is actively manufacturing matrix, as in wound healing. Actin and α-actinin are localized at the periphery of the cell, whereas myosin is present throughout the cytoplasm.

In contrast to active fibroblasts, **Inactive fibroblasts** are smaller, more ovoid, and possess an acidophilic cytoplasm. Their nucleus is smaller, elongated, and more deeply stained. Electron microscopy reveals sparse amounts of RER but an abundance of free ribosomes.

CLINICAL CORRELATIONS

Although considered to be fixed cells in the connective tissues, fibroblasts are capable of some movement. Fibroblasts seldom unergo cell division but may do so during wound healing. These cells, however, may differentiate into adipose cells, chondrocytes (during formation of fibrocartilage), and osteoblasts (under pathological conditions).

Myofibroblasts

Myofibroblasts are modified fibroblasts that demonstrate characteristics similar to those of both fibroblasts and smooth muscle cells.

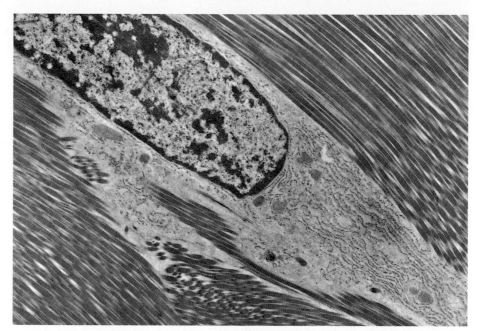

Figure 6–4 Electron micrograph displaying a portion of a fibroblast and the packed collagen fibers in rat tendon. Observe the heterochromatin in the nucleus and the rough endoplasmic reticulum (RER) in the cytoplasm. Banding in the collagen fibers also may be observed. (From Ralphs JR, Benjamin M, Thornett A: Cell and matrix biology of the suprapatella in the rat: A structural and immunocytochemical study of fibrocartilage in a tendon subject to compression. Anat Rec 231:167-177, 1991.)

Histologically, fibroblasts and myofibroblasts are not easily distinguished by routine light microscopy. Electron microscopy, however, reveals that myofibroblasts have bundles of actin filaments and myosin and dense bodies similar to those of smooth muscle cells. Additionally, the surface profile of the nucleus resembles that of a smooth muscle cell. Myofibroblasts differ from smooth muscle cells in that an external lamina (basal lamina) is absent. Myofibroblasts represent transitional modifications of fibroblasts as a result of being contacted by signaling molecules within a regional intercellular matrix. Myofibroblasts are abundant in areas undergoing wound healing, where they function in wound contraction; they also are found in the periodontal ligament, where they probably assist in tooth eruption.

Pericytes

Pericytes surround endothelial cells of capillaries and small venules and technically reside outside the connective tissue compartment, because they possess their own basal lamina.

Pericytes, derived from undifferentiated mesenchymal cells, partly surround the endothelial cells of capillaries and small venules (see Fig. 6-3). These multipotential perivascular cells are outside the connective tissue compartment because they are surrounded by their own basal lamina, which may be fused with that of the endothelial cells. Pericytes possess characteristics of endothelial cells and smooth muscle cells in that they

contain actin, myosin, and tropomyosin, suggesting that they may function in contraction. Under certain conditions, they may differentiate into other cells. Pericytes are discussed more fully in Chapter 11.

Adipose Cells

Adipose cells are fully differentiated cells that function in the synthesis, storage, and release of fat.

Fat cells, or adipocytes, are derived from undifferentiated fibroblast-like mesenchymal cells (Fig. 6-5; see also Figs. 6-1 and 6-3), although under certain conditions histologists believe that fibroblasts may give rise to adipose cells. Adipose cells are fully differentiated and do not undergo cell division. They function in the synthesis and storage of triglycerides. There are two types of fat cells, which constitute two types of adipose tissue. Cells with a single, large lipid droplet, called **unilocular fat cells,** form **white adipose tissue,** and cells with multiple, small lipid droplets, called **multilocular fat cells,** form **brown adipose tissue.** White fat is much more abundant than brown fat. As discussed later, the distribution and histophysiology of the two types of fat tissue differ. Here we describe the histologic characteristics of the adipocytes themselves.

Adipocytes of white fat are large spherical cells, up to 120 μm in diameter, that become polyhedral when crowded into adipose tissue (Fig. 6-6). Unilocular fat cells continuously store fat in the form of a single droplet, which enlarges so much that the cytoplasm and nucleus are displaced peripherally against the plasma

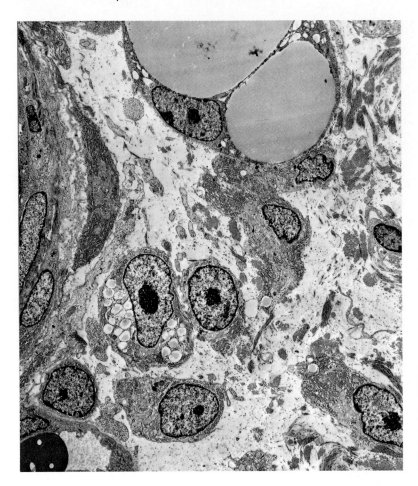

Figure 6–5 Electron micrograph of adipocytes in various stages of maturation in rat hypodermis. Observe the adipocyte at the top of the micrograph with its nucleus and cytoplasm crowded to the periphery by the fat droplet. (From Hausman GJ, Campion DR, Richardson RL, Martin RJ: Adipocyte development in the rat hypodermis. Am J Anat 161:85-100, 1981.)

membrane, thus giving these cells a "signet ring" profile when viewed by light microscopy. Electron micrographs reveal a small Golgi complex situated adjacent to the nucleus, only a few mitochondria, and sparse RER, but an abundance of free ribosomes. That the fat droplet is not bounded by a membrane is clear in electron micrographs but unclear in light micrographs. The external surfaces of the plasma membranes are enveloped by a basal lamina-like substance. Minute pinocytotic vesicles, whose function is unclear, have been noted on the surface of the plasma membrane. During fasting, the cell surface becomes irregular, having pseudopod-like projections.

Multilocular adipocytes contrast with unilocular adipocytes in several ways. First, brown fat cells are smaller and more polygonal than white fat cells. Moreover, because the brown fat cell stores fat in several small droplets rather than a single droplet, the spherical nucleus is not squeezed up against the plasma membrane. Multilocular fat cells contain many more mitochondria but fewer free ribosomes than unilocular fat cells (Fig. 6-7). Although brown fat cells lack RER, they do have smooth endoplasmic reticulum (SER).

Storage and Release of Fat by Adipose Cells

During digestion, fats are broken down in the duodenum by **pancreatic lipase** into **fatty acids** and **glycerol.** The intestinal epithelium absorbs these substances and reesterifies them in the smooth endoplasmic reticulum to **triglycerides,** which then are surrounded by proteins to form **chylomicrons.** Chylomicrons are released into the extracellular space at the basolateral membranes of the surface absorptive cells, enter the lacteals of the villus, and are carried by the lymph to the bloodstream. Additionally, very-low-density lipoprotein (VLDL), which is synthesized by the liver, and albumin-bound fatty acids are present in the bloodstream.

Once in the capillaries of adipose tissue, VLDL, fatty acids, and chylomicrons are exposed to **lipoprotein lipase** (manufactured by fat cells), which breaks them down into free fatty acids and glycerol (Fig. 6-8). The fatty acids enter the connective tissue and diffuse through the cell membranes of adipocytes. These cells then combine their own glycerol phosphate with the

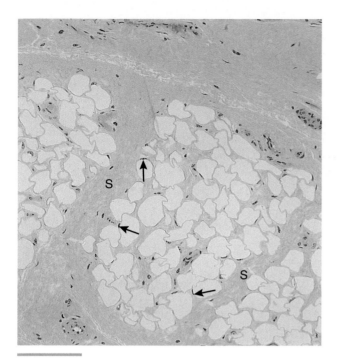

Figure 6–6 Light micrograph of white adipose tissue from monkey hypodermis (×132). The lipid was extracted during tissue processing. Note how the cytoplasm and nuclei *(arrows)* are crowded to the periphery. Septa (S) divide the fat into lobules.

imported fatty acids to form triglycerides, which are added to the forming lipid droplets within the adipocytes until needed. Adipose cells can convert glucose and amino acids into fatty acids when stimulated by insulin.

Norepinephrine is released from nerve endings of postganglionic sympathetic neurons in the vicinity of fat cells. Also, during strenuous exercise, **epinephrine** and norepinephrine are released from the suprarenal medulla. These two hormones bind to their respective receptors of the adipocyte plasmalemma, activating **adenylate cyclase** to form **cyclic adenosine monophosphate (cAMP),** a second messenger, resulting in activation of **hormone-sensitive lipase.** This enzyme cleaves triglycerides into fatty acids and glycerol, which are released into the bloodstream.

Fat cells are found throughout the body in loose connective tissue and are concentrated along blood vessels. They may also accumulate into masses, forming adipose tissue.

Mast Cells

Mast cells arise from bone marrow stem cells and function in mediating the inflammatory process and immediate hypersensitivity reactions.

Mast cells, among the largest of the fixed cells of the connective tissue, are 20 to 30 μm in diameter. They are ovoid and possess a centrally placed, spherical nucleus (Fig. 6-9). Unlike the three types of fixed cells discussed earlier, mast cells probably derive from precursors in the bone marrow (see Fig. 6-1).

The presence of numerous granules in the cytoplasm is the identifying characteristic of mast cells (Fig. 6-10). These membrane-bound granules range in size from 0.3 to 0.8 μm. Because they contain **heparin** (or **chondroitin sulfate**), a sulfated glycosaminoglycan, these granules stain metachromatically with toluidine blue (i.e., toluidine blue stains the granules purple).

Electron microscopic studies of the granules reveal differences in size and form and display variations in ultrastructure even within the same cell. Otherwise, the cytoplasm is unremarkable; it contains several mitochondria, a sparse number of RER profiles, and a relatively small Golgi complex.

In addition to **heparin,** mast cell granules also contain **histamine** (or **chondroitin sulfates**), **neutral proteases** (tryptase, chymase, and carboxypeptidases), **aryl sulfatase** (as well as other enzymes, such as γ-glucuronidase, kininogenase, peroxidase, and superoxide dismutase), **eosinophil chemotactic factor (ECF),** and **neutrophil chemotactic factor (NCF).** These pharmacological agents present in the granules are referred to as the **primary mediators** (also known as **preformed mediators**). Besides the substances found in the granules, mast cells synthesize a number of mediators from membrane arachidonic acid precursors. These newly synthesized mediators include **leukotrienes** (C$_4$, D$_4$, and E$_4$), **thromboxanes** (TXA$_2$ and TXB$_2$), and **prostaglandins** (PGD$_2$). A number of other **cytokines** are also released that are not arachidonic acid precursors, such as **platelet-activating factor (PAF), bradykinins, interleukins (IL-4, IL-5, IL-6),** and **tumor necrosis factor-alpha (TNF-α).** All of these newly synthesized mediators are formed at the time of their release and are collectively referred to as **secondary** (or **newly synthesized) mediators.**

Mast Cell Development and Distribution

Because basophils and mast cells share some characteristics, it was once believed that mast cells were basophils that had left the bloodstream to perform their tasks in the connective tissues. It is now known that basophils and mast cells are different cells and have different precursors (see Fig. 6-1). Mast cell precursors probably originate in the bone marrow, circulate in the blood for a short time, and then enter the connective tissues, where they differentiate into mast cells and acquire their characteristic cytoplasmic granules. These cells have a life span of less than a few months and occasionally undergo cell division.

Mast cells are located throughout the body in the connective tissue proper, where they are concentrated

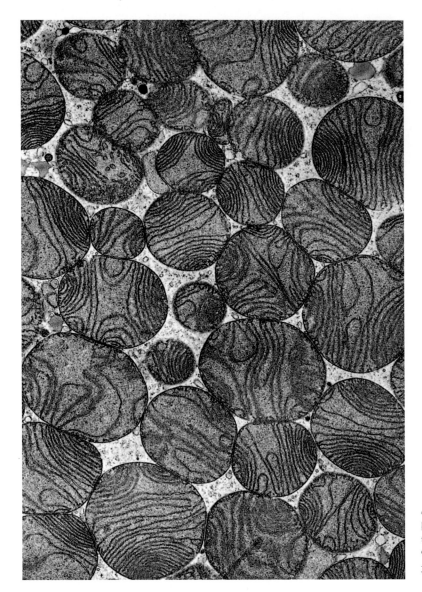

Figure 6–7 Multilocular tissues (brown fat) in the bat (×11,000). Note the numerous mitochondria dispersed throughout the cell. (From Fawcett, DW: An Atlas of Fine Structure. The Cell. Philadelphia, WB Saunders, 1966.)

along small blood vessels. They also are present in the subepithelial connective tissue of the respiratory and digestive systems. Mast cells in connective tissue contain mostly heparin in their granules, whereas those located in the alimentary tract mucosa contain chondroitin sulfate instead of heparin. These latter cells are called **mucosal mast cells.**

The reason for the existence of the two diverse populations of mast cells is not understood. Furthermore, it has been determined that mast cells vary in phenotype, morphology, histochemistry, mediator content, and response. Thus, phenotypically different mast cell populations are thought to function differently in health and disease. For example, mucosal mast cells release histamine to facilitate the activation of parietal cells of the stomach to produce hydrochloric acid.

Mast Cell Activation and Degranulation

Mast cells possess high-affinity cell-surface Fc receptors **(FceRI)** for immunoglobulin E (IgE). They function in the immune system by initiating an inflammatory response known as the **immediate hypersensitivity reaction** (whose systemic form, known as an **anaphylactic reaction,** may have lethal consequences). This response commonly is induced by foreign proteins (antigens) such as bee venom, pollen, and certain drugs, as follows:

1 The first exposure to any of these antigens elicits formation of IgE antibodies, which bind to the FceRI receptors of the plasmalemma of mast cells, thereby **sensitizing** these cells.

2 On subsequent exposure to the *same* antigen, the antigen binds to the IgE on the mast cell surface,

FAT CELL   CAPILLARY

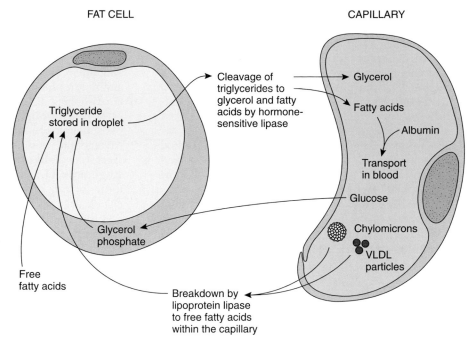

Figure 6–8 Transport of lipid between a capillary and an adipocyte. Lipids are transported in the bloodstream in the form of chylomicrons and very-low-density lipoproteins (VLDLs). The enzyme lipoprotein lipase, manufactured by the fat cell and transported to the capillary lumen, hydrolyzes the lipids to fatty acids and glycerol. Fatty acids diffuse into the connective tissue of the adipose tissue and into the lipocytes, where they are reesterified into triglycerides for storage. When required, triglycerides stored within the adipocyte are hydrolyzed by *hormone-sensitive lipase* into fatty acids and glycerol. These then enter the connective tissue spaces of adipose tissue and from there into a capillary, where they are bound to albumin and transported in the blood. Glucose from the capillary can be transported to adipocytes, which can manufacture lipids from carbohydrate sources.

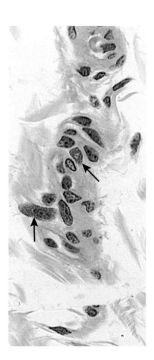

Figure 6–9 Light micrograph of mast cells *(arrows)* in monkey connective tissue (×540). The granules within the mast cells contain histamine and other preformed pharmacological agents.

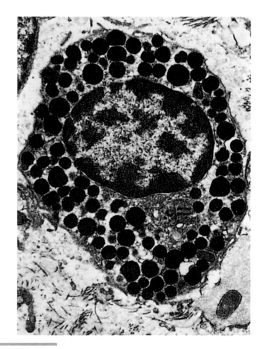

Figure 6–10 Electron micrograph of a mast cell in the rat (×5500). Observe the dense granules filling the cytoplasm. (From Leeson TS, Leeson CR, Paparo AA: Text/Atlas of Histology. Philadelphia, WB Saunders, 1988.)

causing cross-linking of the bound IgE antibodies and clustering of the receptors (Fig. 6-11).

3 Cross-linking and clustering activate membrane-bound **receptor coupling factors,** which in turn initiates at least two independent processes—the release of **primary mediators** from the granules and synthesis and the release of the **secondary mediators** from arachidonic acid precursors as well as from other cytoplasmic or membrane lipid sources.

4 The release of preformed mediators is accomplished by activation of **adenylate cyclase,** the enzyme responsible for the conversion of adenosine diphosphate (ADP) to cAMP.

5 This increase in cAMP levels activates the release of calcium ion (Ca^{2+}) from intracellular storage sites and facilitates an influx from extracellular sources. The resulting increase in cytosolic Ca^{2+} causes the secre-

tory granules to fuse with one another, as well as with the cell membrane. These processes lead to **degranulation,** the release of the granule contents, namely histamine, heparin, neutral proteases, aryl sulfatase and other enzymes, eosinophil chemotactic factor, and neutrophil chemotactic factor.

6 Cross-linking of the membrane-bound IgE also activates **phospholipase A_2,** which acts on membrane phospholipids to form **arachidonic acid**.

7 Arachidonic acid is converted into the secondary mediators **leukotrienes C_4, D_4,** and **E_4, prostaglandin D_2,** and **thromboxane A_2.** Additionally, the mast cell releases other newly formed pharmacological agents and cytokines**.** It is important to note that these secondary mediators are *not* stored in the mast cell granules but are manufactured and immediately released.

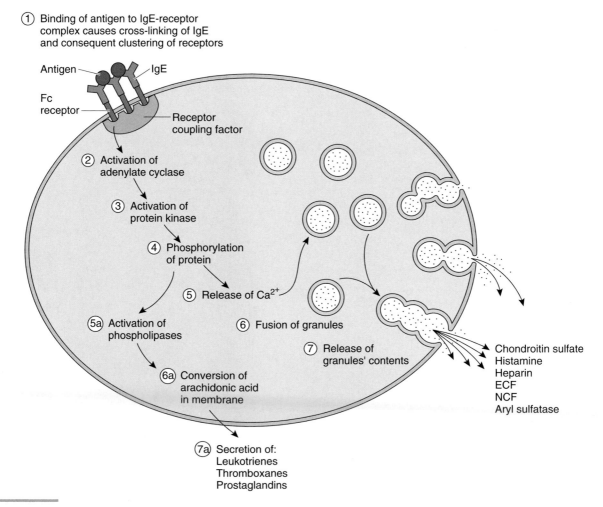

Figure 6–11 Binding of antigens and cross-linking of immunoglobulin E (IgE)-receptor complexes on the mast cell plasma membrane. This event triggers a cascade that ultimately results in the synthesis and release of leukotrienes and prostaglandins as well as in degranulation, thus releasing histamine, heparin, eosinophil chemotactic factor (ECF), and neutrophil chemotactic factor (NCF).

Table 6-1 lists the sources and activities of the principal primary and secondary mediators released from mast cells during immediate hypersensitivity reactions. These mediators initiate the inflammatory response, activate the body's defense system by attracting leukocytes to the site of inflammation, and modulate the degree of inflammation.

SEQUENCE OF EVENTS IN THE INFLAMMATORY RESPONSE

1 **Histamine** causes vasodilation and increases the vascular permeability of blood vessels in the vicinity. It also causes bronchiospasm and increases mucus production in the respiratory tract.
2 Complement components leak out of blood vessels and are cleaved by **neutral proteases** to form additional agents of inflammation.
3 **Eosinophil chemotactic factor** attracts eosinophils to the site of inflammation. These cells phagocytose antigen-antibody complexes, destroy any parasites present, and limit the inflammatory response.
4 **Neutrophil chemotactic factor** attracts neutrophils to the site of inflammation. These cells phagocytose and kill microorganisms, if present.
5 **Leukotrienes C_4, D_4,** and **E_4** increase vascular permeability and cause bronchiospasms. They are several thousand times more potent than histamine in their vasoactive effects.
6 **Prostaglandin D_2** causes bronchiospasm and increases secretion of mucus by the bronchial mucosa.
7 **PAF** causes greater vascular permeability.
8 **Thromboxane A_2** is a vigorous platelet-aggregating mediator and also causes vasoconstriction. It is quickly transformed into thromboxane B_2, its inactive form.
9 **Bradykinin** is a powerful vascular dilator that causes vascular permeability. It is also responsible for pain.

TABLE 6–1 Principal Primary and Secondary Mediators Released by Mast Cells

Substance	Type of Mediator	Source	Action
Histamine	Primary	Granule	Increases vascular permeability, vasodilation, smooth muscle contraction of bronchi, mucus production
Heparin	Primary	Granule	Anticoagulant binds and inactivates histamine
Chondroitin sulfate	Primary	Granule	Binds to and inactivates histamine
Aryl sulfatase	Primary	Granule	Inactivates leukotriene C_4, thus limiting the inflammatory response
Neutral proteases	Primary	Granule	Protein cleavage to activate complement (especially C3a); increases inflammatory response
Eosinophil chemotactic factor	Primary	Granule	Attracts eosinophils to site of inflammation
Neutrophil chemotactic factor	Primary	Granule	Attracts neutrophils to site of inflammation
Leukotrienes C_4, D_4, and E_4	Secondary	Membrane lipid	Vasodilator; increases vascular permeability; bronchial smooth muscle contractant
Prostaglandin D_2	Secondary	Membrane lipid	Causes contraction of bronchial smooth muscle; increases mucus secretion; vasoconstriction
Thromboxane A_2	Secondary	Membrane lipid	Causes platelet aggregation, vasoconstriction
Bradykinins	Secondary	Formed by activity of enzymes located in granules	Causes vascular permeability and is responsible for pain sensation
Platelet-activating factor (PAF)	Secondary	Activated by phospholipase A_2	Attracts neutrophils and eosinophils; causes vascular permeability and contraction of bronchial smooth muscle

CLINICAL CORRELATIONS

Victims of **hay fever** attacks suffer from the effects of **histamine** being released by the mast cells of the nasal mucosa, which causes localized edema from increased permeability of the small blood vessels. The swelling of the mucosa results in feeling "stuffed up" and hinders breathing.

Victims of **asthma** attacks suffer from difficulty in breathing as a result of bronchospasm caused by **leukotrienes** released in the lungs.

Because degranulation of mast cells usually is a localized phenomenon, the typical inflammatory response is mild and site-specific. However, a risk also exists for **hyperallergic persons** who may experience a systemic and severe immediate hypersensitivity reaction **(systemic anaphylaxis)** following a secondary exposure to an allergen (e.g., insect stings, antibiotics). This reaction **(anaphylactic shock),** which includes shortness of breath and a sudden decrease in blood pressure, may occur within seconds to a few minutes and and can result in the person's death (in a matter of a few hours) if left untreated. Persons susceptible to this condition often wear a medical emergency bracelet informing those giving assistance of the need for immediate medical attention.

Macrophages

Macrophages belong to the mononuclear phagocytic system and are subdivided into two groups of cells, phagocytes and antigen-presenting cells.

As noted earlier, some macrophages behave as fixed cells and some as transient cells. Because macrophages are active phagocytes, they function in removing cellular debris and in protecting the body against foreign invaders.

Macrophages measure about 10 to 30 μm in diameter and are irregularly shaped (Fig. 6-12). Their cell surface is uneven, varying from short, blunt projections to finger-like filopodia. More active macrophages have pleats and folds in their plasma membranes as a consequence of cell movement and phagocytosis. Their cytoplasm is basophilic and contains many small vacuoles and small dense granules. The eccentric nucleus of macrophages is smaller and more darkly stained than that of fibroblasts, and it usually does not display nucleoli. The macrophage nucleus is somewhat distinctive in that it is ovoid and usually indented on one side, so that it resembles a kidney. Electron microscopic studies demonstrate a well-developed Golgi apparatus, prominent RER, and an abundance of lysosomes that appear as small, dense granules in light micrographs.

As young macrophages mature they increase in size, and there are concomitant increases in RER profiles, Golgi complex, microtubules, lysosomes, microfilaments, and protein synthesis.

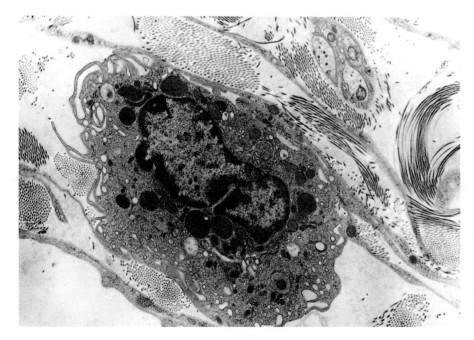

Figure 6–12 Electron micrograph of a macrophage in the rat epididymis. (From Flickinger CJ, Herr CJ, Sisak JR, Howards SS: Ultrastructure of epididymal interstitial reactions following vasectomy and vasovasostomy. Anat Rec 235:61-73, 1993.)

Macrophage Development and Distribution

Histologists once believed that macrophages were derived from precursor cells in the **reticuloendothelial system,** which included nonphagocytic cells such as reticulocytes. This classification has been replaced by the **mononuclear phagocyte system.** All members of the mononuclear phagocyte system arise from a common stem cell in the bone marrow, possess lysosomes, are capable of phagocytosis, and display FcεRI receptors and receptors for complement.

Monocytes develop in the bone marrow and circulate in the blood. At the proper signal, they leave the bloodstream by migrating through the endothelium of capillaries or venules. In the connective tissue compartment they mature into macrophages, which normally have a life span of about 2 months. Macrophages arise from monocytes, activated by the macrophage colony-stimulating factor (M-CSF) (see Chapter 10 and Table 10-6).

Macrophages localized in certain regions of the body were given specific names before their origin was completely understood. Thus, **Kupffer cells** of the liver (Fig. 6-13), **dust cells** of the lung, **Langerhans cells** of the skin, **monocytes** of the blood, and **macrophages** of the connective tissue, spleen, lymph nodes, thymus, and bone marrow are all members of the mononuclear phagocyte system and possess similar morphology and functions. Additionally, **osteoclasts** of bone and **microglia** of the brain, although morphologically different, belong to the mononuclear phagocyte system.

Under chronic inflammatory conditions, macrophages congregate, greatly enlarge, and become polygonal **epithelioid cells.** When the particulate matter to be removed is excessively large, several to many macrophages may fuse to form a **foreign-body giant cell,** a giant multinucleated macrophage.

Macrophages residing in the connective tissues were previously called **fixed macrophages,** and those that developed as a result of an exogenous stimulus and migrated to the particular site were called **free macrophages.** These names have been replaced by the more descriptive terms **resident macrophages** and **elicited macrophages,** respectively.

Macrophage Function

Macrophages phagocytose foreign substances and damaged and senescent cells as well as cellular debris; they also assist in the initiation of the immune response.

Macrophages phagocytose senescent, damaged, and dead cells and cellular debris and digest the ingested material through the action of hydrolytic enzymes in their lysosomes (see Chapter 2). Macrophages also assist in defense of the body by phagocytosing and destroying foreign substances, including microorganisms. During the immune response, factors released by lymphocytes activate macrophages, increasing their phagocytic activity. **Activated macrophages** vary considerably in shape, possess microvilli and lamellipodia, and exhibit more locomotion compared with unactivated macrophages. Macrophages also play a key role in presenting antigens to lymphocytes (see Chapter 12).

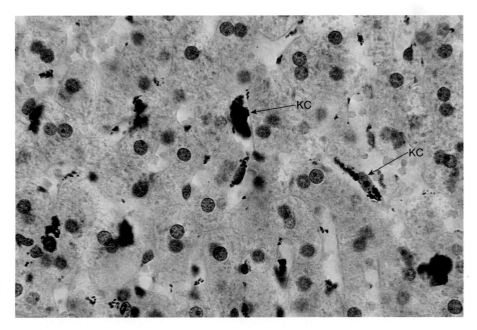

Figure 6–13 Light micrograph of liver of an animal injected with India ink demonstrating the presence of cells known as Kuppfer cells (KC) that preferentially phagocytose the ink (×540).

Transient Connective Tissue Cells

All transient connective tissue cells are derived from precursors in the bone marrow (see Fig. 6-1). These cells are discussed in greater detail in other chapters.

Plasma Cells

> *Plasma cells are derived from B lymphocytes and manufacture antibodies.*

Although plasma cells are scattered throughout the connective tissues, they are present in greatest numbers in areas of chronic inflammation and in areas where foreign substances or microorganisms have entered the tissues. These differentiated cells, which are derived from B lymphocytes that have interacted with antigen, produce and secrete antibodies and are responsible for humorally mediated immunity (see Chapters 10 and 12).

Plasma cells are large, ovoid cells, 20 μm in diameter, with an eccentrically placed nucleus, that have a relatively short life span of 2 to 3 weeks. Their cytoplasm is intensely basophilic as a result of a well-developed RER with closely spaced cisternae (Fig. 6-14). Only a few mitochondria are scattered between the profiles of RER. Electron micrographs display a large, juxtanuclear Golgi complex and a pair of centrioles (Figs. 6-15 and 6-16). In light micrographs, these structures are located in the pale-staining regions adjacent to the nucleus. The spherical nucleus possesses heterochromatin radiating out from the center, giving it a characteristic "clock face" or "spoked" appearance under the light microscope.

Leukocytes

> *Leukocytes exit the bloodstream during inflammation, invasion by foreign elements, and immune responses in order to perform various functions.*

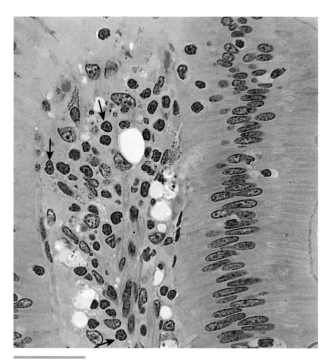

Figure 6–14 Light micrograph of plasma cells in the lamina propria of the monkey jejunum (×540). Observe the "clock face" nucleus (*arrows*).

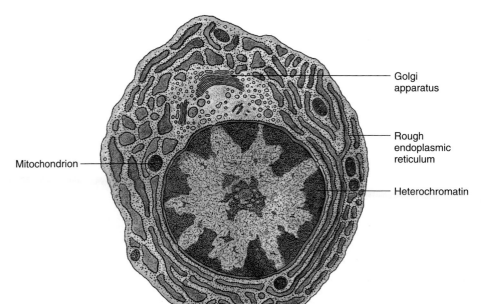

Mitochondrion

Golgi apparatus

Rough endoplasmic reticulum

Heterochromatin

Figure 6–15 Drawing of a plasma cell as seen in an electron micrograph. The arrangement of heterochromatin gives the nucleus a "clock face" appearance. (From Lentz TL: Cell Fine Structure: An Atlas of Drawings of Whole-Cell Structure. Philadelphia, WB Saunders, 1971.)

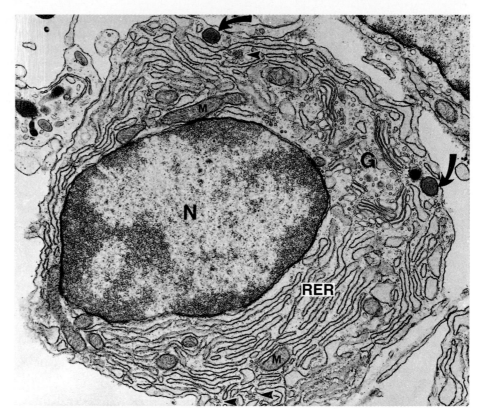

Figure 6–16 Electron micrograph of a plasma cell from the lamina propria of the rat duodenum displaying abundant rough endoplasmic reticulum (RER) and prominent Golgi complex (×10,300). G, Golgi apparatus; M, mitochondria; N, nucleus. *Arrowheads* represent small vesicles; *arrows* represent dense granules. (From Rambourg A, Clermont Y, Hermo L, Chretien M: Formation of secretion granules in the Golgi apparatus of plasma cells in the rat. Am J Anat 184:52-61, 1988.)

Leukocytes are white blood cells that circulate in the bloodstream. However, they frequently migrate through the capillary walls to enter the connective tissues, especially during inflammation, when they carry out various functions. (See Chapter 10 for more comprehensive discussions; also see summary in Table 10-3.)

Monocytes have been discussed under "Macrophages."

Neutrophils phagocytose and digest bacteria in areas of acute inflammation, resulting in formation of **pus,** an accumulation of dead neutrophils and debris.

Eosinophils, like neutrophils, are attracted to areas of inflammation by leukocyte chemotactic factors. Eosinophils combat parasites by releasing cytotoxins. They also are attracted to sites of allergic inflammation, where they moderate the allergic reaction and phagocytose antibody-antigen complexes.

Basophils (similar to mast cells) release preformed and newly synthesized pharmacological agents that initiate, maintain, and control the inflammatory process.

Lymphocytes are present only in small numbers in most connective tissue, except at sites of chronic inflammation, where they are abundant. Chapter 10 describes leukocytes in more detail, and Chapter 12 discusses lymphocytes.

CLASSIFICATION OF CONNECTIVE TISSUE

As noted earlier, connective tissue is classified into connective tissue proper—the major subject of this chapter—and specialized connective tissue, embracing cartilage, bone, and blood. The third recognized category of connective tissue is **embryonic connective tissue.** Table 6-2 summarizes the major classes of connective tissue and their subclasses.

Embryonic Connective Tissue

Embryonic connective tissue includes both mesenchymal tissue and mucous tissue.

Mesenchymal connective tissue is present only in the embryo and consists of mesenchymal cells in a gel-like, amorphous ground substance containing scattered reticular fibers. **Mesenchymal cells** possess an oval nucleus exhibiting a fine chromatin network and prominent nucleoli. The sparse, pale-staining cytoplasm extends small processes in several directions. Mitotic figures frequently are observed in mesenchymal cells because they give rise to most of the cells of loose connective tissue. It is generally believed that most if not

Table 6–2 Classification of Connective Tissues

A. Embryonic connective tissues
  1. Mesenchymal connective tissue
  2. Mucous connective tissue
B. Connective tissue proper
  1. Loose (areolar) connective tissue
  2. Dense connective tissue
    a. Dense irregular connective tissue
    b. Dense regular connective tissue
      (1) Collagenous
      (2) Elastic
  3. Reticular tissue
  4. Adipose tissue
C. Specialized connective tissue
  1. Cartilage
  2. Bone
  3. Blood

all of the mesenchymal cells, once scattered throughout the embryo, are eventually depleted and do not exist as such in the adult except in the pulp of teeth. In adults, however, pluripotential pericytes, which reside along capillaries, can differentiate into other cells of connective tissue.

Mucous tissue is a loose, amorphous connective tissue exhibiting a jelly-like matrix primarily composed of hyaluronic acid and sparsely populated with type I and type III collagen fibers and fibroblasts. This tissue, also known as **Wharton's jelly,** is found only in the umbilical cord and subdermal connective tissue of the embryo.

Connective Tissue Proper

The four recognized types of connective tissue proper (**loose, dense,** and **reticular connective tissues** and **adipose tissue**), differ in their histology, location, and functions.

Loose (Areolar) Connective Tissue

Loose (areolar) connective tissue is composed of a loose arrangement of fibers and dispersed cells embedded in a gel-like ground substance.

Loose connective tissue, also known as **areolar connective tissue,** fills in the spaces of the body just deep to the skin, lies below the mesothelial lining of the internal body cavity, is associated with the adventitia of blood vessels, and surrounds the parenchyma of glands. The loose connective tissue of mucous membranes (as in the alimentary canal) is called the **lamina propria.**

Loose connective tissue is characterized by abundant **ground substance** and tissue fluid (extracellular fluid) housing the fixed connective tissue cells: **fibroblasts, adipose cells, macrophages,** and **mast cells** as well as some **undifferentiated cells.** Also scattered throughout the ground substance are loosely woven **collagen, reticular,** and **elastic fibers.** Coursing in this amorphous tissue are small nerve fibers as well as blood vessels that supply the cells with oxygen and nutrients.

Because this tissue lies immediately beneath the thin epithelia of the digestive and respiratory tracts, this is where the body first attacks antigens, bacteria, and other foreign invaders. Therefore, loose connective tissue contains many transient cells responsible for inflammation, allergic reactions, and the immune response. These cells, which originally circulate in the bloodstream, are released from blood vessels in response to an inflammatory stimulus. Pharmacological agents released by mast cells increase the permeability of small vessels so that excess plasma enters the loose connective tissue spaces, causing it to swell.

CLINICAL CORRELATIONS

Under normal circumstances, extracellular fluid returns to the blood capillaries or enters lymph vessels to be returned to the blood. A potent and prolonged inflammatory response, however, causes accumulation of excess tissue fluid within loose connective tissue beyond what can be returned via the capillaries and lymph vessels. This results in gross swelling, or **edema,** in the affected area. Edema can result from excessive release of histamine and leukotrienes C_4 and D_4, which all increase capillary permeability, as well as from obstruction of venous or lymphatic vessels.

Dense Connective Tissue

Dense connective tissue contains a greater abundance of fibers and fewer cells than loose connective tissue.

Dense connective tissue contains most of the same components found in loose connective tissue, except that it has many more fibers and fewer cells. The orientation and the arrangements of the bundles of collagen fibers in this tissue make it resistant to stress. When the collagen fiber bundles are arranged randomly, the tissue is called dense *irregular* connective tissue. When fiber bundles of the tissue are arranged in parallel or organized fashion, the tissue is called dense *regular* connective tissue, which is divided into collagenous and elastic types.

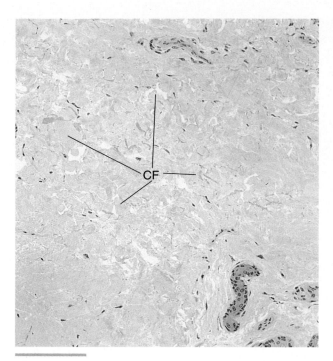

Figure 6–17 Light micrograph of dense irregular collagenous connective tissue from monkey skin (×132). Observe the many bundles of collagen (CF) in random orientation.

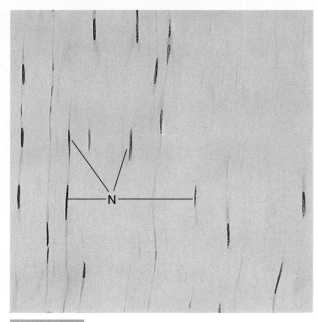

Figure 6–18 Light micrograph of dense regular collagenous connective tissue from monkey tendon (×270). Note the ordered, parallel array of collagen bundles and the elongated nuclei (N) of the fibroblasts lying between collagen bundles.

Dense irregular connective tissue contains mostly coarse collagen fibers interwoven into a meshwork that resists stress from all directions (Fig. 6-17). The collagen bundles are packed so tightly that space is limited for ground substance and cells. Fine networks of elastic fibers are often scattered about the collagen bundles. Fibroblasts, the most abundant cells of this tissue, are located in the interstices between collagen bundles. Dense irregular connective tissue constitutes the dermis of skin, the sheaths of nerves, and the capsules of the spleen, testes, ovary, kidney, and lymph nodes.

Dense regular collagenous connective tissue is composed of coarse collagen bundles densely packed and oriented into parallel cylinders or sheets that resist tensile forces (Fig. 6-18). Because of the tight packing of the collagen fibers, little space can be occupied by ground substance and cells. Thin, sheet-like fibroblasts are located between bundles of collagen with their long axes parallel to the bundles. Tendons (Fig. 6-19), ligaments, and aponeuroses are examples of dense regular collagenous connective tissue.

Dense regular elastic connective tissue possesses coarse branching elastic fibers with only a few collagen fibers forming networks. Scattered throughout the interstitial spaces are fibroblasts. The elastic fibers are arranged parallel to one another and form either thin sheets or fenestrated membranes. The latter are present in large blood vessels, ligamenta flava of the vertebral column, and the suspensory ligament of the penis.

Reticular Tissue

Type III collagen is the major fiber component of reticular tissue. The collagen fibers form mesh-like networks interspersed with fibroblasts and macrophages (Fig. 6-20). It is the fibroblasts that synthesize the type III collagen. Reticular tissue forms the architectural framework of liver sinusoids, adipose tissue, bone marrow, lymph nodes, spleen, smooth muscle, and the islets of Langerhans.

Adipose Tissue

Adipose tissue is classified into two types according to whether it is composed of **unilocular** or **multilocular** adipocytes. Other differences between the two types of adipose tissue are color, vascularity, and metabolic activity.

White (Unilocular) Adipose Tissue

Each *unilocular* fat cell contains a single lipid droplet, giving the adipose tissue composed of such cells a white color. (In a person whose diet is especially rich in foods containing carotenoids, such as carrots, this adipose tissue is yellow.) White adipose tissue is heavily supplied with blood vessels, which form capillary networks

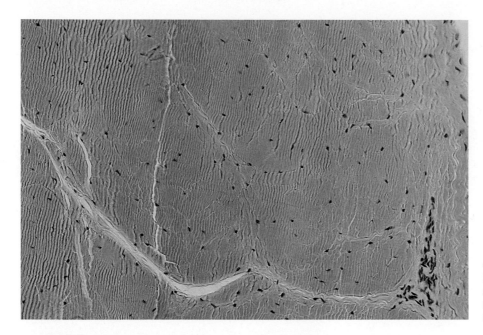

Figure 6–19 Light micrograph of a cross section of monkey tendon. The scattered, small black structures represent nuclei of fibroblasts (×270).

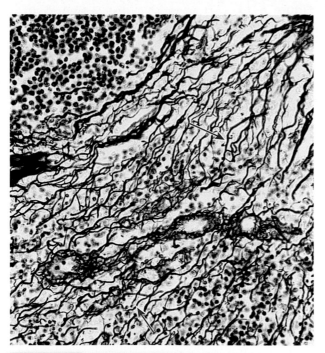

Figure 6–20 Light micrograph of reticular tissue (stained with silver) displaying the networks of reticular fibers (×270). Many lymphoid cells are interspersed between the reticular fibers *(arrows)*.

throughout the tissue. The vessels gain access via connective tissue septa that partition the fat into lobules (see Fig. 6-6). The plasma membranes of the unilocular adipose cells contain receptors for several substances, including **insulin, growth hormone,**

norepinephrine, and **glucocorticoids,** that facilitate the uptake and release of free fatty acids and glycerol.

Unilocular fat is present in the subcutaneous layers throughout the body. It also occurs in masses in characteristic sites influenced by sex and age. In men, fat is stored in the neck, in the shoulders, about the hips, and in the buttocks. As men age, the abdominal wall becomes an additional storage area. In women, fat is stored in the breasts, buttocks, hips, and lateral aspects of the thighs. Additionally, fat is stored in both sexes in the abdominal cavity about the omental apron and the mesenteries.

Brown (Multilocular) Adipose Tissue

Brown adipose tissue (brown fat) is composed of *multilocular* fat cells, which store fat in multiple droplets. This tissue may appear tan to reddish brown because of its extensive vascularity and the chytochromes present in its abundant mitochondria (see Fig. 6-7).

Multilocular adipose tissue has a lobular organization and vascular supply similar to those of a gland. Brown fat tissue is very vascular because the vessels are located near the adipocytes. Unmyelinated nerve fibers enter the tissue, with the axons ending on the blood vessels as well as on fat cells, whereas in white fat tissue, the neurons end only on the blood vessels.

Although it has long been known that multilocular fat is found in many mammalian species, especially those that hibernate, and in the infants of most mammals, it was unclear whether multilocular fat exists in adult humans. However, in the newborn human, brown fat is located in the neck region and in the interscapular region. As humans mature, the fat droplets in

Obesity increases the risks for many health problems, including non–insulin-dependent diabetes mellitus, as well as problems involving the cardiovascular system.

In adults, obesity develops in two ways. **Hypertrophic obesity** results from the accumulation and storage of fat in unilocular fat cells, which may increase their size by as much as four times. **Hypercellular obesity,** as the name implies, results from an overabundance of adipocytes. This type of obesity usually is severe.

Although mature adipocytes do not divide, their precursors proliferate in early postnatal life. There is substantial evidence that overfeeding newborn infants for a few weeks may actually increase the number of adipocyte precursors, leading to an increase in the number of adipocytes and setting the stage for hypercellular obesity in the adult. Overweight infants are at least three times more likely to exhibit obesity as adults than infants of average weight. Presently, it is understood that persons exhibiting severe obesity also exhibit an increase in the adipocyte population, although it is not understood how this recruitment is driven.

There also appears to be a genetic basis in some cases of obesity. Mutations in the gene responsible for the coding for **leptin** produces an inactive form of that hormone. Because leptin regulates the appetite center of the hypothalamus, people who either do not produce leptin or who produce a biologically inactive form of this hormone have a voracious appetite and suffer from an almost uncontrollable weight gain.

These cells can oxidize fatty acids at up to 20 times the rate of white fat, increasing body heat production threefold in cold environments. Sensory receptors in the skin send signals to the temperature-regulating center of the brain, resulting in the relaying of sympathetic nerve impulses directly to the brown fat cells. The neurotransmitter norepinephrine activates the enzyme that cleaves triglycerides into fatty acids and glycerol, initiating heat production by oxidation of fatty acids in the mitochondria. **Thermogenin,** a transmembrane protein located on the inner membrane of mitochondria, permits backflow of protons instead of utilizing them for synthesis of adenosine triphosphate (ATP); as a result of uncoupling oxidation from phosphorylation, the proton flow generates energy that is dispersed as heat.

Histogenesis of Adipose Tissue

It is believed that adipose cells are derived from undifferentiated embryonic stem cells that develop into **preadipocytes,** cells that, under the influence of a series of activating factors, differentiate into adipocytes.

The predominant view is that adipose tissue develops via two separate processes. In **primary fat formation**, which occurs early in fetal life, groups of **epithelioid precursor cells,** probably preadipocytes, are distributed at certain locations in the developing fetus; in these tissues, lipid droplets begin to accumulate in the form of brown adipose tissue. Near the end of fetal life, other **fusiform precursor cells** differentiate in many areas of the connective tissues within the fetus and begin to accumulate lipids that coalesce into the single droplet in each cell, thus forming the unilocular fat cells found in adults. The latter process has been named **secondary fat formation.** It should be understood, however, that brown adipose tissue is present in the embryo but white adipose tissue appears only after birth.

brown fat cells coalesce and form into one droplet (similar to the droplets in white fat cells) and the cells become more like those in unilocular fat tissue. Thus, although adults appear to contain only unilocular fat, there is evidence that they also possess brown fat. This feature can be demonstrated in some of the wasting diseases of older people, in which multilocular fat tissue forms again and in the same areas as in the newborn.

Brown adipose tissue is associated with production of body heat because of the large number of mitochondria in the multilocular adipocytes composing this tissue.

Tumors of the adipose tissues may be benign or malignant. **Lipomas** are common benign tumors of adipocytes, whereas **liposarcomas** are malignant tumors of adipocytes. The latter form most commonly in the leg and in retroperitoneal tissues, although they may form anywhere in the body. The tumor cells may resemble either unilocular adipocytes or multilocular adipocytes, another indication that adult humans do indeed possess the two kinds of adipose tissue.

7

Cartilage and Bone

Cartilage and bone are both specialized connective tissues. Cartilage possesses a firm pliable matrix that resists mechanical stresses. Bone matrix is one of the hardest tissues of the body, and it too resists stresses placed upon it. Both of these connective tissues have cells that are specialized to secrete the matrix in which, subsequently, the cells become trapped. Although cartilage and bone have many varied functions, some of the functions are similar and related. Both are involved in supporting the body because they are intimately associated in the skeletal system. Most of the long bones of the body are formed first in the embryo as cartilage, which then acts as a template that is later replaced by bone; this process is referred to as **endochondral bone formation.** Most of the flat bones are formed within preexisting membranous sheaths; thus this method of osteogenesis is known as **intramembranous bone formation.**

CARTILAGE

Cartilage possesses cells called **chondrocytes,** which occupy small cavities called **lacunae** within the **extracellular matrix** they secreted. The substance of cartilage is neither vascularized nor supplied with nerves or lymphatic vessels; however, the cells receive their nourishment from blood vessels of surrounding connective tissues by diffusion through the matrix. The extracellular matrix is composed of **glycosaminoglycans** and **proteoglycans,** which are intimately associated with the collagen and elastic fibers embedded within the matrix. The flexibility and resistance of cartilage to compression permit it to function as a shock absorber, and its smooth surface permits almost friction-free movement of the joints of the body as it covers the articulating surfaces of the bones.

There are three types of cartilage according to the fibers present in the matrix (Fig. 7-1 and Table 7-1):

- **Hyaline cartilage** contains **type II** collagen in its matrix; it is the most abundant cartilage in the body and serves many functions.
- **Elastic cartilage** contains **type II** collagen and abundant elastic fibers scattered throughout its matrix, giving it more pliability.
- **Fibrocartilage** possesses dense, coarse **type I** collagen fibers in its matrix, allowing it to withstand strong tensile forces.

The **perichondrium** is a connective tissue sheath covering that overlies most cartilage. It has an outer fibrous layer and inner cellular layer whose cells secrete cartilage matrix. The perichondrium is vascular, and its vessels supply nutrients to the cells of cartilage. In areas where the cartilage has no perichondrium (e.g., the articular surfaces of the bones forming a joint), the cartilage cells receive their nourishment from the synovial fluid that bathes the joint surfaces. Perichondria are present in elastic and most hyaline cartilages, but absent in fibrocartilage.

Hyaline Cartilage

Hyaline cartilage, the most abundant cartilage in the body, forms the template for endochondral bone formation.

Hyaline cartilage, a bluish-gray, semitranslucent, pliable substance, is the most common cartilage of the body. It is located in the nose and larynx, on the ventral ends of the ribs where they articulate with the sternum, in the tracheal rings and bronchi, and on the articulating surfaces of the movable joints of the body. Also, it is this cartilage that forms the cartilage template of many of the bones during embryonic development and constitutes the epiphyseal plates of growing bones (see Table 7-1).

HYALINE CARTILAGE

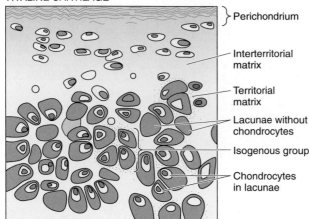

Perichondrium

Interterritorial matrix

Territorial matrix

Lacunae without chondrocytes

Isogenous group

Chondrocytes in lacunae

ELASTIC CARTILAGE

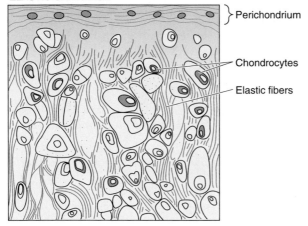

Perichondrium

Chondrocytes

Elastic fibers

FIBROCARTILAGE

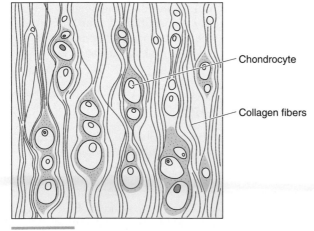

Chondrocyte

Collagen fibers

Figure 7–1 Types of cartilage.

Histogenesis and Growth of Hyaline Cartilage

Cells responsible for hyaline cartilage formation differentiate from mesenchymal cells.

In the region where cartilage is to form, individual mesenchymal cells retract their processes, round up, and congregate in dense masses called **chondrification centers.** These cells differentiate into **chondroblasts** and commence secreting the typical cartilage matrix around themselves. As this process continues, the chondroblasts become entrapped in their own matrix in small individual compartments called **lacunae.** Chondroblasts that are surrounded by this matrix are referred to as **chondrocytes** (Fig. 7-2). These cells are still capable of cell division, forming a cluster of two to four or more cells in a lacuna. These groups are known as **isogenous groups** and represent one, two, or more cell divisions from an original chondrocyte (see Fig. 7-1). As the cells of an isogenous group manufacture matrix, they are pushed away from each other, forming separate lacunae and thus enlarging the cartilage from within. This type of growth is called **interstitial growth.**

Mesenchymal cells at the periphery of the developing cartilage differentiate to form fibroblasts. These cells manufacture a dense irregular collagenous connective tissue, the **perichondrium,** responsible for the growth and maintenance of the cartilage. The perichondrium has two layers, an **outer fibrous layer** composed of type I collagen, fibroblasts, and blood vessels and an **inner cellular layer** composed mostly of **chondrogenic cells.** The chondrogenic cells undergo division and differentiate into chondroblasts, which begin to elaborate matrix. In this way cartilage also grows by adding to its periphery, a process called **appositional growth.**

Interstitial growth occurs only in the early phase of hyaline cartilage formation. Articular cartilage lacks a perichondrium and increases in size only by interstitial growth. This type of growth also occurs in the **epiphyseal plates** of long bones, where the lacunae are arranged in a longitudinal orientation parallel to the long axis of the bone; therefore, interstitial growth serves to lengthen the bone. The cartilage in the remainder of the body grows mostly by apposition, a controlled process that may continue during the life of the cartilage.

It is interesting that mesenchymal cells located within the chondrification centers are induced to become secreting chondroblasts by their attachments and the chemistry of the surrounding extracellular matrix. Also, if chondroblasts are removed from their secreted cartilage matrix and are grown in a monolayer in a low-density substrate, they will cease to secrete "cartilage matrix" containing type II collagen. Instead they will become fibroblast-like and start secreting type I collagen.

TABLE 7–1 Types of Cartilage

Type	Identifying Characteristics	Perichondrium	Location
Hyaline	Type II collagen, basophilic matrix, chondrocytes usually arranged in groups	Perichondrium present in most places (exceptions: articular cartilages and epiphyses)	Articular ends of long bones, nose, larynx, trachea, bronchi, ventral ends of ribs
Elastic	Type II collagen, elastic fibers	Perichondrium present	Pinna of ear, walls of auditory canal, auditory tube, epiglottis, cuneiform cartilage of larynx
Fibrocartilage	Type I collagen, acidophilic matrix; chondrocytes arranged in parallel rows between bundles of collagen; always associated with dense regular collagenous connective tissue or hyaline cartilage	Perichondrium absent	Intervertebral disks, articular disks, pubic symphysis, insertion of some tendons

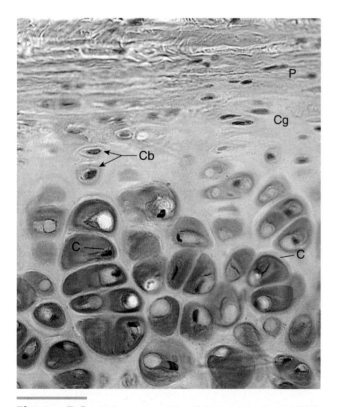

Figure 7–2 Light micrograph of hyaline cartilage (×270). Observe the large ovoid chondrocytes (C) trapped in their lacunae. Above them are the elongated chondroblasts (Cb), and at the very top is the perichondrium (P) and the underlying chondrogenic (Cg) cell layer.

Cartilage Cells

Three types of cells are associated with cartilage: chondrogenic cells, chondroblasts, and chondrocytes (see Fig. 7-2).

Chondrogenic cells are spindle-shaped, narrow cells that are derived from mesenchymal cells. They possess an ovoid nucleus with one or two nucleoli. Their cytoplasm is sparse, and electron micrographs of chondrogenic cells display a small Golgi apparatus, a few mitochondria, some profiles of **rough endoplasmic reticulum (RER),** and an abundance of free ribosomes. These cells can differentiate into both chondroblasts and osteoprogenitor cells.

Chondroblasts are derived from two sources: **mesenchymal cells** located within the center of chondrification and **chondrogenic cells** of the inner cellular layer of the perichondrium (as in appositional growth). Chondroblasts are plump, basophilic cells that display the organelles required for protein synthesis. Electron micrographs of these cells demonstrate a rich network of RER, a well-developed Golgi complex, numerous mitochondria, and an abundance of secretory vesicles.

Chondrocytes are chondroblasts that are surrounded by matrix. Those near the periphery are ovoid, whereas those deeper in the cartilage are more rounded, with a diameter of 10 to 30 μm. Histological processing creates artifactual shrinkage and distortion of the cells. Chondrocytes display a large nucleus with a prominent nucleolus and the usual organelles of protein-secreting cells. Young chondrocytes have a pale-staining cytoplasm with many mitochondria, an elaborate RER, a well-developed Golgi apparatus, and glycogen. Older chondrocytes, which are relatively quiescent, display a greatly reduced complement of organelles, with an abundance of free ribosomes. Thus, these cells can resume active protein synthesis if they revert to chondroblasts.

Matrix of Hyaline Cartilage

The matrix of hyaline cartilage is composed of type II collagen, proteoglycans, glycoproteins, and extracellular fluid.

The semitranslucent blue-gray matrix of hyaline cartilage contains up to 40% of its dry weight in collagen. In addition, it contains proteoglycans, glycoproteins, and extracellular fluid. Because the refractive index of the collagen fibrils and that of the ground substance are nearly the same, the matrix appears to be an amorphous, homogeneous mass with the light microscope.

The matrix of hyaline cartilage contains primarily **type II collagen,** but types IX, X, and XI and other minor collagens are also present in small quantities. Type II collagen does not form large bundles, although the bundle thickness increases with distance from the lacunae. Fiber orientation appears to be related to the stresses placed on the cartilage. For example, in articular cartilage, the fibers near the surface are oriented parallel to the surface, whereas deeper fibers seem to be oriented in curved columns.

The matrix is subdivided into two regions: the territorial matrix, around each lacuna, and the interterritorial matrix (see Fig. 7-1). The **territorial matrix,** a 50-μm-wide band, is poor in collagen and rich in chondroitin sulfate, which contributes to its basophilic and intense staining with periodic acid–Schiff (PAS) reagent. The bulk of the matrix is **interterritorial matrix,** which is richer in type II collagen and poorer in proteoglycans than the territorial matrix.

A small region of the matrix, 1- to 3-mm thick, immediately surrounding the lacuna is known as the **pericellular capsule.** It displays a fine meshwork of collagen fibers embedded in a basal lamina-like substance. These fibers may represent some of the other minor collagens present in hyaline cartilage; it has been suggested that the pericellular capsule may protect chondrocytes from mechanical stresses.

Cartilage matrix is rich in **aggrecans,** large proteoglycan molecules composed of protein cores to which glycosaminoglycan molecules (chondroitin 4-sulfate, chondroitin 6-sulfate, and heparan sulfate) are covalently linked (see Fig. 4-3). As many as 100 to 200 aggrecan molecules are linked noncovalently to hyaluronic acid, forming huge aggrecan composites that can be 3- to 4-μm long. The abundant negative charges associated with these exceedingly large proteoglycan molecules attract cations, predominantly Na^+ ions, which in turn attract water molecules. In this way, the cartilage matrix

becomes hydrated to such an extent that up to 80% of the wet weight of cartilage is water, accounting for the ability of cartilage to resist forces of compression.

Not only do hydrated proteoglycans fill the interstices among the collagen fiber bundles, but their glycosaminoglycan side chains form electrostatic bonds with the collagen. Thus, the ground substance and fibers of the matrix form a cross-linked molecular framework that resists tensile forces.

Cartilage matrix also contains the adhesive glycoprotein **chondronectin.** This large molecule, similar to fibronectin, has binding sites for type II collagen, chondroitin 4-sulfate, chondroitin 6-sulfate, hyaluronic acid, and integrins (transmembrane proteins) of chondroblasts and chondrocytes. Chondronectin thus assists these cells in maintaining their contact with the fibrous and amorphous components of the matrix.

Histophysiology of Hyaline Cartilage

The smoothness of hyaline cartilage and its ability to resist forces of both compression and tension are essential to its function at the articular surfaces of joints. Because cartilage is avascular, nutrients and oxygen must diffuse through the water of hydration present in the matrix. The inefficiency of such a system necessitates a limit on the width of cartilage. There is a constant turnover in the proteoglycans of cartilage that changes with age. Hormones and vitamins also exert influence on the growth, development, and function of cartilage. Many of these substances also affect skeletal formation and growth (Table 7-2).

CLINICAL CORRELATIONS

Hyaline cartilage degenerates when the chondrocytes hypertrophy and die and the matrix begins to calcify. This process is a normal and integral part of endochondral bone formation; however, it is also a natural process of aging, often resulting in less mobility and in joint pain.

Cartilage regeneration is usually poor except in children. Chondrogenic cells from the perichondrium enter the defect and form new cartilage. If the defect is large, the cells form dense connective tissue to repair the scar.

Elastic Cartilage

Elastic cartilage greatly resembles hyaline cartilage, except that its matrix and perichondrium possess elastic fibers.

Elastic cartilage is located in the pinna of the ear, the external and internal auditory tubes, the epiglottis, and

Table 7–2 Effects of Hormones and Vitamins on Hyaline Cartilage

Hormone	Effect
Thyroxine, testosterone, and somatotropin (via insulin-like growth factors)	Stimulate cartilage growth and matrix formation
Cortisone, hydrocortisone, and estradiol	Inhibit cartilage growth and matrix formation

Vitamin	Effect
Hypovitaminosis A	Reduces width of epiphyseal plates
Hypervitaminosis A	Accelerates ossification of epiphyseal plates
Hypovitaminosis C	Inhibits matrix synthesis and deforms architecture of epiphyseal plate, leading to scurvy
Absence of vitamin D, resulting in deficiency in absorption of calcium and phosphorus	Proliferation of chondrocytes is normal but matrix does not become calcified properly, resulting in rickets

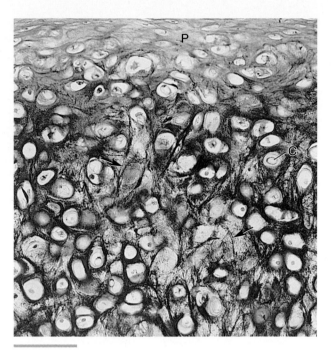

Figure 7–3 Light micrograph of elastic cartilage (×132). Observe the perichondrium (P) and the chondrocytes (C) in their lacunae (shrunken from the walls because of processing), some of which contain more than one cell, evidence of interstitial growth. Elastic fibers (*arrows*) are scattered throughout.

the larynx (cuneiform cartilage). Because of the presence of elastic fibers, elastic cartilage is somewhat yellow and is more opaque than hyaline cartilage in the fresh state (see Table 7-1).

In most respects, elastic cartilage is identical to hyaline cartilage and is often associated with it. The outer fibrous layer of the perichondrium is rich in elastic fibers. The matrix of elastic cartilage possesses abundant, fine to coarse branching elastic fibers interposed with type II collagen fiber bundles, giving it much more flexibility than the matrix of hyaline cartilage (Fig. 7-3). The chondrocytes of elastic cartilage are more abundant and larger than those of hyaline cartilage. The matrix is not as ample as in hyaline cartilage, and the elastic fiber bundles of the territorial matrix are larger and coarser than those of the interterritorial matrix.

Fibrocartilage

Fibrocartilage, unlike hyaline and elastic cartilage, does not possess a perichondrium and its matrix includes type I collagen.

Fibrocartilage is present in intervertebral disks, in the pubic symphysis, in articular disks, and attached to bone. It is associated with hyaline cartilage and with dense connective tissue, which it resembles. Unlike the other two types of cartilage, fibrocartilage does not possess a perichondrium. It displays a scant amount of matrix (rich in chondroitin sulfate and dermatan sulfate), and exhibits bundles of type I collagen, which stain acidophilic (Fig. 7-4). Chondrocytes are often aligned in alternating parallel rows with the thick, coarse bundles of collagen, which parallel the tensile forces attendant on this tissue (see Table 7-1).

Chondrocytes of fibrocartilage usually arise from fibroblasts that begin to manufacture proteoglycans. As the ground substance surrounds the fibroblast, the cell becomes incarcerated in its own matrix and differentiates into a chondrocyte.

Intervertebral disks represent an example of the organization of fibrocartilage. They are interposed between the hyaline cartilage coverings of the articular surface of successive vertebrae. Each disk contains a gelatinous center, called the **nucleus pulposus,** which is composed of cells, derived from the notochord, lying within a hyaluronic acid-rich matrix. These cells disappear by the 20th year of life. Much of the nucleus pulposus is surrounded by the annulus fibrosus, layers of fibrocartilage whose type I collagen fibers run vertically between the hyaline cartilages

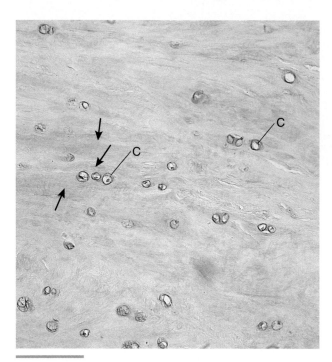

Figure 7–4 Light micrograph of fibrocartilage (×132). Note alignment of the chondrocytes (C) in rows interspersed with thick bundles of collagen fibers (*arrows*).

of the two vertebrae. The fibers of adjacent lamellae are oriented obliquely to each other, providing support to the gelatinous nucleus pulposus. The annulus fibrosus provides resistance against tensile forces, whereas the nucleus pulposus resists forces of compression.

CLINICAL CORRELATIONS

A ruptured disk refers to a tear or break in the laminae of the annulus fibrosus through which the gel-like nucleus pulposus extrudes. This condition occurs more often on the posterior portions of the intervertebral disks, particularly in the lumbar portion of the back, where the disk may dislocate, or slip. A "slipped disk" leads to severe, intense pain in the lower back and extremities as the displaced disk compresses the lower spinal nerves.

BONE

Bone is a specialized connective tissue whose extracellular matrix is calcified, incarcerating the cells that secreted it.

Although bone is one of the hardest substances of the body, it is a dynamic tissue that constantly changes shape in relation to the stresses placed on it. For example, pressures applied to bone lead to its resorption, whereas tension applied to it results in development of new bone. In applying these facts, the orthodontist is able to remodel the bone of the dental arches by moving and straightening the teeth to correct malocclusion, thus providing the patient with a more natural and pleasant smile.

Bone is the primary structural framework for support and protection of the organs of the body, including the brain and spinal cord and the structures within the thoracic cavity, namely the lungs and heart. The bones also serve as levers for the muscles attached to them, thereby multiplying the force of the muscles to attain movement. Bone is a reservoir for several minerals of the body; for example, it stores about 99% of the body's calcium. Bone contains a central cavity, the **marrow cavity,** which houses the **bone marrow,** a hemopoietic organ.

Bone is covered on its external surface, except at synovial articulations, with **periosteum,** which consists of an outer layer of dense fibrous connective tissue and an inner cellular layer containing osteoprogenitor (osteogenic) cells. The central cavity of a bone is lined with **endosteum,** a specialized thin, connective tissue composed of a monolayer of **osteoprogenitor cells** and **osteoblasts.**

Bone is composed of cells lying in an extracellular matrix that has become calcified. The calcified matrix is composed of fibers and ground substance. The fibers constituting bone are primarily type I collagen. The ground substance is rich in proteoglycans with chondroitin sulfate and keratan sulfate side chains. In addition, glycoproteins such as osteonectin, osteocalcin, osteopontin, and bone sialoprotein are present.

The cells of bone include **osteoprogenitor cells,** which differentiate into **osteoblasts.** Osteoblasts are responsible for secreting the matrix. When these cells are surrounded by matrix, they become quiescent and are known as osteocytes. The spaces osteocytes occupy are known as lacunae (Fig. 7-5). Osteoclasts, multinucleated giant cells derived from fused bone marrow precursors, are responsible for bone resorption and remodeling.

Because bone is such a hard tissue, two methods are employed to prepare it for study. **Decalcified sections** can be prepared by decalcifying the bone in an acid solution to remove the calcium salts. The tissue can then be embedded, sectioned, and routinely stained for study. **Ground sections** are prepared by sawing the bone into thin slices, followed by grinding the sections with abrasives between glass plates. When the section is sufficiently thin for study with light microscope, it is mounted for study.

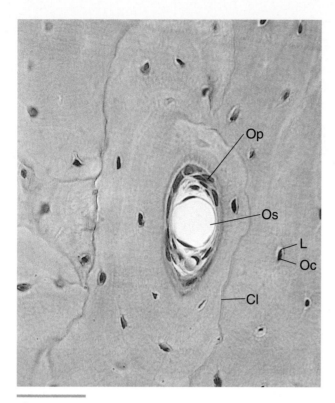

Figure 7–5 Light micrograph of decalcified compact bone (×540). Osteocytes (Oc) may be observed in lacunae (L). Also note the osteon (Os), osteoprogenitor cells (Op), and the cementing lines (Cl).

Each system has disadvantages. In decalcified sections, osteocytes are distorted by the decalcifying acid bath; in ground sections, the cells are destroyed, and the lacunae and canaliculi are filled in with bone debris.

Bone Matrix

Bone matrix has inorganic and organic constituents.

Inorganic Component

The inorganic constituents of bone are crystals of calcium hydroxyapatite, composed mostly of calcium and phosphorus.

The inorganic portion of bone, which constitutes about 65% of its dry weight, is composed mainly of calcium and phosphorus along with other components, including bicarbonate, citrate, magnesium, sodium, and potassium. Calcium and phosphorus exist primarily in the form of **hydroxyapatite crystals** $[Ca_{10}(PO_4)_6(OH)_2]$, but calcium phosphate is also present in an amorphous form. Hydroxyapatite crystals (40-nm long by 25-nm wide by 1.5- to 3-nm thick) are arranged in an ordered fashion along the type I collagen fibers; they are

deposited into the gap regions of the collagen but also are present along the overlap region. The free surface of the crystals is surrounded by amorphous ground substance. The surface ions of the crystals attract H_2O and form a **hydration shell,** which permits ion exchange with the extracellular fluid.

Bone is one of the hardest and strongest substances in the body. Its hardness and strength are due to the association of hydroxyapatite crystals with collagen. If bone is decalcified (i.e., all of the mineral is removed from the bone), it still retains its original shape but becomes so flexible that it can be bent like a piece of tough rubber. If the organic component is extracted from bone, the mineralized skeleton still retains its original shape, but it becomes extremely brittle and can be fractured with ease.

Organic Component

The predominant organic component of bone is type I collagen.

The organic component of bone matrix, constituting approximately 35% of the dry weight of bone, includes fibers that are almost exclusively type I collagen.

Collagen, most of which is type I, makes up about 80% to 90% of the organic component of bone. It is formed in large (50 to 70 nm in diameter) bundles displaying a typical 67-nm periodicity. Type I collagen in bone is highly cross-linked, which prevents it from being easily extracted.

The fact that bone matrix stains with PAS reagent and displays slight metachromasia indicates the presence of sulfated glycosaminoglycans, namely chondroitin sulfate and keratan sulfate. These form small proteoglycan molecules with short protein cores to which the glycosaminoglycans are covalently bound. The proteoglycans are noncovalently bound, via link proteins, to hyaluronic acid, forming very large **aggrecan composites.** The abundance of collagen, however, causes the matrix to be acidophilic.

Several glycoproteins are also present in the bone matrix. These appear to be restricted to bone and include **osteocalcin,** which binds to hydroxyapatite, and **osteopontin,** which also binds to hydroxyapatite but has additional binding sites for other components as well as for integrins present on osteoblasts and osteoclasts. Vitamin D stimulates the synthesis of these glycoproteins. Bone **sialoprotein,** another matrix protein, has binding sites for matrix components and integrins of osteoblasts and osteocytes, suggesting its involvement in the adherence of these cells to bone matrix.

Cells of Bone

The cells of bone are osteoprogenitor cells, osteoblasts, osteocytes, and osteoclasts.

Osteoprogenitor Cells

Osteoprogenitor cells are derived from embryonic mesenchymal cells and retain their ability to undergo mitosis.

Osteoprogenitor cells are located in the inner cellular layer of the periosteum, lining haversian canals, and in the endosteum (see Fig. 7-5). These cells, derived from embryonic mesenchyme, remain in place throughout postnatal life and can undergo mitotic division and have the potential to differentiate into osteoblasts. Moreover, under certain conditions of low oxygen tension, these cells may differentiate into chondrogenic cells. Osteoprogenitor cells are spindle-shaped and have a pale-staining oval nucleus; their scant pale-staining cytoplasm displays sparse RER and a poorly developed Golgi apparatus but an abundance of free ribosomes. These cells are most active during the period of intense bone growth.

Osteoblasts

Osteoblasts not only synthesize the organic matrix of bone but also possess receptors for parathyroid hormone.

Osteoblasts are derived from osteoprogenitor cells and develop under the influence of the **bone morphogenic protein (BMP) family** and **transforming growth factor-β**. Osteoblasts are responsible for the synthesis of the organic protein components of the bone matrix, including type I collagen, proteoglycans, and glycoproteins. Additionally, they produce **RANKL** (receptor for activation of nuclear factor kappa B), **osteocalcin** (for bone mineralization), **osteopontin** (for formation of sealing zone between osteoclasts and the subosteoclastic compartment), **osteonectin** (related to bone mineralization), **bone sialoprotein** (binding osteoblasts to extracellular matrix), and macrophage colony-stimulating factor (**M-CSF**) (discussed later). Osteoblasts are located on the surface of the bone in a sheet-like arrangement of cuboidal to columnar cells (Fig. 7-6). When actively secreting matrix, they exhibit a basophilic cytoplasm.

The organelles of osteoblasts are polarized so that the nucleus is located away from the region of secretory activity, which houses secretory granules believed to contain matrix precursors. The contents of these vesicles stain pink with PAS reagent.

Electron micrographs exhibit abundant RER, a well-developed Golgi complex (Fig. 7-7A), and numerous secretory vesicles containing flocculent material that accounts for the PAS pink-staining vacuoles observed in the light microscope. Osteoblasts extend short processes that make contact with those of neighboring osteoblasts, as well as long processes that make contact

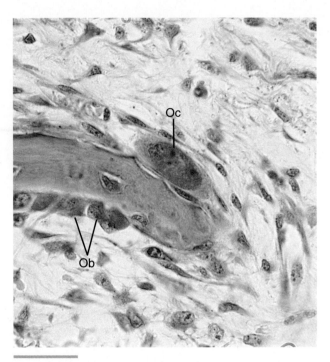

Figure 7–6 Light micrograph of intramembranous ossification (×540). Osteoblasts (Ob) line the bony spicule where they are secreting osteoid onto the bone. Osteoclasts (Oc) may be observed housed in Howship's lacunae.

with processes of osteocytes. Although these processes form **gap junctions** with one another, the number of gap junctions between osteoblasts is much fewer than those between osteocytes.

CLINICAL CORRELATIONS

Osteoblast cell membranes are rich in the enzyme **alkaline phosphatase.** During active bone formation, these cells secrete high levels of alkaline phosphatase, elevating the levels of this enzyme in the blood. Thus, the clinician can monitor bone formation by measuring the blood alkaline phosphatase level.

As osteoblasts exocytose their secretory products, each cell surrounds itself with the bone matrix it has just produced; when this occurs, the incarcerated cell is referred to as an osteocyte, and the space it occupies is known as a **lacuna.** Most of the bone matrix becomes calcified; however, osteoblasts as well as osteocytes are always separated from the calcified substance by a thin, noncalcified layer known as the **osteoid** (uncalcified bone matrix).

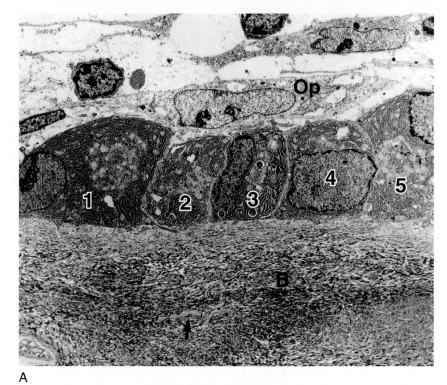

A

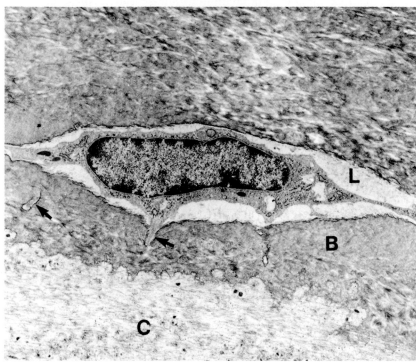

B

Figure 7–7 Electron micrographs of bone-forming cells. **A,** Five osteoblasts (1 to 5) lined up on the surface of bone (B) displaying abundant rough endoplasmic reticulum. Observe the process of an osteocyte in a canaliculus (*arrow*). The cell with the elongated nucleus lying above the osteoblasts is an osteoprogenitor cell (Op) (×2500). **B,** Note the osteocyte in its lacuna (L) with its processes extending into canaliculi (*arrows*) (×1000). B, bone; C, cartilage. (From Marks SC Jr, Popoff SN: Bone cell biology: The regulation of development, structure, and function in the skeleton. Am J Anat 183:1-44, 1988.)

Surface osteoblasts that cease to form matrix revert to a more flattened-shaped quiescent state and are called **bone-lining cells.** Although these cells appear to be similar to osteoprogenitor cells, they are most likely incapable of dividing but can be reactivated to the secreting form with the proper stimulus.

Osteoblasts have several factors on their cell membranes, the most significant of which are integrins and **parathyroid hormone receptors.** When parathyroid hormone binds to these receptors, it stimulates osteoblasts to secrete **osteoprotegerin ligand (OPGL),** a factor that induces the differentiation of preosteoclasts into osteoclasts and it increases RANKL expression. Also osteoblasts secrete an **osteoclast-stimulating factor,** which activates osteoclasts to resorb bone. Osteoblasts also secrete enzymes responsible for removing osteoid so that osteoclasts can make contact with the mineralized bone surface.

Osteocytes

Osteocytes are mature bone cells derived from osteoblasts that became trapped in their lacunae.

Osteocytes are mature bone cells, derived from osteoblasts, that are housed in **lacunae** within the calcified bony matrix (see Figs. 7-5 and 7-7B). There are as many as 20,000 to 30,000 osteocytes per mm^3 of bone. Radiating out in all directions from the lacunaa are narrow, tunnel-like spaces (**canaliculi**) that house cytoplasmic processes of the osteocyte. These processes make contact with similar processes of neighboring osteocytes, forming **gap junctions** through which ions and small molecules can move between the cells. The canaliculi also contain extracellular fluid carrying nutrients and metabolites that nourish the osteocytes.

Osteocytes conform to the shape of their lacunae. Their nucleus is flattened, and their cytoplasm is poor in organelles, displaying scant RER and a greatly reduced Golgi apparatus. Although osteocytes appear to be inactive cells, they secrete substances necessary for bone maintenance. These cells have also been implicated in **mechanotransduction,** in that they respond to stimuli that place tension on bone by releasing cyclic adenosine monophosphate (cAMP), osteocalcin, and insulin-like growth factor. The release of these factors facilitates the recruitment of preosteoblasts to assist in the remodeling of the skeleton (adding more bone) not only during growth and development but also during the long-term redistribution of forces acting on the skeleton. An example of such remodeling is evident in the comparison of male and female skeletons, in which the muscle attachments of the male skeleton are usually better defined than those of the female skeleton.

The interval between the osteocyte plasmalemma and the walls of the lacunae and canaliculi, known as the **periosteocytic space,** is occupied by extracellular fluid. Considering the extensive network of the canaliculi and the sheer number of osteocytes present in the skeleton of an average person, the volume of the periosteocytic space and the surface area of the walls have been calculated to be a staggering 1.3 L and as much as 5000 m^2, respectively. It has been suggested that the 1.3 L of extracellular fluid occupying the periosteocytic space is exposed to as much as 20 g of exchangeable calcium that can be resorbed from the walls of these spaces. The resorbed calcium gains access to the bloodstream and ensures the maintenance of adequate blood calcium levels.

Osteoclasts

Osteoclasts are multinucleated cells originating from granulocyte-macrophage progenitors. They play a role in bone resorption.

The precursor of the osteoclast originates in the bone marrow. Osteoclasts have receptors for osteoclast-stimulating factor, colony-stimulating factor-1, osteoprotegerin (OPG), and calcitonin, among others. Osteoclasts are responsible for resorbing bone, and after they finish doing so, these cells probably undergo apoptosis.

Morphology of Osteoclasts

Osteoclasts are large, motile, multinucleated cells 150 μm in diameter; they contain up to 50 nuclei and have an acidophilic cytoplasm (see Fig. 7-6). Osteoclasts were once thought to be derived from the fusion of many blood-derived monocytes, but the newest evidence shows that they have a bone marrow precursor in common with monocytes termed the **mononuclear-phagocyte system.** These precursor cells are stimulated by macrophage colony–stimulating factor to undergo mitosis. In the presence of bone, these osteoclast precursors fuse to produce the multinucleated osteoclasts.

Osteoblasts secrete three signaling molecules that regulate the differentiation of osteoclasts. The first of these signals, the **macrophage colony–stimulating factor (M-CSF)** binds to a receptor on the macrophage, inducing it to become a proliferating osteoclast precursor, and it induces the expression of the receptor for activation of nuclear factor kappa B (**RANK**) on the precursor. Another osteoblast signaling molecule, RANKL, binds to the RANKL receptor on the osteoclastic precursor, inducing it to differentiate into the multinucleated osteoclast, activating it, and enhancing bone resorption. The third signaling molecule, **OPG,** a member of the **tumor necrosis factor receptor (TNFR)** family, can serve as a decoy by interacting with RANKL, thus prohibiting it from binding to the macrophage and thus inhibiting osteoclast formation. In this way, RANKL, RANK, and OPG regulate bone metabolism and osteoclastic activity. OPG is produced not only by osteoblasts but by cells of many other tissues, including the cardiovascular system, lung, kidney, intestines, as well as hematopoietic and immune cells. Therefore it is not surprising that its expression is modulated by various means by cytokines, peptides, hormones, drugs, and so forth. In bone, OPG not only inhibits the differentiation of precursor cells into osteoclasts but also suppresses the osteoclast's bone resorptive capacities. Also, tensional forces on bone trigger OPG and mRNA synthesis.

Osteoclasts occupy shallow depressions, called **Howship's lacunae,** that identify regions of bone resorption. An osteoclast active in bone resorption may be subdivided into four morphologically recognizable regions:

1 The **basal zone,** located farthest from the Howship lacunae, houses most of the organelles, including the multiple nuclei and their associated Golgi complexes and centrioles. Mitochondria, RER, and polysomes are distributed throughout the cell but are more numerous near the ruffled border.
2 The **ruffled border** is the portion of the cell that is directly involved in resorption of bone. Its finger-like processes are active and dynamic, changing their configuration continuously as they project into the resorption compartment, known as the **subosteoclastic compartment.** The cytoplasmic aspect of the ruffled border plasmalemma displays a regularly spaced, bristle-like coat that increases the thickness of the plasma membrane of this region.

3 The **clear zone** is the region of the cell that immediately surrounds the periphery of the ruffled border. It is organelle-free but contains many actin microfilaments that form an **actin ring** and appear to function in helping integrins of the clear zone plasmalemma maintain contact with the bony periphery of the Howship lacunae. In fact, the plasma membrane of this region is so closely applied to the bone that it forms the **sealing zone** of the subosteoclastic compartment. Thus, the clear zone isolates the subosteoclastic compartment from the surrounding region, establishing a microenvironment whose contents may be modulated by cellular activities. For the osteoclast to be able to resorb bone, the actin ring must first be formed, and its formation may be facilitated by **OPGL.** Then the ruffled border is formed, whose finger-like processes increase the surface area of the plasmalemma in the region of bone resorption, facilitating the resorptive process.
4 The **vesicular zone** of the osteoclast consists of numerous endocytotic and exocytotic vesicles that ferry lysosomal enzymes and metalloproteinases into the subosteoclastic compartment and the products of bone degradation into the cell (Fig. 7-8). The

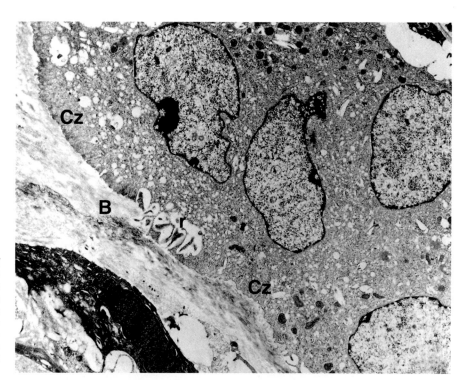

Figure 7–8 Electron micrograph of an osteoclast. Note the clear zone (Cz) on either side of the ruffled border (B) of this multinucleated cell. (From Marks SC Jr, Walker DG: The hematogenous origin of osteoclasts. Experimental evidence from osteopetrotic [microphthalmic] mice treated with spleen cells from beige mouse donors. Am J Anat 161:1-10, 1981.)

vesicular zone is between the basal zone and the ruffled border.

Mechanism of Bone Resorption

Within osteoclasts, the enzyme carbonic anhydrase catalyzes the intracellular formation of carbonic acid (H_2CO_3) from carbon dioxide and water. Carbonic acid dissociates within the cells into H^+ ions and bicarbonate ions, HCO_3^-. The bicarbonate ions, accompanied by Na^+ ions, cross the plasmalemma and enter nearby capillaries. Proton pumps in the plasmalemma of the ruffled border of the osteoclasts actively transport H^+ ions into the subosteoclastic compartment, reducing the pH of the microenvironment (Cl^- ions follow passively). The inorganic component of the matrix is dissolved as the environment becomes acidic; the liberated minerals enter the osteoclast cytoplasm to be delivered to nearby capillaries.

Lysosomal hydrolases and **metalloproteinases,** such as **collagenase** and **gelatinase,** are secreted by osteoclasts into the subosteoclastic compartment to degrade the organic components of the decalcified bone matrix. The degradation products are endocytosed by the osteoclasts and further broken down into amino acids, monosaccharides, and disaccharides, which then are released into nearby capillaries (Fig. 7-9).

CLINICAL CORRELATIONS

Osteopetrosis, not to be confused with osteoporosis, is a genetic disorder where osteoclasts do not possess a ruffled border. Consequently, these osteoclasts cannot resorb bone and persons with osteopetrosis display increased bone density. Individuals suffering from this disease may exhibit anemia resulting from decreased marrow space, as well as blindness, deafness, and cranial nerve involvement because of impingement of the nerves due to narrowing of the foramina.

Hormonal Control of Bone Resorption

The bone-resorbing activity of osteoclasts is regulated by two hormones, parathyroid hormone and calcitonin, produced by the parathyroid and thyroid gland, respectively.

Bone Structure

Bones are classified according to their anatomical shape: long, short, flat, irregular, and sesamoid.

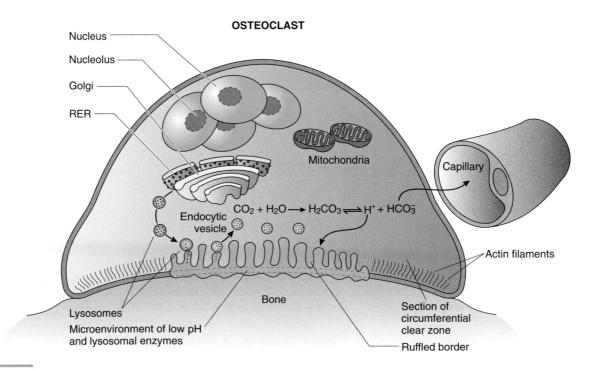

OSTEOCLAST

Nucleus
Nucleolus
Golgi
RER
Mitochondria
Capillary
$CO_2 + H_2O \longrightarrow H_2CO_3 \rightleftharpoons H^+ + HCO_3^-$
Endocytic vesicle
Actin filaments
Lysosomes
Bone
Section of circumferential clear zone
Microenvironment of low pH and lysosomal enzymes
Ruffled border

Figure 7–9 Osteoclastic function. RER, rough endoplasmic reticulum. (From Gartner LP, Hiatt JL, Strum JM: Cell Biology and Histology [Board Review Series]. Philadelphia, Lippincott Williams & Wilkins, 1998, p 100.)

Bones are classified according to their shape:

- **Long bones** display a shaft located between two heads (e.g., tibia).
- **Short bones** have more or less the same width and length (e.g., carpal bones of the wrist).
- **Flat bones** are flat, thin, and plate-like (e.g., bones forming the brain case of the skull).
- **Irregular bones** have an irregular shape that does not fit into the other classes (e.g., sphenoid and ethmoid bones within the skull).
- **Sesamoid bones** develop within tendons, where they increase the mechanical advantage for the muscle (e.g., patella) across a joint.

Gross Observation of Bone

Gross observations of the femur (a long bone) cut in longitudinal section reveal two different types of bone structure. The very dense bone on the outside surface is **compact bone,** whereas the porous portion lining the marrow cavity is **cancellous** or **spongy bone** (Fig. 7-10). Closer observation of the spongy bone reveals branching bony **trabeculae** and **spicules** jutting out from the internal surface of the compact bone into the marrow cavity. There are no haversian systems in spongy bone, but there are irregular arrangements of lamellae. These contain lacunae housing osteocytes that are nourished by diffusion from the marrow cavity, which is filled with bone marrow.

Bone marrow exists as two types: **red bone marrow,** in which blood cells are forming, and **yellow bone marrow,** composed mostly of fat.

The shaft of a long bone is called the **diaphysis,** and the articular ends are called the **epiphyses** (singular, epiphysis). In a person who is still growing, the diaphysis is separated from each epiphysis by the **epiphyseal plate** of cartilage. The articular end of the bone is enlarged and sculpted to articulate with its bony counterpart of the joint. The surface of the articulating end is covered with only a thin layer of compact bone overlying spongy bone. On top of this is the highly polished articular hyaline cartilage, which reduces friction as it moves against the articular cartilage of the bony counterpart of the joint. The area of transition between the epiphyseal plate and the diaphysis is called the **metaphysis,** where columns of spongy bone are located. It is from the epiphyseal plate and the metaphysis that bone grows in length.

The diaphysis is covered by a **periosteum** except where tendons and muscles insert into the bone. There is no periosteum on the surfaces of bone covered by articular cartilage. Periosteum is also absent from sesamoid bones (e.g., patella), which are formed within tendons and function to increase the mechanical advantage across a joint. The periosteum is a noncalcified, dense, irregular, collagenous connective tissue covering the bone on its external surface and inserting into it via **Sharpey's fibers** (see Fig. 7-10). Periosteum is composed of two layers. The **outer fibrous layer** helps distribute vascular and nerve supply to bone, whereas the **inner cellular layer** possesses osteoprogenitor cells and osteoblasts.

The flat bones of the skull develop by a method different from that of most of the long bones of the body. The inner and outer surfaces of the calvaria (**skull cap**) possess two relatively thick layers of compact bone called the **inner** and **outer tables,** which surround the spongy bone (**diploë**) sandwiched between them. The outer table possesses a periosteum, identified as the **pericranium,** whereas internally the inner table is lined with **dura mater,** which serves as a periosteum for the inner table and as a protective covering for the brain.

Bone Types Based on Microscopic Observations

Microscopically, bone is classified as either primary (immature) or secondary (mature) bone.

Microscopic observations reveal two types of bone: primary bone, or immature or woven bone, and secondary bones, or mature or lamellar bone.

Primary bone is immature in that it is the first bone to form during fetal development and during bone repair. It has abundant osteocytes and irregular bundles of collagen, which are later replaced and organized as secondary bone except in certain areas (e.g., at sutures of the calvaria, insertion sites of tendons, and bony alveoli surrounding the teeth). The mineral content of primary bone is also much less than that of secondary bone.

Secondary bone is mature bone composed of parallel or concentric bony lamellae 3- to 7-μm thick. Osteocytes in their lacunae are dispersed at regular intervals between, or occasionally within, lamellae. **Canaliculi,** housing osteocytic processes, connect neighboring lacunae with one another, forming a network of intercommunicating channels that facilitate the flow of nutrients, hormones, ions, and waste products to and from osteocytes. In addition, osteocytic processes within these canaliculi make contact with similar processes of neighboring osteocytes and form gap junctions, permitting these cells to communicate with each other.

Because the matrix of secondary bone is more calcified, it is stronger than primary bone. In addition, the collagen fibers of secondary bone are arranged so that they parallel each other within a given lamella.

Lamellar Systems of Compact Bone

There are four lamellar systems in compact bone: outer circumferential lamellae, inner circumferential lamellae, osteons, and interstitial lamellae.

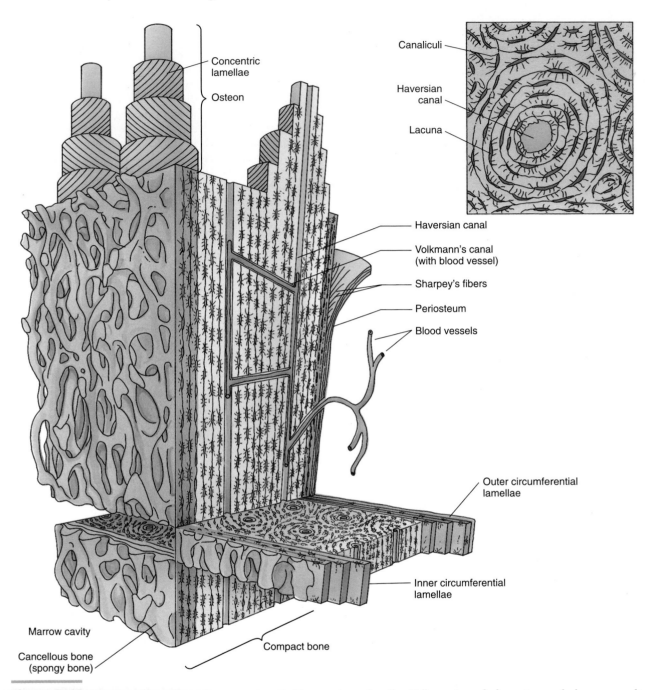

Figure 7–10 Diagram of bone illustrating compact cortical bone, osteons, lamellae, Volkmann's canals, haversian canals, lacunae, canaliculi, and spongy bone.

Compact bone is composed of wafer-like thin layers of bone, **lamellae,** that are arranged in lamellar systems that are especially evident in the diaphyses of long bones. These lamellar systems are the outer circumferential lamellae, inner circumferential lamellae, osteons (haversian canal systems), and interstitial lamellae.

OUTER AND INNER CIRCUMFERENTIAL LAMELLAE

The **outer circumferential lamellae** are just deep to the periosteum, forming the outermost region of the diaphysis, and contain Sharpey's fibers anchoring the periosteum to the bone (see Fig. 7-10).

The **inner circumferential lamellae,** analogous to but not as extensive as outer circumferential lamellae, completely encircle the marrow cavity. Trabeculae of spongy bone extend from the inner circumferential lamellae into the marrow cavity, interrupting the endosteal lining of the inner circumferential lamellae.

HAVERSIAN CANAL SYSTEMS (OSTEONS)

The bulk of compact bone is composed of an abundance of **haversian canal systems (osteons);** each system is composed of cylinders of lamellae, concentrically arranged around a vascular space known as the haversian canal (Fig. 7-11; also see Fig. 7-10). Frequently, osteons bifurcate along their considerable length. Each osteon is bounded by a thin **cementing line,** composed mostly of calcified ground substance with a scant amount of collagen fibers (see Fig. 7-5).

Collagen fiber bundles are parallel to each other within a lamella but are oriented almost perpendicular to those of adjacent lamellae. This arrangement is possible because the collagen fibers follow a helical arrangement around the haversian canal within each lamella but are pitched differently in adjacent lamellae.

Each haversian canal, lined by a layer of osteoblasts and osteoprogenitor cells, houses a neurovascular bundle with its associated connective tissue. Haversian canals of adjacent osteons are connected to each other by **Volkmann's canals** (Fig. 7-12; also see Fig. 7-10). These vascular spaces are oriented oblique to or perpendicular to haversian canals.

The diameter of haversian canals varies from approximately 20 μm to about 100 μm. During the formation of osteons, the lamella closest to the cementing line is the first one to be formed. As additional lamellae are added to the system, the diameter of the haversian canal is reduced, and the thickness of the osteon wall increases. Because nutrients from blood vessels of the haversian canal must traverse canaliculi to reach osteocytes, an inefficient process, most osteons possess only 4 to 20 lamellae.

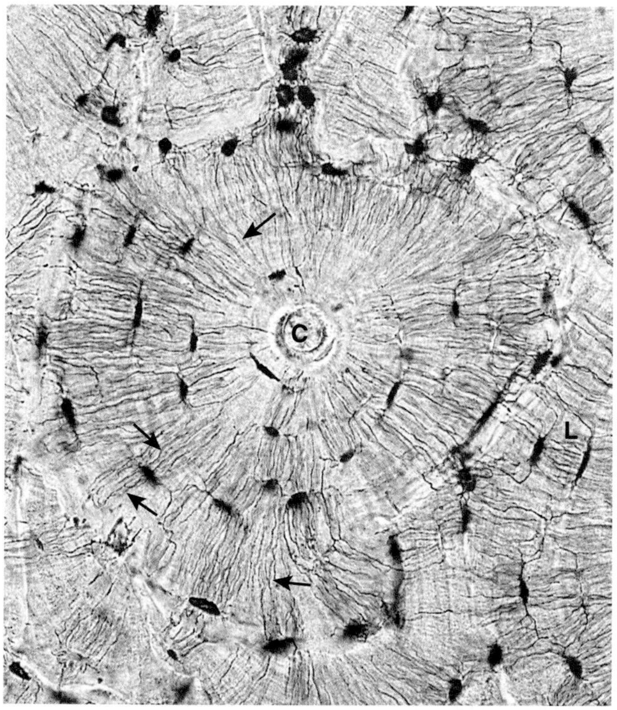

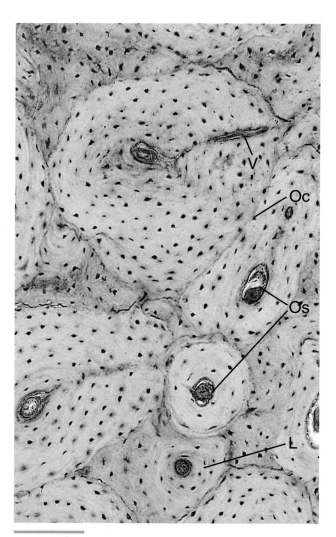

Figure 7–11 Light micrograph of undecalcified ground bone (×270). Observe the haversian system containing the haversian canal (C) and concentric lamellae (L) with lacunae with their canaliculi (*arrows*).

Figure 7–12 Light micrograph of decalcified compact bone (×162). Several osteons (Os) are displayed with their concentric lamellae (L). A Volkmann's canal (V) is also displayed. The dark-staining structures scattered throughout represent nuclei of osteocytes (Oc).

As bone is being remodeled, osteoclasts resorb osteons and osteoblasts replace them. Remnants of osteons remain as irregular arcs of lamellar fragments, known as **interstitial lamellae,** surrounded by osteons. Like osteons, interstitial lamellae are also surrounded by cementing lines.

Histogenesis of Bone

Bone formation during embryonic development may be of two types: **intramembranous** and **endochondral.** Bone that is formed by either of the two methods is identical histologically. The first bone formed is primary bone, which is later resorbed and replaced by secondary bone. Secondary bone continues to be resorbed throughout life, although at a slower rate.

Intramembranous Bone Formation

Intramembranous bone formation occurs within mesenchymal tissue.

Most flat bones are formed by intramembranous bone formation. This process occurs in a richly vascularized mesenchymal tissue, whose cells make contact with each other via long processes.

Mesenchymal cells differentiate into **osteoblasts** that secrete **bone matrix,** forming a network of **spicules** and **trabeculae** whose surfaces are populated by these cells (Figs. 7-13 and 7-14). This region of initial osteogenesis is known as the **primary ossification center.** The collagen fibers of these developing spicules and trabeculae are randomly oriented, as expected in primary bone. Calcification quickly follows osteoid

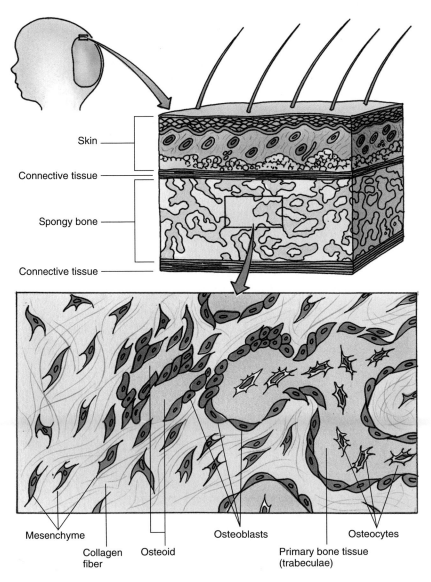

Skin

Connective tissue

Spongy bone

Connective tissue

Mesenchyme

Collagen fiber

Osteoid

Osteoblasts

Osteocytes

Primary bone tissue (trabeculae)

Figure 7–13 Intramembranous bone formation.

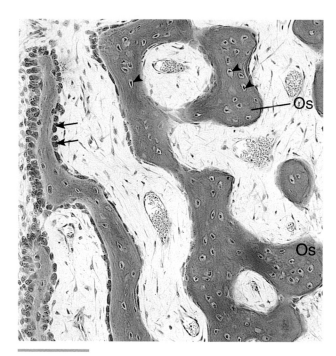

Figure 7–14 Light micrograph of intramembranous bone formation (ossification) (×132). Trabeculae of bone are being formed by osteoblasts lining their surface *(arrows)*. Observe osteocytes trapped in lacunae *(arrowheads)*. Primitive osteons (Os) are beginning to form.

formation, and osteoblasts trapped in their matrices become osteocytes. The processes of these osteocytes are also surrounded by forming bone, establishing a system of canaliculi. Continuous mitotic activity of mesenchymal cells provides a supply of undifferentiated **osteoprogenitor cells,** which form osteoblasts.

As the sponge-like network of trabeculae is established, the vascular connective tissue in their interstices is transformed into bone marrow. The addition of trabeculae to the periphery increases the size of the forming bone. Larger bones, such as the occipital bone of the base of the skull, have several ossification centers, which fuse with each other to form a single bone. The fontanelles ("soft spots") on the frontal and parietal bones of a newborn infant represent ossification centers that are not fused prenatally.

Regions of the mesenchymal tissues that remain uncalcified differentiate into the periosteum and endosteum of developing bone. Moreover, the spongy bone deep to the periosteum and the periosteal layer of the dura mater of flat bones are transformed into compact bone, forming the **inner** and **outer tables** with the intervening diploë.

Endochondral Bone Formation

Endochondral bone formation requires the presence of a cartilage template.

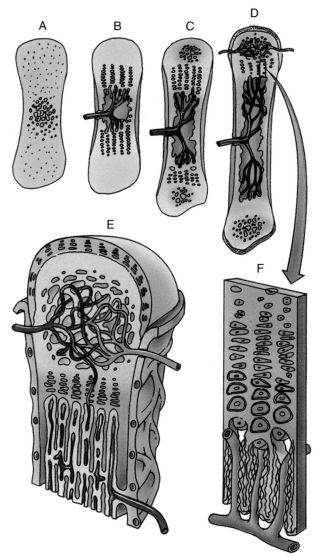

Figure 7–15 Endochondral bone formation. *Blue* represents the cartilage model upon which bone is formed. The bone then replaces the cartilage. **A,** Hyaline cartilage model. **B,** Cartilage at the midriff (diaphysis) is invaded by vascular elements. **C,** Subperiosteal bone collar is formed. **D,** Bone collar prevents nutrients from reaching cartilage cells so they die leaving confluent lacunae. Osteoclasts invade and etch bone to permit periosteal bud to form. **E,** Calcified bone/calcified cartilage complex at epiphyseal ends of the growing bone. **F,** Enlargement of the epiphyseal plate at the end of the bone where bone replaces cartilage.

Most of the long and short bones of the body develop by endochondral bone formation (Table 7-3). This type of bone formation occurs in several phases, the most critical of which are (1) formation of a miniature hyaline cartilage model, (2) continued growth of the model, which serves as a structural scaffold for bone development, and (3) eventual resorption and replacement by bone (Fig. 7-15).

TABLE 7–3 Events in Endochondral Bone Formation

Event	Description
Hyaline cartilage model formed.	Miniature hyaline cartilage model formed in region of developing embryo where bone is to develop; some chondrocytes mature, hypertrophy, and die; cartilage matrix becomes calcified
Primary Center of Ossification	
Perichondrium at the midriff of diaphysis becomes vascularized.	Vascularization of perichondrium changes it to periosteum Chondrogenic cells become osteoprogenitor cells
Osteoblasts secrete matrix, forming subperiosteal bone collar.	The subperiosteal bone collar is formed of primary bone (intramembranous bone formation)
Chondrocytes within the diaphysis core hypertrophy, die, and degenerate.	Presence of periosteum and bone prevents diffusion of nutrients to chondrocytes; their degeneration leaves lacunae, opening large spaces in septa of cartilage
Osteoclasts etch holes in subperiosteal bone collar, permitting entrance of osteogenic bud	Holes permit osteoprogenitor cells and capillaries to invade cartilage model, now calcified, and begin elaborating bone matrix
Calcified cartilage/calcified bone complex is formed.	Bone matrix laid down on septa of calcified cartilage forms this complex (histologically, calcified cartilage stains blue, calcified bone stains red)
Osteoclasts begin resorbing the calcified cartilage/calcified bone complex.	Destruction of the calcified cartilage/calcified bone complex enlarges the marrow cavity
Subperiosteal bone collar thickens, begins growing toward the epiphyses.	This event, over a period of time, completely replaces diaphyseal cartilage with bone
Secondary Center of Ossification	
Ossification begins at epiphysis.	Process begins in same way as at primary center, except that there is no bone collar; osteoblasts lay down bone matrix on calcified cartilage scaffold
Growth of bone occurs at epiphyseal plate.	Cartilaginous articular surface of bone remains; epiphyseal plate persists—growth added at epiphyseal end of plate. Bone is added at diaphyseal end of plate
Epiphysis and diaphysis become continuous.	At the end of bone growth, cartilage of epiphyseal plate ceases proliferation; bone development continues to unite the diaphysis and epiphysis

EVENTS OCCURRING AT THE PRIMARY CENTER OF OSSIFICATION

1 In the region where bone is to grow within the embryo, a **hyaline cartilage model of that bone develops.** This event begins in exactly the same way that hyaline cartilage at any location would develop (discussed earlier). For a period this model grows both appositionally and interstitially. Eventually, the chondrocytes in the center of the cartilage model hypertrophy, accumulate glycogen in their cytoplasm, and become vacuolated (Fig. 7-16). Hypertrophy of the chondrocytes results in enlargement of their lacunae and reduction in the intervening cartilage matrix septae, which become calcified.

2 Concurrently, **the perichondrium at the midriff of the diaphysis of cartilage becomes vascularized** (Fig. 7-17). When this happens, chondrogenic cells become osteoprogenitor cells forming osteoblasts, and the overlying perichondrium becomes a periosteum.

3 The newly formed **osteoblasts secrete bone matrix, forming the subperiosteal bone collar** on the surface of the cartilage template by intramembranous bone formation (see Fig. 7-17).

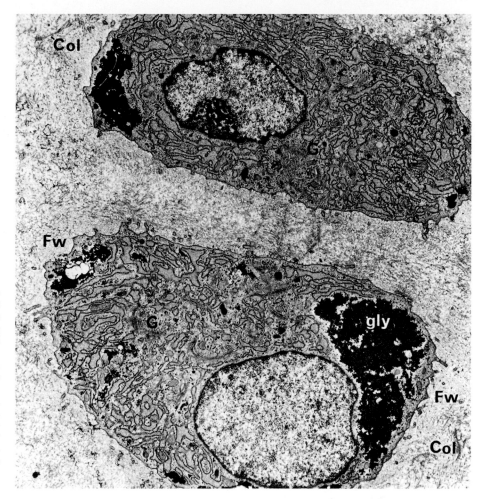

Figure 7–16 Electron micrograph of hypertrophic chondrocytes in the growing mandibular condyle (×83,000). Observe the abundant rough endoplasmic reticulum and developing Golgi apparatus (G). Note also glycogen (gly) deposits in one end of the cells, a characteristic of these cells shortly before death. Col, collagen fibers; Fw, territorial matrix. (From Marchi F, Luder HU, Leblond CP: Changes in cells' secretory organelles and extracellular matrix during endochondral ossification in the mandibular condyle of the growing rat. Am J Anat 190:41-73, 1991.)

4 The bone collar prevents the diffusion of nutrients to the hypertrophied chondrocytes within the core of the cartilage model, causing them to die. This process is responsible for the presence of empty, confluent lacunae forming large concavities—the future marrow cavity in the center of the cartilage model.

5 Holes etched in the bone collar by osteoclasts permit a **periosteal bud** (osteogenic bud), composed of osteoprogenitor cells, hemopoietic cells, and blood vessels, to enter the concavities within the cartilage model (see Fig. 7-15).

6 Osteoprogenitor cells divide to form osteoblasts. These newly formed cells elaborate bone matrix on the surface of the calcified cartilage. The bone matrix becomes calcified to form a **calcified cartilage/calcified bone complex.** This complex can be appreciated in routinely stained histological sections because calcified cartilage stains basophilic, whereas calcified bone stains acidophilic (Figs. 7-18 and 7-19).

7 As the subperiosteal bone becomes thicker and grows in each direction from the midriff of the diaphysis toward the epiphyses, osteoclasts begin resorbing the calcified cartilage/calcified bone complex, enlarging the marrow cavity. As this process continues, the cartilage of the diaphysis is replaced by bone except for the **epiphyseal plates,** which are responsible for the continued growth of the bone for 18 to 20 years.

EVENTS OCCURRING AT SECONDARY CENTERS OF OSSIFICATION

Secondary centers of ossification begin to form at the epiphysis at each end of the forming bone by a process similar to that in the diaphysis, except that a bone collar is not formed. Rather, osteoprogenitor cells invade the cartilage of the epiphysis, differentiate into osteoblasts, and begin secreting matrix on the cartilage scaffold (see Fig. 7-15). These events take place and progress much as they do in the diaphysis, and eventually the cartilage of the epiphysis is replaced with bone except at the articular surface and at the epiphyseal

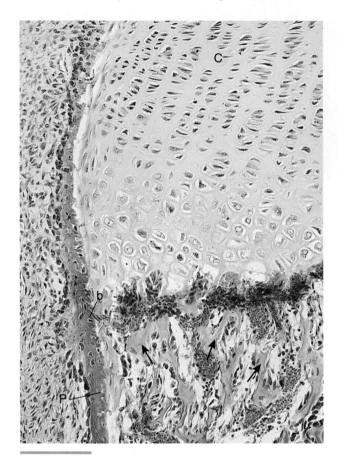

Figure 7–17 Light micrograph of endochondral bone formation (×14). The *upper half* demonstrates cartilage (C) containing chondrocytes that mature, hypertrophy, and calcify at the interface; the *lower half* shows where calcified cartilage/bone complex (*arrows*) is being resorbed and bone (b) is being formed. P, periosteum.

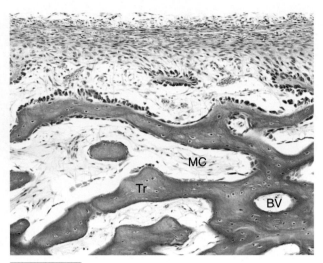

Figure 7–18 Light micrograph of endochondral bone formation (×132). Observe the blood vessel (BV), bone-covered trabeculae (Tr) of calcified cartilage, and medullary cavity (MC).

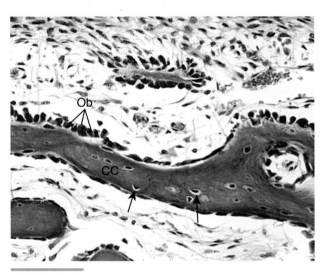

Figure 7–19 Higher magnification of endochondral bone formation (×270). The trabeculae of calcified cartilage (CC) are covered by a thin layer of bone (*darker red*) with osteocytes embedded in it (*arrows*) and with osteoblasts (Ob) lying next to the bone.

plate. The articular surface of the bone remains cartilaginous throughout life. The process at the epiphyseal plate, which controls bone length, is described in the next section.

These events are a dynamic continuum that is completed over a number of years as bone growth and development progress toward the growing epiphyses at each end of the bone (see Table 7-3). At the same time, the bone is constantly being remodeled to meet the changing forces placed on it.

BONE GROWTH IN LENGTH

The continued lengthening of bone depends on the epiphyseal plate.

The chondrocytes of the epiphyseal plate proliferate and participate in the process of endochondral bone formation. Proliferation occurs at the epiphyseal aspect, and replacement by bone takes place at the diaphyseal side of the plate. Histologically, the epiphyseal plate is divided into five recognizable zones. These zones, beginning at the epiphyseal side, are as follows:

- **Zone of reserve cartilage:** Chondrocytes randomly distributed throughout the matrix are mitotically active.
- **Zone of proliferation:** Chondrocytes, rapidly proliferating, form rows of isogenous cells that parallel the direction of bone growth.

- **Zone of maturation and hypertrophy:** Chondrocytes mature, hypertrophy, and accumulate glycogen in their cytoplasm (see Fig. 7-16). The matrix between their lacunae narrows with a corresponding growth of lacunae.
- **Zone of calcification:** Lacunae become confluent, hypertrophied chondrocytes die, and cartilage matrix becomes calcified.
- **Zone of ossification:** Osteoprogenitor cells invade the area and differentiate into osteoblasts, which elaborate matrix that becomes calcified on the surface of calcified cartilage. This is followed by resorption of the calcified cartilage/calcified bone complex.

As long as the rate of mitotic activity in the zone of proliferation equals the rate of resorption in the zone of ossification, the epiphyseal plate remains the same width and the bone continues to grow longer. At about the 20th year of age, the rate of mitosis decreases in the zone of proliferation and the zone of ossification overtakes the zones of proliferation and cartilage reserve. The cartilage of the epiphyseal plate is replaced by a plate of calcified cartilage/calcified bone complex, which is resorbed by osteoclastic activity, and the marrow cavity of the diaphysis becomes confluent with the bone marrow cavity of the epiphysis. Once the epiphyseal plate is resorbed, growth in length is no longer possible.

BONE GROWTH IN WIDTH

Bone growth in width takes place by appositional growth.

The events just described detail how bone lengthening is accomplished by the proliferation and interstitial growth of cartilage, which is eventually replaced by bone. Growth of the diaphysis in girth, however, takes place by **appositional growth.** The **osteoprogenitor cells** of the osteogenic layer of the periosteum proliferate and differentiate into osteoblasts that begin elaborating bone matrix on the subperiosteal bone surface. This process occurs continuously throughout the total period of bone growth and development, so that in a mature long bone the shaft is built via subperiosteal intramembranous bone formation.

During bone growth and development, bone resorption is as important as bone deposition. Formation of bone on the outside of the shaft must be accompanied by osteoclastic activity internally so that the marrow space can be enlarged.

Calcification of Bone

Calcification begins when there are deposits of calcium phosphate on the collagen fibril.

Exactly how calcification occurs is unclear, although it is known to be stimulated by certain proteoglycans and the Ca^{2+}-binding glycoprotein **osteonectin** as well as **bone sialoprotein.** One theory, called **heterogeneous nucleation,** is that collagen fibers in the matrix are nucleation sites for the metastable calcium and phosphate solution and that the solution begins to crystallize into the gap region of the collagen. Once this region has "nucleated," calcification proceeds.

The most commonly accepted theory of calcification is based on the presence of matrix vesicles within the osteoid. Osteoblasts release these small, membrane-bounded matrix vesicles, 100 to 200 nm in diameter, which contain a high concentration of Ca^{2+} and PO_4^{3-} ions, cAMP, adenosine triphosphate (ATP), adenosine triphosphatase (ATPase), alkaline phosphatase, pyrophosphatase, calcium-binding proteins, and phosphoserine. The matrix vesicle membrane possesses numerous calcium pumps, which transport Ca^{2+} ions into the vesicle. As the concentration of calcium Ca^{2+} ions within the vesicle increases, crystallization occurs and the growing calcium hydroxyapatite crystal pierces the membrane, bursting the matrix vesicle and releasing its contents.

Alkaline phosphatase cleaves pyrophosphate groups from the macromolecules of the matrix. The liberated pyrophosphate molecules are inhibitors of calcification, but they are cleaved by the enzyme pyrophosphatase into PO_4^{3-} ions, increasing the concentration of this ion in the microenvironment.

The calcium hydroxyapatite crystals released from the matrix vesicles act as **nidi of crystallization.** The high concentration of ions in their vicinity, along with the presence of calcification factors and calcium-binding proteins, fosters the calcification of the matrix. As crystals are deposited into the gap regions on the surface of collagen molecules, water is resorbed from the matrix.

Mineralization occurs around numerous closely spaced nidi of crystallization; as it progresses, these centers enlarge and fuse with each other. In this fashion, an increasingly large region of the matrix is dehydrated and calcified.

Bone Remodeling

In the adult, bone development is balanced with bone resorption as bone is remodeled to meet stresses placed on it.

In a young person, bone development exceeds bone resorption because new haversian systems are being developed much faster than old ones are being resorbed. Later, in adulthood, when the epiphyseal plates close and bone growth has been attained, new bone development is balanced with bone resorption.

Growing bones largely retain their general architectural shape from the beginning of bone development in the fetus to the end of bone growth in the adult. This is accomplished by **surface remodeling,** a process involving bone deposition under certain regions of the periosteum with concomitant bone resorption under other regions of the periosteum. Similarly, bone is being deposited in certain regions of the endosteal surface, whereas it is being resorbed in other regions. The bones of the calvarium are being reshaped in a similar way to accommodate the growing brain; however, how this process is regulated is unclear.

Cortical bone and cancellous bone, however, are not remodeled in the same fashion, probably because osteoblasts and osteoprogenitor cells of cancellous bone are located within the confines of bone marrow and, therefore, they are under the direct, paracrine influence of nearby bone marrow cells. The factors produced by these bone marrow cells include interleukin-1 (IL-1), tumor necrosis factor, colony-stimulating factor-1, osteoprotegrin (OPG), osteoprotegrin ligand (OPGL), and transforming growth factor-β. The osteoprogenitor cells and osteoblasts of compact bone are located in the cellular layer of the periosteum and in the lining of haversian canals and thus are too far from the cells of bone marrow to be under their paracrine influence. Instead, these cells of compact bone respond to systemic factors, such as calcitonin and parathyroid hormone.

The internal structure of adult bone is continually being remodeled as new bone is formed and dead and dying bone is resorbed; for example,

■ Haversian systems are continually being replaced.
■ Bone must be resorbed from one area and added to another to meet changing stresses placed on it (e.g., weight, posture, fractures).

As haversian systems are resorbed, their osteocytes die; in addition, osteoclasts are recruited to the area to resorb the bone matrix, forming **absorption cavities.** Continual osteoclastic activity increases the diameter and length of these cavities, which are invaded by blood vessels. At this point, bone resorption ceases and osteoblasts deposit new concentric lamellae around the blood vessels, forming new haversian systems. Although primary bone is remodeled in this fashion, which strengthens the bone by ordered collagen alignment about the haversian system, remodeling continues throughout life as resorption is replaced by deposition and the formation of new haversian systems. This process of bone resorption, followed by bone replacement, is known as **coupling.** The interstitial lamellae observed in adult bone are remnants of remodeled haversian systems.

Bone Repair

Bone repair involves both intramembranous and endochondral bone formation.

A bone fracture causes damage and destruction to the bone matrix, death to cells, tears in the periosteum and endosteum, and possible displacement of the ends of the broken bone (fragments). Blood vessels are severed near the break, and localized hemorrhaging fills in the zone of the break, resulting in blood clot formation at the site of injury. Soon the blood supply is shut down in a retrograde fashion from the injury site back to regions of anastomosing vessels, which can establish a new circulation route. As a consequence there is a widening zone of injury, on either side of the original break, resulting in a lack of a blood supply to many haversian systems, thus causing the zone of dead and dying osteocytes to increase appreciably. Because bone marrow and the periosteum are highly vascularized, the initial injury site in either of these two areas does not grow significantly, nor is there a notable increase in dead and dying cells much beyond the original injury site. Whenever the bone's haversian systems are without a blood supply, osteocytes become pyknotic and undergo lysis, leaving empty lacunae.

The blood clot filling the site of the fracture is invaded by small capillaries and fibroblasts from the surrounding connective tissue, forming **granulation tissue.** A similar event occurs in the marrow cavities as a clot forms; the clot is soon invaded by osteoprogenitor cells of the endosteum and multipotential cells of the bone marrow, forming an **internal callus** of bony trabeculae within a week or so (Fig. 7-20). Within 48 hours after injury, osteoprogenitor cells build up because of increased mitotic activity of the osteogenic layer of the periosteum and the endosteum and from undifferentiated cells of the bone marrow. The deepest layer of proliferating osteoprogenitor cells of the periosteum (those closest to the bone), which are in the vicinity of capillaries, differentiate into osteoblasts and begin elaborating a collar of bone, cementing it to the dead bone about the injury site.

Although the capillaries are growing, their rate of proliferation is much slower than that of the osteoprogenitor cells; thus the osteoprogenitor cells in the middle of the proliferating mass are now without a profuse capillary bed. This results in lowered oxygen tension, and these cells become chondrogenic cells, giving rise to chondroblasts that form cartilage in the outer parts of the collar.

The outermost layer of the proliferating osteoprogenitor cells (those adjacent to the fibrous layer of the periosteum), having some capillaries in their midst, continue to proliferate as osteoprogenitor cells. Thus, the collar exhibits three zones that blend together: (1) a

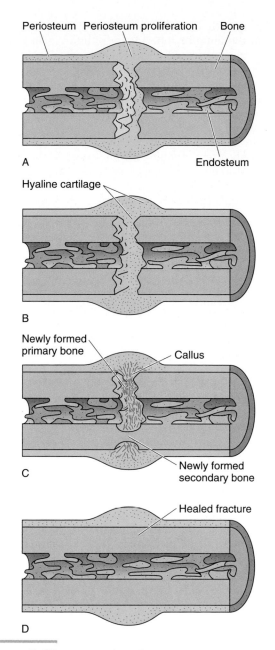

Periosteum Periosteum proliferation   Bone

A

Endosteum

Hyaline cartilage

B

Newly formed
primary bone

Callus

C

Newly formed
secondary bone

Healed fracture

D

Figure 7–20 Events in bone fracture repair.

layer of new bone cemented to the bone of the fragment, (2) an intermediate layer of cartilage, and (3) a proliferating osteogenic surface layer. In the meantime, the collars formed on the ends of each fragment fuse into one collar, known as the **external callus,** leading to union of the fragments. Continued growth of the external collar is derived mainly from proliferation of osteoprogenitor cells and, to some degree, from interstitial growth of the cartilage in its intermediate zone.

The cartilage matrix adjacent to the new bone formed in the deepest region of the collar becomes calcified and is eventually replaced with cancellous bone. Ultimately, all of the cartilage is replaced with primary bone by endochondral bone formation.

Once the fragments of bone are united by bridging with cancellous bone, it is necessary to remodel the injury site by replacing the primary bone with secondary bone and resolving the callus.

The first bone elaborated against injured bone develops by intramembranous bone formation, and the new trabeculae become firmly cemented to the injured or dead bone. Matrices of dead bone, located in the empty spaces between newly developing bony trabeculae, are resorbed, and the spaces are filled in by new bone. Eventually, all of the dead bone is resorbed and replaced by new bone formed by the osteoblasts that invade the region. These events are concurrent, resulting in repair of the fracture with cancellous bone surrounded by a bony callus.

Through the events of remodeling, the primary bone of intramembranous bone formation is replaced with secondary bone, further reinforcing the mended fracture zone; at the same time, the callus is resorbed. It appears that the healing and remodeling processes at the fracture site are in direct response to the stresses placed on it; eventually, the repaired zone is restored to its original shape and strength. It is interesting that bone repair involves cartilage formation and both intramembranous and endochondral bone formation.

CLINICAL CORRELATIONS

If segments of bone are lost or damaged so severely that they have to be removed, a **"bony union"** is not possible; that is, the process of bone repair cannot occur because a bony callus does not form. In cases of this sort, a bone graft is required. Since the 1970s, bone banks have become available to supply viable bone for grafting purposes. The bone fragments are harvested and frozen to preserve their osteogenic potential and are then utilized as transplants by orthopedic surgeons. **Autografts** are the most successful because the transplant recipient is also the donor. **Homografts** are from different individuals of the same species and may be rejected because of immunological response. **Heterografts,** grafts from different species, are least successful, although it has been shown that calf bone loses some of its antigenicity after being refrigerated, making it a worthy bone graft when necessary.

Histophysiology of Bone

Bone supports soft tissues of the body and protects the central nervous system and hemopoietic tissue. It also is the site for attachment of the tendons of muscle that use the bone as levers to increase the mechanical advantage needed for locomotion. Just as important, bone serves as a reservoir of calcium and phosphate for maintaining adequate levels of these elements in the blood and other tissues of the body.

Maintenance of Blood Calcium Levels

Calcium is vital for the activity of many enzymes and also functions in membrane permeability, cell adhesion, blood coagulation, nerve impulse transmission, muscle contraction, among other bodily processes. To fulfill all of the necessary functional requirements for which calcium is responsible, a tightly controlled blood plasma concentration of 9 to 11 mg/dL must be maintained.

Because 99% of the calcium in the body is stored in bone as hydroxyapatite crystals, the remaining 1% must be available for mobilization from the bone on short notice. Indeed, there is a constant turnover between the calcium ions in bone and in blood. The calcium ions retrieved from bone to maintain blood calcium levels come from new and young osteons, where mineralization is incomplete. Because bone remodeling is constant, new osteons are always forming where labile calcium ions are available for this purpose. It seems that older osteons are more heavily mineralized; because of this, their calcium ions are less available.

Hormonal Effects

Osteoclastic activity is necessary for maintaining a constant supply of calcium ions for the body. Parenchymal cells of the parathyroid gland are sensitive to the blood calcium level; when calcium levels fall below normal, parathyroid hormone (PTH) is secreted. As discussed earlier, this hormone activates receptors on osteoblasts, suppressing matrix formation and initiating manufacture and secretion of **OPGL** and **osteoclast-stimulating factor** by the osteoblasts. These factors induce osteoclast formation and stimulate quiescent osteoclasts to become active, leading to bone resorption and the release of calcium ions.

Parafollicular cells (C cells) of the thyroid gland also monitor calcium ion levels in the plasma. When calcium ion levels become elevated, these cells secrete **calcitonin,** a polypeptide hormone that activates receptors on osteoclasts, inhibiting them from resorbing bone. Additionally, osteoblasts are stimulated to increase osteoid synthesis and calcium deposition is increased.

The growth hormone **somatotropin,** secreted by cells in the anterior lobe of the pituitary gland, influences bone development via somatomedins (insulin-like growth factors), especially stimulating growth of the epiphyseal plates. Children deficient in this hormone exhibit dwarfism, whereas persons with an excess of somatotropin in their growing years display **pituitary gigantism.**

Many additional factors are involved in bone metabolism, only a few of which are indicated in the following list. Moreover, many of these factors are released by a variety of cells and have numerous target cells; however, only their bone-related functions are listed:

- **Interleukin-1,** released by osteoblasts, activates osteoclast precursors to proliferate; it also has an indirect role in osteoclast stimulation.
- **Tumor necrosis factor,** released by activated macrophages, acts in a fashion similar to interleukin-1.
- **Colony-stimulating factor-1,** released by bone marrow stromal cells, induces osteoclast formation.
- **OPG** inhibits osteoclast differentiation.
- **Interleukin-6,** released by various bone cells, especially by osteoclasts, stimulates the formation of other osteoclasts.
- **Interferon-γ,** released by T lymphocytes, inhibits differentiation of osteoclast precursors into osteoclasts.
- **Transforming growth factor-β,** liberated from bone matrix during osteoclasia, induces osteoblasts to manufacture bone matrix and enhances the process of matrix mineralization; also, it inhibits proliferation of osteoclast precursors and their differentiation into mature osteoclasts.

CLINICAL CORRELATIONS

Acromegaly occurs in adults who produce an excess of somatotropin, causing an abnormal increase in bone deposition without normal bone resorption. This condition creates thickening of the bones, especially those of the face, in addition to disfiguring soft tissue.

Skeletal maturation is also influenced by hormones produced in the male and female gonads. Closure of the epiphyseal plates is normally rather stable and constant and is related to sexual maturation. Precocious sexual maturation stunts skeletal development because the epiphyseal plates are stimulated to close too early. In other people whose sexual maturation is retarded, skeletal growth continues beyond normal limits because the epiphyseal plates do not close.

CLINICAL CORRELATIONS

Osteoporosis affects about 10 million chronically immobilized Americans. It often affects women older than 40 years of age, especially postmenopausal women. Osteoporosis is related to decreasing bone mass, which becomes more serious after menopause, when estrogen secretion drops appreciably. Binding of estrogen to specific receptors on osteoblasts activates the cells to manufacture and secrete bone matrix. With diminished secretion of estrogen, osteoclastic activity is greater than bone deposition, potentially reducing bone mass to the point at which the bone cannot withstand stresses and breaks easily.

For decades estrogen replacement therapy coupled with calcium supplements and painkillers were used to alleviate or eliminate this condition. However, in 2004 it was determined that estrogen replacement therapy increases the risk for heart disease, stroke, breast cancer, and blood clots. A newly developed group of drugs called the bisphosphonates reduces the incidence of osteoporosis fractures without the risks of estrogen replacement therapy. An early diagnostic tool, dual-energy x-ray absorptiometry (DEXA), is being employed as a reliable method for assessing increasing bone density even in individuals with osteoporosis.

Nutritional Effects

Normal bone growth is sensitive and dependent on several nutritional factors. Unless a person's intake of protein, minerals, and vitamins is sufficient, the amino acids essential for collagen synthesis by osteoblasts are lacking and collagen formation is reduced. Insufficient intake of calcium or phosphorus leads to poorly calcified bone, which is subject to fracture. A deficiency of vitamin D prevents calcium absorption from the intestines, causing rickets in children. Vitamins A and C are also necessary for proper skeletal development (Table 7-4).

CLINICAL CORRELATIONS

Rickets is a disease in infants and children who are deficient in vitamin D. Without vitamin D, the intestinal mucosa cannot absorb calcium even though there may be adequate dietary intake. This results in disturbances in ossification of the epiphyseal cartilages and disorientation of the cells at the metaphysis, giving rise to poorly calcified bone matrix. Children with rickets display deformed bones, particularly in the legs, simply because the bones cannot bear their weight.

Osteomalacia, or adult rickets, results from prolonged deficiency of vitamin D. When this occurs, the newly formed bone in the process of remodeling does not calcify properly. This condition may become severe during pregnancy because the fetus requires calcium, which must be supplied by the mother.

Scurvy is a condition resulting from a deficiency of vitamin C. One effect is deficient collagen production, causing a reduction in formation of bone matrix and bone development. Healing is also delayed.

TABLE 7–4 Vitamins Affecting Skeletal Development

Deficiency/Excess	Effect
Vitamin A deficiency	Inhibits proper bone formation as coordination of osteoblast and osteoclast activities fails; failure of resorption and remodeling of cranial vault to accommodate the brain results in serious damage to the central nervous system
Hypervitaminosis A	Erosion of cartilage columns without increases of cells in proliferation zone; epiphyseal plates may become obliterated, ceasing growth prematurely
Vitamin C deficiency	Mesenchymal tissue is affected because connective tissue is unable to produce and maintain extracellular matrix; deficient production of collagen and bone matrix results in retarded growth and delayed healing (scurvy)
Vitamin D deficiency	Ossification of epiphyseal cartilages is disturbed; cells become disordered at metaphysis, leading to poorly calcified bones, which become deformed by weight bearing (in children, termed rickets; in adults, osteomalacia)

Joints

Bones articulate or come into close proximity with one another at joints, which are classified according to the degree of movement available between the bones of the joint. Those that are closely bound together with only a minimum of movement between them are called **synarthroses;** joints in which the bones are free to articulate over a fairly wide range of motion are classified as **diarthroses.**

There are three types of **synarthrosis joints** according to the tissue making up the union:

1 **Synostosis.** There is little if any movement, and joint-uniting tissue is bone (e.g., skull bones in adults).
2 **Synchondrosis.** There is little movement, and joint-uniting tissue is hyaline cartilage (e.g., joint of first rib and sternum).
3 **Syndesmosis.** There is little movement, and bones are joined by dense connective tissue (e.g., pubic symphysis).

Most of the joints of the extremities are **diarthroses** (Fig. 7-21). The bones making up these joints are covered by persistent **hyaline cartilage,** or **articular cartilage.** Usually, ligaments maintain the contact between the bones of the joint, which is sealed by the **joint capsule.** The **capsule** is composed of an outer **fibrous layer** of dense connective tissue, which is continuous with the periosteum of the bones, and an inner cellular **synovial layer,** which covers all non-articular surfaces. Some prefer to call this a **synovial membrane.**

Two kinds of cells are located in the synovial layer:

1 **Type A cells** are macrophages displaying a well-developed Golgi apparatus and many lysosomes but only a small amount of RER. These phagocytic cells are responsible for removing debris from the joint space.

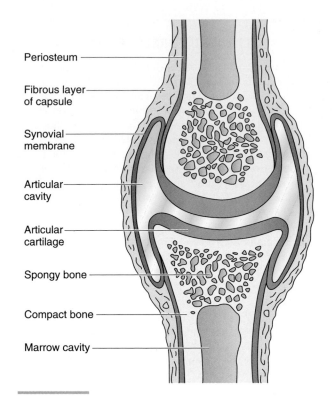

Figure 7–21 Anatomy of a diarthrodial joint.

2 **Type B cells** resemble fibroblasts, exhibiting a well-developed RER; these cells are thought to secrete the **synovial fluid.**

Synovial fluid contains a high concentration of **hyaluronic acid** and the glycoprotein **lubricin** combined with filtrate of plasma. In addition to supplying nutrients and oxygen to the chondrocytes of the articular cartilage, this fluid has a high content of hyaluronic acid and lubricin that permits it to function as a lubricant for the joint. Moreover, macrophages in the synovial fluid act to phagocytose debris in the joint space.

8

Muscle

Although many cells of multicellular organisms have limited contractile abilities, it is the capability of muscle cells, which are specialized for contraction, that permits animals to move. Organisms harness the contraction of muscle cells and the arrangement of the extracellular components of muscle to permit locomotion, constriction, pumping, and other propulsive movements.

Cells of muscle are elongated and are called either striated muscle cells or smooth muscle cells, depending on the respective presence or absence of a regularly repeated arrangement of myofibrillar contractile proteins, the myofilaments. **Striated muscle cells** display characteristic alternations of light and dark cross-bands, which are absent in smooth muscle (Fig. 8-1). There are *two types* of striated muscle: **skeletal,** accounting for most of the voluntary muscle mass of the body, and involuntary **cardiac,** limited almost exclusively to the heart.

Smooth muscle cells are located in the walls of blood vessels and the viscera as well as in the dermis of the skin.

Unique terms are often used to describe the components of muscle cells. Thus, muscle cell membrane is referred to as **sarcolemma;** the cytoplasm, as **sarcoplasm;** the smooth endoplasmic reticulum, as **sarcoplasmic reticulum;** and occasionally, the mitochondria, as **sarcosomes.** Because they are much longer than they are wide, muscle cells frequently are called **muscle fibers;** unlike collagen fibers, however, they are *living* entities.

All three muscle types are derived from mesoderm. Cardiac muscle originates in splanchnopleuric mesoderm, most smooth muscle is derived from splanchnic and somatic mesoderm, and most skeletal muscles originate from somatic mesoderm.

SKELETAL MUSCLE

Skeletal muscle is composed of long, cylindrical, multinucleated cells that undergo voluntary contraction to facilitate movement of the body or its parts.

During embryonic development, several hundred **myoblasts,** precursors of skeletal muscle fibers, line up end to end, fusing with one another to form long multinucleated cells known as **myotubes.** These newly formed myotubes manufacture cytoplasmic constituents as well as contractile elements, called **myofibrils.** Myofibrils are composed of specific arrays of **myofilaments**, the proteins responsible for the contractile capability of the cell.

Muscle fibers are arranged parallel to one another, with their intervening intercellular spaces housing parallel arrays of **continuous capillaries.** Each skeletal muscle fiber is long, cylindrical, multinucleated, and striated. The diameters of the fibers vary, ranging from 10 to 100 µm, although hypertrophied fibers may exceed the latter figure. The relative strength of a muscle fiber directly depends on its diameter, whereas the strength of the entire muscle is a function of the number and thickness of its component fibers.

Skeletal muscle is pink to red because of its rich vascular supply as well as the presence of **myoglobin pigments,** oxygen-transporting proteins that resemble, but are smaller than, hemoglobin. Depending on the fiber diameter, quantity of myoglobin, number of mitochondria, extensiveness of the sarcoplasmic reticulum, concentration of various enzymes, and rate of contraction, the muscle fiber may be classified as **red, white,** or **intermediate** (Table 8-1).

Usually, a gross anatomical muscle (e.g., biceps) contains all three types of muscle fibers (red, white, and intermediate) in relatively constant proportions that are characteristic of that particular muscle. In chickens, for instance, thigh muscle fibers are predominantly red, and breast muscle fibers are predominantly white. The innervation of the muscle fiber appears to be the factor that determines fiber type. If the innervation is experimentally switched, the fiber accommodates itself to the new nerve supply.

TABLE 8–1 Comparison of Types of Skeletal Muscle Fibers*

Characteristics	Red Muscle Fibers	White Muscle Fibers
Vascularization	Rich vascular supply	Poorer vascular supply
Innervation	Smaller nerve fibers	Larger nerve fibers
Fiber diameter	Smaller	Larger
Contraction	Slow but repetitive; not easily fatigued; weaker contraction	Fast but easily fatigued; stronger contraction
Sarcoplasmic reticulum	Not extensive	Extensive
Mitochondria	Numerous	Few
Myoglobin	Rich	Poor
Enzymes	Rich in oxidative enzymes; poor in adenosine triphosphatase	Poor in oxidative enzymes; rich in phosphorylases and adenosine triphosphatase

*Intermediate muscle fibers have characteristics between those of red and white fibers.

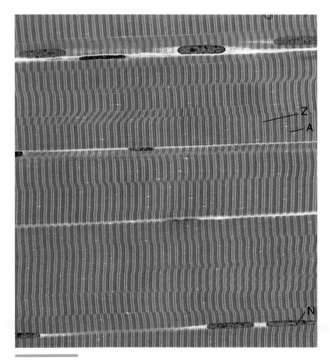

Figure 8–1 Light micrograph of a longitudinal section of skeletal muscle (×540). Note the peripherally located nuclei (N) as well as the very fine connective tissue elements between individual muscle fibers. A, band; Z, disk.

Investments

The investments of skeletal muscle are the epimysium, perimysium, and endomysium.

The entire muscle is surrounded by **epimysium,** a dense irregular collagenous connective tissue. **Perimysium,** a less dense collagenous connective tissue derived from epimysium, surrounds bundles (**fascicles**) of muscle fibers. **Endomysium,** composed of reticular fibers and an **external lamina** (basal lamina), surrounds each muscle cell (Fig. 8-2).

Because these connective tissue elements are interconnected, contractile forces exerted by individual muscle cells are transferred to them. Tendons and aponeuroses, which connect muscle to bone and to other tissues, are continuous with the connective tissue encasements of muscle and, therefore, act in harnessing the contractile forces for motion.

Light Microscopy

Light microscopy of skeletal muscle fibers displays long, cylindrical, multinucleated cells whose nuclei are peripherally located.

Skeletal muscle fibers are multinucleated cells, with their numerous nuclei peripherally located just beneath the cell membrane (Fig. 8-3). Each cell is surrounded by endomysium, whose fine reticular fibers intermingle with those of neighboring muscle cells. Small **satellite cells,** which have a single nucleus and act as regenera-

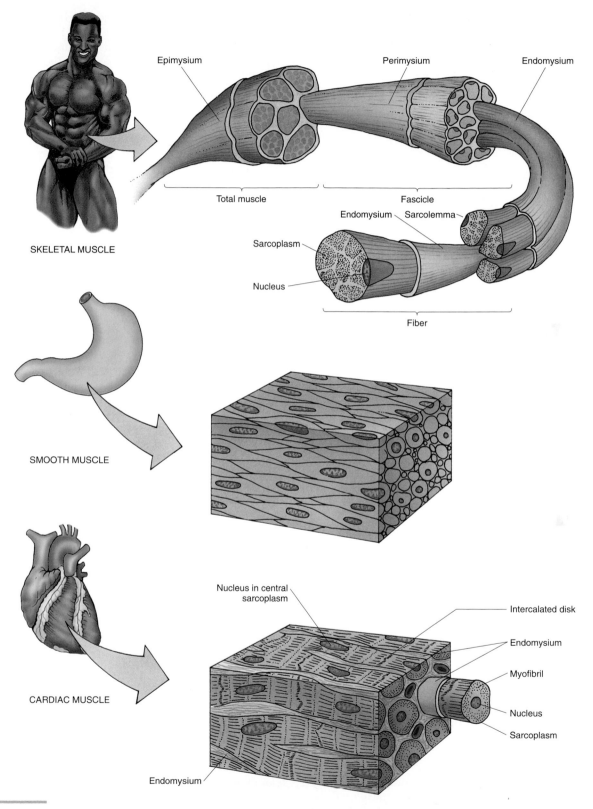

Figure 8–2 Three types of muscle. *Top,* Skeletal muscle; *center,* smooth muscle; *bottom,* cardiac muscle.

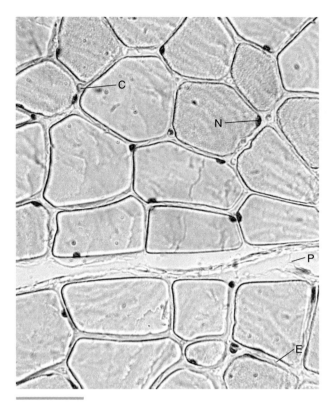

Figure 8–3 Light micrograph of a cross section of skeletal muscle (×540). Note the peripheral location of the nuclei (N) as well as the capillary (C) located in the slender connective tissue elements of the endomysium (E). Also observe the perimysium (P) that envelops bundles of muscle fibers.

tive cells, are located in shallow depressions on the muscle cell's surface, sharing the muscle fiber's external lamina. The chromatin network of the satellite cell nucleus is denser and coarser than that of the muscle fiber.

Much of the skeletal muscle cell is composed of longitudinal arrays of cylindrical **myofibrils,** each 1 to 2 μm in diameter (Fig. 8-4). They extend the entire length of the cell and are aligned precisely with their neighbors. This strictly ordered parallel arrangement of the myofibrils is responsible for the cross-striations of light and dark banding that are characteristic of skeletal muscle viewed in longitudinal section (see Fig. 8-1).

The dark bands are known as **A bands** (*a*nisotropic with polarized light) and the light bands as **I bands** (*i*sotropic with polarized light). The center of each A band is occupied by a pale area, the **H band**, which is bisected by a thin **M line.** Each I band is bisected by a thin dark line, the **Z disk (Z line).** The region of the myofibril between two successive Z disks, known as a **sarcomere,** is 2.5 μm in length and is considered the contractile unit of skeletal muscle fibers (Fig. 8-5; also see Fig. 8-4).

During muscle contraction, the various transverse bands behave characteristically. The I band becomes narrower, the H band is extinguished, and the Z disks move closer together (approaching the interface between the A and I bands), but the width of the A bands remains unaltered.

Fine Structure of Skeletal Muscle Fibers

Electron microscopy has helped reveal the functional and morphological significance of skeletal muscle cross-striations and other structural components.

T Tubules and Sarcoplasmic Reticulum

T tubules and sarcoplasmic reticulum are essential components involved in skeletal muscle contraction.

The fine structure of the sarcolemma is similar to that of other cell membranes. A distinguishing feature of this membrane, however, is that it is continued within the skeletal muscle fiber as numerous **T tubules (transverse tubules),** long, tubular invaginations that intertwine among the myofibrils (see Fig. 8-5).

In mammalian skeletal muscle, T tubules pass transversely across the fiber and lie specifically in the plane of the junction of the A and I bands. These tubules branch and anastomose but usually remain in a single plane; hence, each sarcomere possesses two sets of T tubules, one at each interface of the A and I bands. Thus, T tubules extend deep into the interior of the fiber and facilitate the conduction of waves of depolarization along the sarcolemma (Figs. 8-6 and 8-7).

Associated with this system of T tubules is the **sarcoplasmic reticulum,** which is maintained in close register with the A and I bands as well as with the T tubules. The sarcoplasmic reticulum, which stores intracellular calcium, forms a meshwork around each myofibril and displays dilated **terminal cisternae** at each A–I junction. Thus, two of these cisternae are always in close apposition to a T tubule, forming a **triad** in which a T tubule is flanked by two terminal cisternae. This arrangement permits a wave of depolarization to spread, almost instantaneously, from the surface of the sarcolemma throughout the cell, reaching the terminal cisternae, which have **voltage-gated** calcium release channels (**junctional feet**) in their membrane.

The sarcoplasmic reticulum regulates muscle contraction through controlled sequestering (leading to relaxation) and release (leading to contraction) of calcium ions (Ca^{2+}) within the sarcoplasm. The trigger for the calcium ion release is the wave of depolarization transmitted by T tubules, which causes opening of the

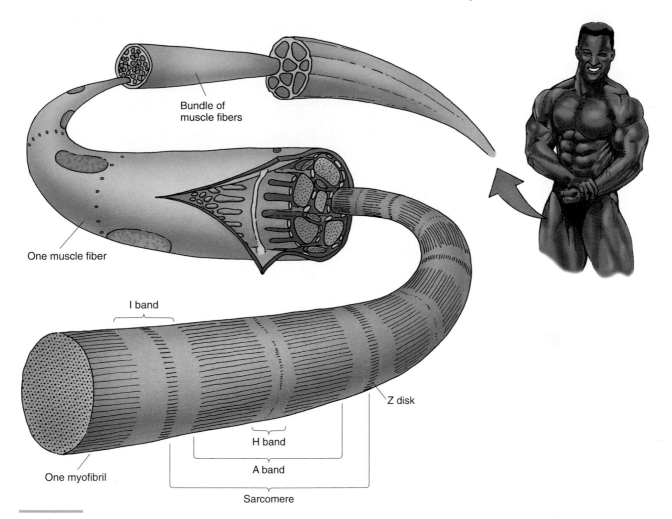

Figure 8–4 Organization of myofibrils and sarcomeres within a skeletal muscle cell. Note that the entire gross muscle is surrounded by a thick connective tissue investment, known as the epimysium, which provides finer connective tissue elements (the perimysium) that surround bundles of skeletal muscle fibers. Individual muscle cells are surrounded by still finer connective tissue elements, the endomysium. Individual skeletal muscle fibers possess a sarcolemma that has tubular invaginations (T tubules) that course through the sarcoplasm and are flanked by terminal cisternae of the sarcoplasmic reticulum. The contractile elements of the skeletal muscle fiber are organized into discrete cylindrical units called myofibrils. Each myofibril is composed of thousands of sarcomeres with their characteristic A, I, and H bands and Z disk.

calcium release channels of the terminal cisternae, resulting in release of calcium ions into the cytosol in the vicinity of the myofibrils.

Myofibrils are held in register with one another by the intermediate filaments desmin and vimentin, which secure the periphery of the Z disks of neighboring myofibrils to each other. These bundles of myofibrils are attached to the cytoplasmic aspect of the sarcolemma by various proteins, including **dystrophin,** a protein that binds to actin.

Deep to the sarcolemma and interspersed between and among myofibrils are numerous elongated mitochondria with many highly interdigitating cristae. The mitochondria may either parallel the longitudinal axis of the myofibril or wrap around the myofibril. Moreover, numerous mitochondria are located just deep to the sarcoplasm.

Structural Organization of Myofibrils

Myofibrils are composed of interdigitating thick and thin myofilaments.

Electron microscopy reveals the same banding as noted by light microscopy but also demonstrates the presence of parallel, interdigitating, rod-like **thick myofilaments** and **thin myofilaments.** The thick filaments (15 nm in diameter and 1.5 μm long) are composed of **myosin II,** whereas the thin filaments (7 nm in diameter and 1.0 μm long) are composed primarily of **actin.**

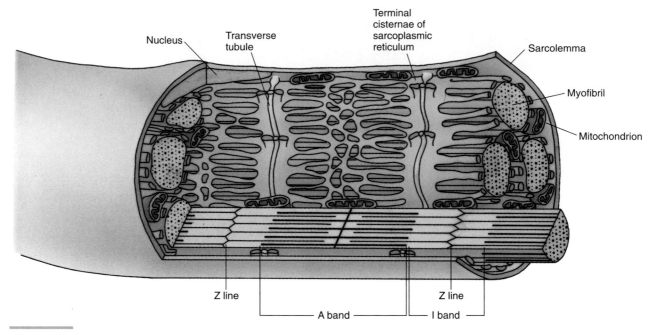

Figure 8–5 Organization of triads and sarcomeres of skeletal muscle. Note that in skeletal muscle the triad is always located at the junction of the A and I bands, permitting the quick release of calcium ions from the terminal cisternae of the sarcoplasmic reticulum just in the region where the interaction of the thick and thin filaments can produce efficient sarcomere shortening. Observe the presence of mitochondria around the periphery of the myofibrils.

Thin filaments originate at the Z disk and project toward the center of the two adjacent sarcomeres, thus pointing in opposite directions. Hence, a single sarcomere has two groups of parallel arrays of thin filaments, each attached to one Z disk, with all of the filaments in each group pointing toward the middle of the sarcomere (Fig. 8-8). Thick filaments also form parallel arrays, interdigitating with the thin filaments in a specific fashion.

In a relaxed skeletal muscle fiber, the thick filaments do not extend the entire length of the sarcomere, and the thin filaments projecting from the two Z disks of the sarcomere do not meet in the midline. Therefore, there are regions of each sarcomere, on either side of each Z disk, where only thin filaments are present. These adjacent portions of two successive sarcomeres correspond to the I band seen by light microscopy; for instance, the region of each sarcomere that encompasses the entire length of the thick filaments is the A band, and the zone in the middle of the A band, which is devoid of thin filaments, is the H band. As noted earlier, the H band is bisected by the M line, which consists of **myomesin, C protein,** and other as yet poorly characterized proteins that interconnect thick filaments to maintain their specific lattice arrangement (Table 8-2).

During contraction, individual thick and thin filaments do not shorten; instead, the two Z disks are brought closer together as the thin filaments slide past the thick filaments **(Huxley's sliding filament theory).** Thus, when contraction occurs, the motion of the thin filaments toward the center of the sarcomere creates a greater overlap between the two groups of filaments, effectively reducing the widths of the I and H bands without influencing the width of the A band.

The arrangement of the thick and thin filaments bears a specific and constant relationship. In mammalian skeletal muscle, each thick filament is surrounded equidistantly by six thin filaments. Cross sections through the region of overlapping thin and thick filaments display a hexagonal pattern, with thin filaments for the apices of each hexagon, the center of which is occupied by a thick filament (Fig. 8-9; also see Fig. 8-8). Thick filaments are separated from each other by a distance of 40 to 50 nm, whereas the distance between thick and thin filaments is only 15 to 20 nm.

The structural organization of myofibrils is maintained largely by five proteins:

- Titin
- α-Actinin
- Cap Z
- Nebulin
- Tropomodulin

Thick filaments are positioned precisely within the sarcomere with the assistance of **titin,** a large, linear,

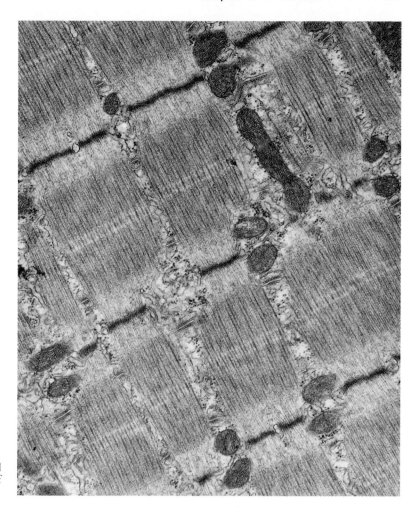

Figure 8–6 Electron micrograph of longitudinal section of rat skeletal muscle (×19,330). (Courtesy of Dr. J. Strum.)

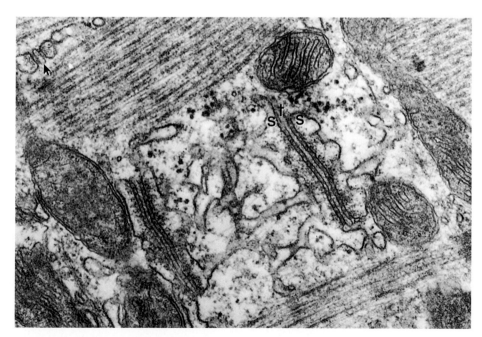

Figure 8–7 Electron micrograph of triads and sarcoplasmic reticulum in skeletal muscle (×57,847). Evident are a T tubule (t) and terminal cisternae of the sarcoplasmic reticulum (S). Note the cross-section of a T tubule flanked by terminal cisternae *(arrow)*. (From Leeson TS, Leeson CR, Papparo AA. Text/Atlas of Histology. Philadelphia, WB Saunders, 1988.)

Sarcomere

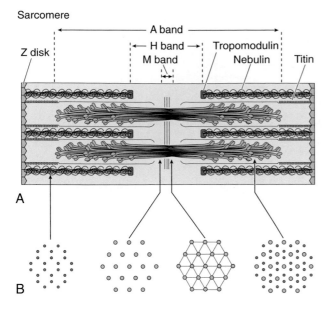

A

B

Myofilaments

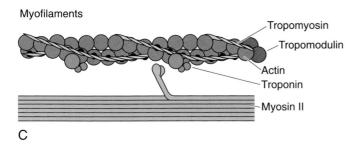

Tropomyosin

Tropomodulin

Actin

Troponin

Myosin II

C

Myosin II molecule

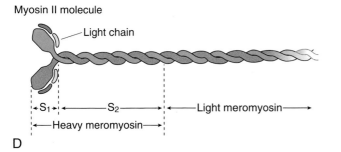

Light chain

S₁ — S₂ — Light meromyosin

Heavy meromyosin

D

Figure 8–8 The sarcomere and its components. **A,** The myosin molecules are arranged in an antiparallel fashion so that their heads are projecting from each end of the thick filament, and each thick filament is anchored in position by four titin molecules that extend from the Z disk to the center of the thick filament at the M line. Additionally, each thin filament is fixed in place by nebulin molecules that extend from the Z disk to the distal end of the thin filament. **B,** Cross-sectional profiles of a sarcomere at indicated regions. Each thick filament is surrounded equidistally by six thin filaments, so that there are always two thin filaments between neighboring thick filaments. **C,** Myofilaments (thick and thin filaments). Each thin filament is composed of two chains of F-actins, where each F-actin is composed of numerous G-actin molecules assembled head to toe. Each groove of a thin filament is occupied by a linear protein called tropomyosin; these proteins are positioned in such a fashion that they block the myosin-binding site of each G-actin molecule. Additionally the tripartite molecule, troponin, is associated with each tropomyosin molecule. When the troponin C moiety of troponin binds calcium, the conformational change in the troponin molecule pushes the tropomyosin deeper into the groove, unmasking the myosin-binding site of the G-actin and permitting muscle contraction to occur. **D,** Myosin II molecule. Each myosin II molecule is composed of two light chains and two heavy chains. The heavy chains can be cleaved by trypsin into light and heavy meromyosin, and each heavy meromyosin can be cleaved by papain into S1 and S2 fragments.

elastic protein. Two titin molecules extend from each half of a thick filament to the adjacent Z disk; thus four titin molecules anchor a thick filament between the two Z disks of each sarcomere.

Thin filaments are held in register by the rod-shaped protein **α-actinin,** a component of the Z disk that can bind thin filaments in parallel arrays. The plus end of the thin filament is held in place by a protein known as **Cap Z** that also prevents the addition or subtraction of G-actin molecules to or from the thin filament, thus assisting in the maintenance of its precise length. In

addition, two molecules of **nebulin,** a long, nonelastic protein, are wrapped around the entire length of each thin filament, further anchoring it in the Z disk and ensuring the maintenance of the specific array of the thin filaments. Moreover, nebulin acts as a "ruler," ensuring the precise length of the thin filament. It is assisted in this function by the protein **tropomodulin,** a cap on the minus end of the thin filament that, similarly to Cap Z, prevents the addition or the deletion of G-actin molecules to or from the thin filament (see Table 8-2 and Fig. 8-8).

TABLE 8–2 Proteins Associated with Skeletal Muscle

Protein	Molecular Weight (kD)	Subunits and Their Molecular Weight	Function
Myosin II	510	2 heavy chains, 222 kD each; 2 pairs of light chains, 18 kD and 22 kD	Major protein of thick filament; its interaction with actin hydrolyzes ATP and produces contraction
Myomesin	185	None	Cross-links thick filaments that are next to each other at M line
Titin	2500	None	Forms an elastic lattice that anchors thick filaments to Z disks
C protein	140	None	Binds to thick filaments at the M line
G actin	42	None	Polymerizes to form thin filaments of F-actin; interaction of G-actin with myosin II assists in hydrolyzing ATP, resulting in contraction
Tropomyosin	64	2 chains, 32 kD each	Occupies grooves of the thin filaments
Troponin	78	TnC, 18 kD TnT, 30 kD TnI, 30 kD	Binds calcium Binds to tropomyosin Binds to actin, thus inhibiting actinmyosin interaction
α-Actinin	190	2 units, each 95 kD	Anchors plus ends of thin filaments to Z disk
Nebulin	600	None	Z disk protein that may assist α-actinin to anchor thin filaments to Z disk
Cap Z			Forms part of the Z disk and caps the plus end of the thick filament
Tropomodulin	43 kD		Caps the minus end of the thin filament

ATP, adenosine triphosphate; kD, kilodalton.

THICK FILAMENTS

Thick filaments are composed of myosin II molecules aligned end to end.

Every thick filament consists of 200 to 300 myosin II molecules. Each **myosin II** molecule (150 nm in length; 2 to 3 nm in diameter) is composed of two identical **heavy chains** and two pairs of **light chains.** The heavy chains resemble two golf clubs, whose rod-like polypeptide chains are wrapped around each other in an α-helix. The heavy chains can be cleaved by trypsin into:

■ **Light meromyosin,** a rod-like tail composed of most of the two rod-like polypeptide chains wrapped around each other
■ **Heavy meromyosin,** the two globular heads with the attendant short proximal portions of the two rod-like polypeptide chains wrapped around each other

Light meromyosin functions in the proper assembly of the molecules into the bipolar thick filament. Heavy meromyosin is cleaved by papain into two globular (S_1) moieties and a short, helical, rod-like segment (S_2) (see Fig. 8-8). The S_1 subfragment binds **adenosine triphosphate (ATP)** and functions in the formation of cross-bridges between the thick and thin myofilaments. Light chains (not to be confused with light meromyosin) are of two types, and one of each type is associated with each S_1 subfragment of the myosin II molecule. For each heavy chain, therefore, there are two light chains. A myosin II molecule is composed of two heavy chains and four light chains.

Myosin II molecules are closely packed in a specific fashion in the thick filament. They are lined up in a parallel but staggered manner, spaced at regular intervals, lying arranged head to tail, so that the middle of each thick filament is composed solely of tail regions, whereas the two ends of the thick filament consist of both heads

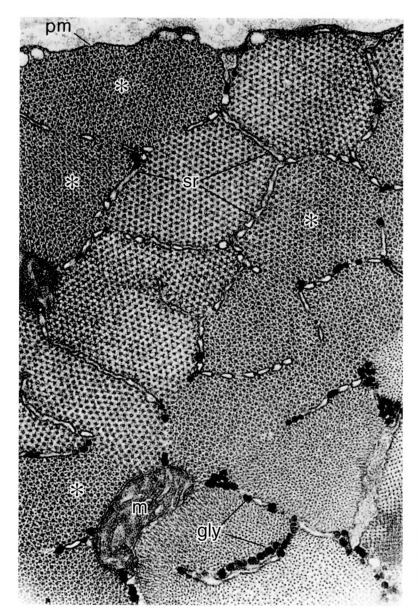

Figure 8–9 Electron micrograph of cross section of skeletal muscle fiber. *Asterisks* represent thick and thin filaments. gly, glycogen; m, mitochondria; pm, plasma membrane. (Electron micrograph courtesy of Dr. C. Peracchia; in Hopkins CR: Structure and Function of Cells. Philadelphia, WB Saunders, 1978.)

and tails. The spatial orientation of the myosin II molecules permits the heavy meromyosin portion to project from the thick filament at a 60-degree angle relative to neighboring heavy meromyosin, so that the head regions are always in register with the thin filaments.

Each myosin II molecule appears to have two flexible regions, one at the junction of the heavy meromyosin and the light meromyosin and the other at the junction of the S_1 and S_2 subfragments. The flexible region between the heavy and light meromyosins permits each myosin II molecule to contact the thin filament, forming a cross-bridge between the two filament types. As discussed later, the flexible region between the S_1 and S_2 subfragments enables the myosin II molecule to drag the thin filament, incrementally, toward the middle of the sarcomere.

THIN FILAMENTS

Thin filaments are composed of two chains of F-actin filaments wrapped around each other in association with tropomyosin and troponin.

The major component of each thin filament is **F-actin,** a polymer of globular **G-actin** units. Although G-actin molecules are globular, they all polymerize in the same spatial orientation, imparting a distinct polarity to the filament. The **plus end** of each filament is bound to the Z disk by α-actinin; the **minus end** extends toward the center of the sarcomere. Each G-actin molecule also contains an **active site,** where the head region (S_1 subfragment) of myosin II binds. Two chains of F-actin are wound around each other in a tight helix (36-nm periodicity) like two strands of pearls (see Fig. 8-8).

Running along the length of the F-actin double-stranded helix are two shallow grooves. Pencil-shaped **tropomyosin molecules,** about 40-nm long, polymerize to form head-to-tail filaments that occupy the shallow grooves of the double-stranded actin helix. Bound tropomyosin masks the active sites on the actin molecules by partially overlapping them.

Approximately 25 to 30 nm from the beginning of each tropomyosin molecule is a single **troponin molecule,** composed of three globular polypeptides: TnT, TnC, and TnI. The **TnT** subunit binds the entire troponin molecule to tropomyosin; **TnC** has a great affinity for calcium; and **TnI** binds to actin, preventing the interaction between actin and myosin II. Binding of calcium by **TnC** induces a conformational shift in tropomyosin, exposing the previously blocked active sites on the actin filament so that myosin II molecules can flex, forming cross-bridges, and so that the S_1 moieties (myosin heads) can bind to the active site on the actin molecule (see later).

Muscle Contraction and Relaxation

Muscle contraction obeys the "all-or-none law" and is followed by muscle relaxation.

Contraction effectively reduces the resting length of the muscle fiber by an amount that is equal to the sum of all shortenings that occur in all sarcomeres of that particular muscle cell. The process of contraction, usually triggered by neural impulses, obeys the **all-or-none law,** in that a single muscle fiber either contracts as a result of stimulation or does not respond at all. The strength of contraction of a gross anatomical muscle, such as the biceps, is a function of the number of muscle fibers that undergo contraction. The stimulus is transferred at the neuromuscular junction. During muscle contraction, the thin filaments slide past the thick filaments, as proposed by **Huxley's sliding filament theory.**

The following sequence of events leads to contraction in skeletal muscle:

1 An impulse, generated along the sarcolemma, is transmitted into the interior of the fiber via the T tubules, where it is conveyed to the terminal cisternae of the sarcoplasmic reticulum (see Fig. 8-5).
2 Calcium ions leave the terminal cisternae through **voltage-gated calcium release channels,** enter the cytosol, and bind to the TnC subunit of troponin, altering its conformation.
3 Conformational change in troponin shifts the position of tropomyosin deeper into the groove, unmasking the active site (myosin-binding site) on the actin molecule.
4 ATP present on the S_1 subfragment of myosin II is hydrolyzed, but both adenosine diphosphate (ADP)

and inorganic phosphate (P_i) remain attached to the S_1 subfragment, and the complex binds to the active site on actin (Fig. 8-10).
5 P_i is released, resulting not only in a greater bond strength between the actin and myosin II but also in a conformational alteration of the S_1 subfragment.
6 ADP is also released, and the thin filament is dragged toward the center of the sarcomere ("power stroke").
7 A new ATP molecule binds to the S_1 subfragment, causing the release of the bond between actin and myosin II.

The attachment and release cycles must be repeated numerous times for contraction to be completed. Each attachment and release cycle requires ATP for the conversion of chemical energy into motion.

CLINICAL CORRELATIONS

Shortly after the death of an animal, or of a human being, the joints become immoveable. This stiffening of the joints is referred to as **rigor mortis** and, depending on the ambient temperature, it may last as long as three days. Because the dead cells are unable to manufacture ATP, the dissociation of the thick and thin filaments cannot occur, and the myosin heads will remain bound to the active site of the actin molecule until the muscle begins to decompose. The time of death may be estimated by the state of rigor mortis, when it is correlated with the record of the ambient temperature fluctuations. It is interesting to note that the facial muscles are the first to undergo rigor mortis and that the maximal rigor occurs 12 to 24 hours after death.

As long as the cytosolic calcium concentration is high enough, actin filaments remain in the active state and contraction cycles continue. Once the stimulating impulses cease, however, muscle relaxation occurs, involving a reversal of the steps that led to contraction.

First, calcium pumps in the membrane of the sarcoplasmic reticulum actively drive Ca^{2+} back into the terminal cisternae, where the ions are bound by the protein calsequestrin. The reduced levels of Ca^{2+} in the cytosol cause TnC to lose its bound Ca^{2+}; tropomyosin then reverts to the position in which it masks the active site of actin, preventing the interaction of actin and myosin II.

Energy Sources for Muscle Contraction

Energy sources for muscle contraction are the phosphogen energy system, glycolysis, and the aerobic energy system.

Because the process of muscle contraction consumes a great deal of energy, skeletal muscle cells maintain a high concentration of the energy-rich compounds ATP

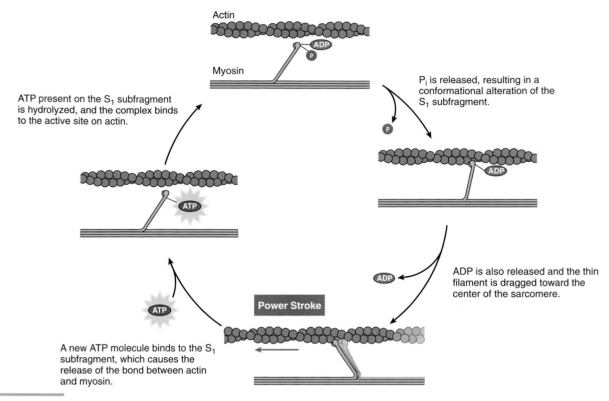

Actin

Myosin

ATP present on the S$_1$ subfragment is hydrolyzed, and the complex binds to the active site on actin.

P$_i$ is released, resulting in a conformational alteration of the S$_1$ subfragment.

ADP is also released and the thin filament is dragged toward the center of the sarcomere.

Power Stroke

A new ATP molecule binds to the S$_1$ subfragment, which causes the release of the bond between actin and myosin.

Figure 8–10 The role of adenosine triphosphate (ATP) in muscle contraction. ADP, adenosine diphosphate; P, phosphate; P$_i$, inorganic phosphate; S$_1$ subfragment, fragment of myosin. (Modified from Alberts B, Bray D, Lewis J, et al: Molecular Biology of the Cell. New York, Garland Publishing, 1994.)

and creatine phosphate (or phosphocreatine). Because both ATP and creatine phosphate contain high-energy phosphate bonds, they constitute the **phosphogen energy system,** and can provide enough energy for about a total of 9 seconds of maximal muscle activity (3 seconds for ATP and 6 seconds for creatine phosphate).

Additional energy can be derived from anaerobic metabolism of glycogen **(glycolysis),** which results in the formation and buildup of lactic acid. This is known as the glycogen-lactic acid system. This system provides about 90 to 100 seconds' worth of energy at almost maximal muscle activity.

The third system, known as the **aerobic energy system,** uses the normal diet for the manufacture of ATP. The aerobic system does not support maximal muscle activity, but it can sustain normal muscle activity indefinitely if the dietary intake is maintained and the nutrients persist.

ATP is manufactured via oxidative phosphorylation within the abundant mitochondria of muscle cells during periods of inactivity or low activity. Lipid droplets and glycogen, which abound in the sarcoplasm, also are readily converted into energy sources. The three metabolic systems of skeletal muscle are harnessed to supply the energy requirement of the muscle according to their activ-

ity modalities. During bursts of muscle contraction, the ADP that is generated is rephosphorylated by two means: (1) **glycolysis,** leading to accumulation of lactic acid, and (2) transfer of high-energy phosphate from creatine phosphate (phosphogen system) catalyzed by **phosphocreatine kinase.** During prolonged muscle activity, however, the aerobic system of energy production is employed.

Myotendinous Junctions

The connective tissue elements of the muscle fiber are continuous with the tendon to which the muscle is attached. At the myotendinous junctions, the cells become tapered and highly fluted. Collagen fibers of the tendon penetrate deep into these infoldings and probably become continuous with the reticular fibers of the endomysium. Within the cell, the myofilaments are anchored to the internal aspect of the sarcolemma so that the force of contraction is transmitted to the collagen fibers of the tendon.

Innervation of Skeletal Muscle

Skeletal muscle cells and the single motor neuron that innervates them constitute a motor unit.

Each skeletal muscle receives at least two types of nerve fibers: **motor** and **sensory.** The motor nerve functions in eliciting contraction, whereas the sensory fibers pass to muscle spindles (see later). Additionally, autonomic fibers supply the vascular elements of skeletal muscle. The specificity of motor innervation is a function of the muscle innervated. If the muscle acts fastidiously, as do some muscles of the eye, a single motor neuron may be responsible for as few as 5 to 10 skeletal muscle fibers, whereas a muscle located in the abdominal wall may have as many as 1000 fibers under the control of a single motor neuron. Each motor neuron and the muscle fibers it controls form a **motor unit.** The muscle fibers of a motor unit contract in unison and follow the all-or-none law of muscle contraction.

Impulse Transmission at the Neuromuscular Junction

Impulse transmission from the motor neuron to the skeletal muscle fiber occurs at the neuromuscular junction.

Motor fibers are **myelinated axons** of **α-motor neurons,** which pass in the connective tissue of the muscle. The axon arborizes, eventually losing its myelin sheath (but not its Schwann cells). The terminal of each arborized twig becomes dilated and overlies the **motor end plates** of individual muscle fibers. Each of these muscle–nerve junctions, known as a **neuromuscular junction,** is composed of an axon terminal, a synaptic cleft, and the muscle cell membrane (Figs. 8-11 to 8-13).

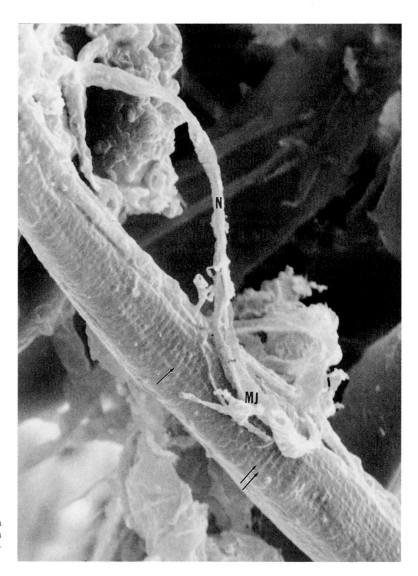

Figure 8–11 Scanning electron micrograph of a neuromuscular junction (MJ) from the tongue of a cat (×2315). N, nerve fiber. *Arrows* indicate striations. (Courtesy of Dr. L. Litke.)

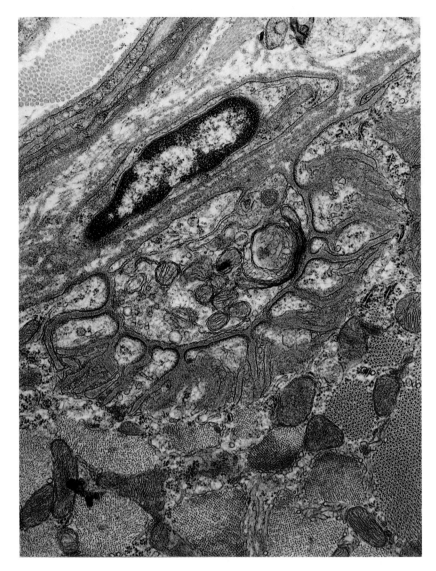

Figure 8–12 Electron micrograph of a mouse neuromuscular junction. (From Feczko D, Klueber KM: Cytoarchitecture of muscle in a genetic model of murine diabetes. Am J Anat 182:224-240, 1988.)

The muscle cell membrane **(postsynaptic membrane)** is modified, forming the **primary synaptic cleft**, a trough-like structure occupied by the **axon terminal**. Opening into the primary synaptic clefts are numerous **secondary synaptic clefts (junctional folds),** a further modification of the sarcolemma. Both the primary synaptic cleft and the junctional folds are lined by a basal lamina–like **external lamina**. The sarcoplasm in the vicinity of the secondary synaptic cleft is rich in glycogen, nuclei, ribosomes, and mitochondria.

The axon terminal, covered by Schwann cells, houses mitochondria, smooth endoplasmic reticulum, and as many as 300,000 **synaptic vesicles** (each 40 to 50 nm in diameter) containing the neurotransmitter **acetylcholine.** The function of the neuromuscular junction is to transmit a stimulus from the nerve fiber to the muscle cell.

Stimulus transmission across a synaptic cleft involves the following sequence of events (Fig. 8-14):

1 A stimulus, traveling along the axon, depolarizes the membrane of the axon terminal, thus opening the voltage-gated calcium channels, located in the vicinity of linearly arranged structures known as **dense bars.**

2 The influx of calcium into the axon terminal results in the fusion of about 120 synaptic vesicles per nerve impulse with the axon terminal's membrane **(presynaptic membrane)** and subsequent release of acetylcholine (along with proteoglycans and ATP) into the primary synaptic cleft. Fusion occurs along specific regions of the presynaptic membrane, known as **active sites,** adjoining the dense bars.

3 The neurotransmitter acetylcholine (ligand) is liberated in large quantities, known as **quanta** (equal

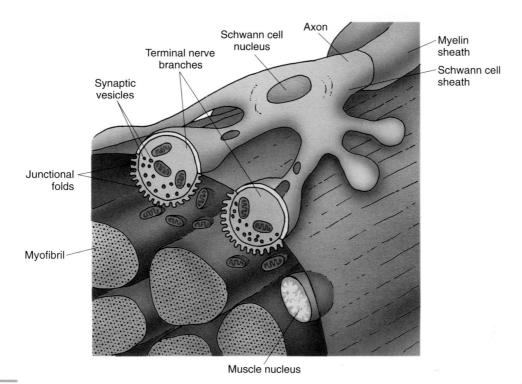

Figure 8–13   Neuromuscular junction. Note that the myelin sheath stops as the axon arborizes over the skeletal muscle fiber, but the Schwann cell sheath continues to insulate the nerve fiber. The terminal nerve branches expand to form axon terminals that overlie the motor endplates of individual muscle fibers.

to 10,000 to 20,000 molecules), from the nerve terminal.

4 Acetylcholine then diffuses across the synaptic cleft and binds to postsynaptic **acetylcholine receptors** in the muscle cell membrane. These receptors, located in the vicinity of the presynaptic active sites, are ligand-gated ion channels, which open in response to the binding of acetylcholine. The resulting ion influx leads to **depolarization** of the sarcolemma and generation of an **action potential** (see Chapter 9).

5 The impulse generated spreads quickly throughout the muscle fiber via the system of T tubules, initiating muscle contraction.

To prevent a single stimulus from eliciting multiple responses, **acetylcholinesterase,** an enzyme located in the external lamina lining the primary and secondary synaptic clefts, degrades acetylcholine into acetate and choline, thus permitting the reestablishment of the **resting potential.** Degradation is so rapid that all of the released acetylcholine is cleaved within a few hundred milliseconds.

Choline is transported back into the axon terminal by a sodium-choline symport protein powered by the sodium concentration gradient. Within the axon termi-nal, the acetylcholine is synthesized from activated acetate (produced in mitochondria) and the recycled choline, a reaction catalyzed by **choline acetyl transferase.** The newly formed acetylcholine is transported, through the use of an antiport system powered by a proton concentration gradient, into newly formed synaptic vesicles.

In addition to the recycling of choline, the synaptic vesicle membrane is recycled to conserve the surface area of the presynaptic membrane. This membrane recycling is accomplished by the formation of clathrin-coated endocytotic vesicles, which become the newly formed synaptic vesicles.

Muscle Spindles and Golgi Tendon Organs

Muscle spindles and Golgi tendon organs are sensory receptors that monitor muscle contraction.

The neural control of muscle function requires not only the capability of inducing or inhibiting muscle contraction but also the ability to monitor the status of the muscle and its tendon during muscle activity. This monitoring is performed by two types of sensory receptors:

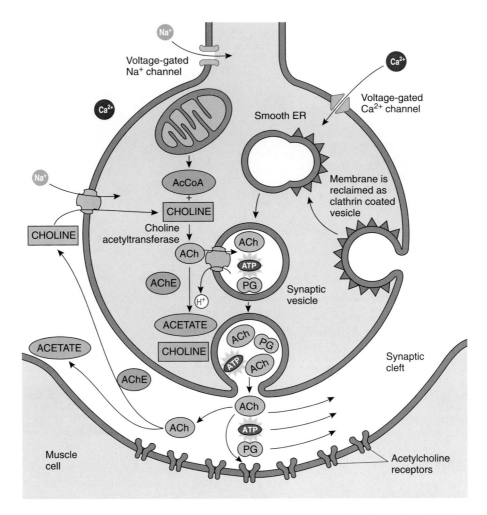

Figure 8–14 Diagram depicting events occurring at the neuromuscular junction during the release of acetylcholine. AcCoA, acetyl CoA; Ach, acetylcholine; AchE, acetylcholinesterase; ATP, adenosine triphosphate; PG, proteoglycan. (Modified from Katzung BG: Basic and Clinical Pharmacology, 4th ed. East Norwalk, Conn, Appleton & Lange, 1989.)

- **Muscle spindles,** which provide feedback about the changes in muscle length as well as the rate of alteration in muscle length
- **Golgi tendon organs,** which monitor the tension as well as the rate at which the tension is being produced during movement

Information from these two sensory structures is generally processed at unconscious levels, within the spinal cord. The information also reaches the cerebellum and even the cerebral cortex, however, so a person may sense muscle position.

Muscle Spindles

Muscle spindles continuously monitor the length and the changes in length of the muscle.

When muscle is stretched, it normally undergoes reflex contraction, or **stretch reflex.** This proprioceptive response is initiated by the muscle spindle, an encapsulated sensory receptor located among, and in parallel with, the muscle cells (Fig. 8-15). Each muscle spindle is composed of 8 to 10 elongated, narrow, very small, modified muscle cells called **intrafusal fibers,** surrounded by the fluid-containing **periaxial space,** which in turn is enclosed by the capsule. The connective tissue elements of the capsule are continuous with the collagen fibers of the perimysium and endomysium. The skeletal muscle fibers surrounding the muscle spindle are unremarkable and are called **extrafusal fibers.**

Intrafusal fibers are of two types: **nuclear bag fibers** and the more numerous, thinner **nuclear chain fibers.** Furthermore, there are two categories of

CLINICAL CORRELATIONS

Botulism is usually caused by ingestion of improperly preserved canned foods. The toxin, produced by the microbe *Clostridium botulinum*, interferes with the release of acetylcholine, with resultant muscle paralysis and, without treatment, death.

Myasthenia gravis is an autoimmune disease in which autoantibodies attach to acetylcholine receptors, blocking their availability to acetylcholine. Receptors thus inactivated are endocytosed and replaced by new receptors, which are also inactivated by the autoantibodies. Thus, the number of locations for the initiation of muscle depolarization is reduced and the skeletal muscles (including the diaphragm) weaken gradually. Certain **neurotoxins,** such as the bungarotoxin of some poisonous snakes, also bind to acetylcholine receptors, causing paralysis and eventual death due to respiratory compromise.

Botulinum toxin type A, produced by *Clostridium botulinum,* is an inhibitor of acetylcholine release by motor fibers that cause skeletal muscle contraction. For cosmetic purposes, **"Botox"** is injected into the procerus and corrugator muscles to diminish the frown lines that the contraction of those facial muscles otherwise produces. By eradicating these "wrinkles," the face appears smoother and younger looking. In 2001, almost 2 million people were injected with Botox for cosmetic purposes. The effect lasts for less than 3 months, and many patients repeat the procedure two to three times per year. There appear to be no serious side effects, but if injected into the wrong muscles, ptosis of the eyelids could persist for several months. Occasionally individuals suffer headaches, cold-like symptoms, and nausea, as well as muscle weakness, pain, and inflammation in the area of the injection for as long as 4 months.

nuclear bag fibers: **static** and **dynamic.** The nuclei of both types of fibers occupy the centers of the cells; their myofibrils are located on either side of the nuclear region, limiting contraction to the polar regions of these spindle-shaped cells. The central regions of the intrafusal fibers do not contract. The nuclei are aggregated in the nuclear bag fibers, whereas they are aligned in a single row in nuclear chain fibers.

Within a specific muscle spindle, a single, myelinated, large, sensory nerve fiber **(group Ia)** wraps spirally around the nuclear regions of each of the three types of intrafusal fibers, forming the **primary sensory endings** (also known as **dynamic** and **Ia** sensory endings). Additionally, **secondary sensory nerve endings** (also known as **static** and **II** sensory nerve endings) are formed by **group II** nerve fibers, which wrap around every nuclear chain fiber as well as around the static nuclear bag fibers.

The contractile regions of the intrafusal fibers receive two types of γ-motor neurons. Dynamic nuclear bag fibers are innervated by a **dynamic γ-motor neuron,** whereas all nuclear chain fibers as well as all of the static nuclear bag fibers are innervated by a **static γ-motor neuron.**

The extrafusal fibers receive their normal nerve fibers, which are the large, rapidly conducting axons of **α-efferent (motor) neurons.**

As a muscle is stretched, the intrafusal muscle fibers of its muscle spindle are also stretched, causing the primary (group Ia, dynamic) and secondary (group II, static) sensory nerve fibers to initiate an action potential; with increased stretching, these nerve fibers accelerate their rate of firing. Group Ia and group II fibers both respond to a stretching of the muscle at a constant rate. Only group Ia fibers, however, respond to a *change in the rate* at which stretching occurs, thus furnishing information concerning both the rapidity of movement and unanticipated stretching of the muscle.

Firing of the γ-motor neurons causes the polar regions of the intrafusal fibers to contract. When this occurs, the noncontractile regions of the intrafusal fibers are stretched from both directions, resulting in activation of the primary and secondary sensory nerve endings. Modulation of γ-motor neuron activity sensitizes the muscle spindle so that it can react even to a small degree of muscle stretching, as follows:

- Firing of dynamic γ-motor neurons primes the dynamic nerve endings but not the static nerve endings (because their firing does not cause contraction of the static nuclear bag fibers).
- Firing of static γ-motor neurons increases the continuous, steady response of both group Ia and group II sensory fibers (because both fibers form sensory nerve endings on static nuclear bag and all nuclear chain intrafusal fibers). However, the dynamic sensory fiber response decreases (because static γ-motor neurons do not innervate dynamic nuclear bag fibers).

Thus, modulation of the γ-motor neuron activity gives the nervous system the ability to adjust the sensitivity of the muscle spindle.

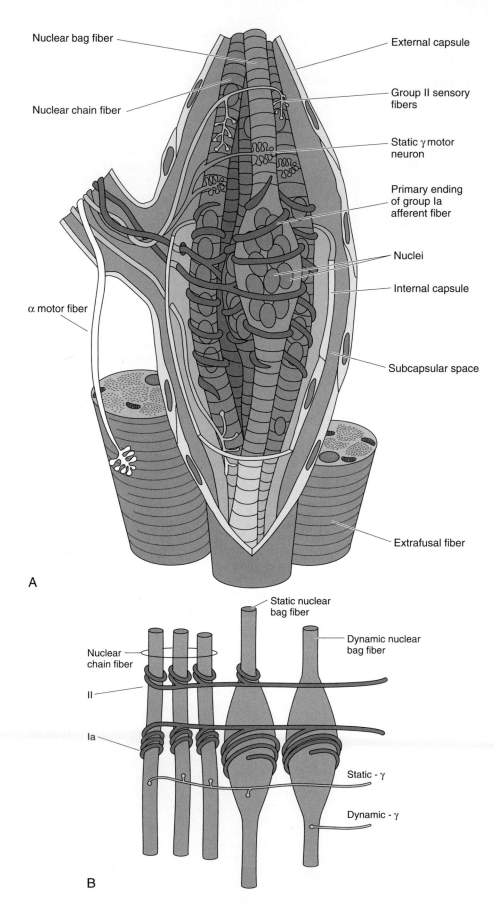

Figure 8–15 Muscle spindle. **A,** Schematic diagram showing components of a muscle spindle. **B,** The various fiber types of a muscle spindle and their innervation are presented in a spread-out fashion. Ia, group Ia sensory fiber; II, group II sensory fiber. (**A,** Modified from Krstic RV: Die Gewebe des Menschen und der Saugertiere. Berlin, Springer-Verlag, 1978. **B,** Modified from Hulliger M: The mammalian muscle spindle and its central control. Rev Physiol Biochem Pharmacol 101:1-110, 1984.)

Golgi Tendon Organs (Neurotendinous Spindles)

Golgi tendon organs monitor the intensity of muscle contraction.

Golgi tendon organs, also called neurotendinous spindles, are cylindrical structures about 1 mm in length and 0.1 mm in diameter. They are located at the juncture of a muscle with its tendon and are positioned in series with the muscle fibers. Golgi tendon organs are composed of **wavy collagen fibers** and the nonmyelinated continuation of a single **type Ib axon** that ramifies as free nerve endings in the interstices between the collagen fibers. When the muscle contracts, it places tensile forces on the collagen fibers, straightening them, with a consequent compression and firing of the entwined nerve endings. The rate of firing is directly related to the amount of tension placed on the tendon.

When a muscle undergoes strenuous contraction, it may generate a great amount of force. To protect the muscle, bone, and tendon, Golgi tendon organs provide an inhibitory feedback to the γ-motor neuron of the muscle, resulting in relaxation of the contracting tendon's muscle. Thus, the Golgi tendon organs monitor the force of muscle contraction, whereas muscle spindles monitor the stretching of the muscle in which they are located. These two sensory organs act in concert to integrate spinal reflex systems.

CARDIAC MUSCLE

Cardiac muscle is nonvoluntary striated muscle limited to the heart and the proximal portions of the pulmonary veins.

Cardiac muscle (heart muscle), another form of striated muscle, is found only in the heart and in pulmonary veins where they join the heart. Cardiac muscle is derived from a strictly defined mass of splanchnic mesenchyme, the **myoepicardial mantle,** whose cells give rise to the epicardium and **myocardium.**

The adult myocardium consists of an anastomosing network of branching cardiac muscle cells arranged in layers **(laminae).** Laminae are separated from one another by slender connective tissue sheets that convey blood vessels, nerves, and the conducting system of the heart. Capillaries, derived from these branches, invade the intercellular connective tissue, forming a rich, dense network of capillary beds surrounding every cardiac muscle cell.

Cardiac muscle differs from skeletal and smooth muscles in that it possesses an **inherent rhythmicity** as well as the ability to **contract spontaneously.** A system of modified cardiac muscle cells has been adapted to ensure the coordination of its contractile actions. This specialized system, as well as the associated autonomic nerve supply, is discussed in Chapter 11.

Almost half the volume of the cardiac muscle cell is occupied by mitochondria, attesting to its great energy consumption. Glycogen, to a certain extent, but mostly triglycerides (~60% during basal rate) form the energy supply of the heart. Because the oxygen requirement of cardiac muscle cells is high, they contain an abundant supply of myoglobin.

Although the resting lengths of individual cardiac muscle cells vary, on average they are 15 μm in diameter and 80 μm in length. Each cell possesses a single, large, oval, centrally placed nucleus, although two nuclei are occasionally present (Figs. 8-16 to 8-18).

Muscle cells of the atria are somewhat smaller than those of the ventricles. These cells also house granules (especially in the right atrium) containing **atrial natriuretic peptide,** a substance that functions to lower blood pressure (Fig. 8-19). This peptide acts by decreasing the capabilities of renal tubules to resorb (conserve) sodium and water.

Intercalated Disks

Cardiac muscle cells form highly specialized end-to-end junctions, referred to as intercalated disks (Figs. 8-20 to 8-22; also see Fig. 8-16). The cell membranes involved in these junctions approximate each other, so that in most areas they are separated by a space of less than 15 to 20 nm.

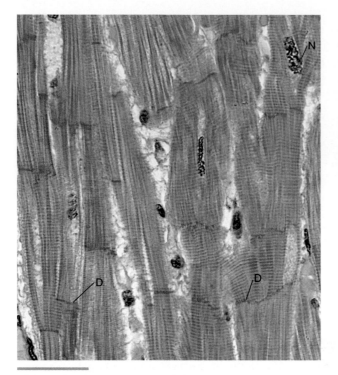

Figure 8–16 Light micrograph of cardiac muscle in longitudinal section (×540). Note the nucleus (N) and the presence of intercalated disks, regions where the cardiac muscle cells form desmosomes (D), fasciae adherents, and gap junctions with each other.

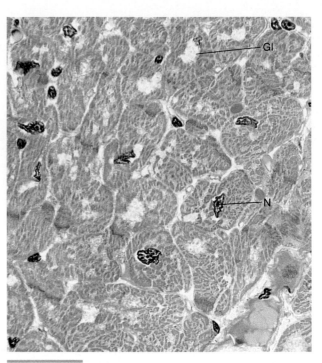

Figure 8–17 Light micrograph of cardiac muscle in cross-section (×540). The nucleus (N) is centrally located, and at each pole of the nucleus the glycogen deposits (Gl) have been extracted during the histological preparation.

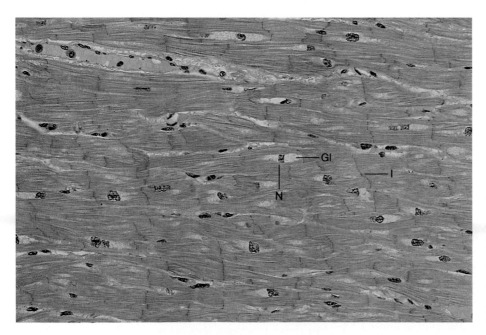

Figure 8–18 Light micrograph of cardiac muscle cells in longitudinal section, displaying their characteristic branching patterns and glycogen deposits (Gl) (×270). The branching of the cardiac muscle fibers, the central location of the nuclei (N), and the presence of intercalated disks (I) are identifying characteristics of cardiac muscle.

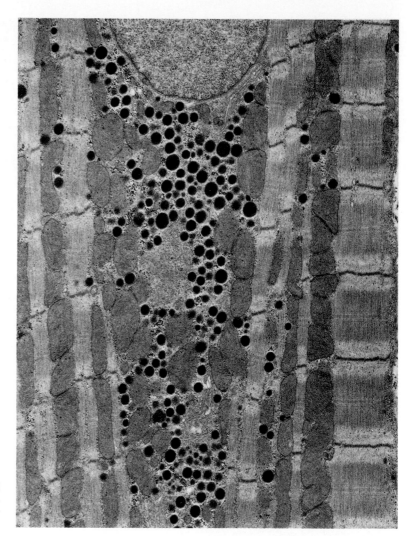

Figure 8–19 Electron micrograph of a rat atrial muscle cell (×14,174). Observe the secretory granules containing atrial natriuretic peptide. (Courtesy of Dr. Stephen C. Pang.)

Intercalated disks have **transverse portions,** where fasciae adherentes and desmosomes abound, as well as **lateral portions** rich in gap junctions (see Figs. 8-20 to 8-22). On the cytoplasmic aspect of the sarcolemma of intercalated disks, **thin myofilaments** attach to the fasciae adherens, which are thus analogous to Z disks. Gap junctions, which function in permitting rapid flow of information from one cell to the next, also form in regions where cells lying side by side come in close contact with each other.

Organelles

The extracellular fluid is the primary calcium source for cardiac muscle contraction.

The bandings of cardiac muscle fibers are identical with those of skeletal muscle, including alternating I and A bands. Each sarcomere possesses the same substructure as its skeletal muscle counterpart; therefore, the mode and mechanism of contraction are virtually identical in the two striated muscles. Several major differences should be noted, however; they are found in the sarcoplasmic reticulum, the arrangement of T tubules, the Ca^{2+} supply of cardiac muscle, the ion channels of the plasmalemma, and the duration of the action potential.

The sarcoplasmic reticulum of cardiac muscle does not form terminal cisternae and is not nearly as extensive as in skeletal muscle; instead, small terminals of sarcoplasmic reticulum approximate the **T tubules.** These structures do not normally form a triad, as in skeletal muscle; rather, the association is usually limited to two partners, resulting in a **dyad.** Unlike in skeletal muscle, where the triads are located at the A-I interfaces, the dyads in cardiac muscle cells are located in the vicinity of the Z line. The T tubules of cardiac muscle cells are

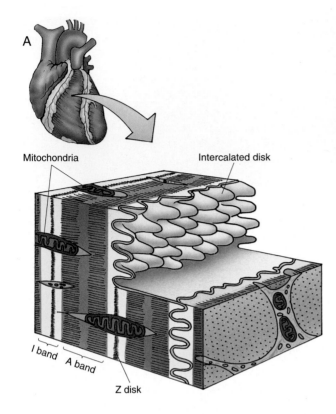

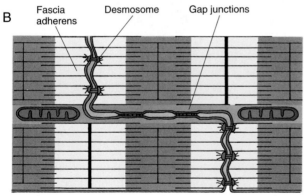

Figure 8–20 Cardiac muscle. **A,** Three-dimensional view of an intercalated disk. **B,** Two-dimensional view of the intercalated disk with a display of adhering and communicating junctions. The transverse portions of the intercalated disk act as a Z plate, and thin filaments are embedded in them.

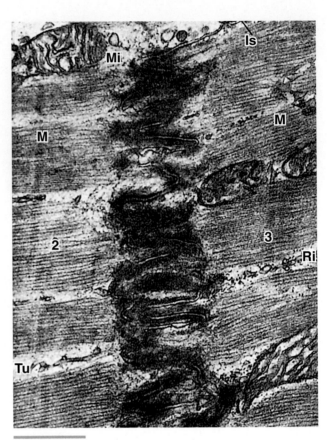

Figure 8–21 Electron micrograph of an intercalated disk from a steer heart (×29,622). Is, intercellular space; M, M-line; Mi, mitochondrion; Ri, ribosomes; Tu, sarcoplasmic reticulum. The numerals 2 and 3 denote the two cardiac muscle cells, one on either side of the intercalated disk. (From Rhodin JAG: An Atlas of Ultrastructure. Philadelphia, WB Saunders, 1963.)

almost two and one-half times the diameter of those in skeletal muscle and are lined by an **external lamina.**

Because the sarcoplasmic reticulum is relatively sparse, it cannot store enough calcium to accomplish a forceful contraction; therefore, additional sources of calcium are available. Because the T tubules open into the extracellular space and have a relatively large bore, extracellular calcium flows through the T tubules and

enters the cardiac muscle cells at the time of depolarization. Moreover, the negatively charged external lamina coating of the T tubule stores calcium for instantaneous release. An additional method whereby calcium can enter the cardiac muscle cells is through the large calcium-sodium channels described later.

Skeletal muscle cell action potential is achieved by an abundance of **fast sodium channels,** which open and close within a few ten-thousandths of a second, leading to the generation of very rapid action potentials. In addition to fast sodium channels, cardiac muscle cell membranes possess **calcium-sodium channels (slow sodium channels).** Although these channels are slow to open initially, they remain open for a considerable time (several tenths of a second). During this time, a tremendous number of sodium and calcium ions enter the cardiac muscle cell cytoplasm, thus increasing the calcium ion concentration supplied by the T tubule and the sarcoplasmic reticulum. An additional difference between the movement of ions in skeletal and cardiac

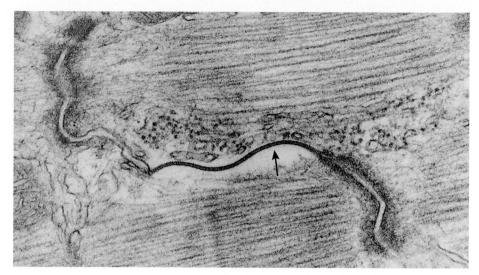

Figure 8–22 Electron micrograph of an intercalated disk from the atrium of a mouse heart (×57,810). Observe the gap junctions *(arrow).* (From Forbes MS, Sperelakis N: Intercalated disks of mammalian heart: A review of structure and function. Tissue Cell 17:605, 1985.)

muscle cells is that potassium ions can leave the skeletal muscle cells extremely quickly, thus reestablishing the resting membrane potential; in cardiac muscle cells, the egress of potassium ions is retarded, thus contributing to the protracted action potential.

CLINICAL CORRELATIONS

During **cardiac hypertrophy,** the number of myocardial fibers is not increased; instead, the cardiac muscle cells become longer and larger in diameter. Damage to the heart does not result in regeneration of muscle tissue; instead, the dead muscle cells are replaced by fibrous connective tissue.

Lack of Ca^{2+} in the extracellular compartment results in cessation of cardiac muscle contraction within 1 minute, whereas skeletal muscle fibers can continue to contract for several hours.

Although a small amount of energy production may be achieved by anaerobic metabolism (up to 10% during hypoxia), totally anaerobic conditions cannot sustain ventricular contraction.

SMOOTH MUSCLE

The cells of the third type of muscle exhibit no striations; therefore, they are referred to as smooth muscle. Additionally, smooth muscle cells do not possess a system of T tubules (Table 8-3). Smooth muscle is found in the walls of hollow viscera (e.g., the gastrointestinal tract, some of the reproductive tract, and the urinary tract), walls of blood vessels, larger ducts of compound glands, respiratory passages, and small bundles within the dermis of skin. Smooth muscle is not under voluntary control; it is regulated by the autonomic nervous system, hormones (such as bradykinins), and local physiological conditions. Hence, smooth muscle is also referred to as **involuntary muscle.**

There are two types of smooth muscle:

■ Cells of **multiunit smooth muscle** can contract independently of one another, because each muscle cell has its own nerve supply.
■ Cell membranes of **unitary (single-unit, vascular) smooth muscle** form gap junctions with those of contiguous smooth muscle cells, and nerve fibers form synapses with only a few of the muscle fibers. Thus, cells of unitary smooth muscle cannot contract independently of one another.

In addition to its contractile functions, some smooth muscle is capable of exogenous **protein synthesis.** Among the substances manufactured by smooth muscle cells for extracellular utilization are collagen, elastin, glycosaminoglycans, proteoglycans, and growth factors.

Light Microscopy of Smooth Muscle Fibers

Light microscopy reveals that smooth muscle fibers are short, spindle-shaped cells with a centrally placed nucleus.

Smooth muscle fibers are **fusiform,** elongated cells whose average length is about 0.2 mm with a diameter of 5 to 6 μm. The cells taper at either end, and the central portion contains an oval nucleus housing two

TABLE 8–3 Comparison of the Three Types of Muscle

Feature	Skeletal Muscle	Cardiac Muscle	Smooth Muscle
Sarcomeres and myofibrils	Yes	Yes	No
Nuclei	Multinucleated; peripherally located	One (or two); centrally located	One; centrally located
Sarcoplasmic reticulum	Well-developed with terminal cisterns	Poorly defined; some small terminals	Some smooth endoplasmic reticulum
T tubules	Yes; small, involved in triad formation	Yes; large, involved in dyad formation	No
Cell junctions	No	Intercalated disks	Nexus (gap junctions)
Contraction	Voluntary; "all or none"	Involuntary; rhythmic and spontaneous	Involuntary; slow and forceful; not "all or none"
Calcium control	Calsequestrin in terminal cisternae	Calcium from extracellular sources and the sarcoplasmic reticulum	Calcium from extracellular sources (via caveolae) and the sarcoplasmic/endoplasmic reticulum
Calcium binding	Troponin C	Troponin C	Calmodulin
Regeneration	Yes, via satellite cells	No	Yes
Mitosis	No	No	Yes
Nerve fibers	Somatic motor	Autonomic	Autonomic
Connective tissue	Epimysium, perimysium, and endomysium	Connective tissue sheaths and endomysium	Connective tissue sheaths and endomysium
Distinctive features	Long; cylinder-shaped; many peripheral nuclei	Branched cells; intercalated disks; one or two nuclei	Fusiform cells with no striations; single nucleus

or more nucleoli (Figs. 8-23 and 8-24; also see Fig. 8-2). During muscle shortening, the nucleus assumes a characteristic "corkscrew appearance," as a result of the method of smooth muscle contraction (Fig. 8-25).

Each smooth muscle cell is surrounded by an **external lamina,** which invariably separates the sarcolemma of contiguous muscle cells (Fig. 8-26). Embedded in the external lamina are numerous **reticular fibers,** which appear to envelop individual smooth muscle cells and function in harnessing the force of contraction.

With hematoxylin and eosin (H&E) staining, the cytoplasm of smooth muscle fibers appears unremarkable; however, iron hematoxylin stain demonstrates the presence of **dense bodies** adhering to the cytoplasmic aspect of the cell membrane. In addition to dense bodies, thin, longitudinal striations may be evident in the sarcoplasm of smooth muscle cells, representing clumped associations of **myofilaments.**

Smooth muscle cells usually form sheets of various thicknesses, although they may also occur as individual cells. When they form sheets, the cells are arranged so that they form a continuous network in which their tapered portions fit almost precisely into existing spaces between the expanded regions of neighboring smooth muscle cells (see Fig. 8-2). In cross section, outlines of various diameters may be noted, some containing nuclei, some not (see Fig. 8-24). Cross sections without nuclei represent the tapered ends of smooth muscle cells as they interdigitate with the other smooth muscle fibers.

Sheets of smooth muscle cells are frequently arranged in two layers perpendicular to each other, as in the digestive and urinary systems. This arrangement permits waves of peristalsis.

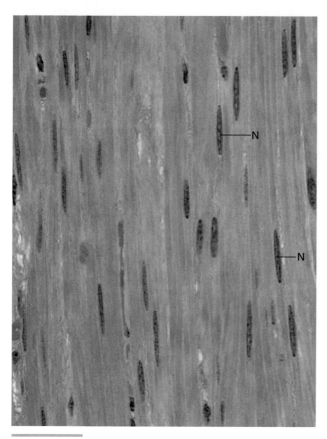

Figure 8–23 Light micrograph of smooth muscle in longitudinal section (×540). The nuclei (N) are located in the midline of the cell but off-center, so that they are closer to one lateral cell membrane than to the other. The nuclei are not corkscrew-shaped, indicating that the muscle is not undergoing contraction.

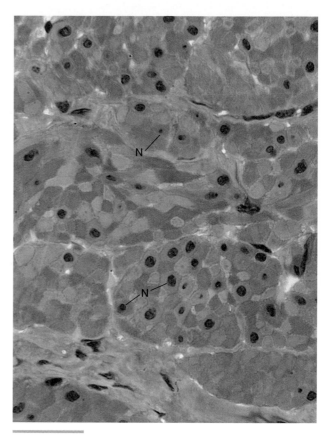

Figure 8–24 Light micrograph of smooth muscle in cross section (×540). The nuclei (N) are of various diameters, indicating that they are spindle-shaped and that they have been sectioned at various regions along their length. Also, knowing that the nucleus of the cell is located at its center and that the cell is much longer than the nucleus, it is reasonable to expect that there will be many smooth muscle cells in the field that do not display their nuclei, because they have been sectioned along regions of the cell that are away from the center.

Fine Structure of Smooth Muscle

The perinuclear cytoplasm of smooth muscle cells, especially the regions adjacent to the two poles of the nucleus, contains numerous mitochondria, Golgi apparatus, rough endoplasmic reticulum (RER), smooth endoplasmic reticulum (SER), and inclusions such as glycogen (see Fig. 8-26). Additionally, an extensive array of interweaving **thin filaments** (7 nm) and **thick filaments** (15 nm) is present. The thin filaments are composed of actin (with its associated **caldesmon,** a protein that blocks the active site of F-actin, and **tropomyosin,** with the notable absence of **troponin**). The thick filaments are composed of the same **myosin II** that is present in skeletal muscle.

Myofilaments of smooth muscle are not arranged in the paracrystalline fashion of striated muscle, and the organization of the thick filaments is not the same. Instead, the myosin II molecules are lined up so that the **heavy meromyosin heads** (S_1) project from the

thick filaments throughout the length of the filament, with the two ends lacking heavy meromyosin. The middle of the filament, unlike that of striated muscle, also possesses heavy meromyosin, resulting in the availability of a larger surface area for the interaction of actin with myosin II and permitting **contractions of long duration.**

The all-or-none law for striated muscle contraction does not apply to smooth muscle. The entire cell, or only a portion of the cell, may contract at a given instant even though the method of contraction probably follows the sliding filament theory of contraction.

The contractile forces are harnessed intracellularly by an additional system of intermediate filaments, which consist of **vimentin** and **desmin** in unitary smooth muscle and **desmin** (only) in multiunit smooth muscle. These intermediate filaments as well as thin

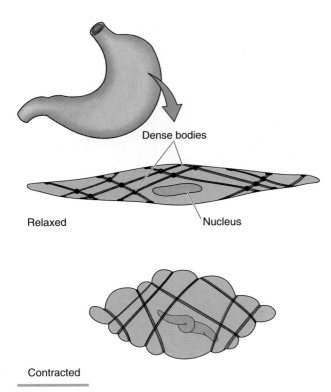

Figure 8–25 A relaxed smooth muscle cell and a contracted smooth muscle cell. Note that in a contracted smooth muscle cell the nucleus appears corkscrew-shaped.

filaments insert into **dense bodies,** formed of **α-actinin** and other Z disk–associated proteins. Dense bodies may be located in the cytoplasm or associated with the cytoplasmic aspect of the smooth muscle sarcolemma. They are believed to resemble Z disks in function and in three dimensions may even be more extensive than formerly assumed, in that they form interconnected branching networks that extend throughout the cytoplasm. The force of contraction is relayed, through the association of myofilaments with dense bodies, to the intermediate filaments, which act to twist and shorten the cell along its longitudinal axis.

Associated with the cell membrane domains are structures known as caveolae that act, among other functions, as T tubules of skeletal and cardiac muscle in regulating the cytosolic free calcium ion concentration.

Control of Smooth Muscle Contraction

Although the regulation of contraction in smooth muscle depends on Ca^{2+}, the control mechanism differs from that encountered in striated muscle because smooth muscle thin filaments are devoid of troponin. Additionally, myosin II molecules assume a different configuration, in that their actin-binding site is masked by their light meromyosin moiety (Fig. 8-27), and also their light chains are different from those of striated muscle.

Contraction of smooth muscle fibers proceeds as follows:

1 Calcium ions, released from the sarcoplasmic reticulum as well as entering the cell at plasma membrane caveolae, bind to **calmodulin** (a regulatory protein ubiquitous in living organisms), thereby altering its conformation. The Ca^{2+}-calmodulin complex binds to caldesmon, causing its release from the active site of F-actin, and then activates **myosin light chain kinase.**
2 Myosin light chain kinase phosphorylates one of the myosin light chains, known as the **regulatory chain,** permitting the unfolding of the light meromyosin moiety to form the typical, "golf club"–shaped myosin II molecule (see Fig. 8-27).
3 The phosphorylated light chain permits the interaction between actin and the S$_1$ subfragment of myosin II that results in contraction.

Because both phosphorylation and the attachment-detachment of the myosin cross-bridges occur slowly, the process of smooth muscle contraction takes longer than skeletal or cardiac muscle contraction. It is interesting that ATP hydrolysis also occurs much more slowly and the myosin heads remain attached to the thin filaments for a longer time in smooth muscle than in striated muscle. Thus, smooth muscle contraction not only is *prolonged* but also requires *less energy*.

Decrease in the sarcoplasmic calcium level results in the dissociation of the **calmodulin-calcium complex,** causing inactivation of myosin light chain kinase. The subsequent dephosphorylation of myosin light chain, catalyzed by the enzyme **myosin phosphatase,** brings about **masking** of the myosin's actin binding site and the subsequent **relaxation** of the muscle.

Innervation of Smooth Muscle

Neuromuscular junctions in smooth muscle are not as specifically organized as those in skeletal muscle. The synapses may vary from 15 to 100 nm in width. The neural component of the synapse is the **en passant** type, which occurs as axonal swellings that contain **synaptic vesicles,** housing either **norepinephrine** for sympathetic innervation or **acetylcholine** for parasympathetic innervation.

In certain cases, every smooth muscle cell receives individual innervation, as in the iris and the vas deferens. As indicated previously, smooth muscle innervated in this fashion is referred to as **multiunit.**

Other smooth muscle cells, such as those of the gastrointestinal tract and uterus, do not possess individual

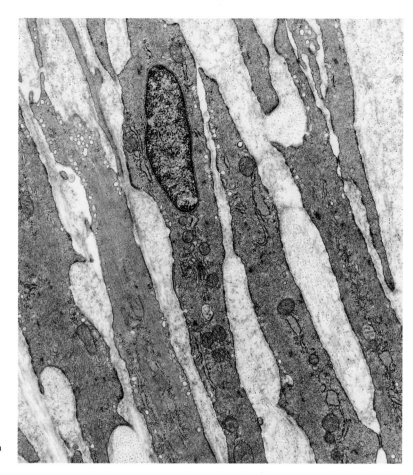

Figure 8–26 Electron micrograph of smooth muscle cells. (Courtesy of Dr. J. Strum.)

innervation; rather, only a few muscle cells are equipped with neuromuscular junctions. As discussed previously, impulse transmission in these muscles, referred to as **unitary** (**single-unit** or **visceral smooth muscles**), occurs via **nexus** (gap junctions) formed between neighboring smooth muscle cells. Visceral smooth muscle may also be regulated by humoral or microenvironmental factors, such as oxytocin in the uterus or stretching of the muscle fibers in the intestines.

Still other smooth muscles of the body are of an **intermediate** type, in which a certain percentage (30% to 60%) of the cells receive individual innervation.

REGENERATION OF MUSCLE

Although **skeletal muscle** cells do not have the capability of mitotic activity, the tissue can regenerate because of the presence of satellite cells. These cells may undergo mitotic activity, resulting in **hyperplasia,** subsequent to muscle injury. Under certain other conditions, such as "muscle building," satellite cells may fuse with existing muscle cells, thus increasing muscle mass during skeletal muscle **hypertrophy.** Skeletal

muscle cells regulate their number and their size by the secretion of a member of the transforming growth factor-β (TGF-β) superfamily of extracellular signaling molecules, **myostatin.** Certain mutant mice, whose skeletal muscle fibers cannot produce myostatin have enormous muscles that not only have many more cells but whose muscle cells are much larger than those of normal mice.

Cardiac muscle is incapable of regeneration. Following damage, such as a myocardial infarct, **fibroblasts** invade the damaged region, undergo cell division, and form fibrous connective tissue (scar tissue) to repair the damage.

Smooth muscle cells retain their mitotic capability to form more smooth muscle cells. This ability is especially evident in the pregnant uterus, where the muscular wall becomes thicker both by hypertrophy of individual cells and by hyperplasia derived from mitotic activity of the smooth muscle cells. Small defects, subsequent to injury, may result in formation of new smooth muscle cells. These new cells may be derived via mitotic activity of existing smooth muscle cells, as in the gastrointestinal and urinary tracts, or from

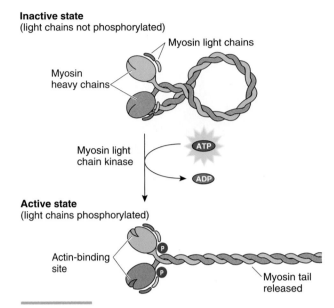

Inactive state
(light chains not phosphorylated)

Myosin light chains

Myosin
heavy chains

Myosin light
chain kinase

ATP

ADP

Active state
(light chains phosphorylated)

Actin-binding
site

P

P

Myosin tail
released

Figure 8–27 Activation of a myosin molecule of smooth muscle. ADP, adenosine diphosphate; ATP, adenosine triphosphate; P, myosin light chain–bound phosphate. (Modified from Alberts B, Bray D, Lewis J, et al.: Molecular Biology of the Cell. New York, Garland Publishing, 1994.)

differentiation of relatively undifferentiated **pericytes** accompanying some blood vessels.

MYOEPITHELIAL CELLS AND MYOFIBROBLASTS

Certain cells associated with glandular secretory units possess contractile capabilities. These myoepithelial cells are modified to assist in the delivery of the secretory products into the ducts of the gland. Myoepithelial cells are flattened and possess long processes that wrap around the glandular units (see Chapter 5, Figs. 5-24 and 5-25). Myoepithelial cells contain both actin and myosin. Mechanisms and control of contraction in myoepithelial cells resemble, but are not identical to, those in smooth muscle.

In lactating mammary glands, myoepithelial cells contract upon the release of **oxytocin;** in the lacrimal gland, they contract because of the action of **acetylcholine.**

Myofibroblasts resemble fibroblasts but have abundant actin and myosin. They can contract and are especially prominent in wound contraction and tooth eruption.

9

Nervous Tissue

Nervous tissue, composed of as many as a trillion neurons with multitudes of interconnections, forms the complex system of neuronal communication within the body. Certain neurons have **receptors,** elaborated on their terminals, that are specialized for receiving different types of stimuli (e.g., mechanical, chemical, thermal) and transducing them into nerve impulses that may eventually be conducted to nerve centers. These impulses are then transferred to other neurons for processing and transmission to higher centers for perceiving sensations or for initiating motor responses.

To accomplish these functions, the nervous system is organized anatomically into the **central nervous system (CNS),** which comprises the brain and spinal cord, and the **peripheral nervous system (PNS).** The PNS, located outside the CNS, includes cranial nerves, emanating from the brain; spinal nerves, emanating from the spinal cord; and their associated ganglia.

Functionally, the PNS is divided into a **sensory (afferent) component,** which receives and transmits impulses to the CNS for processing, and a **motor (efferent) component,** which originates in the CNS and transmits impulses to effector organs throughout the body. The motor component is further subdivided as follows:

- In the **somatic system,** impulses originating in the CNS are transmitted directly, via a single neuron, to skeletal muscles.
- In the **autonomic system,** in contrast, impulses from the CNS first are transmitted to an autonomic **ganglion** via one neuron; a second neuron originating in the autonomic ganglion then transmits the impulses to smooth muscles, cardiac muscles, or glands.

In addition to neurons, nervous tissue contains numerous other cells, collectively called **neuroglial cells,** which do not receive or transmit impulses; instead, these cells support neurons in various ways.

DEVELOPMENT OF NERVOUS TISSUE

The nervous system develops from the ectoderm of the embryo in response to signaling molecules from the notochord.

As the notochord develops early in embryonic life, it releases signaling molecules that induce the overlying ectoderm to form **neuroepithelium,** which thickens and forms the **neural plate.** As the margins of this plate continue to thicken, the plate buckles, forming a **neural groove** whose edges continue to grow toward each other until they come together, forming the **neural tube.** The rostral (anterior) end of this structure develops into the brain; the remaining (caudal) portion of the neural tube develops into the spinal cord. Additionally, the neural tube gives rise to the neuroglia, ependyma, neurons, and choroid plexus.

A small mass of cells at the lateral margins of the neural plate, which does not become incorporated into the neural tube, forms the **neural crest cells.** This group of cells begins to migrate away from the developing neural tube early in development. Once they reach their destinations, these cells eventually form many structures, including the following:

- Most of the sensory components of the PNS
- Sensory neurons of cranial and spinal sensory ganglia (dorsal root ganglia)
- Autonomic ganglia and the postganglionic autonomic neurons originating in them
- Much of the mesenchyme of the anterior head and neck
- Melanocytes of the skin and oral mucosa
- Odontoblasts (cells responsible for production of dentin)
- Chromaffin cells of the adrenal medulla

185

- Cells of the arachnoid and pia mater
- Satellite cells of peripheral ganglia
- Schwann cells

CLINICAL CORRELATIONS

Abnormal organogenesis of the CNS results in various types of congenital malformations. **Spina bifida** is a defective closure of the spinal column. In severe cases, the spinal cord and meninges may protrude through the unfused areas. **Spina bifida anterior** is a defective closure of the vertebrae. Severe cases may be associated with defective development of the viscera of the thorax and abdomen.

    Anencephaly is failure of the developmental anterior neuropore to close, with a poorly formed brain and absence of the cranial vault. It usually is not compatible with life.

    Epilepsy may result from abnormal migration of cortical cells, which disrupts normal interneuronal functioning.

    Hirschsprung disease, also known as **congenital megacolon,** is caused by failure of the neural crest cells to invade the wall of the gut. The wall lacks **Auerbach's plexus,** a portion of the parasympathetic system innervating the distal end of the colon. Absence of the plexus leads to dilatation and hypertrophy of the colon.

CELLS OF THE NERVOUS SYSTEM

The cells of the nervous system are divided into **two categories:** neurons, which are responsible for the receptive, integrative, and motor functions of the nervous system; and neuroglial cells, which support and protect neurons.

Neurons

The cells responsible for the reception and transmission of nerve impulses to and from the CNS are the neurons. Ranging in diameter from 5 to 150 mm, neurons are among both the smallest and the largest cells in the body.

Structure and Function of Neurons

Neurons are composed of a cell body, dendrites, and an axon.

Most neurons are composed of three distinct parts: a cell body, multiple dendrites, and a single axon. The **cell**

body of a neuron, also known as the **perikaryon** or **soma,** is the central portion of the cell where the nucleus and perinuclear cytoplasm are contained. Generally, neurons in the CNS are polygonal (Fig. 9-1), with concave surfaces between the many cell processes, whereas neurons in the dorsal root ganglion (a sensory ganglion of the PNS) have a round cell body from which only one process exits (Fig. 9-2). Cell bodies exhibit different sizes and shapes that are characteristic for their type and location. These different morphologies are described later in the discussion of the various regions of the nervous system.

Projecting from the cell body are the **dendrites,** processes specialized for receiving stimuli from sensory cells, axons, and other neurons (Fig. 9-3). Often the dendrites are multibranched. They are arborized so that they can receive multiple stimuli from many other neurons simultaneously. The nerve impulses received by the dendrites are then transmitted toward the soma.

Each neuron possesses a single **axon,** a process of varying diameter and up to 100 cm in length, which usually has terminal dilatations, known as **axon terminals,** at or near its end. The axon conducts impulses away from the soma to other neurons, muscles, or glands, but it may also receive stimuli from other neurons, which may modify its behavior. Like dendrites, the axon arborizes. These axon terminals, also known as

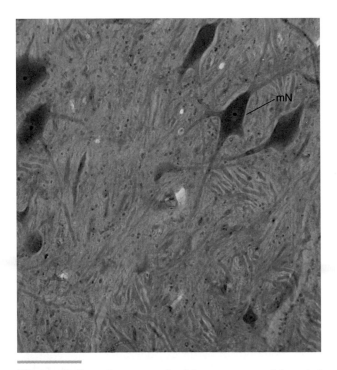

Figure 9–1 Light micrograph of the gray matter of the spinal cord (×270). Observe the multipolar neuron (mN) cell bodies and their processes.

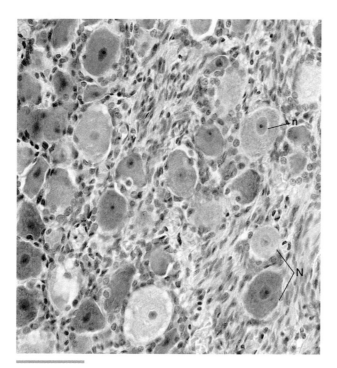

Figure 9–2 Light micrograph of a sensory ganglion (×270). Observe the large neuronal cell bodies (N) with singular nucleoli (n).

end bulbs (terminal boutons), approach other cells to form a **synapse,** the region where impulses can be transmitted between cells. Neurons can be classified according to their shape and the arrangement of their processes (Fig. 9-4).

Neuronal Cell Body (Soma, Perikaryon)

The cell body is the region of the neuron containing the large, pale-staining nucleus and the perinuclear cytoplasm.

The cell body is the most conspicuous region of the neuron, but the largest volume of the neuron's cytoplasm is located in the processes originating from the cell body. The **nucleus** is large, usually spherical to ovoid, and centrally located. It contains finely dispersed chromatin, indicative of a rich synthetic activity, although smaller neurons may present some condensed, inactive heterochromatin. A well-defined nucleolus is also common.

The **cytoplasm** of the cell body has abundant rough endoplasmic reticulum (RER) with many cisternae in parallel arrays, a characteristic especially prominent in large motor neurons. Polyribosomes are also scattered throughout the cytoplasm. When these stacked RER cisternae and polyribosomes are stained with basic dyes, they appear as clumps of basophilic material called **Nissl bodies,** which are visible with the light micro-

scope. RER is also present in the dendritic region of the neuron, but only as scattered short or branching cisternae. RER is absent at the **axon hillock,** the region on the cell body where the axon arises; however, smooth endoplasmic reticulum (SER) is present in the axon.

Although Nissl bodies in each type of neuron have a characteristic size, shape, and form, no pattern has been observed. Generally, small neurons display small granular Nissl bodies, but not all large neurons display larger Nissl bodies. These differences may be related to changing physiological and pathological conditions within the neuron.

Most neurons have abundant SER throughout the cell body; this reticulum extends into the dendrites and the axon, forming **hypolemmal cisternae** directly beneath the plasmalemma. These cisternae are continuous with the RER in the cell body and weave between the Nissl bodies on their way into the dendrites and axon. Although it is unclear how they function, it is known that hypolemmal cisternae sequester calcium and contain protein. These cisternae may serve as a conduit for the distribution of protein throughout the cell. Some authors theorize that transport and synaptic vesicles bud from these cisternae, but much of this issue is still unclear.

A prominent juxtanuclear **Golgi complex** is present, composed of several closely associated cisternae exhibiting a dilated periphery, characteristic of protein-secreting cells. The Golgi complex is thought to be responsible for the packaging of neurotransmitter substances or enzymes essential for their production in the axon.

Numerous **mitochondria** are scattered throughout the cytoplasm of the soma, dendrites, and axon, but they are most abundant at the axon terminals. Generally, the mitochondria in neurons are more slender than those in other cells, and occasionally their cristae are oriented longitudinally rather than transversely. It has been shown that neuronal mitochondria are constantly moving along microtubules in the cytoplasm.

Most adult neurons display only one **centriole** associated with a basal body of a cilium; it possesses the 9 + 0 arrangement of microtubules (see Chapter 2 concerning microtubule structure). Because neurons do not undergo cell division, their centrioles are believed to be vestigial structures.

INCLUSIONS

Inclusions located in neuronal cell bodies encompass nonliving substances such as melanin and lipofuscin pigments as well as lipid droplets.

Dark brown to black **melanin granules** are found in neurons in certain regions of the CNS (e.g., mostly in the substantia nigra and locus ceruleus, with lesser

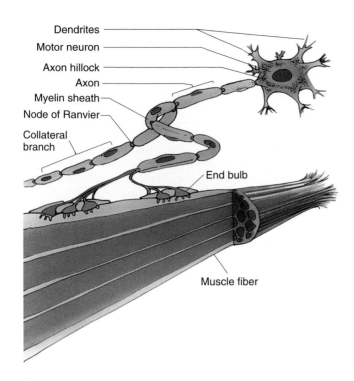

Dendrites

Motor neuron

Axon hillock

Axon

Myelin sheath

Node of Ranvier

Collateral branch

End bulb

Muscle fiber

A

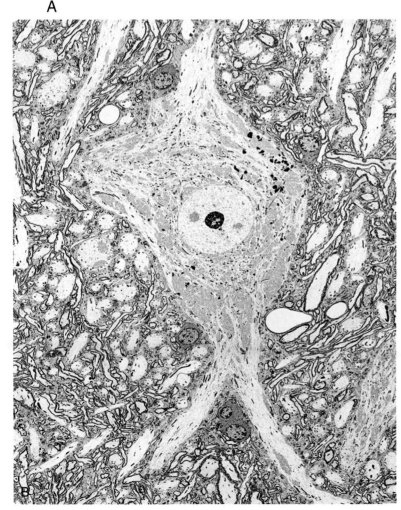

B

Figure 9–3 **A,** Typical motor neuron. **B,** Electron micrograph of a ventral horn neuron with several of its dendrites (×1300). (**B,** From Ling EA, Wen CY, Shieh JY, et al: Neuroglial response to neuron injury: A study using intraneural injection of *Ricinus communis* agglutinin-60. J Anat 164:201-213, 1989.)

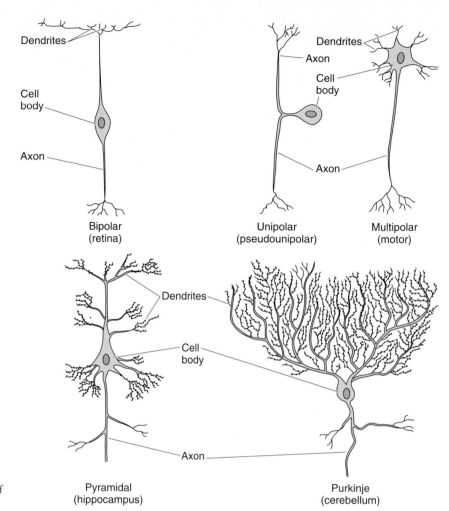

Figure 9–4 The various types of neurons.

amounts in the dorsal motor nucleus of the vagus and the spinal cord) and in the sympathetic ganglia of the PNS. The function of these granules in these various locations is unknown. However, dihydroxyphenylalanine (DOPA), or methyldopa, the precursor of this pigment, is also the precursor of the neurotransmitters dopamine and noradrenaline. It has been suggested, therefore, that melanin may accumulate as a by-product of the synthesis of these neurotransmitters.

Lipofuscin, an irregularly shaped, yellowish brown pigment granule, is more prevalent in the neuronal cytoplasm of older adults and is thought to be the remnant of lysosomal enzymatic activity. Lipofuscin granules increase in number with advancing age and may even crowd the organelles and nucleus to one side in the cell, possibly affecting cellular function. It is interesting that certain cells (e.g., Purkinje cells of the cerebellar cortex) do not accumulate lipofuscin. Iron-containing pigments also may be observed in certain neurons of the CNS and may accumulate with age.

Lipid droplets sometimes are observed in the neuronal cytoplasm and may be the result of faulty metabolism or from energy reserves. **Secretory granules** are observed in neurosecretory cells; many of them contain signaling molecules.

CYTOSKELETAL COMPONENTS

When prepared by silver impregnation for visualization with light microscopy, the neuronal cytoskeleton exhibits **neurofibrils** (up to 2 mm in diameter) coursing through the cytoplasm of the soma and extending into the processes. Electron microscopic studies reveal three different filamentous structures: **microtubules** (24 nm in diameter), **neurofilaments** (intermediate filaments 10 nm in diameter), and **microfilaments** (6 nm in diameter). The neurofibrils observed with light microscopy possibly represent clumped bundles of neurofilaments, a suggestion supported by the fact that neurofilaments are stained by silver nitrate. Microfilaments (actin filaments) are associated with the plasma membrane. The microtubules in neurons are identical to those in other cells, except that the **microtubule-associated protein MAP-2** is found in the cytoplasm of the cell body and dendrite, whereas MAP-3 is present only in the axon.

Dendrites

Dendrites receive stimuli from other nerve cells.

Dendrites are elaborations of the receptive plasma membrane of the neuron. In some neurons, however, the cell body and the proximal end of the axon may also serve in a receptive capacity. Most neurons possess multiple dendrites, each of which arises from the cell body, usually as a single, short trunk that ramifies several times into smaller and smaller branches, tapering at the ends like branches of a tree. Each kind of neuron has a characteristic dendrite branching pattern. The base of the dendrite arises from the cell body and contains the usual complement of organelles except for Golgi complexes (Fig. 9-5). Farther away from the base, toward the distal end of the dendrite, many of the organelles become sparse or are absent.

In the dendrites of most neurons, neurofilaments are reduced to small bundles or single filaments, which may be cross-linked to microtubules. Mitochondria, however, are abundant in dendrites. The branching of dendrites, which results in numerous synaptic terminals, permits a neuron to receive and integrate multiple, perhaps even hundreds of thousands, of impulses. **Spines** located on the surfaces of some dendrites permit them to form synapses with other neurons.

These spines diminish with age and poor nutrition, and they may exhibit structural changes in persons with trisomy 13 and trisomy 21 (Down syndrome). Dendrites sometimes contain vesicles and transmit impulses to other dendrites.

Axons

Axons transmit impulses to other neurons or effector cells, namely cells of muscle and glands.

The axon arises from the cell body at the axon hillock as a single, thin process extending longer distances from the cell body than does the dendrite. In some instances, axons of motor neurons may be 1 meter or more in length. Axon thickness is directly related to conduction velocity, so that velocity increases as axon diameter increases. Although axon thickness varies, it is constant for a particular type of neuron. Some axons possess **collateral branches,** which arise at right angles from the axonal trunk (see Fig. 9-3A). As the axon terminates, it may ramify, forming many small branches (**terminal arbor**).

The **axon hillock,** a pyramid-shaped region of the soma, is devoid of ribosomes and is usually located on the opposite side of the soma from the dendrites. The portion of the axon from its origin to the beginning of the myelin sheath is called the **initial segment.** Deep to the **axolemma** (plasmalemma) of the initial segment is a thin, electron-dense layer whose function is not known but that resembles the layer located at the nodes of Ranvier. This area of the soma lacks RER and ribosomes but houses abundant microtubules and neurofilaments that are believed to facilitate the regulation

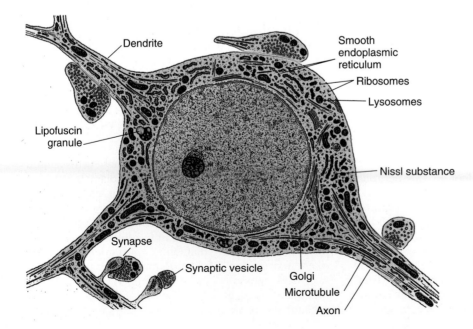

Figure 9–5 Ultrastructure of a neuronal cell body. (From Lentz TL: Cell Fine Structure: An Atlas of Drawings of Whole-Cell Structure. Philadelphia, WB Saunders, 1971.)

of the axon's diameter. In some neurons, the number of neurofilaments may increase three-fold in the initial segment, whereas the number of microtubules increases only slightly. It is in this initial segment, referred to as the **spike trigger zone,** where excitatory and inhibitory impulses are summed to determine whether propagation of an action potential is to occur.

The axoplasm contains short profiles of SER and remarkably long, thin mitochondria and many microtubules; however, it lacks RER and polyribosomes. Thus, the axon relies on the soma for its maintenance. Microtubules are grouped in small bundles at the origin of the axon and in its initial segment; distally, however, they become arranged as uniformly spaced, single microtubules interspersed with neurofilaments.

The plasmalemma of certain neuroglial cells forms a **myelin sheath** around some axons in both the CNS and the PNS, referred to as **myelinated axons** (Figs. 9-6 and 9-7) (the process of myelination is described in detail later). Axons lacking myelin sheaths are called **unmyelinated axons** (Fig. 9-8). Nerve impulses are conducted much faster along myelinated axons than along unmyelinated axons. In the fresh state, the myelin sheath imparts a white, glistening appearance to the axon. The presence of myelin permits the subdivision of the CNS into **white matter** and **gray matter.**

In addition to impulse conduction, an important function of the axon is **axonal transport** of materials between the soma and the axon terminals. In **anterograde transport,** the direction is from the cell body to the axon terminal; in **retrograde transport,** the direction is from the axon terminal to the cell body. Axonal transport is crucial to **trophic relationships** within the axon because it is located between neurons and muscles or glands. If these relationships are interrupted, the target cells atrophy.

Axonal transport occurs at three velocities: fast, intermediate, and slow. The most rapid transport (up to 400 mm/day) takes place in anterograde transport of organelles, which move more rapidly in the cytosol. In retrograde transport, the fastest speed is less than half that observed in anterograde transport, with the slowest being only about 0.2 mm/day. Axonal transport speeds between these two extremes are considered intermediate.

Anterograde transport is used in the translocation of organelles and vesicles as well as of macromolecules such as actin, myosin, and clathrin and of some enzymes necessary for neurotransmitter synthesis at the axon terminals. Items returned to the cell body from the axon in **retrograde transport** include protein building blocks of neurofilaments, subunits of microtubules, soluble enzymes, and materials taken up by endocytosis (e.g., viruses and toxins). Additionally, small molecules and proteins destined for degradation are transported to endolysosomes of the soma.

CLINICAL CORRELATIONS

Retrograde axonal transport is used by certain viruses (e.g., herpes simplex and rabies virus) to spread from one neuron to the next in a chain of neurons. It is also the method whereby toxins (e.g., tetanus) are transported from the periphery into the CNS.

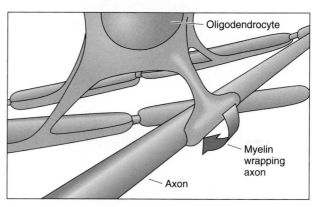

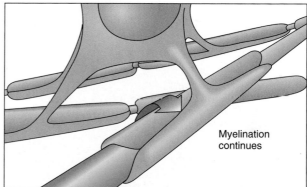

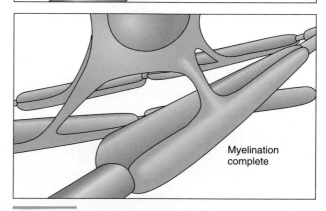

Figure 9–6 Process of myelination in the central nervous system. Unlike the Schwann cell of the peripheral nervous system, each oligodendroglion is capable of myelinating several axons.

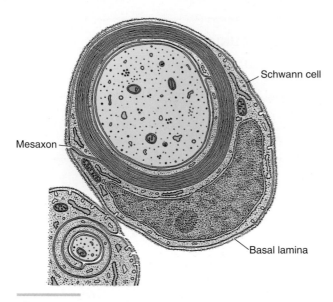

Figure 9–7 The fine structure of a myelinated nerve fiber and its Schwann cell. (From Lentz TL: Cell Fine Structure: An Atlas of Drawings of Whole-Cell Structure. Philadelphia, WB Saunders, 1971.)

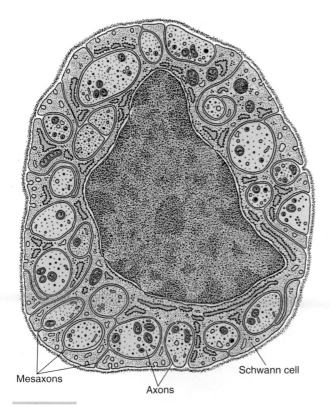

Figure 9–8 The fine structure of an unmyelinated nerve fiber. (From Lentz TL: Cell Fine Structure. An Atlas of Drawings of Whole-Cell Structure. Philadelphia, WB Saunders, 1971.)

Axonal transport not only distributes materials for nerve conduction and neurotransmitter synthesis but also serves to provide and ensure general maintenance of the axon cytoskeleton.

Since the 1970s, much has been learned about the nature and functioning of the neuron through study of the mechanism of axonal retrograde transport with the use of the enzyme **horseradish peroxidase.** When this enzyme is injected into the axon terminal, it can be detected later by histochemical techniques that mark its pathway to the cell body. In studying anterograde axonal transport, researchers inject radiolabeled amino acids into the cell body and then later determine the radioactivity at the axon terminals using autoradiography.

Microtubules are important in fast anterograde transport because they exhibit a polarity, with their plus ends directed toward the axon terminal. **Tubulin dimers,** reaching the axoplasm via anterograde transport, are assembled onto the microtubules at their plus ends and depolymerized at their minus ends. The mechanism for anterograde transport involves **kinesin,** a microtubule-associated protein, because one end attaches to a vesicle and the other end interacts in a cyclical fashion with a microtubule, thus permitting the kinesin to transport the vesicle at a speed of about 3 mm/second. **Dynein,** another microtubule-associated protein, is responsible for moving vesicles along the microtubules in retrograde transport.

CLINICAL CORRELATIONS

Although **neurological tumors** account for about 50% of intracranial tumors, those of neurons of the CNS are rare. Most intracranial tumors originate from neuroglial cells (e.g., **benign oligodendrogliomas** and fatal **malignant astrocytomas).** Tumors that arise from cells of connective tissue associated with nervous tissue (e.g., **benign fibroma** or **malignant sarcoma)** are connective tissue tumors and are not related to the nervous system. Tumors of neurons in the PNS may be extremely malignant (e.g., **neuroblastoma** in the suprarenal gland, which attacks mostly infants and young children).

Classification of Neurons

Neurons are classified morphologically into three major types according to their shape and the arrangement of their processes.

There are three major types of neurons (see Fig. 9-4):

■ **Bipolar neurons** possess two processes emanating from the soma, a single dendrite and a single axon.

Bipolar neurons are located in the vestibular and cochlear ganglia and in the olfactory epithelium of the nasal cavity.

■ **Unipolar neurons** (formerly called **pseudounipolar neurons**) possess only one process emanating from the cell body, but this process branches later into a peripheral branch and a central branch. The central branch enters the CNS, and the peripheral branch proceeds to its destination in the body. Each of the branches is morphologically axonal and can propagate nerve impulses, although the very distal aspect of the peripheral branch arborizes and displays small dendritic ends, indicating its receptor function. Unipolar neurons develop from embryonic bipolar neurons whose processes migrate around the cell body during development and eventually fuse into a single process. During impulse transmission, the impulse passes from the dendritic (receiving) end of the peripheral process to the central process without involving the cell body. Unipolar neurons are present in the dorsal root ganglia and in some of the cranial nerve ganglia.

■ **Multipolar neurons,** the most common type, possess various arrangements of multiple dendrites emanating from the soma and a single axon. They are present throughout the nervous system, and most of them are motor neurons. Some multipolar neurons are named according to their morphology (e.g., pyramidal cells) or after the scientist who first described them (e.g., Purkinje cells).

Neurons also are classified into three general groups according to their function:

■ **Sensory (afferent) neurons** receive sensory input at their dendritic terminals and conduct impulses to the CNS for processing. Those located in the periphery of the body monitor changes in the environment, and those within the body monitor the internal environment.

■ **Motor (efferent) neurons** originate in the CNS and conduct their impulses to muscles, glands, and other neurons.

■ **Interneurons,** located completely in the CNS, function as interconnectors or integrators that establish networks of neuronal circuits between sensory and motor neurons and other interneurons. With evolution, the number of neurons in the human nervous system has grown enormously, but the greatest increase has involved the interneurons, which are responsible for the complex functioning of the body.

Neuroglial Cells

Neuroglial cells function in the physical and metabolic support of neurons.

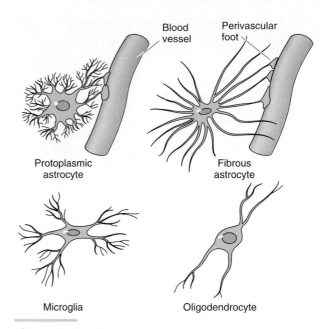

Figure 9–9 The various types of neuroglial cells.

Cells whose function is the metabolic and mechanical support and protection of neurons collectively form the neuroglia (Fig. 9-9). There may be as many as 10 times more neuroglial cells than neurons in the nervous system. Neuroglial cells undergo mitosis, whereas neurons cannot—only their progenitors can. Although neuroglial cells form gap junctions with other neuroglial cells, they do not react to or propagate nerve impulses. Neuroglial cells that reside exclusively in the CNS include astrocytes, oligodendrocytes, microglia (microglial cells), and ependymal cells. Schwann cells, although located in the PNS, are now also considered neuroglial cells.

Astrocytes

Astrocytes provide structural and metabolic support to neurons and act as scavengers of ions and neurotransmitters released into the extracellular space.

Astrocytes are the largest of the neuroglial cells and exist as two distinct types: (1) protoplasmic astrocytes in the gray matter of the CNS and (2) fibrous astrocytes present mainly in the white matter of the CNS. It is difficult to distinguish the two types of astrocytes in light micrographs. Some researchers have suggested that they may be the same cells functioning in different environments. Electron micrographs display distinct cytoplasmic bundles of intermediate filaments 8- to 11-nm in diameter composed of **glial fibrillar acidic protein,** which is unique to astrocytes.

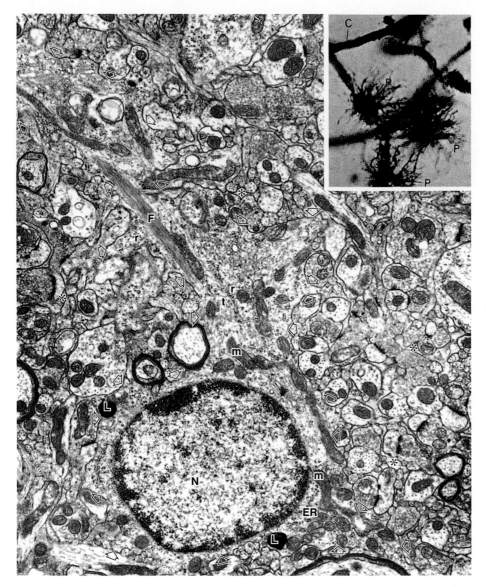

Figure 9–10 Electron micrograph of protoplasmic astrocyte (×11,400). Observe the nucleus (N), filaments (F), mitochondria (m), microtubules (t), free ribosomes (r), and granular endoplasmic reticulum (ER). Two lysosomes (L) are also identified in the processes of the neuroglia. Note the irregular cell boundary (*arrowheads*) and processes of other neuroglial cells of the neuropil (*asterisks*). *Inset*, Light micrograph of three highly branched protoplasmic astrocytes (P) surrounding capillaries (C). (*Large image*, From Peters A, Palay SL, Webster HF: The Fine Structure of the Nervous System. Philadelphia, WB Saunders, 1976. *Inset*, From Leeson TS, Leeson CR, Paparo AA: Text/Atlas of Histology. Philadelphia, WB Saunders, 1988.)

Protoplasmic astrocytes are stellate cells displaying abundant cytoplasm, a large nucleus, and many short branching processes (Fig. 9-10). The tips of some processes end as **pedicels (vascular feet)** that come into contact with blood vessels. Other astrocytes lie adjacent to blood vessels with the cell body apposed to the vessel wall. Still other protoplasmic astrocytes near the brain or surface of the spinal cord exhibit pedicel-tipped processes that contact the pia mater, forming the **pia-glial membrane.** Some smaller protoplasmic astrocytes located adjacent to neuronal cell bodies are a form of satellite cells.

Fibrous astrocytes possess a euchromatic cytoplasm containing only a few organelles, free ribosomes, and glycogen (Fig. 9-11). The processes of these cells

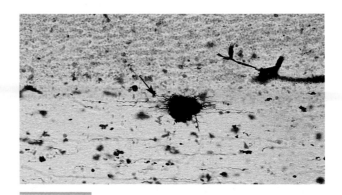

Figure 9–11 Light micrograph of a fibrous astrocyte (*arrow*) in the human cerebellum (×132).

are long and mostly unbranched. These processes are closely associated with the pia mater and blood vessels but are separated from these structures by their own basal lamina.

Astrocytes function in scavenging ions, neurotransmitters, and remnants of neuronal metabolism, such as potassium ions (K⁺), glutamate, and γ-aminobutyric acid (GABA), accumulated in the microenvironment of the neurons, especially at the nodes of Ranvier, where they provide a cover for the axon. These cells also contribute to energy metabolism within the cerebral cortex by releasing glucose from their stored glycogen when induced by the neurotransmitters norepinephrine and vasoactive intestinal peptide. Astrocytes located at the periphery of the CNS form a continuous layer over the blood vessels and may assist in maintaining the **blood-brain barrier.** Astrocytes are also recruited to damaged areas of the CNS, where they form cellular scar tissue.

Oligodendrocytes

Oligodendrocytes function in electrical insulation and in myelin production in the CNS.

Oligodendrocytes resemble astrocytes but are smaller and contain fewer processes with sparse branching. The darkest-staining neuroglial cells, oligodendrocytes are located in both the gray and the white matter of the CNS. Their dense cytoplasm contains a relatively small nucleus, abundant RER, many free ribosomes and mitochondria, and a conspicuous Golgi complex (Fig. 9-12). Microtubules also are present, especially in the perinuclear zone and in the processes.

Interfascicular oligodendrocytes, located in rows beside bundles of axons, are responsible for manufacturing and maintaining **myelin** about the axons of the CNS, serving to insulate them (see Fig. 9-6). In producing myelin, oligodendrocytes function similarly to

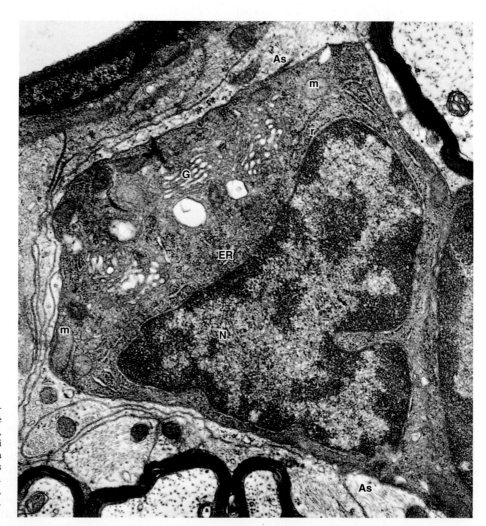

Figure 9–12 Electron micrograph of an oligodendrocyte (×2925). Note the nucleus (N), endoplasmic reticulum (ER), Golgi apparatus (G), and mitochondria (m). Processes of fibrous astrocytes (As) contact the oligodendrocyte. (From Leeson TS, Leeson CR, Paparo AA: Text/Atlas of Histology. Philadelphia, WB Saunders, 1988.)

the Schwann cells of the PNS, except that a single oligo-dendrocyte may wrap several axons with segments of myelin, whereas a single Schwann cell wraps only one axon with myelin. Schwann cells also differ from inter-fascicular oligodendrocytes in the following ways: Schwann cells possess a basal lamina and retain some cytoplasm within the intracellular domains of the myelin lamellae, and connective tissue invests the myelin sheaths and their surrounding Schwann cells.

Satellite oligodendrocytes are closely applied to cell bodies of large neurons; their function is not clear.

Microglial Cells

Microglia are members of the mononuclear phagocyte system.

Scattered throughout the CNS, microglial cells are small, dark-staining cells that faintly resemble oligo-dendrocytes. These cells exhibit scant cytoplasm, an oval to triangular nucleus, and irregular short processes. Spines also adorn the cell body and processes. These cells function as phagocytes in clearing debris and damaged structures in the CNS. Microglial cells also protect the nervous system from viruses, microorgan-isms, and tumor formation. When activated, they act as antigen-presenting cells and secrete cytokines. Unlike the other neuroglial cells, which are derived embry-ologically from the neural tube, microglial cells originate in the bone marrow and are part of the mononuclear phagocytic cell population.

CLINICAL CORRELATIONS

Large populations of microglial cells are pre-sent in the brains of patients with acquired immunodeficiency syndrome (AIDS) and human immunodeficiency virus-1 (HIV-1). Although HIV-1 does not attack neurons, it does attack microglial cells, which then produce cytokines that are toxic to neurons.

Ependymal Cells

Ependymal cells form limiting membranes and also may function in the transportation of cerebrospinal fluid.

Ependymal cells (ependymocytes) are low columnar to cuboidal epithelial cells lining the ventricles of the brain and central canal of the spinal cord. They are derived from embryonic neuroepithelium of the developing nervous system. Their cytoplasm contains abundant mitochondria and bundles of intermediate filaments. In some regions, these cells are ciliated, a feature

that facilitates the movement of **cerebrospinal fluid (CSF).** In the embryo, processes emanating from the cell body reach the surface of the brain, but in the adult the processes are reduced, ending on nearby cells.

Where the neural tissue is thin, ependymal cells form an **internal limiting membrane** lining the ventricle and an **external limiting membrane** beneath the pia, both formed by thin fused pedicels. Modifications of some of the ependymal cells in the ventricles of the brain participate in the formation of the **choroid plexus,** which is responsible for secreting and main-taining the chemical composition of the CSF.

Tanycytes, specialized ependymal cells, extend processes into the hypothalamus, where they terminate near blood vessels and neurosecretory cells. It is believed that tanycytes transport CSF to these neu-rosecretory cells and, possibly under control from the anterior lobe of the pituitary, may respond to changes in hormone levels in the CSF by discharging secretory products into capillaries of the median eminence.

Schwann Cells

Schwann cells form both myelinated and unmyelinated coverings over axons of the PNS.

Unlike other neuroglial cells, **Schwann cells** are located in the PNS, where they envelop axons. They can form either myelinated or unmyelinated coverings over axons. Axons that have myelin wrapped around them are referred to as **myelinated nerves.**

Schwann cells are flattened cells whose cytoplasm contains a flattened nucleus, a small Golgi apparatus, and a few mitochondria. Electron microscopy has revealed that myelin is the plasmalemma of the Schwann cell organized into a sheath that is wrapped several times around the axon. Interruptions occur in the myelin sheath at regular intervals along the length of the axon, exposing the axon; these interruptions are called **nodes of Ranvier** (Fig. 9-13). Each node indi-cates an interface between the myelin sheaths of two different Schwann cells located along the axon.

The outer portion of Schwann cells is covered by a basal lamina that dips into the nodes of Ranvier, cover-ing the overlapped areas of the myelin sheath lamellae of adjacent Schwann cells. Thus, each Schwann cell is covered by a basal lamina, as is the axon at the node of Ranvier. After nerve injury, the regenerating nerve is guided by the basal lamina to its location.

Areas of the axon covered by concentric lamellae of myelin and the single Schwann cell that produced the myelin are called **internodal segments,** which range in length from 200 to 1000 μm. Light microscopy has revealed several cone-shaped, oblique clefts in the myelin sheath of each internodal segment called **clefts (incisures) of Schmidt-Lanterman.** These clefts,

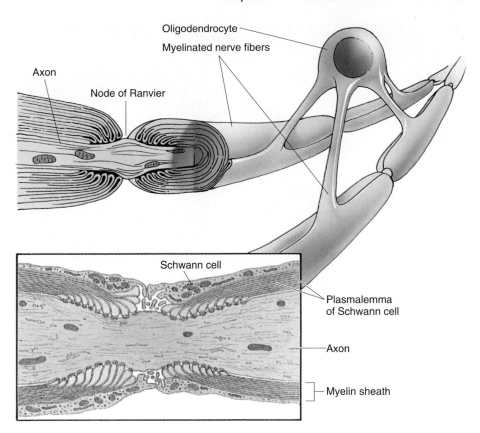

Figure 9–13 Diagrammatic representation of the myelin structure at the nodes of Ranvier of axons in the central nervous system and (*inset*) in the peripheral nervous system.

viewed with the electron microscope, are demonstrated to be Schwann cell cytoplasm trapped within the lamellae of myelin.

As the membrane spirals around the axon, it produces a series of alternating wide, dense lines with narrower, less dense lines occurring at 12-nm intervals. The wider line (3 nm in width) is known as the **major dense line.** It represents the fused cytoplasmic surfaces of the Schwann cell plasma membrane. The narrower **intraperiod line** represents the apposing outer leaflets of the Schwann cell plasma membrane. High-resolution electron microscopy has revealed small gaps within the intraperiod line between spiraled layers of the myelin sheath called **intraperiod gaps.** These gaps are thought to provide access for small molecules to reach the axon. The region of the intraperiod line that is in intimate contact with the axon is known as the **internal mesaxon,** whereas its outermost aspect, which is in contact with the body of the Schwann cell, is the **external mesaxon** (Fig. 9-14; also see Fig. 9-7).

The mechanism of **myelination,** that is, the process whereby the Schwann cell located in the PNS (or oligodendrocyte, located in the CNS) concentrically wraps its membrane around the axon to form the myelin sheath, is unclear. It is believed to begin when a Schwann cell envelops an axon and somehow wraps its membrane around the axon. The wrapping may continue for more than 50 turns. During this process, the cytoplasm is squeezed back into the body of the Schwann cell, bringing the cytoplasmic surfaces of the membranes in contact with each other, thus forming the major dense line that spirals through the myelin sheath. A single Schwann cell can myelinate only one internode of a single axon (and only in the PNS), whereas oligodendrocytes can myelinate an internode of several axons (and only in the CNS).

Nerves are not myelinated simultaneously during development. Indeed, the onset and completion of myelination vary considerably in different areas of the nervous system. This variation seems to be correlated with function. For example, motor nerves are nearly completely myelinated at birth, whereas sensory roots are not myelinated for several months thereafter. Some CNS nerve tracts and commissural axons are not fully myelinated until several years after birth.

Some axons in the PNS are not wrapped with the many layers of myelin typical of myelinated axons. These unmyelinated axons are surrounded by a single layer of Schwann cell plasma membrane and cytoplasm of the Schwann cell (see Fig. 9-8). Although a single Schwann cell can myelinate only one axon, several unmyelinated axons may be enveloped by a single Schwann cell.

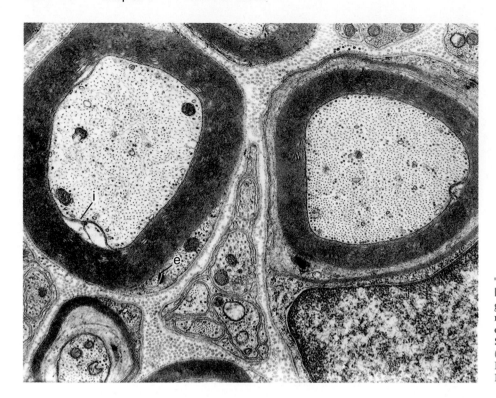

Figure 9–14 Electron micrograph of a myelinated peripheral nerve. Note the internal (i) and external (e) mesaxons as well as the Schwann cell cytoplasm and nucleus. (From Jennes L, Traurig HH, Conn PM: Atlas of the Human Brain. Philadelphia, Lippincott-Raven, 1995.)

GENERATION AND CONDUCTION OF NERVE IMPULSES*

Nerve impulses are generated in the spike trigger zone of the neuron and are conducted along the axon to the axon terminal.

Nerve impulses are electrical signals that are generated in the spike trigger zone of a neuron as the result of **membrane depolarization** and are conducted along the axon to the axon terminal. Transmission of impulses from the terminals of one neuron to another neuron, a muscle cell, or a gland occurs at synapses (see Synapses and the Transmission of the Nerve Impulse).

Neurons and other cells are electrically **polarized** with a **resting potential** of about −90 mV (the inside of the cell being less positive than the outside) across the plasma membrane, although in smaller muscle cells and small nerve fibers, this differential may be as low as −40 to −60 mV. This potential arises because of the difference between ion concentrations inside and outside the cell. In mammalian cells, the concentration of

*Although negatively charged proteins within the cytoplasm of the neuron do not cross the cell membrane, they do affect the behavior of the various charged species. However, their role in the generation and conduction of nerve impulses is not described here. The interested reader is referred to textbooks of physiology or neuroscience for an in-depth explanation of these phenomena.

potassium ions (K^+) is much higher inside the cell than outside the cell, whereas the concentration of sodium ions (Na^+) and chloride ions (Cl^-) is much higher outside the cells than inside the cell.

K^+ leak channels in the plasmalemma permit a relatively free flow of potassium ions out of a cell down its concentration gradient (Fig. 9-15). Although the K^+ leak channel allows sodium ions to enter the cell, the ratio of potassium to sodium is 100:1, so that many more potassium ions leave the cell than sodium ions enter; thus, a small net positive charge accumulates on the outside of the plasma membrane. Although maintenance of the resting potential depends primarily on K^+ leak channels, **Na^+-K^+ pumps** in the plasma membrane assist by actively pumping Na^+ out of the cell and K^+ into the cell. For every three sodium ions pumped out, two potassium ions enter the cell, also making a minor contribution to the potential difference between the two sides of the membrane.

In most cells, the potential across the plasma membrane is generally constant. In neurons and muscle cells, however, the membrane potential can undergo controlled changes, making these cells capable of conducting an electrical signal, as follows:

1 Stimulation of a neuron causes opening of voltage-gated Na^+ channels in a small region of the membrane, leading to an influx of Na^+ into the cell at that site (Fig. 9-16). Eventually, the overabundance of

CLINICAL CORRELATIONS

Multiple sclerosis (MS), a relatively common disease affecting myelin, is 1.5 times more common in females than in males. It usually occurs between 15 and 45 years of age, and its principal pathological feature is demyelination in the CNS (optic nerve, cerebellum, and white matter of the cerebrum, spinal cord, and cranial and spinal nerves). The disease is distinguished by episodes of random, multifocal inflammation, edema, and subsequent demyelination of axons in the CNS, followed by periods of remission that may last for several months to decades. Each episode may further jeopardize the patient's vitality. Any single episode of demyelination may cause deterioration or malignancy of the affected nerves and may lead to death in a matter of months. Because this demyelination is thought to result from an autoimmune disease with inflammatory features (which may manifest as a possible aftermath of an infectious agent), immunosuppression with corti-costeroids is the most common therapy for multiple sclerosis, although the anti-inflammatory activity of the therapy is thought to be most beneficial.

Radiation therapy can lead to demyelination of the brain or spinal cord when these structures are in the radiation field during therapy. Toxic agents, such as those used in **chemotherapy** for cancer, may also lead to demyelination, resulting in neurological problems.

Guillain-Barré Syndrome is an immune disorder that produces inflammation and rapid demyelination within the peripheral nerves and the motor nerves arising from the ventral roots. This disease is associated with recent respiratory and/or gastrointestinal infection. A symptom of this disease is muscle weakness in the extremities, reaching a high point within just a few weeks. Early recognition is followed by physical therapy and respiratory and autoimmune globulin treatments.

Na^+ inside the cell causes a reversal of the resting potential (i.e., the cytoplasmic aspect of the plasma membrane becomes positive relative to its extracytoplasmic aspect), and the membrane is said to be **depolarized.**

2 As a result, the Na^+ channels become inactivated for 1 to 2 msec, a condition known as the **refractory period.** During this period the Na^+ channels are inactive; that is, they cannot open or close and Na^+ cannot traverse them. The presence of the refractory period is due to the specialized construction of the voltage-gated Na^+ channels. These channels have two gates: an extracytoplasmic gate **(activation gate)** that opens as a result of the depolarization of the cell membrane and remains open as long as the membrane is depolarized; and an intracytoplasmic gate **(inactivation gate)** that closes within a few ten-thousandths of a second after the opening of the activation gate. Therefore, even though the activation gate remains open, Na^+ can no longer enter or leave the cell through these channels.

3 During the refractory period, **voltage-gated K^+ channels** open, permitting an efflux of K^+ into the extracellular fluid that eventually restores the resting membrane potential; however, there may be a brief period of hyperpolarization.

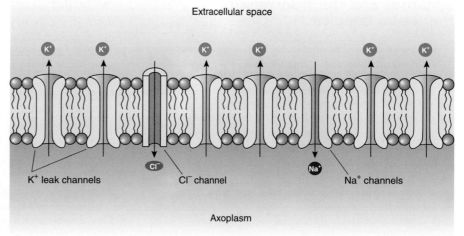

Figure 9–15 Schematic diagram of the establishment of the resting potential in a typical neuron. Observe that the potassium ion (K^+) leak channels outnumber the sodium ion (Na^+) and calcium ion (Cl^-) channels; consequently, more K^+ can leave the cell than Na^+ or Cl^- can enter. Because there are more positive ions outside than inside the cell, the outside is more positive than the inside, establishing a potential difference across the membrane. Ion channels and ion pumps not directly responsible for the establishment of resting membrane potential are not shown.

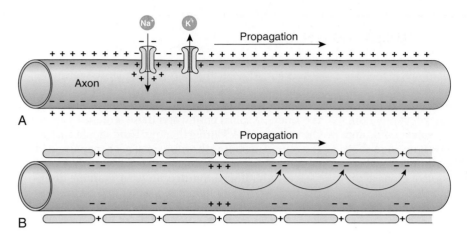

Figure 9–16 Schematic diagram of the propagation of an action potential in an unmyelinated (**A**) and a myelinated (**B**) axon (see text).

4 Once the resting potential is restored, the voltage-gated K⁺ channels close, and the refractory period is ended with the closing of the activation gate and the opening of the inactivation gate of the voltage-gated Na⁺ channel.

The cycle of membrane depolarization, hyperpolarization, and return to the resting membrane potential is called the **action potential,** an all-or-none response that can occur at rates of 1000 times per second. The membrane depolarization that occurs with the opening of voltage-gated Na⁺ channels at one point on an axon spreads passively for a short distance and triggers the opening of adjacent channels, resulting in the generation of another action potential. In this manner, the **wave of depolarization,** or **impulse,** is conducted along the axon. In vivo, an impulse is conducted in only one direction, from the site of initial depolarization to the axon terminal. The inactivation of the Na⁺ channels during the refractory periods prevents retrograde propagation of the depolarization wave.

Synapses and the Transmission of the Nerve Impulse

Synapses are the sites of impulse transmission between the presynaptic and postsynaptic cells.

Synapses are the sites where nerve impulses are transmitted from a presynaptic cell (a neuron) to a postsynaptic cell (another neuron, muscle cell, or cell of a gland). Synapses thus permit neurons to communicate with each other and with effector cells (muscles and glands). Impulse transmission at synapses can occur electrically or chemically.

Although **electrical synapses** are uncommon in mammals, they are present in the brain stem, retina, and cerebral cortex. Electrical synapses are usually represented by gap junctions that permit free movement of ions from one cell to another. When this ion movement occurs between neurons, there is a flow of current. Impulse transmission is much faster across electrical synapses than across chemical synapses.

Chemical synapses are the most common mode of communication between two nerve cells. The **presynaptic membrane** releases one or more **neurotransmitters** into the **synaptic cleft,** a small gap (20 to 30 nm), located between the presynaptic membrane of the first cell and the **postsynaptic membrane** of the second cell (Fig. 9-17). The neurotransmitter diffuses across the synaptic cleft to **gated ion-channel receptors** on the postsynaptic membrane. Binding of the neurotransmitter to these receptors initiates the opening of ion channels, which permits the passage of certain ions, altering the permeability of the postsynaptic membrane and reversing its membrane potential. Neurotransmitters do not accomplish the reaction events at the postsynaptic membrane; they only activate the response.

When the stimulus at a synapse results in depolarization of the postsynaptic membrane to a threshold value that initiates an action potential, it is called an **excitatory postsynaptic potential.** A stimulus at the synapse that results in maintaining a membrane potential or increasing its hyperpolarization is called an **inhibitory postsynaptic potential.**

Various types of synaptic contacts between neurons have been observed. The following synapses are the most common (Fig. 9-18; also see Fig. 9-17):

- **Axodendritic synapse**—between an axon and a dendrite
- **Axosomatic synapse**—between an axon and a soma
- **Axoaxonic synapse**—between two axons
- **Dendrodendritic synapse**—between two dendrites

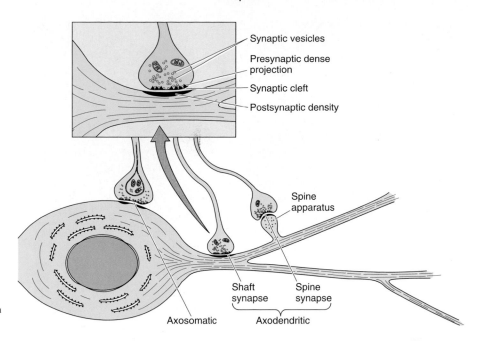

Synaptic vesicles
Presynaptic dense projection
Synaptic cleft
Postsynaptic density

Spine apparatus

Shaft synapse
Spine synapse

Axosomatic
Axodendritic

Figure 9–17 Schematic diagram of the various types of synapses.

Synaptic Morphology

Terminals of axons vary according to the type of synaptic contact. Often the axon forms a bulbous expansion at its terminal end called **bouton terminal.** Other forms of synaptic contacts in axons are derived from swellings along the axon called **boutons en passage,** where each bouton may serve as a synaptic site.

The cytoplasm at the **presynaptic membrane** contains mitochondria, a few elements of SER, and an abundance of synaptic vesicles assembled around the presynaptic membrane (Fig. 9-19). **Synaptic vesicles** are spherical structures (40 to 60 nm in diameter) filled with neurotransmitter substance that usually was manufactured and packaged near the axon terminal. Peptide neurotransmitters, however, are manufactured and packaged in the cell body and are transported to the axon terminal via anterograde transport. Enzymes located in the axoplasm protect neurotransmitters from degradation.

Also located on the cytoplasmic side of the presynaptic membrane are cone-shaped densities that project from the membrane into the cytoplasm; they appear to be associated with many of the synaptic vesicles, forming the **active site** of the synapse. Those synaptic vesicles associated with the active site are released at stimulation. **Cell adhesion molecules** (CAMs) are known to play an additional role in this location as signaling molecules at both the presynaptic and postsynaptic aspects of the synapse. Other synaptic vesicles, forming a reserve pool, adhere to actin microfilaments.

Synapsin-I, a small protein that forms a complex with the vesicle surface, appears to assist in the clustering of synaptic vesicles held in reserve. When synapsin-I is phosphorylated, these synaptic vesicles become free to move to the active zone in preparation for release of the neurotransmitter; dephosphorylation of synapsin-I reverses the process.

Synapsin-II and **rab3a,** another small protein, control association of the vesicles with actin microfilaments. Docking of the synaptic vesicles with the presynaptic membrane is under control of two additional synaptic vesicle proteins: **synaptotagmin** and **synaptophysin.** When an action potential reaches the presynaptic membrane, it initiates opening of the **voltage-gated calcium ion (Ca^{2+}) channels,** permitting Ca^{2+} to enter. This Ca^{2+} influx causes synaptic vesicles, under the influence of SNARE (SNAP receptor) proteins (including synaptobrevin, syntaxin, and soluble N-ethylmaleimide-sensitive fusion protein attachment protein-25 [SNAP-25]) to fuse with the presynaptic membrane, emptying neurotransmitter into the synaptic cleft via exocytosis.

Excess membrane is recaptured via **clathrin-mediated endocytosis.** Recycling of synaptic vesicles involves interactions between synaptotagmin and **vesicle coat protein AP-2.** The endocytic vesicle fuses with the smooth endoplasmic reticulum, where new membrane is continuously recycled. It is interesting that the target protein for tetanus toxin and *Clostridium botulinum* neurotoxin B is synaptobrevin, the synaptic vesicle protein. Thus, these toxins selectively block

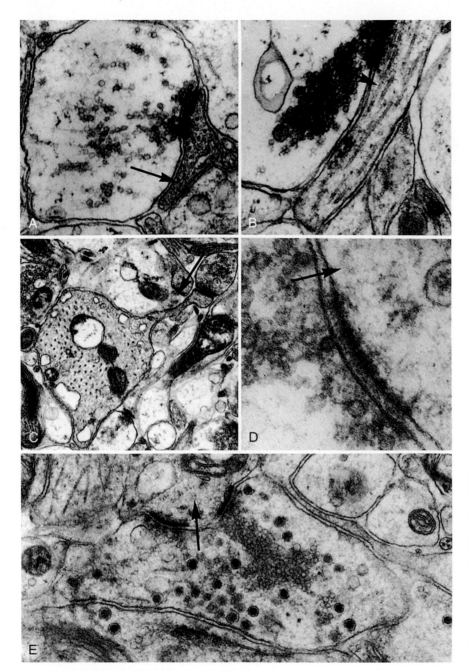

Figure 9–18 Electron micrographs of synapses. The *arrow* indicates transmission direction. **A,** Axodendritic synapse (×37,600). Presynaptic vesicles are located to the left **B,** Axodendritic synapse (×43,420). Note neurotubules in dendrite. **C,** Dendrite in cross section (×43,420). Note the synapse. **D,** Axodendritic synapse (×76,000). Note presynaptic vesicle fusing with the axolemma. **E,** Axon terminal with clear synaptic vesicles and dense-cored vesicles (×31,000). (From Leeson TS, Leeson CR, Paparo AA: Text/Atlas of Histology. Philadelphia, WB Saunders, 1988.)

synaptic vesicle exocytosis without affecting any other aspect of nerve function.

The **postsynaptic membrane,** a thickened portion of the plasma membrane of the postsynaptic cell, contains neurotransmitter receptors, and the cytoplasmic area contains some dense material. Coupling of the neurotransmitter with the receptors in the plasmalemma initiates depolarization (an excitatory response) or hyperpolarization (an inhibitory response) of the postsynaptic membrane. Glial cells have been shown to

increase synaptogenesis, synaptic efficacy, and action-potential firing.

The relative thicknesses and densities of the pre-synaptic and postsynaptic membranes, coupled with the width of the synaptic cleft, generally correlate with the nature of the response. A thick postganglionic density and a 30-nm-wide synaptic cleft constitutes an **asymmetric synapse,** which is usually the site of **excitatory responses.** A thin postsynaptic density and a 20-nm-wide synaptic cleft constitutes a **symmetric**

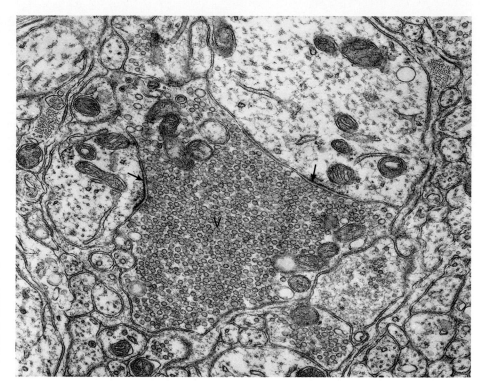

Figure 9–19 Electron micrograph of an axodendritic synapse. Observe the numerous synaptic vesicles (V) within the axon terminal synapsing with dendrites and the synaptic clefts at these sites (*arrows*). (From Jennes L, Traurig HH, Conn PM: Atlas of the Human Brain. Philadelphia, Lippincott-Raven, 1995.)

synapse, which is usually the site of **inhibitory responses.**

Neurotransmitters

Neurotransmitters are signaling molecules that are released at the presynaptic membranes and activate receptors on postsynaptic membranes.

Cells of the nervous system communicate mostly by the release of signaling molecules. The released molecules contact receptor molecules protruding from the plasmalemma of the target cell, eliciting a response from the target cell. These signaling molecules were called neurotransmitters (Table 9-1). However, such molecules may act on two types of receptors: (1) those directly associated with ion channels and (2) those associated with G proteins or receptor kinases, which activate a second messenger. Therefore, signaling molecules that act as "first messenger systems" (i.e., act on receptors directly associated with ion channels) retain the name **neurotransmitters,** and signaling molecules that invoke the "second messenger system" now are referred to as **neuromodulators** or **neurohormones.** Because neurotransmitters act directly, the entire process is fast, lasting usually less than 1 msec. Events utilizing neuromodulators are much slower and may last as long as a few minutes.

There are perhaps 100 known neurotransmitters (and neuromodulators), represented by the following three groups:

- Small-molecule transmitters
- Neuropeptides
- Gases

Small-molecule transmitters are of three major types:

- *Acetylcholine* (the only one in this group that is not an amino acid derivative)
- The *amino acids:* glutamate, aspartate, glycine, and γ-aminobutyric acid (GABA)
- The *biogenic amines:* (monoamines) serotonin and the three catecholamines: dopamine, norepinephrine (noradrenaline), and epinephrine (adrenaline).

Neuropeptides, many of which are neuromodulators, form a large group. They include:

- The *opioid peptides*: enkephalins and endorphins
- *Gastrointestinal peptides*, which are produced by cells of the diffuse neuroendocrine system: substance P, neurotensin, and vasoactive intestinal peptide
- *Hypothalamic-releasing hormones*, such as thyrotropin-releasing hormone and somatostatin
- *Hormones* stored in and released from the neurohypophysis (antidiuretic hormone and oxytocin).

Gases may act as neuromodulators. The ones that do are nitric oxide (NO) and carbon monoxide (CO).

TABLE 9–1 Common Neurotransmitters and Functions Elicited by Their Receptor

Neurotransmitter	Compound Group	Function
Acetylcholine	Small molecule transmitter; not derived from amino acids	Myoneural junctions, all parasympathetic synapses, and preganglionic sympathetic synapses
Norepinephrine	Small molecule transmitter; biogenic amine; catecholamine	Postganglionic sympathetic synapses (except for eccrine sweat glands)
Glutamate	Small molecule transmitter; amino acid	Presynaptic sensory and cortex: most common excitatory neurotransmitter of CNS
γ-Aminobutyric acid (GABA)	Small molecule transmitter; amino acid	Most common inhibitory neurotransmitter of CNS
Dopamine	Small molecule transmitter; biogenic amine; catecholamine	Basal ganglia of CNS; inhibitory or excitatory, depending on receptor
Serotonin	Small molecule transmitter; biogenic amine	Inhibits pain; mood control; sleep
Glycine	Small molecule transmitter; amino acid	Brain stem and spinal cord; inhibitory
Endorphins	Neuropeptide; opioid peptide	Analgesic; inhibit pain transmission?
Enkephalins	Neuropeptide; opioid peptide	Analgesic; inhibit pain transmission?

CNS, central nervous system.

CLINICAL CORRELATIONS

Huntington's chorea is a hereditary condition with an onset in the third or fourth decade of life. It begins as flicking of the joints that progresses to severe distortions, dementia, and motor dysfunction. The condition is thought to be related to loss of cells producing **GABA,** an inhibitory neurotransmitter. Without it, outbursts are uncontrolled. The dementia associated with this disease is thought to be related to subsequent loss of acetylcholine-secreting cells.

Parkinson's disease, a crippling disease related to the absence of **dopamine** in certain regions of the brain, is characterized by muscular rigidity, constant tremor, bradykinesia (slow movement), and, finally, a mask-like face and difficult voluntary movement. Because dopamine cannot cross the blood-brain barrier, therapy is administered as L-dopa (levodopa), which relieves the motor abnormalities temporarily, although the neurons in the affected area continue to die. Efforts to transplant fetal adrenal gland tissue into persons with this disease have provided only transient relief. The therapeutic grafting of genetically modified cells capable of secreting dopamine will perhaps allow the establishment of synaptic connections to cells in the corpus striatum of the brain where dopamine is needed.

Several principles appear to describe the functioning of neurotransmitters. First, a specific neurotransmitter may elicit different actions under varied circumstances. Second, the nature of the postsynaptic receptors determines the effect of a neurotransmitter on postsynaptic cells. Synaptic communication commonly involves multiple neurotransmitters. Additionally, there is mounting evidence for **volume transmission** as a method of communication between brain cells. According to this concept, chemical and electrical "neurotransmitters," believed to exist in the intercellular fluid–filled spaces between brain cells, activate groups or fields of cells that contain appropriate receptors rather than individual cells. Whereas synaptic communication is fast-acting, volume transmission is thought to be slow and may be related to such conditions as autonomic function, alertness, awareness, changes in brain patterns during sleep, sensitivity to pain, and moods.

PERIPHERAL NERVOUS SYSTEM

The peripheral nervous system includes the peripheral nerves and nerve cell bodies located outside the central nervous system (CNS).

Peripheral nerves are bundles of nerve fibers (axons), located outside the central nervous system and surrounded by several investments of connective tissue sheaths (Figs. 9-20 through 9-22). These bundles (**fascicles**) may be observed with the unaided eye; those that

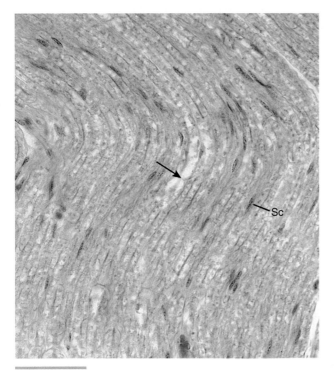

Figure 9–20 Light micrograph of a longitudinal section of a peripheral nerve (×270). Myelin and nodes of Ranvier (*arrow*) as well as the lightly stained oval nuclei of Schwann cells (Sc) may be observed.

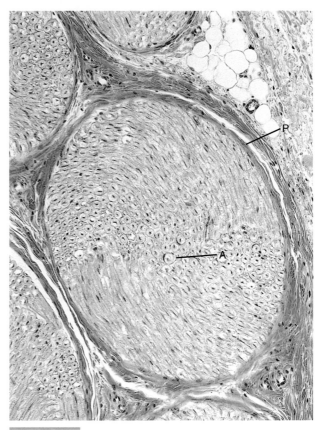

Figure 9–21 Light micrograph of a cross-section of a peripheral nerve (×132). Observe the axons (A) and the perineurium (P) surrounding the fascicle.

are myelinated appear white because of the presence of myelin. Usually, each bundle of nerve fibers, regardless of size, has both sensory and motor components.

Connective Tissue Investments

Connective tissue investments of peripheral nerves include the epineurium, perineurium, and endoneurium.

Epineurium is the outermost layer of the three connective tissue investments covering nerves (see Fig. 9-22). The epineurium is composed of dense, irregular, collagenous connective tissue containing thick elastic fibers that completely ensheathe the nerve. Collagen fibers within the sheath are aligned and oriented to prevent damage by overstretching of the nerve bundle. The epineurium is thickest where it is continuous with the dura covering the CNS at the spinal cord or brain, where the spinal or cranial nerves originate, respectively. The epineurium becomes progressively thinner as the nerves branch into smaller nerve components, eventually disappearing.

Perineurium, the middle layer of connective tissue investments, covers each bundle of nerve fibers (fascicle) within the nerve. The perineurium is composed of dense connective tissue but is thinner than epineurium. Its inner surface is lined by several layers of epithelioid

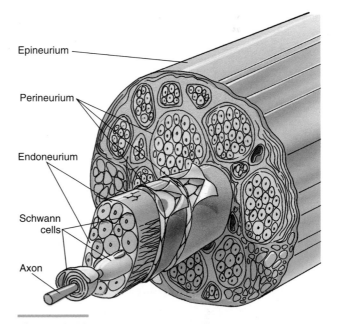

Figure 9–22 Structure of a nerve bundle.

cells joined by zonulae occludentes and surrounded by a basal lamina that isolates the neural environment. Between the layers of epithelioid cells are sparse collagen fibers oriented longitudinally and intertwined with a few elastic fibers. The thickness of the perineurium is progressively reduced to a sheet of flattened cells.

Endoneurium, the innermost layer of the three connective tissue investments of a nerve, surrounds individual nerve fibers (axons). A loose connective tissue composed of a thin layer of reticular fibers (produced by the underlying Schwann cells), scattered fibroblasts, fixed macrophages, capillaries, and perivascular mast cells in extracellular fluid, the endoneurium is in contact with the basal lamina of the Schwann cells. Thus, the endoneurium is housed in a compartment completely isolated from the perineurium and Schwann cells, an important factor in regulation of the microenvironment of the nerve fiber. Near the distal terminus of the axon, the endoneurium is reduced to a few reticular fibers surrounding the basal lamina of the Schwann cells of the axon.

Functional Classification of Nerves

Functionally, nerve fibers are classified as sensory (afferent) or motor (efferent).

Nerve fibers are segregated functionally into sensory (**afferent**) fibers and motor (**efferent**) fibers. Sensory nerve fibers carry sensory input from the cutaneous areas of the body and from the viscera back to the CNS for processing. Motor nerve fibers originate in the CNS and carry motor impulses to the effector organs. The sensory roots and motor roots of the spinal cord unite to form **mixed peripheral nerves,** the **spinal nerves,** which carry both sensory and motor fibers.

Conduction Velocity

The conduction velocity of peripheral nerve fibers depends on the extent of their myelination. In myelinated nerves, ions can cross the axonal plasma membrane, initiating depolarization, only at the nodes of Ranvier, for two reasons:

1 Voltage-gated Na^+ channels of the axon plasmalemma are clustered mostly at the nodes of Ranvier.
2 The myelin sheath covering the internodes prevents the outward movement of the excess Na^+ in the axoplasm associated with the action potential.

Therefore, the excess positive ions can diffuse only through the axoplasm to the next node, triggering depolarization there. In this way, the action potential "jumps" from node to node, a process called **saltatory conduction** (see Fig. 9-16B).

As noted earlier, unmyelinated fibers lack a thick myelin sheath and nodes of Ranvier. These fibers are surrounded by a single layer of Schwann cell plasma membrane and cytoplasm, which provides little insulation. Moreover, voltage-gated Na^+ channels are distributed along the entire length of the axon plasma membrane. Therefore, impulse propagation in unmyelinated fibers occurs by **continuous conduction,** which is slower and requires more energy than the saltatory conduction occurring in myelinated fibers.

As shown in Table 9-2, peripheral nerve fibers are classified into three major groups according to their conduction velocity. In thin unmyelinated fibers, the conduction velocity ranges from about 0.5 to 2 m/sec, whereas in heavily myelinated fibers, it ranges from 15 to 120 m/sec.

The sensory component of the peripheral nervous system is presented in the various chapters related to function.

SOMATIC MOTOR AND AUTONOMIC NERVOUS SYSTEMS

Functionally, the motor component is divided into the somatic and autonomic nervous systems.

The somatic nervous system provides motor impulses to the skeletal muscles, whereas the autonomic nervous

---

TABLE 9–2 Classification of Peripheral Nerve Fibers

Fiber Group	Diameter (μm)	Conduction Velocity (m/sec)	Function
Type A fibers—heavily myelinated	1-20	15-120	High-velocity fibers: acute pain, temperature, touch, pressure, proprioception, somatic efferent fibers
Type B fibers—less heavily myelinated	1-3	3-15	Moderate-velocity fibers: visceral afferents, preganglionic autonomics
Type C fibers—unmyelinated	0.5-1.5	0.5-2	Slow-velocity fibers: postganglionic autonomics, chronic pain

system provides motor impulses to the smooth muscles of the viscera, cardiac muscle of the heart, and secretory cells of the exocrine and endocrine glands, thus helping to maintain homeostasis.

Motor Component of the Somatic Nervous System

Motor innervation to skeletal muscles is provided by somatic nerves.

Skeletal muscles receive motor nerve impulses conducted to them by spinal and selected cranial nerves of the somatic nervous system. The cell bodies of these nerve fibers originate in the CNS. The cranial nerves containing **somatic efferent components** are cranial nerves III, IV, VI, and XII (excluding those nerves supplying muscles of branchiomeric origin). Most of the 31 pairs of spinal nerves contain somatic efferent components to skeletal muscles.

Cell bodies of neurons of the somatic nervous system originate in motor nuclei of the cranial nerves embedded within the brain or in the ventral horn of the spinal cord. These neurons are multipolar, and their axons

leave the brain or spinal cord and travel to the skeletal muscle via the cranial nerves or spinal nerves (Fig. 9-23). They synapse with the skeletal muscle at the motor end plate (see Chapter 8).

Autonomic Nervous System

Autonomic nerves provide motor innervation to smooth muscle and cardiac muscle and supply secretomotor innervation to glands.

The autonomic (**involuntary, visceral**) nervous system is generally defined as a motor system; although agreement on this point is not universal, it is regarded as a motor system in this discussion. The autonomic nervous system controls the viscera of the body by supplying the **general visceral efferent (visceral motor)** component to smooth muscle, cardiac muscle, and glands.

In contrast to the somatic system, in which one neuron originating in the CNS acts directly on the effector organ, the autonomic nervous system possesses two neurons between the CNS and the effector organ.

Cell bodies of the first neurons in the chain lie in the CNS and their axons are usually myelinated. These **pre-**

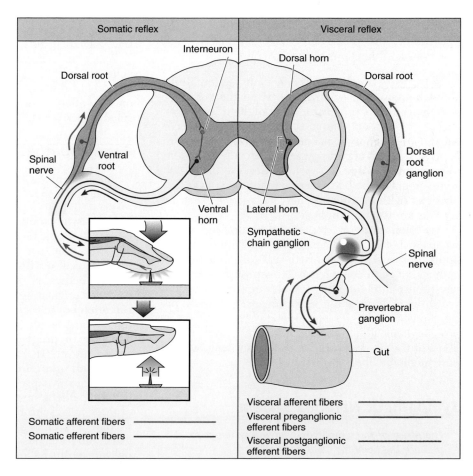

Figure 9–23 Comparison of somatic and visceral reflexes.

ganglionic fibers (axons) seek an autonomic ganglion located outside the CNS, where they synapse on multipolar cell bodies of postganglionic neurons. Postganglionic fibers, which are usually unmyelinated although they always are enveloped by Schwann cells, exit the ganglion to terminate on the effector organ (smooth muscle, cardiac muscle, gland).

Also unlike the somatic system, the autonomic system has postganglionic synapses that branch out, and the neurotransmitter diffuses out for some distance to the effector cells, thus contributing to more prolonged and widespread effects than in the somatic system. Smooth muscle cells stimulated by the neurotransmitter activate adjacent smooth muscle cells to contract by relaying the information via gap junctions.

The autonomic nervous system is subdivided into two functionally different divisions (Fig. 9-24):

- In general, the sympathetic nervous system prepares the body for action by increasing respiration, blood pressure, heart rate, and blood flow to the skeletal muscles, dilating pupils of the eyes and generally slowing down visceral function.
- The parasympathetic nervous system tends to be functionally antagonistic to the sympathetic system in that it decreases respiration, blood pressure, and heart rate, reduces blood flow to skeletal muscles, constricts the pupils, and generally increases the actions and functions of the visceral system.

Thus, the parasympathetic nervous system brings about homeostasis, whereas the sympathetic nervous system prepares the body for "fight or flight" (see later).

The sympathetic nervous system is broadly considered to function in vasoconstriction, whereas the parasympathetic nervous system is broadly considered to be secretomotor in function. Because the visceral components of the body receive innervation from both divisions of the autonomic nervous system, these two systems are balanced in health.

Acetylcholine is the neurotransmitter at all synapses between preganglionic and postganglionic fibers and between parasympathetic postganglionic endings and effector organs. Norepinephrine is the neurotransmitter at synapses between postganglionic sympathetic fibers and effector organs. Generally, preganglionic fibers of the sympathetic system are short but postganglionic fibers are long. In contrast, preganglionic fibers of the parasympathetic system are long, whereas postganglionic fibers are short.

Sympathetic Nervous System

The effect of the sympathetic nervous system is to prepare the body for "flight or fight."

The sympathetic nervous system originates in the spinal cord from segments of the thoracic spinal cord and upper lumbar spinal cord (T1 to L2). Thus, the sympathetic nervous system is sometimes called the thoracolumbar outflow (see Fig. 9-24). Cell bodies of preganglionic neurons are small, spindle-shaped cells that originate in the lateral horn of the spinal cord; their axons exit the cord via the ventral roots to join the spinal nerve. After a short distance, the fibers leave the peripheral nerve, via white rami communicantes, to enter one of the paravertebral chain ganglia.

Typically, the preganglionic neuron either synapses on a cell body of one of the multipolar postganglionic neurons residing in the ganglion associated with that spinal cord segment or ascends or descends in the sympathetic trunk to synapse on a cell in another of the chain ganglia. However, certain preganglionic fibers do not synapse in the chain ganglia; instead, they pass through to enter the abdominal cavity as splanchnic nerves. Here they seek collateral ganglia located along the abdominal aorta for synapsing on cell bodies of postganglionic fibers residing there.

Axons of postganglionic neurons housed in the chain ganglia exit the ganglia, via gray rami communicantes, to reenter the peripheral nerve for distribution to effector organs in the periphery (i.e., sweat glands, blood vessels, dilator pupillae muscles, cardiac muscle, bronchial tree, salivary glands, and arrector muscles of hair).

Axons of postganglionic neurons housed in the collateral ganglia exit the ganglia and accompany the myriad blood vessels to the viscera, where they synapse on the effector organs (i.e., blood vessels and the smooth muscles and glands of the viscera).

Parasympathetic Nervous System

The effect of the parasympathetic nervous system is to prepare the body to "rest or digest."

The parasympathetic nervous system originates in the brain and the sacral segments of the spinal cord (S2 to S4); thus, the parasympathetic system is called the craniosacral outflow (see Fig. 9-24).

Cell bodies of preganglionic parasympathetic neurons originating in the brain lie in the visceromotor nuclei of the four cranial nerves that carry visceral motor components (cranial nerves III, VII, IX, and X).

Axons of preganglionic parasympathetic fibers of cranial nerves III, VII, and IX seek parasympathetic (terminal) ganglia located outside the brain case, where they synapse on cell bodies of postganglionic parasympathetic neurons housed in the ganglia. Axons of these nerves are usually delivered by cranial nerve V to the effector organs they serve, including salivary glands and mucous glands, whereas cranial nerve III delivers postganglionic parasympathetic fibers to the

Sympathetic division

Parasympathetic division

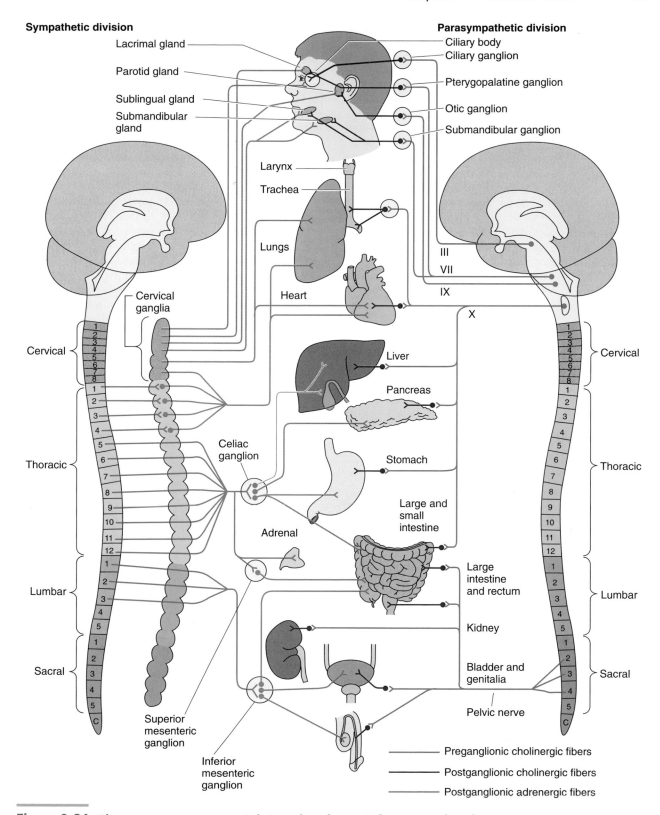

Figure 9–24 The autonomic nervous system. *Left*, Sympathetic division. *Right*, Parasympathetic division.

ciliary muscle and the sphincter pupillae muscles of the eye.

Axons of preganglionic parasympathetic fibers in cranial nerve X travel to the thorax and abdomen before synapsing in the terminal ganglia within the respective viscera.

Axons of **postganglionic parasympathetic nerves** synapse on the glands, smooth muscles, and cardiac muscle.

Cell bodies of preganglionic parasympathetic nerves originating in segments of the sacral spinal cord are located in the lateral segment of the ventral horn and leave via the ventral root with the sacral nerves. From here, the axons project to terminal ganglia (**Meissner's** and **Auerbach's plexuses**) in the walls of the lower gastrointestinal tract, where they synapse on cell bodies of postganglionic parasympathetic neurons.

Axons of postganglionic neurons synapse on the effector organs in the viscera of the lower abdominal wall and the pelvis.

GANGLIA

Ganglia are aggregations of cell bodies of neurons located outside the CNS. There are two types of ganglia: **sensory** and **autonomic.**

Sensory Ganglia

Sensory ganglia house cell bodies of sensory neurons.

Sensory ganglia are associated with cranial nerves V, VII, IX, and X and with each of the spinal nerves originating from the spinal cord. A sensory ganglion of a cranial nerve appears as a swelling of the nerve either inside the cranial vault or at its exit. Ganglia are usually identified with specific names that relate to the nerves. Sensory ganglia of the spinal nerves are called **dorsal root ganglia.** Sensory ganglia house unipolar (pseudounipolar) cell bodies of the sensory nerves enveloped by cuboidal **capsule cells.** These capsule cells are then surrounded by a connective tissue capsule composed of **satellite cells** and collagen. The endoneurium of each axon becomes continuous with the connective tissue surrounding the ganglia. Peripheral processes of the neurons possess specialized receptors at their terminals to transduce various types of stimuli from the internal and external environments. Central processes pass from the ganglion unsynapsed to the brain within the cranial nerves or to the spinal cord within the spinal nerves, where they terminate on other neurons for processing.

Autonomic Ganglia

Autonomic ganglia house cell bodies of postganglionic autonomic nerves.

By definition, nerve cell bodies of autonomic ganglia are motor in function because they cause smooth or cardiac muscle contraction or glandular secretion. In the *sympathetic system,* preganglionic sympathetic fibers synapse on postganglionic sympathetic cell bodies in the sympathetic ganglia located in either the **sympathetic chain ganglia,** adjacent to the spinal cord, or the **collateral ganglia,** along the abdominal aorta in the abdomen. Postganglionic sympathetic nerves originating in these ganglia are then distributed, for the most part, by peripheral nerves that they join after exiting the ganglia. They then terminate in the effector organs that they innervate.

In the *parasympathetic system,* **preganglionic parasympathetic** fibers originate in one of two places: in certain cranial nerves or, as previously described, in certain segments of the sacral spinal cord. These fibers synapse on postganglionic cell bodies (Fig. 9-25) located in **terminal ganglia.** Preganglionic parasympathetic fibers originating in the nuclei (term for a cluster of nerve cell bodies located in the CNS) of the cranial nerves conducting parasympathetic fibers synapse in one of the four terminal ganglia located in the head (except those of cranial nerve X). Terminal ganglia associated with cranial nerve X and for preganglionic fibers arising from the sacral spinal cord are located in the walls of the viscera.

Postganglionic parasympathetic nerves originating in the terminal ganglia within the head exit the ganglia and usually join the trigeminal nerve (cranial nerve V) to be distributed to the effector organs. Those postganglionic parasympathetic nerves originating in the ganglia located in the walls of the viscera pass directly to the effector organs located within the viscera.

CENTRAL NERVOUS SYSTEM

The CNS, composed of the brain and the spinal cord, consists of white matter and gray matter without intervening connective tissue elements; therefore, the CNS has the consistency of a semifirm gel.

White matter is composed mostly of myelinated nerve fibers along with some unmyelinated fibers and neuroglial cells; its white color results from the abundance of myelin surrounding the axons.

Gray matter consists of aggregations of neuronal cell bodies, dendrites, and unmyelinated portions of axons as well as neuroglial cells; the absence of myelin causes these regions to appear gray in live tissue.

Axons, dendrites, and neuroglial processes form a tangled network of neural tissue called the **neuropil** (Fig. 9-26). In certain regions, aggregations of neuron cell bodies embedded in white matter are called **nuclei,** whereas their counterparts in the peripheral nervous system are called ganglia.

Gray matter in the brain is located at the periphery (**cortex**) of the cerebrum and cerebellum and forms the deeper basal ganglia, whereas the white matter lies deep to

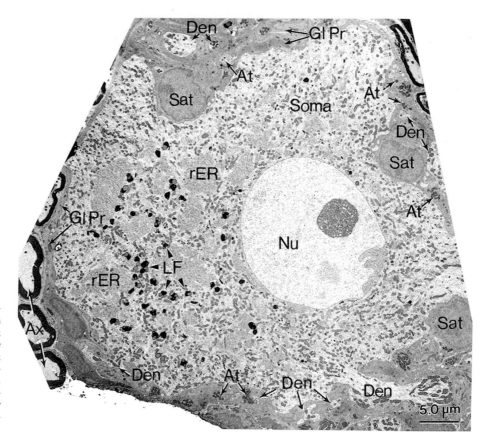

Figure 9–25 Electron micrograph of the ciliary ganglion. At, axon terminal; Ax, axon; Den, dendrite; GIPr, gastric inhibitory peptide receptor; LF, lipofuscin granules; Nu, nucleus; rER, rough endoplasmic reticulum; Sat, satellite cells. (From May PJ, Warren S: Ultrastructure of the macaque ciliary ganglion. J Neurocytol 22:1073-1095, 1993.)

the cortex and surrounds the basal ganglia. The reverse is true in the spinal cord; white matter is located in the periphery of the spinal cord, whereas gray matter lies deep in the spinal cord, where it forms an **H** shape in cross section. A small **central canal,** lined by **ependymal cells** and representing the lumen of the original neural tube, lies in the center of the crossbar of the **H.** The upper vertical bars of the **H** represent the **dorsal horns** of the spinal cord, which receive central processes of the sensory neurons whose cell bodies lie in the **dorsal root ganglion.** Cell bodies of interneurons are also located in the dorsal horns. Cell bodies of **interneurons (internuncial neurons** or **intercalated neurons)** originate in the CNS and are entirely confined there, where they form networks of communication for integration between sensory and motor neurons. Interneurons constitute the vast majority of the neurons of the body. The lower vertical bars of the **H** represent the **ventral horns** of the spinal cord, which house cell bodies of large multipolar motor neurons whose axons exit the spinal cord via the ventral roots.

Meninges

The three connective tissue coverings of the brain and spinal cord are the meninges. The outermost layer of the meninges is the **dura mater,** the intermediate layer

is the **arachnoid,** and the innermost or intimate layer of the meninges is the **pia mater** (Fig. 9-27).

Dura Mater

The dura mater is the dense outermost layer of the meninges.

The dura mater covering the brain is a dense, collagenous connective tissue composed of two layers that are closely apposed in the adult. **Periosteal dura mater,** the outer layer, is composed of osteoprogenitor cells, fibroblasts, and organized bundles of collagen fibers that are loosely attached to the inner surface of the skull, except at the sutures and base of the skull, where the attachment is firm. As the name implies, periosteal dura mater serves as the periosteum of the inner surface of the skull, and as such it is well vascularized.

The inner layer of the dura, **meningeal dura mater,** is composed of fibroblasts displaying dark-staining cytoplasm, elongated processes, ovoid nuclei, and sheet-like layers of fine collagen fibers. This layer also contains small blood vessels.

A layer of cells internal to the meningeal dura mater, called the **border cell layer,** is composed of flattened fibroblasts exhibiting long processes that are

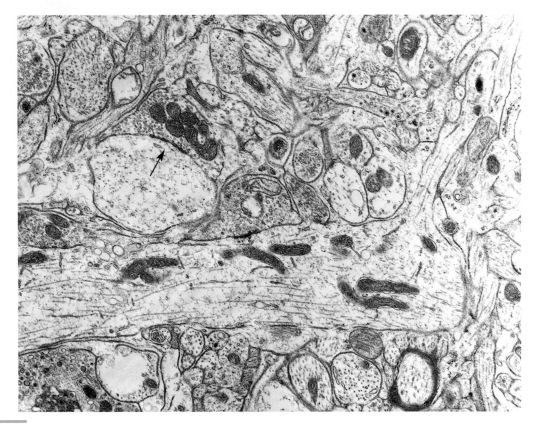

Figure 9–26 Electron micrograph of axodendritic synapses (*arrow*). (From Jennes L, Traurig HH, Conn PM: Atlas of the Human Brain. Philadelphia, Lippincott-Raven, 1995.)

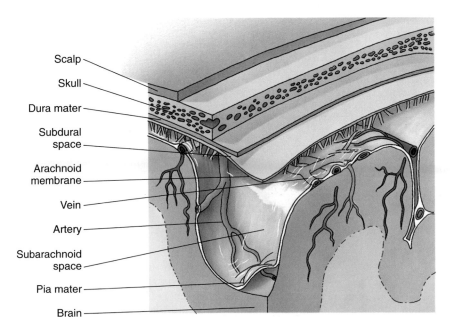

Scalp
Skull
Dura mater
Subdural space
Arachnoid membrane
Vein
Artery
Subarachnoid space
Pia mater
Brain

Figure 9–27 The skull and the layers of the meninges covering the brain.

occasionally attached to one another by desmosomes and gap junctions. Collagen fibers are lacking in this layer, but in their place an extracellular, amorphous, flocculent material (thought to be a proteoglycan) surrounds the fibroblasts and extends into the interface between this layer and the meningeal dura.

Spinal dura mater does not adhere to the walls of the vertebral canal; rather, it forms a continuous tube from the foramen magnum to the second segment of the sacrum and is pierced by the spinal nerves. The **epidural space,** the space between the dura and the bony walls of the vertebral canal, is filled with epidural fat and a venous plexus.

Arachnoid

The arachnoid is the intermediate layer of the meninges.

The arachnoid layer of the meninges is avascular, although blood vessels course through it. This intermediate layer of the meninges consists of fibroblasts, collagen, and some elastic fibers. The fibroblasts form gap junctions and desmosomes with one another. The arachnoid is composed of two regions. The first is a flat, sheet-like membrane in contact with the dura mater. The second is a deeper, gossamer-like region composed of loosely arranged **arachnoid trabecular cells** (modified fibroblasts), along with a few collagen fibers, which form trabeculae that contact the underlying pia mater. These arachnoid trabeculae span the **subarachnoid space,** the space between the sheet-like portion of the arachnoid and the pia. The arachnoid trabecular cells have long processes that attach to one another via desmosomes and communicate with one another by gap junctions.

The interface between the dura and arachnoid, the **subdural space,** is considered a "potential space" because it appears only as the aftermath of injury resulting in subdural hemorrhage, when blood forces these two layers apart.

Blood vessels from the dura pierce the arachnoid on their way to the vascular pia mater. However, these vessels are isolated both from the arachnoid and from the subarachnoid space by a close investment of arachnoid-derived, modified fibroblasts. In certain regions, the arachnoid extends through the dura to form **arachnoid villi,** which protrude into the spaces connected to the lumina of the dural venous sinuses. These specialized regions of the arachnoid function in transporting CSF from the subarachnoid space into the venous system. In later life, the villi enlarge and become sites for calcium deposits.

The interface between the arachnoid mater and pia mater is difficult to distinguish; therefore, the two layers are often called the **pia-arachnoid,** with both surfaces being covered by a thin layer of squamous epithelioid cells composed of modified fibroblasts.

Pia Mater

Pia mater, the innermost highly vascular layer of the meninges, is in close contact with the brain.

The pia mater is the innermost layer of the meninges and is intimately associated with the brain tissue, following closely all of its contours. The pia mater does not quite come into contact with the neural tissue, however, because a thin layer of neuroglial processes is always interposed between them.

The pia mater is composed of a thin layer of flattened, modified fibroblasts that resemble arachnoid trabecular cells. Blood vessels, abundant in this layer, are surrounded by pial cells interspersed with macrophages, mast cells, and lymphocytes. Fine collagenous and elastic fibers lie between the pia and neural tissue.

CLINICAL CORRELATIONS

Meningiomas are slow growing tumors of the meninges that are usually benign and produce clinical effects by compressing the brain and increasing intracranial pressure. **Meningitis** is an inflammation of the meninges resulting from bacterial or viral infection in the CSF.

Viral meningitis is not as severe a condition as *bacterial* meningitis, which is contagious and can be quite a severe condition leading to brain damage, hearing loss, learning disability, and death, if untreated. Presently, in the United States, all children 4 years of age or younger are vaccinated for the most prevalent form of this disease. Major symptoms of bacterial meningitis include fever, headache, stiff neck, and alteration of consciousness. Diagnosis is based on spinal fluid culture to determine the bacterial species involved, followed by treating with a specific antibiotic. Bacterial meningitis can be spread by respiratory and throat secretions (e.g., coughing, kissing).

The pia mater is completely separated from the underlying neural tissue by neuroglial cells. Blood vessels penetrate the neural tissues and are covered by pia mater until they form the **continuous capillaries** characteristic of the CNS. End-feet of astrocytes, pedicels, rather than pia mater, cover capillaries within the neural tissue.

Blood-Brain Barrier

Endothelial cells of CNS capillaries prevent the free passage of selective blood-borne substances into the neural tissue.

A highly selective barrier, known as the blood-brain barrier, exists between specific blood-borne substances and the neural tissue of the CNS. This barrier is established by the endothelial cells lining the **continuous capillaries** that course through the CNS. These endothelial cells form fasciae occludentes with one another, retarding the flow of materials between cells. Additionally, these endothelial cells have relatively few pinocytotic vesicles, and vesicular traffic is almost completely restricted to **receptor-mediated transport.**

Macromolecules injected into the vascular system cannot enter the intercellular spaces of the CNS; conversely, macromolecules injected into the intercellular spaces of the CNS cannot enter the capillary lumen. Certain substances, however, such as oxygen, water, and carbon dioxide, and other small, lipid-soluble materials, including some drugs, can easily penetrate the blood-brain barrier. Molecules such as glucose, amino acids, certain vitamins, and nucleosides are transferred across the blood-brain barrier by specific carrier proteins, many via facilitated diffusion. Ions are also transported across the blood-brain barrier through ion channels via active transport. The energy requirement for this process is satisfied by the presence of large numbers of mitochondria within the endothelial cell cytoplasm.

Capillaries of the CNS are invested by well-defined basal laminae, which in turn are almost completely surrounded by the end-feet of numerous astrocytes, collectively called the **perivascular glia limitans.** It is believed that these astrocytes help convey metabolites from blood vessels to neurons. Additionally, astrocytes remove excess K⁺ and neurotransmitters from the neuron's environment, thus maintaining the neurochemical balance of the CNS extracellular milieu.

CLINICAL CORRELATIONS

Because the blood-brain barrier is very selective, antibiotics, some therapeutic drugs, and certain neurotransmitters (e.g., dopamine) cannot pass across it. Perfusion of a hypertonic solution of **mannitol** transiently opens the tight junctions of the capillary endothelial cells for administration of therapeutic drugs. Therapeutic drugs can also be bound to antibodies developed against **transferrin receptors** in the endothelial cells of the capillaries, permitting their transport across the blood-brain barrier and into the CNS.

In some diseases of the CNS (e.g., stroke, infection, tumors), the integrity of the blood-brain barrier is compromised, resulting in the accumulation of toxins and extraneous metabolites in the extracellular environment.

Choroid Plexus

The choroid plexus, composed of folds of pia mater within the ventricles of the brain, produces CSF.

Folds of pia mater housing an abundance of fenestrated capillaries and invested by the simple cuboidal (ependymal) lining extend into the third, fourth, and lateral ventricles of the brain, forming the choroid plexus (Fig. 9-28). The choroid plexus produces **cerebrospinal fluid (CSF),** which fills the ventricles of the brain and central canal of the spinal cord. The CSF bathes the CNS as it circulates through the subarachnoid space. Although more than half of the CSF is produced by the choroid plexus, there is evidence that parenchyma in several other regions of the brain produce a substantial amount of CSF, which diffuses through the ependymal lining to enter the ventricles.

Cerebrospinal Fluid

Cerebrospinal fluid bathes, nourishes, and protects the brain and spinal cord.

CSF is produced by the choroid plexus at the rate of about 14 to 36 mL/hour, replacing its total volume about four to five times daily. CSF circulates through the ventricles of the brain, the subarachnoid space, the perivascular space, and the central canal of the spinal cord. CSF is low in protein but rich in sodium, potassium, and

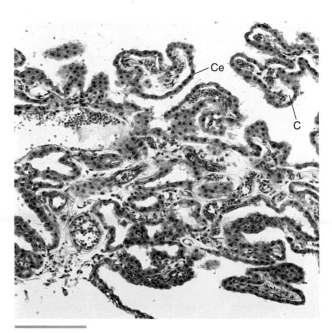

Figure 9–28 Light micrograph of the choroid plexus (×270). Observe capillaries (C) and the simple cuboidal epithelium of the choroid plexus (Ce).

chloride ions. It is clear and has a low density. Consisting of about 90% water and ions, it may also contain a few desquamated cells and occasional lymphocytes.

CSF is important to the metabolic activity of the CNS because brain metabolites diffuse into the CSF as it passes through the subarachnoid space. It also serves as a liquid cushion for protection of the CNS. CSF is able to flow by diffusion and is reabsorbed through the thin cells of the arachnoid villi in the superior sagittal venous sinus from where the CSF is returned to the bloodstream.

CLINICAL CORRELATIONS

Because CSF is constantly being produced by the choroid plexus, any decrease in absorption of the fluid by the arachnoid villi or blockage within the ventricles of the brain causes swelling in the brain tissue. This condition, called **hydrocephalus,** leads to enlargement of the head in the fetus and neonate, impairment of mental and muscular functions, and death if left untreated.

TABLE 9–3 Comparison of Serum and Cerebrospinal Fluid (CSF)

Constituent	Serum	CSF
White blood cells (cells/mL)	0	0-5
Protein (g/L)	60-80	Negligible
Glucose (mMol/L)	4.0-5.5	2.1-4.0
Na^+ (mMol/L)	135-150	135-150
K^+ (mMol/L)	4.0-5.1	2.8-3.2
Cl^- (mMol/L)	100-105	115-130
Ca^{2+} (mMol/L)	2.1-2.5	1.0-1.4
Mg^{2+} (mMol/L)	0.7-1.0	0.8-1.3
pH	7.4	7.3

The chemical stability of the CSF is maintained by the **blood-CSF barrier,** which is composed of zonulae occludentes between the cells of the simple cuboidal epithelium. These tight junctions impede the movement of substances between cells, compelling the substances to take the transcellular route. The production of CSF thus depends on facilitated and active transport across the simple cuboidal epithelium, resulting in differences in composition between CSF and plasma (Table 9-3).

Cerebral Cortex

The cerebral cortex is responsible for learning, memory, sensory integration, information analysis, and initiation of motor responses.

Gray matter at the periphery of the cerebral hemispheres is folded into many **gyri** and **sulci** called the cerebral cortex. This portion of the brain is responsible for learning, memory, information analysis, initiation of motor response, and integration of sensory signals.

The cerebral cortex is divided into six layers composed of neurons that exhibit a morphology unique to the particular layer. The most superficial layer lies just deep to the pia mater; the sixth, or deepest, layer of the cortex is bordered by white matter of the cerebrum. The six layers and their components are as follows:

1 The **molecular layer** is composed mostly of nerve terminals originating in other areas of the brain, **horizontal cells,** and neuroglia.

2 The **external granular layer** contains mostly **granule** (stellate) **cells** and neuroglial cells.
3 The **external pyramidal layer** contains neuroglial cells and large **pyramidal cells,** which become increasingly larger from the external to the internal border of this layer.
4 The **internal granular layer** is a thin layer characterized by closely arranged, small **granule cells** (stellate cells), **pyramidal cells,** and neuroglia. This layer has the greatest cell density of the cerebral cortex.
5 The **internal pyramidal layer** contains the largest **pyramidal cells** and neuroglia. This layer has the lowest cell density of the cerebral cortex.
6 The **multiform layer** consists of cells of various shapes (**Martinotti cells),** and neuroglia.

Cerebellar Cortex

The cerebellar cortex is responsible for balance, equilibrium, muscle tone, and muscle coordination.

The layer of gray matter located in the periphery of the cerebellum is called the cerebellar cortex (Fig. 9-29). This portion of the brain is responsible for maintaining balance and equilibrium, muscle tone, and coordination of skeletal muscles. Histologically, the cerebellar cortex is divided into three layers:

1 The **molecular layer** lies directly below the pia mater and contains superficially located stellate cells, dendrites of **Purkinje cells,** basket cells, and unmyelinated axons from the granular layer.
2 The **Purkinje cell layer** contains the large, flask-shaped Purkinje cells, which are present only in the

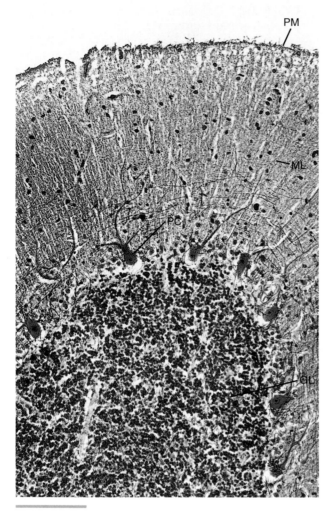

Figure 9–29 Light micrograph of the cerebellum showing its layers: the pia mater (PM), molecular layer (ML), and granular layer (GL) (×132). Especially note the prominent Purkinje cells (PC).

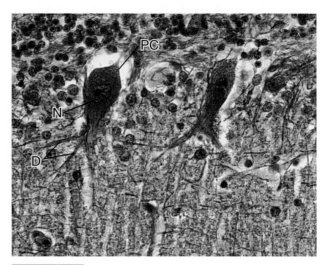

Figure 9–30 Higher-magnification light micrograph of the granular layer of the cerebellum illustrating Purkinje cells (x540). The multi-polar Purkinji cells (PC) display a nucleus (N) and a dentritic tree (D).

NERVE REGENERATION

Nerve cells, unlike neuroglial cells, cannot proliferate but can regenerate their axons, located in the PNS.

When a traumatic event destroys neurons, they are not replaced because neurons cannot proliferate (although some suggest that proliferation of certain neurons may take place even within the CNS); therefore, the damage to the CNS is permanent. However, if a peripheral nerve fiber is injured or transected, the neuron attempts to repair the damage, regenerate the process, and restore function by initiating a series of structural and metabolic events, collectively called the **axon reaction.**

Axon Reaction

The reactions to the trauma are characteristically localized in three regions of the neuron: (1) at the site of damage (**local changes**); (2) distal to the site of damage (**anterograde changes**); and (3) proximal to the site of damage (**retrograde changes**). Some of the changes occur simultaneously, whereas others may occur weeks or months apart. The following description of nerve regeneration assumes that the cut ends remain near each other; otherwise, regeneration is unsuccessful (Fig. 9-31).

Local Reaction

Local reaction to injury involves repair and removal of debris by neuroglial cells.

cerebellum (Fig. 9-30; also see Figs. 9-4 and 9-29). Their arborized dendrites project into the molecular layer, and their myelinated axons project into the white matter. Each Purkinje cell receives hundreds of thousands of excitatory and inhibitory synapses that it must integrate to form the proper response. The Purkinje cell is the only cell of the cerebellar cortex that sends information to the outside, and it is always an **inhibitory output** using GABA as the neurotransmitter.

3 The **granular layer** (the deepest layer) consists of small granule cells and **glomeruli (cerebellar islands).** Glomeruli are regions of the cerebellar cortex where synapses are taking place between axons entering the cerebellum and the granule cells.

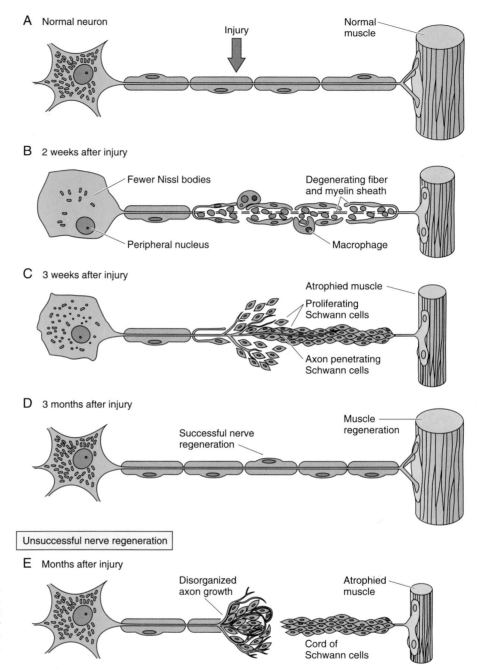

Figure 9–31 Schematic diagram of nerve regeneration. **A,** Normal neuron. Appearance 2 weeks (**B**), 3 weeks (**C**), and 3 months (**D**) after injury. Appearance several months after injury of neuron with unsuccessful nerve regeneration is shown in **E.**

In local reaction, the severed ends of the axon retract away from each other, and the cut membrane of each stump fuses to cover the open end, preventing loss of axoplasm. Each severed end begins to expand as material delivered by axoplasmic flow accumulates. Macrophages and fibroblasts infiltrate the damaged area, secrete cytokines and growth factors, and up-regulate the expression of their receptors. Macrophages invade the basal lamina and, assisted to a certain limited extent by Schwann cells, phagocytose the debris.

Anterograde Reaction

In the anterograde reaction process, that portion of the axon distal to an injury undergoes degeneration and is phagocytosed.

The axon undergoes anterograde changes as follows:

1 The axon terminal becomes hypertrophied and degenerates within a week; as a result, contact with the postsynaptic membrane is terminated. Schwann cells proliferate and phagocytose the remnants of the axon terminal, and the newly formed Schwann cells occupy the synaptic space.

2 The distal portion of the axon undergoes **wallerian degeneration (orthograde degeneration),** whereby, distal to the lesion, the axon and the myelin disintegrate, Schwann cells dedifferentiate, and myelin synthesis is discontinued. Moreover, macrophages and, to a certain extent, Schwann cells phagocytose the disintegrated remnants.

3 Schwann cells proliferate, forming a column of Schwann cells (**Schwann tubes**) enclosed by the original basal lamina of the endoneurium.

Retrograde Reaction and Regeneration

In retrograde reaction and regeneration process, the proximal portion of the injured axon undergoes degeneration followed by sprouting of a new axon whose growth is directed by Schwann cells.

The portion of the axon proximal to the damage undergoes the following changes:

1 The perikaryon of the damaged neuron becomes hypertrophied, its Nissl bodies disperse, and its nucleus is displaced. These events, called **chromatolysis,** may last several months. Meanwhile, the soma is actively producing free ribosomes and synthesizing proteins and various macromolecules, including ribonucleic acid (RNA). During this time, the proximal axon stump and surrounding myelin sheath degenerate as far proximally as the nearest collateral axon.

2 Several "sprouts" of axons emerge from the proximal axon stump, enter the endoneurium, and are guided by the Schwann cells to their target cell. For regeneration to occur, the Schwann cells, macrophages, and fibroblasts as well as the basal lamina must be present. These cells manufacture growth factors and cytokines and up-regulate the expression for the receptors of these signaling molecules.

3 The sprout is guided by the Schwann cells that redifferentiate and either begin to manufacture myelin around the growing axon or, in nonmyelinated axons, form a Schwann cell sheath. The sprout that reaches the target cell first forms a synapse, whereas the other sprouts degenerate. The process of regeneration proceeds at about 3 to 4 mm/day.

Transneuronal Degeneration

The nerve cell has a **trophic influence** on the cells it contacts. If the neuron dies, sometimes its target cells atrophy and degenerate or other cells targeting that particular neuron also atrophy and degenerate. This process, called transneuronal degeneration, may thus be anterograde or retrograde but occurs only infrequently.

Regeneration in the Central Nervous System

Regeneration in the CNS is much less likely than in the PNS because connective tissue sheaths are absent in the CNS. Injured cells within the CNS are phagocytosed by special macrophages, known as **microglia,** and the space liberated by the phagocytosis is occupied by proliferation of glial cells, which form a cell mass called a **glial scar.** It is believed that the glial cell masses hinder the process of repair. Thus, generally, neuronal damage within the CNS appears to be irreparable.

Although neurons do not divide, there is evidence that there are neural stem cells within the adult mammalian and human brain that, when provided the proper stimulus, could be activated to replace lost or injured neurons. Some of these cells have the capacity to produce glial cells and others to differentiate into neurons. These neural stem cells exhibit multi-potential ability to differentiate into the cells of the tissue into which they were introduced.

It has been shown recently that reducing additional cell damage or death within 1 hour of injury increases the survivability of neurons in the vicinity of the lesion. This information—coupled with results of recent investigations concerning growth factors, applications of embryonic neural stem cells, reducing neuron growth inhibitors, applying axon grafts and grafting axons directly into the gray matter of the spinal cord—is providing promising results for the future in spinal cord therapy.

Neuronal Plasticity

Plasticity is evident during development because those neurons that are present in excess and/or not making correct connections must be destroyed. However, it has been shown in adult mammals that after injury neuronal circuits may be reestablished from the growth of neuronal processes located at some distance away from the lesion; these neuronal circuits are able to provide at least some functional recovery. Regeneration of this sort relies on growth factors called **neurotrophins** produced by neurons, glial cells, Schwann cells, and certain target cells. Evidence for neuronal plasticity in humans may be observed in stroke victims as well as in victims of other neurological injuries.

Blood and Hemopoiesis

10

Blood is a bright to dark red, viscous, slightly alkaline fluid (pH, 7.4) that accounts for approximately 7% of the total body weight. The total volume of blood of an average adult is about 5 L, and it circulates throughout the body within the confines of the circulatory system. Blood is a specialized connective tissue composed of formed elements—**red blood cells (RBCs; erythrocytes), white blood cells (WBCs; leukocytes),** and **platelets**—suspended in a fluid component (the extracellular matrix), known as **plasma** (Figs. 10-1 and 10-2).

Because blood circulates throughout the body, it is an ideal vehicle for the transport of materials. The primary functions of blood include conveying nutrients from the gastrointestinal system to all of the cells of the body and subsequently delivering the waste products of these cells to specific organs for elimination. Numerous other metabolites, cellular products (e.g., hormones and other signaling molecules), and electrolytes are also ferried by the bloodstream to their final destinations. Oxygen (O_2) is carried by hemoglobin within erythrocytes from the lungs for distribution to the cells of the organism, and carbon dioxide (CO_2) is conveyed both by hemoglobin and by the fluid component of plasma (as bicarbonate ion, HCO_3^-, and in its free form) for elimination by the lungs.

Blood also helps to regulate body temperature and to maintain the acid-base and osmotic balance of the body fluids. Finally, blood acts as a pathway for migration of white blood cells between various connective tissue compartments of the body.

The fluid state of blood necessitates the presence of a protective mechanism, **coagulation,** to stop its flow in case of damage to the vascular tree. The process of coagulation is mediated by platelets and bloodborne factors that transform blood from a sol to a gel state.

When blood is removed from the body and placed in a test tube, clotting occurs unless the tube is coated with an anticoagulant such as heparin. Upon centrifugation, the formed elements settle to the bottom of the tube as a red precipitate (44%) covered by a thin translucent layer, the **buffy coat** (1%), and the fluid plasma remains on top as the supernatant (55%). The red precipitate is composed of red blood cells, and the total red blood cell volume is known as the **hematocrit;** the buffy coat consists of white blood cells and platelets.

The finite life span of blood cells requires their constant renewal to maintain a steady circulating population. This process of blood cell formation from established blood cell precursors is called **hemopoiesis** (also referred to as hematopoiesis).

BLOOD

Blood is composed of a fluid component (plasma) and formed elements consisting of the various types of blood cells as well as platelets.

Light microscopic examination of circulating blood cells is performed by evenly smearing a drop of blood on a glass slide, air-drying the preparation, and staining it with mixtures of dyes specifically designed to demonstrate distinctive characteristics of the cells. The current methods are derived from the technique developed in the late 19th century by Romanovsky, who used a mixture of methylene blue and eosin. Most laboratories now use either the Wright or Giemsa modifications of the original procedure, and identification of blood cells is based on the colors produced by these stains. Methylene blue stains acidic cellular components blue, and eosin stains alkaline components pink. Still other components are colored a reddish blue by binding to **azures,** substances formed when methylene blue is oxidized.

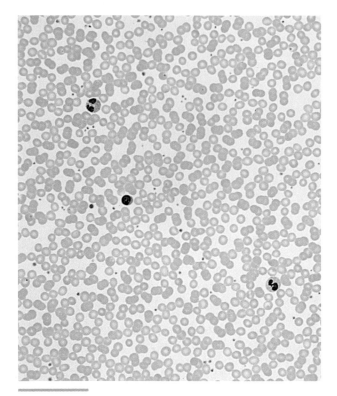

Figure 10–1 Light micrograph of circulating blood (×270). Note the abundance of erythrocytes as well as the three leukocytes. Also observe the presence of numerous platelets that appear as small dots interspersed among the erythrocytes.

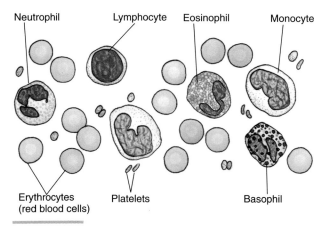

Figure 10–2 Cells and platelets of circulating blood.

Plasma

> *Plasma is a yellowish fluid in which cells, platelets, organic compounds, and electrolytes are suspended and/or dissolved.*

During coagulation, some of the organic and inorganic components leave the plasma to become integrated into the clot. The remaining fluid, which no longer has those components dissolved or suspended in it, differs from plasma, is straw-colored, and is known as **serum.**

The major component of plasma is water, constituting about 90% of its volume. Proteins constitute 9%, and inorganic salts, ions, nitrogenous compounds, nutrients, and gases constitute the remaining 1%. The types, origins, and functions of the blood proteins are listed in Table 10-1.

The fluid component of blood leaves the capillaries and small venules to enter the connective tissue spaces as **extracellular fluid,** which has a composition of electrolytes and small molecules similar to that in plasma. The concentration of proteins in extracellular fluid is much lower than that in plasma, however, because it is difficult even for small proteins, such as albumin, to traverse the endothelial lining of a capillary. In fact, albumin is chiefly responsible for the establishment of blood's **colloid osmotic pressure,** the force that maintains normal blood and interstitial fluid volumes.

Formed Elements

> *Red blood cells, white blood cells, and platelets constitute the formed elements of blood.*

Erythrocytes

> *Erythrocytes (red blood cells), the smallest and most numerous cells of blood, have no nuclei and are responsible for the transport of oxygen and carbon dioxide to and from the tissues of the body.*

Each erythrocyte resembles a biconcave-shaped disk 7.5 μm in diameter, 2.0 μm thick at its widest region, and less than 1 μm thick at its center (Figs. 10-3 and 10-4). This shape provides the cell with a large surface area relative to its volume, thus enhancing its capability for gaseous exchange. Although erythrocyte precursor cells within the bone marrow possess nuclei, during development and maturation the precursor cells or erythrocytes expel not only their nuclei but also all of their organelles before entering the circulation. Thus, mature erythrocytes have no nuclei. When stained with Giemsa or Wright stain, erythrocytes display a salmon-pink color.

Although erythrocytes possess no organelles, they do have soluble enzymes in their cytosol. Within the erythrocyte, the enzyme **carbonic anhydrase** facilitates the formation of carbonic acid from CO_2 and water. This acid dissociates to form bicarbonate (HCO_3^-) and hydrogen (H^+). It is as bicarbonate that most of the CO_2 is ferried to the lungs for exhalation. The ability of bicarbonate to cross the erythrocyte cell membrane is medi-

TABLE 10–1 Proteins of Plasma

Protein	Size	Source	Function
Albumin	60,000-69,000 Da	Liver	Maintains colloid osmotic pressure and transports certain insoluble metabolites
Globulins α- and β-Globulins	80,000-1 × 10⁶ Da	Liver	Transport metal ions, protein-bound lipids, and lipid-soluble vitamins
γ-Globulin		Plasma cells	Antibodies of immune defense
Clotting proteins (e.g., prothrombin, fibrinogen, accelerator globulin)	Varied	Liver	Formation of fibrin threads
Complement proteins C1 through C9	Varied	Liver	Destruction of microorganisms and initiation of inflammation
Plasma lipoproteins Chylomicrons	100-500 μm	Intestinal epithelial cells	Transport of triglycerides to liver
Very-low-density lipoprotein (VLDL)	25-70 nm	Liver	Transport of triglycerides from liver to body cells
Low-density lipoprotein (LDL)	3 × 10⁶ Da	Liver	Transport of cholesterol from liver to body cells

ated by the integral membrane protein **band 3,** a coupled anion transporter that exchanges intracellular bicarbonate for extracellular chloride; this exchange is known as the **chloride shift.** Additional enzymes include those of the glycolytic pathway (Embden-Meyerhoff pathway) as well as enzymes that are responsible for the pentose monophosphate shunt (hexose monophosphate shunt) for the production of the high-energy molecule reduced nicotinamide adenine dinucleotide phosphate (NADPH), a reducing agent. The glycolytic pathway does not require the presence of oxygen and is the chief method whereby the erythrocyte produces adenosine triphosphate (ATP), necessary for its energy requirement.

Males have more erythrocytes per unit volume of blood than do females (5×10^6 versus 4.5×10^6 per mm³), and members of both sexes living at higher altitudes have correspondingly more red blood cells than residents living at lower altitudes.

Human erythrocytes have an average life span of 120 days; when they reach that age, they display on their surface a group of oligosaccharides. Red blood cells bearing these sugar groups are destroyed by macrophages of the spleen, bone marrow, and liver.

Hemoglobin

Hemoglobin is a large protein composed of four polypeptide chains, each of which is covalently bound to a heme group.

Red blood cells are packed with hemoglobin, a large tetrameric protein (68,000 Da) composed of four polypeptide chains, each of which is covalently bound to an iron-containing **heme;** this molecule is bound within a hydrophobic depression, the heme pocket, of the globin chain which protects the iron from being oxidized while permitting the binding of oxygen to it. It is hemoglobin that provides the *unstained* cell with its pale yellow color. The globin moiety of hemoglobin releases CO_2, and, in regions of high oxygen concentration, such as in the lungs, O_2 binds to the iron of each heme. When oxygen is bound to the heme, the hemoglobin molecule is in the relaxed state [(R⁻) Hb], the globin moieties of the molecule are less constrained and can move with respect to each other, and the O_2 can easily be released. When O_2 is released, its place becomes occupied by 2,3-diphosphoglycerate and the hemoglobin becomes known as deoxyhemoglobin,

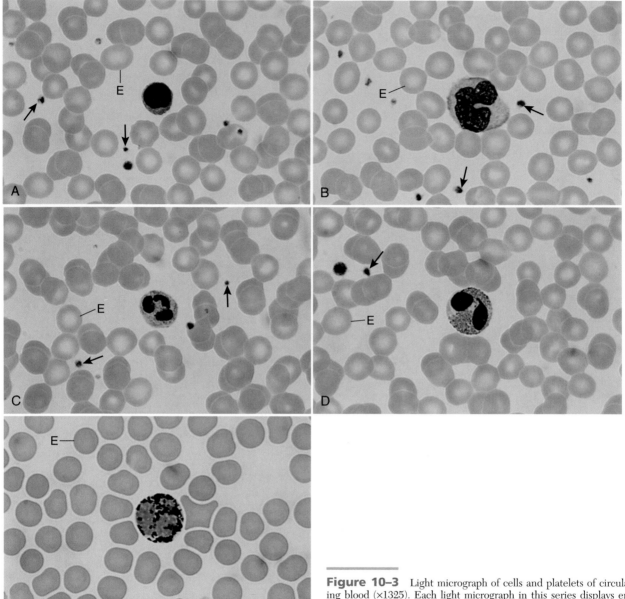

Figure 10–3 Light micrograph of cells and platelets of circulating blood (×1325). Each light micrograph in this series displays erythrocytes (E), platelets (*arrows*), and a single white blood cell. **A,** Lymphocyte; **B,** monocyte; **C,** neutrophil; **D,** eosinophil; **E,** basophil.

or taut hemoglobin [(T^-) Hb]. The number of ionic and H bonds between the globin chains of (T^-) Hb is greater than that of (R^-) Hb, and the movement of the globin chains with respect to each other is reduced. However, in oxygen-poor regions, as in tissues, hemoglobin releases O_2 and binds CO_2. This property of hemoglobin makes it ideal for the conveyance of respiratory gases. Hemoglobin carrying O_2 is known as **oxyhemoglobin,** and hemoglobin

carrying CO_2 is called **carbaminohemoglobin** (or **carbamylhemoglobin**). Hypoxic tissues release 2,3-diphosphoglyceride, a carbohydrate that facilitates the release of oxygen from the erythrocyte. Hemoglobin also binds nitric oxide (NO), a neurotransmitter substance that causes dilation of blood vessels, permitting red blood cells to release more oxygen and pick up more CO_2 within the tissues of the body.

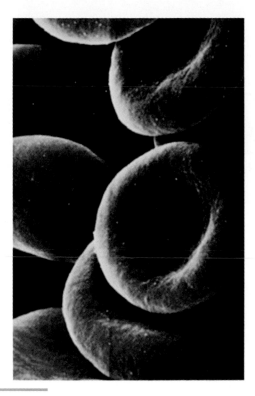

Figure 10–4 Scanning electron micrograph of circulating red blood cells displaying their biconcave disk shape (×5850). (From Leeson TS, Leeson CR, Paparo AA: Text/Atlas of Histology. Philadelphia, WB Saunders, 1988.)

CLINICAL CORRELATIONS

Carbon monoxide (CO) has a much greater affinity than O_2 for the heme portion of hemoglobin, and when CO binds to the iron of the heme, the hemoglobin molecule is transformed to its (R^-) Hb form and will increase its affinity to oxygen so that it cannot be released to the tissues even in hypoxic regions. People who are trapped in areas of poor ventilation with a running gasoline-powered engine or in a building on fire frequently succumb to CO poisoning. Many such victims, if fair-skinned, instead of being cyanotic (with a bluish pallor) present with healthy-looking, cherry-red skin because of the color of the CO-hemoglobin complex (**carbon monoxy-hemoglobin**).

On the basis of the amino acid sequences, there are four normal, human polypeptide chains of hemoglobin, designated α, β, γ, and δ. The principal hemoglobin of the fetus, **fetal hemoglobin (HbF),** composed of two α-chains and two γ-chains, is replaced shortly after birth by adult hemoglobin (HbA). There are two types of normal adult hemoglobin, HbA_1 ($\alpha_2\beta_2$) and the much rarer form, HbA_2 ($\alpha_2\delta_2$). In the adult, approximately 96% of the hemoglobin is HbA_1, 2% is HbA_2, and the remaining 2% is HbF.

CLINICAL CORRELATIONS

Several hereditary diseases result from defects in the genes encoding the hemoglobin polypeptide chains. Diseases referred to as **thalassemia** are marked by decreased synthesis of one or more hemoglobin chains. In β-thalassemia, synthesis of the β-chains is impaired. In the homozygous form of this disease, which is most prevalent among persons of Mediterranean descent, HbA is missing and high levels of HbF persist after birth.

Sickle cell anemia is the result of a point mutation at a single locus of the β-chain (valine is incorporated into the sequence instead of glutamate), forming the abnormal hemoglobin HbS. When the oxygen tension is reduced (e.g., during strenuous exercise), HbS changes shape, producing abnormally shaped (crescent-shaped) erythrocytes that are less pliant, more fragile, and more prone to hemolysis than normal cells. Sickle cell anemia is prevalent in the black population, especially in those whose ancestors lived in regions of Africa where malaria is endemic. In the United States, about 1 of 600 newborn African-American babies is stricken with this condition.

Erythrocyte Cell Membrane

The cell membrane of the erythrocyte and the underlying cytoskeleton are highly pliable and can withstand great shear forces.

The red blood cell plasma membrane, a typical lipid bilayer, is composed of about 50% protein, 40% lipids, and 10% carbohydrates. Most of the proteins are transmembrane proteins, principally **glycophorin A** (as well as lesser quantities of glycophorins B, C, and D), ion channels (calcium-dependent potassium channels and Na^+-K^+ adenosine triphosphatase), and the anion transporter **band 3 protein,** which transports Cl^- and HCO_3^-; it also acts as an anchoring site for **ankyrin,** band 4.1 protein, hemoglobin, and glycolytic enzymes (Fig. 10-5). Additionally, the red blood cell membrane also possesses the peripheral proteins band 4.1 protein, spectrin, ankyrin, and actin. **Band 4.1 protein** acts as an anchoring site for spectrin, band 3 protein, and

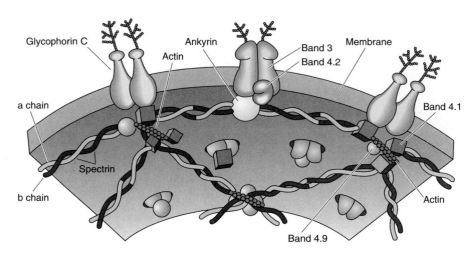

Figure 10–5 The cytoskeleton and integral proteins of the erythrocyte plasmalemma. Spectrin forms a hexagonal latticework that is anchored to the erythrocyte plasma membrane by band 4.1 and band 3 proteins as well as by ankyrin.

glycophorins. Thus, ankyrin, band 3 protein, and band 4.1 protein anchor the cytoskeleton, a hexagonal lattice composed chiefly of **spectrin tetramers**, **actin**, and **adducin**, to the cytoplasmic aspect of the red blood cell plasmalemma (see Chapter 2). This subplasmalemmal cytoskeleton helps to maintain the biconcave disk shape of the erythrocyte.

During its 120-day life, each erythrocyte negotiates the entire circulatory system at least 100,000 times and therefore must pass through innumerable capillaries whose lumen is smaller than the cell's diameter. To navigate through such small-bore vessels, the erythrocyte undergoes deformations of its shape and becomes subject to tremendous shear forces. It is the erythrocyte cell membrane and the underlying cytoskeleton that contribute to the ability of the red blood cell to maintain its structural and functional integrity.

CLINICAL CORRELATIONS

Defects in the cytoskeletal components of erythrocytes result in various conditions marked by abnormally shaped cells. **Hereditary spherocytosis,** for instance, is caused by synthesis of an abnormal spectrin that exhibits defective binding to band 4.1 protein. Red blood cells of patients with this condition are more fragile and transport less oxygen compared with normal erythrocytes. Moreover, these spherocytes are preferentially destroyed in the spleen, leading to **anemia.**

Deficiency of glycophorin C is responsible for **elliptocytic red blood cells** without the resultant hemolytic anemia. These cells are unstable and fragile and are less capable of deformation than normal erythrocytes.

TABLE 10–2 ABO Blood Group System

Blood Group	Antigens Present	Miscellaneous
A	Antigen A	
B	Antigen B	
AB	Antigens A and B	Universal acceptor
O	Neither antigen A nor B	Universal donor

The extracellular surface of the red blood cell plasmalemma has specific inherited carbohydrate chains that act as antigens and determine the blood group of an individual for the purposes of blood transfusion. The most notable of these are the **A and B antigens,** which determine the four primary blood groups, **A, B, AB, and O** (Table 10-2). People who lack either the A or B antigen, or both, have antibodies against the missing antigen in their blood; if they undergo transfusion with blood containing the missing antigen, the donor erythrocytes are attacked by the recipient's serum antibodies and are eventually lysed.

Another important blood group, the **Rh group,** is so-named because it was first identified in rhesus monkeys. This complex group comprises more than two dozen antigens, although many are relatively rare. Three of the Rh antigens (C, D, and E) are so common in the human population that the erythrocytes of 85% of Americans have one of these antigens on their surface, and these individuals are thus said to be **Rh-positive (Rh⁺).** Individuals lacking these antigens are RH-negative (RH⁻).

CLINICAL CORRELATIONS

When an Rh⁻ pregnant woman delivers her first Rh⁺ baby, enough of the baby's blood is likely to enter her circulation to induce the formation of anti-Rh antibodies. During a subsequent pregnancy with an Rh⁺ fetus, these antibodies attack the erythrocytes of the fetus, causing **erythroblastosis fetalis,** a condition that may be fatal to the newborn. Prenatal and postnatal transfusions to the fetus are necessary to prevent brain damage and death of the newborn unless the mother has been treated with anti-Rh agglutinins—$Rh_0(D)$ immune globulin (RhoGAM)—before or shortly after the birth of the first Rh⁺ baby.

Leukocytes

Leukocytes are white blood cells that are classified into two major categories: granulocytes and agranulocytes.

The number of leukocytes is much smaller than that of red blood cells; in fact, in a healthy adult there are only 6500 to 10,000 white blood cells per mm^3 of blood. Unlike erythrocytes, leukocytes do not function within the bloodstream but use it as a means of traveling from one region of the body to another. When leukocytes reach their destination, they leave the bloodstream by migrating between the endothelial cells of the blood vessels **(diapedesis),** enter the connective tissue spaces, and perform their function. Within the bloodstream as well as in smears, leukocytes are round; in connective tissue, they are pleomorphic. They generally defend the body against foreign substances.

White blood cells are classified into two groups (Table 10-3):

- Granulocytes, which have specific granules in their cytoplasm
- Agranulocytes, which lack specific granules.

Both granulocytes and agranulocytes possess nonspecific (azurophilic) granules, now known to be **lysosomes.**

There are three types of **granulocytes,** differentiated according to the color of their specific granules after application of Romanovsky-type stains:

- Neutrophils
- Eosinophils
- Basophils.

There are two types of **agranulocytes:**

- Lymphocytes
- Monocytes.

Neutrophils

Neutrophils compose most of the white blood cell population; they are avid phagocytes, destroying bacteria that invade connective tissue spaces.

Polymorphonuclear leukocytes (polys, neutrophils) are the most numerous of the white blood cells, constituting 60% to 70% of the total leukocyte population. In blood smears, neutrophils are 9 to 12 μm in diameter and have a multilobed nucleus (see Figs. 10-2 and 10-3). The lobes, connected to each other by slender chromatin threads, increase in number with the age of the cell. In females, the nucleus presents a characteristic small appendage, the "drumstick," which contains the condensed, inactive second X chromosome. It is also called the **Barr body** or **sex chromosome** but is not always evident in every cell. Neutrophils are among the first cells to appear in acute bacterial infections. The neutrophil plasmalemma possesses complement receptors as well as Fc receptors for IgG.

NEUTROPHIL GRANULES

Neutrophils possess specific, azurophilic, and tertiary granules.

Three types of granules are present in the cytoplasm of neutrophils:

- Small, specific granules (0.1 μm in diameter)
- Larger azurophilic granules (0.5 μm in diameter)
- Tertiary granules.

Specific granules contain various enzymes and pharmacological agents that aid the neutrophil in performing its antimicrobial functions (see Table 10-3). In electron micrographs these granules appear somewhat oblong (Fig. 10-6).

Azurophilic granules, as already indicated, are lysosomes, containing acid hydrolases, myeloperoxidase, the antibacterial agent lysozyme, bactericidal permeability-increasing (BPI) protein, cathepsin G, elastase, and nonspecific collagenase.

Tertiary granules contain gelatinase and cathepsins as well as glycoproteins that are inserted into the plasmalemma.

NEUTROPHIL FUNCTIONS

Neutrophils phagocytose and destroy bacteria by using the contents of their various granules.

Neutrophils interact with chemotactic agents to migrate to sites invaded by microorganisms. They accomplish this by entering postcapillary venules in the region of inflammation and adhering to the various

TABLE 10–3　Leukocytes

Features	GRANULOCYTES			AGRANULOCYTES	
	Neutrophils	**Eosinophils**	**Basophils**	**Lymphocytes**	**Monocytes**
Number/mm^3 % of WBCs	3500-7000 60-70	150-400 2-4	50-100 <1	1500-2500 20-25	200-800 3-8
Diameter (μm) 　Section 　Smear	 8-9 9-12	 9-11 10-14	 7-8 8-10	 7-8 8-10	 10-12 12-15
Nucleus	Three to four lobes	Two lobes (sausage shaped)	S-shaped	Round	Kidney-shaped
Specific granules	0.1 μm, light pink°	1-1.5 μm, dark pink°	0.5 μm, blue/black°	None	None
Contents of specific granules	Type IV collagenase, phospholipase A$_2$, lactoferrin, lysozyme, phagocytin, alkaline phosphatase, vitamin B$_{12}$-binding protein	Aryl sulfatase, histaminase, β-glucuronidase, acid phosphatase, phospholipase, major basic protein, eosinophil cationic protein, neurotoxin, ribonuclease, cathepsin, peroxidase	Histamine, heparin, eosinophil chemotactic factor, neutrophil chemotactic factor, peroxidase, neutral proteases, chondroitin sulfate	None	None
Surface markers	Fc receptors, platelet-activating factor receptor, leukotriene B$_4$ receptor, leukocyte cell adhesion molecule-1	IgE receptors, eosinophil chemotactic factor receptor	IgE receptors	*T cells:* T-cell receptors, CD molecules, IL receptors *B cells:* surface immunoglobulins	Class II HLA, Fc receptors
Life span	<1 week	<2 weeks	1-2 years (in murines)	Few months to several years	Few days in blood, several months in connective tissue
Function	Phagocytosis and destruction of bacteria	Phagocytosis of antigen-antibody complex; destruction of parasites	Similar to mast cells to mediate inflammatory responses	*T cells:* cell-mediated immune response *B cells:* humorally mediated immune response	Differentiate into macrophage: phagocytosis, presentation of antigens

°Using Romanovsky-type stains (or their modifications).
CD, cluster of differentiation; HLA, human leukocyte antigen; IgE, immunoglobulin E; IL, interleukin; WBC, white blood cell.

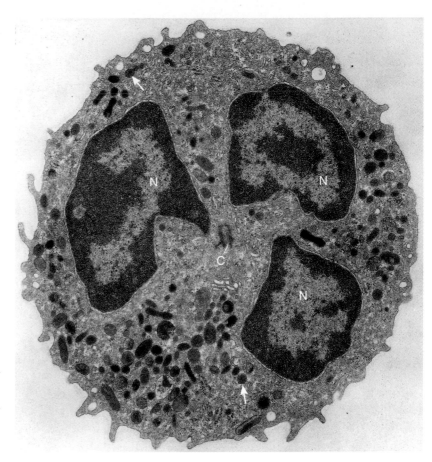

Figure 10–6 Electron micrograph of a human neutrophil. Note the three lobes of the nucleus (N), the presence of granules (arrows) throughout the cytoplasm, and the centrally located centriole (C). Although it appears as if there are three distinct nuclei in this image, they are merely lobes of the same nucleus, and the connections are outside the present field of view. (From Zucker-Franklin D, et al [eds]: Atlas of Blood Cells. Vol 1. Milan, Edi Ermes, 1981.)

selectin molecules of endothelial cells of these vessels by use of their **selectin receptors.** The interaction between the neutrophil's selectin receptors and the selectins of the endothelial cells causes the neutrophils to roll slowly along the vessel's endothelial lining. As the neutrophils are slowing their migrations, **interleukin-1** (**IL-1**) and **tumor necrosis factor** (**TNF**) induce the endothelial cells to express intercellular adhesion molecule type 1 (**ICAM-1),** to which the **integrin molecules** of neutrophils avidly bind.

When binding occurs, the neutrophils stop migrating in preparation for their passage through the endothelium of the postcapillary venule to enter the connective tissue compartment. Once there, they destroy the microorganisms by phagocytosis and by the release of hydrolytic enzymes (and **respiratory burst**). In addition, by manufacturing and releasing **leukotrienes,** neutrophils assist in the initiation of the inflammatory process. The sequence of events is:

1 The binding of neutrophil chemotactic agents to the neutrophil's plasmalemma facilitates the release of the contents of tertiary granules into the extracellular matrix.

2 Gelatinase degrades the basal lamina, facilitating neutrophil migration. Glycoproteins that become inserted in the cell membrane aid the process of phagocytosis.

3 The contents of the specific granules are also released into the extracellular matrix, where they attack the invading microorganisms and aid neutrophil migration.

4 Microorganisms, phagocytosed by neutrophils, become enclosed in **phagosomes** (Fig. 10-7A and B). Enzymes and pharmacological agents of the azurophilic granules are usually released into the lumina of these intracellular vesicles, where they destroy the ingested microorganisms. Because of their phagocytic functions, neutrophils are also known as **microphages** to distinguish them from the larger phagocytic cells, the **macrophages.**

5 Bacteria are killed not only by the action of enzymes but also by the formation of reactive oxygen compounds within the phagosomes of neutrophils. These are **superoxide** (O_2^-), formed

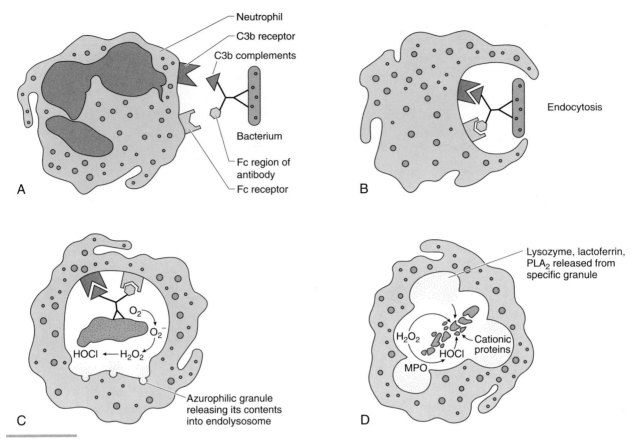

Figure 10–7 Bacterial phagocytosis and destruction by a neutrophil. These actions are dependent on the ability of the neutrophil to recognize the bacterium via the presence of complement and/or antibody attached to the microorganism. H_2O_2, hydrogen peroxide; HOCl, hypochlorous acid; MPO, myeloperoxidase, O_2^-, superoxide, PLA_2, phospholipase A_2.

by the action of NADPH oxidase on O_2 in a respiratory burst; **hydrogen peroxide** (H_2O_2), formed by the action of superoxide dismutase on superoxide; and **hypochlorous acid** (HOCl), formed by the interaction of myeloperoxidase (MPO) and chloride ions with hydrogen peroxide (see Fig. 10-7C and D).

6 Frequently, the contents of the azurophilic granules are released into the extracellular matrix, causing tissue damage, but usually **catalase** and **glutathione peroxidase** limit the tissue injury by degrading hydrogen peroxide.

7 Once neutrophils perform their function of killing microorganisms, they also die, resulting in the formation of **pus,** the accumulation of dead leukocytes, bacteria, and extracellular fluid.

8 Not only do neutrophils destroy bacteria, they also synthesize **leukotrienes** from arachidonic acids in their cell membranes. These newly formed leukotrienes aid the initiation of the inflammatory process.

CLINICAL CORRELATIONS

Children with **hereditary deficiency of NADPH oxidase** are subject to persistent bacterial infections because their neutrophils cannot form a respiratory burst response to the bacterial challenge. Their neutrophils cannot generate superoxide, hydrogen peroxide, or hypochlorous acid during phagocytosis of bacteria.

Eosinophils

Eosinophils phagocytose antigen-antibody complexes and kill parasitic invaders.

Eosinophils constitute less than 4% of the total white blood cell population. They are round cells in suspension and in blood smears, but they may be pleomorphic during their migration through connective tissue. Their cell membrane has receptors for immunoglobulin G (IgG), IgE, and complement. Eosinophils are 10 to 14 μm in diameter (in blood smears) and have a sausage-shaped, bilobed nucleus in which the two lobes are connected by a thin chromatin strand and surrounding nuclear envelope (see Figs. 10-2 and 10-3). Electron micrographs display a small, centrally located Golgi apparatus, a limited amount of rough endoplasmic reticulum (RER), and only a few mitochondria, usually in the vicinity of the centrioles near the cytocenter. Eosinophils are produced in the bone marrow, and it is **interleukin-5 (IL-5)** that causes proliferation of their precursors and their differentiation into mature cells.

EOSINOPHIL GRANULES

The specific granules of eosinophils possess an externum and an internum.

Eosinophils possess specific granules and azurophilic granules. Specific granules are oblong (1.0 to 1.5 μm in length, <1.0 μm in width) and stain deep pink with Giemsa and Wright stains. Electron micrographs show that specific granules have a crystal-like, electron-dense center, the **internum,** surrounded by a less electron-dense **externum** (Fig. 10-8). The internum contains **major basic protein**, **eosinophilic cationic protein,** and **eosinophil-derived neurotoxin,** the first two of

which are highly efficacious agents in combating parasites. The externum also contains the enzymes listed in Table 10-3.

The nonspecific azurophilic granules are lysosomes (0.5 μm in diameter) containing hydrolytic enzymes similar to those found in neutrophils. These function both in the destruction of parasitic worms and in the hydrolysis of antigen-antibody complexes internalized by eosinophils.

EOSINOPHIL FUNCTIONS

Eosinophils help to eliminate antibody-antigen complexes and to destroy parasitic worms.

Eosinophils are associated with these functions:

■ Binding of histamine, leukotrienes, and eosinophil chemotactic factor (released by mast cells, basophils, and neutrophils) to eosinophil plasmalemma receptors, which results in the migration of eosinophils to the site of allergic reaction, inflammatory reaction, or parasitic worm invasion
■ Degranulation of their major basic protein or eosinophil cationic protein on the surface of parasitic worms, killing them by forming pores in their pellicles, thus facilitating access of agents such as **superoxides** and **hydrogen peroxide** to the parasite
■ Release of substances that inactivate the pharmacological initiators of the inflammatory response, such as **histamine** and **leukotriene C**

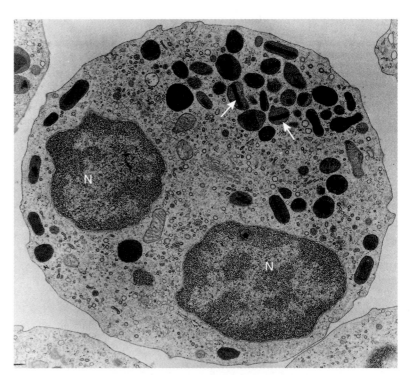

Figure 10–8 Electron micrograph of a human eosinophil. Note the electron-dense internum (*arrows*) of the eosinophilic granules and the two lobes of the nucleus (N). (From Zucker-Franklin D: Eosinophil function and disorders. Adv Intern Med 19:1-25, 1974.)

▪ Engulfing of antigen-antibody complexes, which pass into the **endosomal** compartment for eventual degradation.

CLINICAL CORRELATIONS

Connective tissue cells in the vicinity of antigen-antibody complexes release the pharmacological agents histamine and IL-5, causing increased formation and release of eosinophils from the bone marrow. In contrast, elevation of blood corticosteroid levels depresses the number of eosinophils in circulation.

Basophils

Basophils are similar to mast cells in function even though they have different origins.

Basophils constitute less than 1% of the total leukocyte population. They are round cells in suspension but may be pleomorphic during migration through connective tissue. They are 8 to 10 μm in diameter (in blood smears) and have an **S-shaped nucleus**, which is commonly masked by the large specific granules present in the cytoplasm (see Figs. 10-2 and 10-3). In electron micrographs, the small Golgi apparatus, a few mitochondria, extensive RER, and occasional glycogen deposits are clearly evident. Basophils have several surface receptors on their plasmalemma, including **immunoglobulin E (IgE) receptors (FcεRI).**

BASOPHIL GRANULES

Basophils possess specific and azurophilic granules.

The **specific granules** of basophils stain dark blue to black with Giemsa and Wright stains. They are approximately 0.5 μm in diameter and frequently press against the periphery of the cell, creating the basophil's characteristic "roughened" perimeter, as seen by light microscopy. The granules contain heparin, histamine, eosinophil chemotactic factor, neutrophil chemotactic factor, neutral proteases, chondroitin sulfate, and peroxidase (see Table 10-3). The nonspecific **azurophilic granules** are lysosomes, which contain enzymes similar to those of neutrophils.

BASOPHIL FUNCTIONS

Basophils function as initiators of the inflammatory process

In response to the presence of some antigens in certain individuals, plasma cells manufacture and release a par-

ticular class of immunoglobulin, IgE. The Fc portions of the IgE molecules become attached to the **FcεRi** of basophils and mast cells without any apparent effect. However, the next time the same antigens enter the body, they bind to the IgE molecules on the surface of these cells. Although mast cells and basophils appear to have similar functions, they are different cells and have different origins.

Although the following sequence of steps occurs in both mast cells and basophils, the basophil is used here for descriptive purposes:

1 Binding of antigens to the IgE molecules on the surface of a basophil causes the cell to release the contents of its specific granules into the extracellular space.
2 In addition, the enzyme **phospholipase A** generates arachidonic acid residues from the plasma membrane which then are fed into the cyclooxigenase or the lipoxigenase pathway to produce chemical factors that mediate the inflammatory response. These factors are platelet activating factor, leukotriene B_4, prostaglandin D_2, thromboxane A_2, leukotriene C_4, leukotriene D_4, leukotriene E_4 (formerly called slow-reacting substance of anaphylaxis, or SRS-A), adenosine, bradykinin, superoxide, TNF factor α, IL4, IL5, IL6, and granulocyte-monocyte colony-stimulating factor.
3 The release of histamine causes vasodilation, smooth muscle contraction (in the bronchial tree), and leakiness of blood vessels.
4 Leukotrienes have similar effects, but these actions are slower and more persistent than those associated with histamine. In addition, leukotrienes activate leukocytes, causing them to migrate to the site of antigenic challenge.

CLINICAL CORRELATIONS

In certain hyperallergic individuals, a second exposure to the same allergen may result in an intense generalized response. A large number of basophils (and mast cells) degranulate, resulting in widespread vasodilation and sweeping reduction in blood volume (because of vessel leakiness). Thus, the person goes into circulatory shock. The smooth muscles of the bronchial tree constrict, causing respiratory insufficiency. The combined effect is a life-threatening condition known as **anaphylactic shock.**

Monocytes

Monocytes, the largest of the circulating blood cells, enter the connective tissue spaces, where they are known as macrophages.

Monocytes are the largest of the circulating blood cells (12 to 15 μm in diameter in blood smears) and constitute 3% to 8% of the leukocyte population. They have a large, acentric, kidney-shaped nucleus that frequently has a "moth-eaten," soap-bubble" appearance and whose lobe-like extensions seem to overlap one another. The chromatin network is coarse but not overly dense, and typically two nucleoli are present, although they are not always evident in smears. The cytoplasm is bluish gray and has numerous azurophilic granules (lysosomes) and occasional vacuole-like spaces (see Figs. 10-2 and 10-3).

Electron micrographs display both heterochromatin and euchromatin in the nucleus as well as two nucleoli. The Golgi apparatus is usually near the indentation of the kidney-shaped nucleus. The cytoplasm contains deposits of glycogen granules, a few profiles of RER, some mitochondria, free ribosomes, and numerous lysosomes. The periphery of the cell displays microtubules, microfilaments, pinocytotic vesicles, and filopodia.

Monocytes stay in circulation for only a few days; they then migrate through the endothelium of venules and capillaries into the connective tissue, where they differentiate into **macrophages.** Macrophages are discussed in greater detail in Chapter 12; an introduction to their properties and functions follows here.

FUNCTION OF MACROPHAGES

Macrophages phagocytose unwanted particular matter, produce cytokines that are required for the inflammatory and immune responses, and present epitopes to T lymphocytes.

Macrophages are avid phagocytes and, as members of the **mononuclear phagocyte system,** they phagocytose and destroy dead and defunct cells (such as senescent erythrocytes) as well as antigens and foreign particulate matter (such as bacteria). The destruction occurs within the phagosomes through both enzymatic digestion and the formation of superoxide, hydrogen peroxide, and hypochlorous acid.

Macrophages produce cytokines that activate the inflammatory response as well as the proliferation and maturation of other cells.

Certain macrophages, known as **antigen-presenting cells,** phagocytose antigens and present their most antigenic portions, the **epitopes,** in conjunction with the integral proteins, **class II human leukocyte antigen (class II HLA;** also known as **major histocompatibility complex antigens [MHC II]),** to immunocompetent cells.

In response to large foreign particulate matter, macrophages fuse with one another, forming **foreign-body giant cells** that are large enough to phagocytose the foreign particle.

Lymphocytes

Lymphocytes are agranulocytes and form the second largest population of white blood cells.

Lymphocytes constitute 20% to 25% of the total circulating leukocyte population. They are round cells in blood smears, but they may be pleomorphic as they migrate through connective tissue. Lymphocytes are somewhat larger than erythrocytes, 8 to 10 μm in diameter (in blood smears), and have a slightly indented, round nucleus that occupies most of the cell. The nucleus is dense, rich in heterochromatin, and is acentrically located. The peripherally situated cytoplasm stains a light blue and contains a few azurophilic granules. On the basis of size, lymphocytes may be described as small (8 to 10 μm in diameter), medium (12 to 15 μm), or large (15 to 18 μm), although the latter two are much less numerous (see Figs. 10-2 and 10-3).

Electron micrographs of lymphocytes display a scant amount of peripheral cytoplasm housing a few mitochondria, a small Golgi apparatus, and a few profiles of RER. A small number of lysosomes, representing azurophilic granules 0.5 μm in diameter, and an abundant supply of ribosomes also are evident (Fig. 10-9).

Lymphocytes are discussed in greater detail in Chapter 12; an introduction to their properties and functions follows here.

Lymphocytes are subdivided into **three functional categories:**

- B lymphocytes (B cells)
- T lymphocytes (T cells)
- Null cells.

Although morphologically they are indistinguishable from each other, they can be recognized immunocytochemically by the differences in their surface markers (see Table 10-3). Approximately 80% of the circulating lymphocytes are T cells, about 15% are B cells, and the remainder are null cells. Their life spans also differ widely: some T cells may live for years, whereas some B cells may die in a few months.

FUNCTIONS OF B AND T CELLS

In general, B cells are responsible for the humorally mediated immune system, whereas T cells are responsible for the cellularly mediated immune system.

Lymphocytes have no function in the bloodstream, but in the connective tissue these cells are responsible for the proper functioning of the immune system. To be immunologically competent, they migrate to specific body compartments to mature and to express specific surface markers and receptors. B cells enter as yet unidentified regions of the **bone marrow,** whereas T

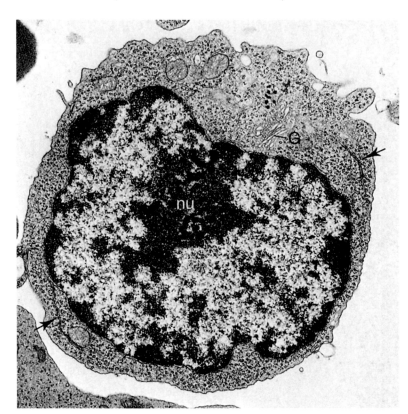

Figure 10–9 Electron micrograph of a lymphocyte (×14,173). *Arrows* point to the rough endoplasmic reticulum. G, Golgi apparatus; nu, nucleus. (From Hopkins CR: Structure and Function of Cells. Philadelphia, WB Saunders, 1978.)

cells migrate to the cortex of the **thymus.** Once they have become immunologically competent, lymphocytes leave their respective sites of maturation, enter the lymphoid system, and undergo mitosis, forming a group of identical cells, known as a **clone.** All members of a particular clone can recognize and respond to the same antigen.

After stimulation by a specific antigen, both B and T cells proliferate and differentiate into two subpopulations:

- **Memory cells** do not participate in the immune response but remain as part of the clone with an "immunological memory," ready to undergo cell division and mount a response against a subsequent exposure to a particular antigen or foreign substance.
- **Effector cells** are classified as B cells and T cells (and their subtypes).

Effector cells are immunocompetent lymphocytes that can perform lymphocyte immune functions; that is, eliminating antigens. B cells are responsible for the **humorally mediated immune system;** that is, they differentiate into **plasma cells,** which produce **antibodies** against **antigens.** T cells are responsible for the **cellularly mediated immune system.** Some T cells differentiate into **cytotoxic T cells (CTLs; T killer cells),** which make physical contact with and kill

foreign or **virally altered cells.** In addition, certain T cells are responsible for the initiation and development (**T helper cells**) or for the suppression (**regulatory T cells,** formerly known as T suppressor cells) of most humorally and cellularly mediated immune responses. They accomplish this by releasing signaling molecules known as **cytokines (lymphokines)** that elicit specific responses from other cells of the immune system (see Chapter 12).

FUNCTIONS OF NULL CELLS

Null cells are composed of two distinct populations:

- Circulating **stem cells,** which give rise to all of the formed elements of blood
- **Natural killer (NK) cells,** which can kill some foreign and virally altered cells without the influence of the thymus or T cells.

Platelets

Platelets (thromboplastids) are small, disk-shaped, nonnucleated cell fragments derived from megakaryocytes in the bone marrow.

Platelets are about 2 to 4 μm in diameter in blood smears (see Figs. 10-2 and 10-3). In light micrographs, they display a peripheral clear region, the **hyalomere,** and a central darker region, the **granulomere.** The platelet plasmalemma has numerous receptor molecules as well as a relatively thick (15 to 20 nm) glycocalyx. There are between 250,000 and 400,000 platelets per mm³ of blood, each with a life span of less than 14 days.

Platelet Tubules and Granules

Platelets possess three types of granules (alpha, delta, lambda) as well as two tubular systems (dense and surface opening).

Electron micrographs of platelets display 10 to 15 microtubules arranged parallel to each other and forming a ring within the hyalomere. The microtubules assist platelets in maintaining their diskoid morphology. Associated with this bundle of microtubules are actin and myosin monomers, which can rapidly assemble to form a contractile apparatus. In addition, two tubular systems are present in the hyalomere, the **surface-opening (connecting)** and the **dense tubular systems** (Figs. 10-10 and 10-11). The surface-opening system is coiled, forming a labyrinthine complex within the platelet. Because this system communicates with the outside, the luminal aspect of this tubular system is a continuation of the outer surface of the platelet, thus increasing the platelet surface area by a factor of seven or eight.

The ultrastructure of the granulomere displays the presence of a small number of mitochondria, glycogen deposits, peroxisomes, and three types of granules: alpha granules (*a-granules*), **delta granules (δ-granules),** and **lambda granules (λ-granules)** (lysosomes). The tubules and granules, as well as their contents and functions, are listed in Table 10-4. The granulomere also houses a system of enzymes that permits platelets to catabolize glycogen, consume oxygen, and generate ATP.

Platelet Function

Platelets function in limiting hemorrhage to the endothelial lining of the blood vessel in case of injury.

If the endothelial lining of a blood vessel is disrupted and platelets come in contact with the subendothelial collagen, they become **activated,** release the contents of their granules, adhere to the damaged region of the vessel wall **(platelet adhesion),** and adhere to each other **(platelet aggregation).** Interactions of tissue factors, plasma-borne factors, and platelet-derived factors form a blood clot (Figs. 10-12 and 10-13). Although the mechanism of platelet aggregation, adhesion, and blood clotting is beyond the scope of histology, some of its salient features are as follows:

1 Normally the intact endothelium produces **prostacyclins** and **NO,** which inhibit platelet aggregation. It also blocks coagulation by the presence of **thrombomodulin** and **heparin-like molecule** on its luminal plasmalemma. These two membrane-associated molecules inactivate specific coagulation factors.

2 Injured endothelial cells cease the production and expression of the inhibitors of coagulation and platelet aggregation and they release **von Willebrand factor** and **tissue thromboplastin.** They also release **endothelin,** a powerful vasoconstrictor that reduces the loss of blood.

3 Platelets avidly adhere to subendothelial collagen, especially in the presence of von Willebrand factor, release the contents of their granules, and adhere to one another. These three events are collectively called **platelet activation.**

4 The release of some of their granular contents, especially **adenosine diphosphate (ADP)** and **thrombospondin,** makes platelets "sticky," causing

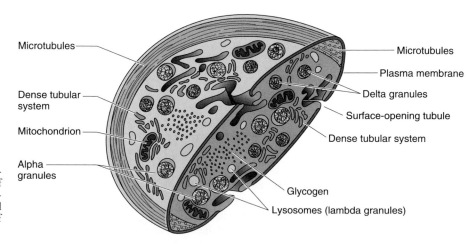

Figure 10–10 Platelet ultrastructure. Note that the periphery of the platelet is occupied by actin filaments that encircle the platelet and maintain the discoid morphology of this structure.

Microtubules

Dense tubular system

Mitochondrion

Alpha granules

Microtubules

Plasma membrane

Delta granules

Surface-opening tubule

Dense tubular system

Glycogen

Lysosomes (lambda granules)

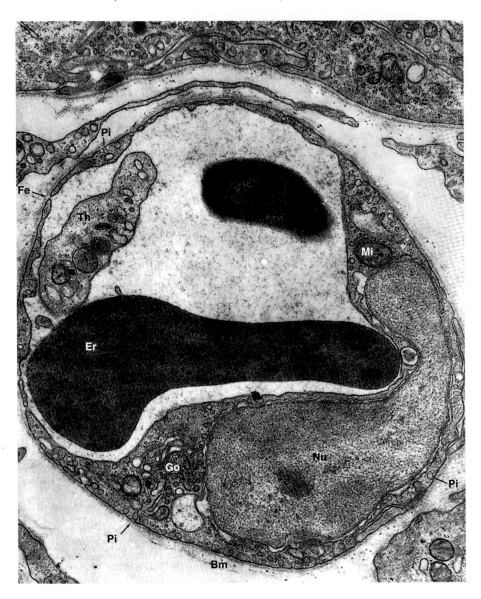

Figure 10–11 Electron micrograph of a platelet and two erythrocytes in the gastric mucosa capillary (×22,100). Th, platelet; Bm, basal lamina; Er, erythrocyte; Fe, fenestra; Go, Golgi apparatus; Mi, mitochondrion; Nu, nucleus of the capillary; Pi, pinocytotic vesicles; Th, platelet. (From Rhodin JAG: An Atlas of Ultrastructure. Philadelphia, WB Saunders, 1963.)

circulating platelets to adhere to the collagen-bound platelets and to degranulate.

5 Arachidonic acid, formed in the activated platelet plasmalemma, is converted to **thromboxane A₂,** a potent vasoconstrictor and platelet activator.

6 The aggregated platelets act as a plug, blocking hemorrhage. In addition, they express **platelet factor 3** on their plasmalemma, providing the necessary phospholipid surface for the proper assembly of the coagulation factors (especially of **thrombin**).

7 As part of the complex cascade of reactions involving the various **coagulation factors,** tissue thromboplastin and platelet thromboplastin both act on circulating **prothrombin,** converting it into **thrombin.** Thrombin is an enzyme that facilitates

platelet aggregation. In the presence of calcium (Ca^{2+}), it also converts **fibrinogen** to **fibrin.**

8 The fibrin monomers thus produced polymerize and form a **reticulum of clot,** entangling additional platelets, erythrocytes, and leukocytes into a stable, gelatinous **blood clot (thrombus).** The erythrocytes facilitate platelet activation, whereas neutrophils and endothelial cells limit both platelet activation and thrombus size.

9 Approximately 1 hour after clot formation, actin and myosin monomers form thin and thick filaments, which interact by utilizing ATP as their energy source. As a result, the clot contracts to about half its previous size, pulling the cut edges of the damaged vessel closer together and minimizing blood loss.

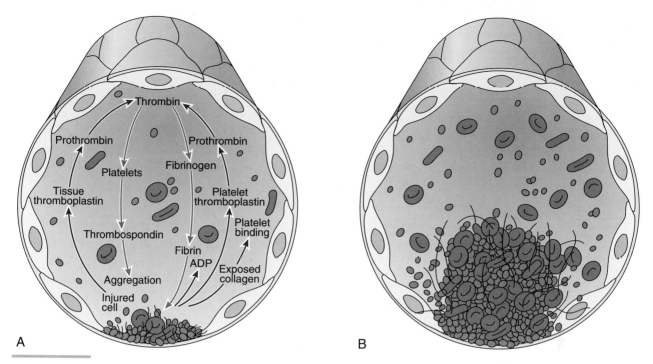

Figure 10–12 Clot formation. **A,** Injury to the endothelial lining releases various clotting factors and ceases the release of inhibitors of clotting. **B,** The increase in the size of the clot plugs the defect in the vessel wall and stops the loss of blood. (Modified from Fawcett DW: Bloom and Fawcett's A Textbook of Histology, 12th ed. New York, Chapman and Hall, 1994.)

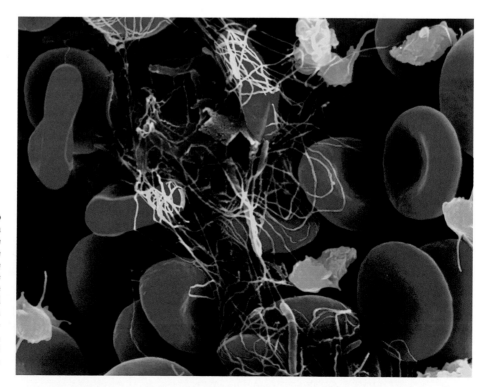

Figure 10–13 This close-up view of a clot forming in human blood shows beautifully how the different blood components are crammed into the plasma. (The scanning electron micrographs have been colored to emphasize the different structures.) Red blood cells are entangled with the fibrin (*yellow*) that makes up the scaffolding of the clot. The platelets (*blue*), which initiate clotting, are fragments of larger cells (megakaryocytes). (© 2000 by Dennis Kunkel, Ph.D.)

TABLE 10–4 Platelet Tubules and Granules

Structure (Size)	Location	Contents	Function
Surface-opening tubule system	Hyalomere		Expedites rapid uptake and release of molecules from activated platelets
Dense tubular system	Hyalomere		Probably sequesters calcium ions to prevent platelet "stickiness"
α-Granules (300-500 nm)	Granulomere	Fibrinogen, platelet-derived growth factor, platelet thromboplastin, thrombospondin, coagulation factors	Contained factors facilitate vessel repair, platelet aggregation, and coagulation of blood
δ-Granules (dense bodies) (250-300 nm)	Granulomere	Calcium, ADP, ATP, serotonin, histamine, pyrophosphatase	Contained factors facilitate platelet aggregation and adhesion, as well as vasoconstriction
λ-Granules (lysosomes) (200-250 nm)	Granulomere	Hydrolytic enzymes	Contained enzymes aid clot resorption

ADP, adenosine diphosphate; ATP, adenosine triphosphate.

10 When the vessel is repaired, the endothelial cells release **plasminogen activators,** which convert circulating plasminogen to **plasmin,** the enzyme that initiates lysis of the thrombus. The hydrolytic enzymes of λ-granules assist in this process.

BONE MARROW

Bone marrow, a gelatinous, vascular connective tissue located in the marrow cavity, is richly endowed with cells that are responsible for hemopoiesis.

The medullary cavity of long bones and the interstices between trabeculae of spongy bones house the soft, gelatinous, highly vascular, and cellular tissue known as marrow. Bone marrow is isolated from bone by the endosteum (composed of osteoprogenitor cells, osteoblasts, and occasional osteoclasts). Bone marrow constitutes almost 5% of the total body weight. It is responsible for the formation of blood cells (**hemopoiesis**) and their delivery into the circulatory system, and it performs this function from the fifth month of prenatal life until the person dies. Bone marrow also provides a microenvironment for much of the maturation process of B lymphocytes and for the initial maturation of T lymphocytes.

The marrow of the newborn is called **red marrow** because of the great number of erythrocytes being produced there. By age 20 years, however, the diaphyses of long bones house only **yellow marrow** because of the accumulation of large quantities of fat and the absence of hemopoiesis in the shafts of these bones.

The vascular supply of bone marrow is derived from the nutrient arteries that pierce the diaphysis via the nutrient foramina, tunnels leading from the outside surface of bone into the medullary cavity. These arteries enter the marrow cavity and give rise to a number of small, peripherally located vessels that provide numerous branches both centrally, to the marrow, and peripherally, to the cortical bone. Vessels entering the cortical bone are distributed through the haversian and Volkmann canals to serve the compact bone.

The centrally directed branches deliver their blood to the extensive network of large **sinusoids** (45 to 80 μm in diameter). The sinusoids drain into a **central longitudinal vein,** which is drained by veins leaving the bone via the nutrient canal.

It is interesting that the veins are *smaller* than the arteries, thus establishing high hydrostatic pressure within the sinusoids, thus preventing their collapse. The veins, arteries, and sinusoids form the **vascular compartment,** and the intervening spaces are filled with pleomorphic **islands of hemopoietic cells** that merge with each other, forming the **hemopoietic compartment** (Fig. 10-14).

The sinusoids are lined by endothelial cells and are surrounded by slender threads of **reticular fibers** and a large number of **adventitial reticular cells.** Processes of adventitial reticular cells touch the sparse basement membrane of the endothelial cells, covering a large portion of the sinusoidal surface. Additional processes of

CLINICAL CORRELATIONS

In a patient with a **thromboembolism,** the most common type of embolism, clots break free and circulate in the bloodstream until they reach a vessel whose lumen is too small to accommodate them. If a clot is large enough to occlude the bifurcation of the pulmonary artery **(saddle embolus),** it can result in sudden, unexpected death. If a clot obstructs branches of the coronary artery, a **myocardial infarct** may occur.

Several types of coagulation disorders that result in excessive bleeding are known. The disorder may be acquired (as in vitamin K deficiency) or hereditary (as in hemophilia) or may be caused by low levels of blood platelets (thrombocytopenia). **Vitamin K** is required by the liver as a cofactor in the synthesis of the **clotting factors VII, IX,** and **X** and **prothrombin.** Absence of or reduced levels of these factors result in partial or complete dysfunction of the clotting process.

The most common type of **hemophilia** is due to factor VIII deficiency **(classic hemophilia),** a recessive hereditary trait transmitted by mothers to their male children. Because the trait is carried on the X chromosomes, girls are not affected unless both parents have deficient X chromosomes. Affected persons are likely to bleed after trauma, usually involving damage to larger vessels.

In patients with **thrombocytopenia,** the blood level of platelets is decreased. The condition becomes serious when the platelet level is below 50,000/mm^3. Although bleeding is common in these patients, the bleeding is generalized and occurs from small vessels, resulting in purplish splotches on the skin. This condition is believed to be an **autoimmune disease,** in which antibodies are formed to one's own platelets and these antibodies destroy the platelets.

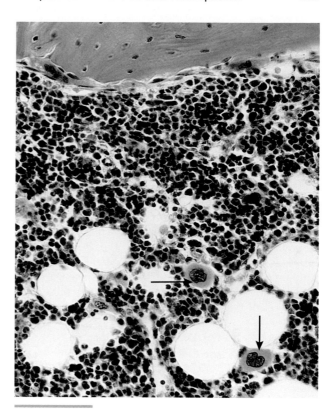

Figure 10–14 Light micrograph of human bone marrow displaying two megakaryocytes (*arrows*) (×270). Observe that marrow has a much greater population of nucleated cells than does peripheral blood. Also note the presence of epithelial reticular cells that resemble adipocytes. The decalcified bone with osteocytes located in lacunae is evident at the *top* of the photomicrograph.

processes of macrophages penetrate the spaces between endothelial cells to enter the sinusoidal lumina.

As adventitial reticular cells accumulate fat in their cytoplasm, they begin to resemble adipose cells. The volume occupied by these very large cells reduces the hemopoietic compartment in size, transforming the red marrow to yellow marrow.

CLINICAL CORRELATIONS

In certain leukemias or in severe bleeding, adventitial reticular cells may lose their lipids and decrease in size, transforming yellow marrow to red marrow, thus making more space available for hemopoiesis.

these cells are directed away from the sinusoids and are in contact with similar processes of other adventitial reticular cells, forming a three-dimensional network surrounding discrete **hemopoietic cords (islands).**

The islands of hemopoietic cells are composed of blood cells in various stages of maturation as well as **macrophages,** which not only destroy the extruded nuclei of erythrocyte precursors, malformed cells, and excess cytoplasm but also regulate hemopoietic cell differentiation and maturation, as well as transmit iron to developing erythroblasts to be utilized in the synthesis of the heme portion of hemoglobin. Frequently,

Prenatal Hemopoiesis

Prenatally, hemopoiesis is subdivided into four phases: mesoblastic, hepatic, splenic, and myeloid.

Blood cell formation begins 2 weeks after conception (**mesoblastic phase**) in the mesoderm of the yolk sac, where mesenchymal cells aggregate into clusters known as **blood islands.** The peripheral cells of these islands form the vessel wall, and the remaining cells become **erythroblasts,** which differentiate into nucleated **erythrocytes.**

The mesoblastic phase begins to be replaced by the **hepatic phase** by the 6th week of gestation. The erythrocytes still have nuclei, and leukocytes appear by the 8th week of gestation. The **splenic phase** begins during the second trimester, and both hepatic and splenic phases continue until the end of gestation.

Hemopoiesis begins in the bone marrow (**myeloid phase**) by the end of the second trimester. As the skeletal system continues to develop, the bone marrow assumes an increasing role in blood cell formation. Although postnatally the liver and the spleen are not active in hemopoiesis, they can revert to forming new blood cells if the need arises.

Postnatal Hemopoiesis

Postnatal hemopoiesis occurs almost exclusively in bone marrow.

Because all blood cells have a finite life span, they must be replaced continuously. This replacement is accomplished by hemopoiesis, starting from a common population of stem cells within the bone marrow (Fig. 10-15). On a daily basis, more than 10^{11} blood cells are produced in the marrow to replace cells that leave the bloodstream, die, or are destroyed. During hemopoiesis, stem cells undergo multiple cell divisions and differentiate through several intermediate stages, eventually giving rise to the mature blood cells discussed earlier. Table 10-5 outlines the numerous intermediate cells in the formation of each type of mature blood cell. The entire process is regulated by various growth factors and cytokines that act at different steps to control the type of cells formed and their rate of formation.

Stem Cells, Progenitor Cells, and Precursor Cells

The least differentiated of the cells responsible for the formation of the formed elements of blood are stem cells; stem cells give rise to progenitor cells whose progeny are the precursor cells.

All blood cells arise from **pluripotential hemopoietic stem cells (PHSCs),** which account for about 0.1% of the nucleated cell population of bone marrow. They are usually amitotic but may undergo bursts of cell division, giving rise to more PHSCs as well as to two types of **multipotential hemopoietic stem cells (MHSCs):**

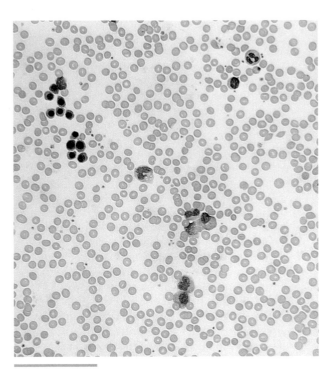

Figure 10–15 Light micrograph of a human bone marrow smear (×270).

colony-forming unit-lymphocyte (CFU-Ly) cells and **colony-forming unit-granulocyte, erythrocyte, monocyte, megakaryocyte (CFU-GEMM) cells**, previously known as colony-forming unit-spleen [CFU-S] cells. These two populations of MHSCs are responsible for the formation of various progenitor cells. CFU-GEMM cells are predecessors of the **myeloid cell lines** (erythrocytes, granulocytes, monocytes, and platelets); CFU-Ly cells are predecessors of the **lymphoid cell lines** (T cells and B cells). Both PHSCs and MHSCs resemble lymphocytes and constitute a small fraction of the null-cell population of circulating blood.

Stem cells are commonly in the G_0 stage of the cell cycle but can be driven into the G_1 stage by various growth factors and cytokines. Early stem cells may be recognized because they express the specific marker molecules CD34, p170 pump, and c-*kit* on their plasma membranes. **Homeobox genes** may be active in the differentiation of the early stages of hemopoietic cells, specifically *Hox1* in the myeloid (but not erythroid) cell lines and certain members of the *Hox2* group in the erythroid (but not myeloid) cell lines.

Progenitor cells also resemble small lymphocytes but are **unipotential** (i.e., committed to forming a single cell line, such as eosinophils). Their mitotic activity and differentiation are controlled by specific hemopoietic factors. These cells have only limited capacity for self-renewal.

TABLE 10-5 Cells of Hemopoiesis

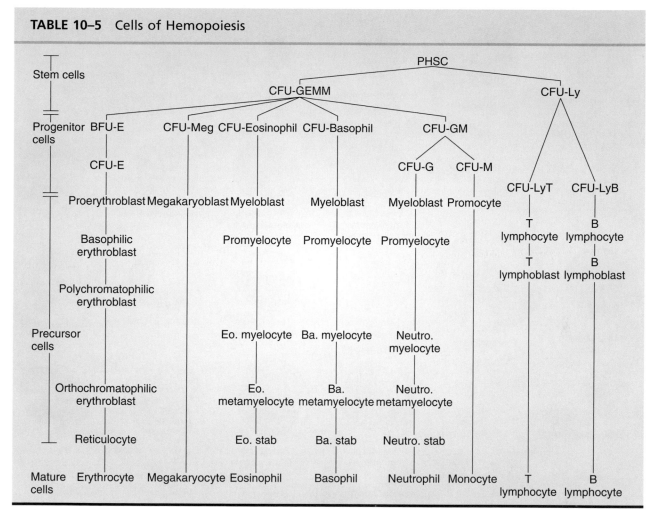

Ba., basophil; BFU, burst-forming unit (E, erythrocyte); CFU, colony-forming unit (E, erythrocyte); G, granulocyte; GEMM, granulocyte, erythrocyte, monocyte, megakaryocyte; GM, granulocyte-monocyte; Ly, lymphocyte; LyB, B cell; LyT, T cell; M, monocyte; Meg, megakaryoblast); Eo., eosinophil; Neutro., neutrophil; PHSC, pluripotential hemopoietic stem cell.
Modified from Gartner LP, Hiatt JL, Strum J: Histology. Baltimore, Williams & Wilkins, 1988.

Precursor cells arise from progenitor cells and are incapable of self-renewal. They have specific morphological characteristics that permit them to be recognized as the first cell of a particular cell line. Precursor cells undergo cell division and differentiation, eventually giving rise to a clone of mature cells. As cell maturation and differentiation proceed, succeeding cells become smaller, their nucleoli disappear, their chromatin network becomes denser, and the morphological characteristics of their cytoplasm approximate those of the mature cells (Fig. 10-16).

Researchers studying hemopoiesis have isolated individual lymphocyte-like cells that, under proper conditions, occasionally give rise to groups (*colonies*) of cells composed of granulocytes, erythrocytes, monocytes, lymphocytes, and platelets. Thus, it has been shown that all blood cells are derived from a single **pluripotential stem cell.** More frequently, however, isolated individual cells give rise to only erythrocytes or eosinophils or another type of blood cell. Because these experiments used the spleen as the site of hemopoiesis, the individual lymphocyte-like cells were originally called colony-forming units-spleen (CFU-S), but have been renamed to describe their function to CFU-GEMM. Careful observations have shown that, as stated previously, there are two types of multipotential cells (CFU-GEMM and CFU-Ly) that give rise to the myeloid series of cells and lymphocytes, respectively. Newer research has demonstrated that each precursor cell has a unipotential CFU as its predecessor (see Table 10-5). Precursor cells undergo a series of cell divisions and differentiations to yield the mature cell.

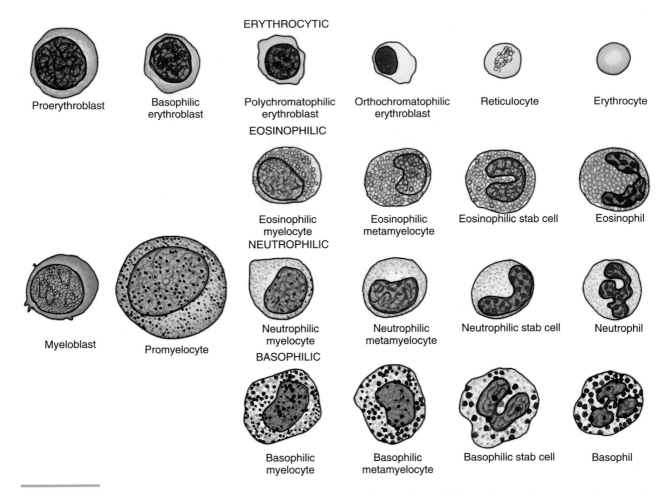

ERYTHROCYTIC

Proerythroblast — Basophilic erythroblast — Polychromatophilic erythroblast — Orthochromatophilic erythroblast — Reticulocyte — Erythrocyte

EOSINOPHILIC

Eosinophilic myelocyte — Eosinophilic metamyelocyte — Eosinophilic stab cell — Eosinophil

NEUTROPHILIC

Myeloblast — Promyelocyte — Neutrophilic myelocyte — Neutrophilic metamyelocyte — Neutrophilic stab cell — Neutrophil

BASOPHILIC

Basophilic myelocyte — Basophilic metamyelocyte — Basophilic stab cell — Basophil

Figure 10–16 Precursor cells in the formation of erythrocytes and granulocytes. The myeloblast and promyelocyte intermediaries in the formation of eosinophils, neutrophils, and basophils are indistinguishable for the three cell types.

CLINICAL CORRELATIONS

Patients who require bone marrow transplants after therapeutic procedures (such as irradiation or chemotherapy) must be matched for the major histocompatibility complex of the donor. Unless an identical twin is available for the transplantation, grafting failure is common. This can be circumvented by freezing the patient's own bone marrow in liquid nitrogen and reintroducing it (as in an **autologous transplant**) in the patient after treatment with irradiation or chemotherapy. Because the number of stem cells per unit volume of bone marrow is relatively small, large volumes of marrow have to be harvested from the patient. Newer procedures that permit the isolation of pluripotential hemopoietic stem cells (PHSCs) by the use of monoclonal antibodies against the CD34 molecule, which is expressed only by these cells, permit the use of small volumes of bone marrow enriched in PHSCs. These procedures are being investigated clinically, involving patients with various types of malignancies.

Perhaps in the relatively near future, people with hereditary blood cell disorders (e.g., sickle cell anemia) may be treated by the use of genetically engineered stem cells. PHSCs isolated from the patient may be transfected with the normal gene (e.g., for hemoglobin) and reintroduced as an autologous transplant. These genetically engineered cells bearing the normal gene would proliferate, and their progeny would produce normal blood cells. Although the patient would still be producing some defective cells, it is hoped that enough normal cells would be produced to minimize the hereditary defect.

Hemopoietic Growth Factors (Colony-Stimulating Factors)

Hemopoiesis is regulated by a number of cytokines and growth factors, such as interleukins, colony-stimulating factors, macrophage inhibiting protein-a, and steel factor.

Hemopoiesis is regulated by numerous growth factors produced by various cell types. Each factor acts on specific stem cells, progenitor cells, and precursor cells, generally inducing rapid mitosis, differentiation, or both (Table 10-6). Some of these growth factors also promote the functioning of mature blood cells. Most hemopoietic growth factors are glycoproteins.

Three routes are used to deliver growth factors to their target cells: (1) transport via the bloodstream (as endocrine hormones), (2) secretion by stromal cells of the bone marrow near the hemopoietic cells (as paracrine hormones), and (3) direct cell-to-cell contact (as surface signaling molecules).

Certain growth factors—principally, **steel factor** (also known as **stem cell factor**), **granulocyte-macrophage colony-stimulating factor (GM-CSF)** and two **interleukins (IL-3 and IL-7)**—stimulate proliferation of pluripotential and multipotential stem cells, thus maintaining their populations. Additional cytokines, such as granulocyte colony-stimulating factor (G-CSF), monocyte colony-stimulating factor (M-CSF), IL-2, IL-5, IL-6, IL-11, IL-12, macrophage inhibitory protein-α (MIP-α), and erythropoietin, are believed to be responsible for the mobilization and differentiation of these cells into unipotential progenitor cells.

Colony-stimulating factors (CSFs) are also responsible for the stimulation of cell division and for the differentiation of unipotential cells of the granulocytic and monocytic series. **Erythropoietin** activates cells of the erythrocytic series, whereas **thrombopoietin** stimulates platelet production. **Steel factor (stem cell factor),** which, as discussed previously, acts on pluripotential, multipotential, and unipotential stem cells, is produced by stromal cells of the bone marrow and is inserted into their cell membranes. Stem cells must come in contact with these stromal cells before they can become mitotically active. It is believed that hemopoiesis cannot occur without the presence of cells that express stem cell factors, which is why postnatal blood cell formation is restricted to the bone marrow (and liver and spleen, if necessary).

Hemopoietic cells are programmed to die by undergoing **apoptosis** unless they come into contact with growth factors. Such dying cells display clumping of the chromatin in their shrunken nuclei and a dense, granular-appearing cytoplasm. On their cell surface, they express specific macromolecules that are recog-nized by receptors of the macrophage plasma membrane. These phagocytic cells engulf and destroy the apoptotic cells.

It has been suggested that there are factors responsible for the release of mature (and almost mature) blood cells from the marrow. These proposed factors have not yet been characterized completely, but they include interleukins, CSF, and steel factor.

CLINICAL CORRELATIONS

Pathologically increased secretion of erythropoietin can cause **secondary polycythemia,** an increase in the total number of red blood cells in the blood, increasing its viscosity, reducing its flow rate, and thus impeding circulation. The increased secretion is usually caused by tumors of erythropoietin-secreting cells. Patients may have an erythrocyte count of 10 million red blood cells/mm^3.

Erythropoiesis

Erythropoiesis, the formation of red blood cells, is under the control of several cytokines, namely steel factor, IL-3, IL-9, GM-CSF, and erythropoietin.

The process of erythropoiesis, red blood cell formation, generates 2.5×10^{11} erythrocytes every day. In order to produce such a tremendous number of cells, two types of unipotential progenitor cells arise from the CFU-GEMM: the **burst-forming units-erythrocyte (BFU-E)** and **colony-forming units-erythrocyte (CFU-E)**.

If the circulating red blood cell level is low, the kidney produces a high concentration of **erythropoietin,** which, in the presence of IL-3, IL-9, steel factor, and GM-CSF, induces CFU-GEMM to differentiate into BFU-E. These cells undergo a "burst" of mitotic activity, forming a large number of CFU-E. Interestingly, this transformation requires the loss of IL-3 receptors.

CFU-E require a low concentration of erythropoietin not only to survive but also to form the first recognizable erythrocyte precursor, the **proerythroblast** (Fig. 10-17; also see Fig. 10-16). The proerythroblasts and their progeny (Figs. 10-18 and 10-19) form spherical clusters around macrophages **(nurse cells)** which phagocytose extruded nuclei and excess or deformed erythrocytes. Nurse cells may also provide growth factors to assist erythropoiesis. The properties of the cells in the erythropoietic series are presented in Table 10-7.

TABLE 10–6 Hemopoietic Growth Factors

Factors	Principal Action	Site of Origin
Stem cell factor	Promotes hemopoiesis	Stromal cells of bone marrow
GM-CSF	Promotes CFU-GM mitosis and differentiation; facilitates granulocyte activity	T cells; endothelial cells
G-CSF	Promotes CFU-G mitosis and differentiation; facilitates neutrophil activity	Macrophages; endothelial cells
M-CSF	Promotes CFU-M mitosis and differentiation	Macrophages; endothelial cells
IL-1	In conjunction with IL-3 and IL-6, it promotes proliferation of PHSC, CFU-GEMM, CFU-S, and CFU-Ly; suppresses erythroid precursors	Monocytes; macrophages, endothelial cells
IL-2	Stimulates activated T- and B-cell mitosis; induces differentiation of NK cells	Activated T cells
IL-3	In conjunction with IL-1 and IL-6, it promotes proliferation of PHSC, CFU-GEMM, CFU-S, and CFU-Ly as well as all unipotential precursors (except for LyB and LyT)	Activated T and B cells
IL-4	Stimulates T- and B-cell activation and development of mast cells and basophils	Activated T cells
IL-5	Promotes CFU-Eo mitosis and activates eosinophils	T cells
IL-6	In conjunction with IL-1 and IL-3, it promotes proliferation of PHSC, CFU-GEMM, CFU-S, and CFU-Ly; also facilitates CTL and B-cell differentiation	Monocytes and fibroblasts
IL-7	Promotes differentiation of CFU-LyB; enhances differentiation of NK cells	Stromal cells, adventitial reticular cells?
IL-8	Induces neutrophil migration and degranulation	Leukocytes, endothelial cells, and smooth muscle cells
IL-9	Induces mast cell activation and proliferation; modulates IgE production; promotes T helper cell proliferation	T helper cells
IL-10	Inhibits cytokine production by macrophages, T cells, and NK cells; facilitates CTL differentiation and proliferation of B cells and mast cells	Macrophages and T cells
IL-12	Stimulates NK cells; enhances TCL and NK cell function	Macrophages
γ-Interferons	Activate B cells and monocytes; enhance CTL differentiation; augment the expression of class II HLA	T cells and NK cells
Erythropoietin	CFU-E differentiation; BFU-E mitosis	Endothelial cells of the peritubular capillary network of kidney; hepatocytes
Thrombopoietin	Proliferation and differentiation of CFU-meg and megakaryoblasts	Not known

BFU-E, burst-forming unit-erythrocyte; CTL, cytotoxic T cell; CFU, colony-forming unit (E, erthrocyte; Eo., eosinophil; G, granulocyte; GEMM, granulocyte, erythrocyte, monocyte, megakaryocyte; GM, granulocyte-monocyte; Meg, megakaryoblast; Ly, lymphocyte; LyB, B cell; LyT, T cell; S, spleen); CSF, colony-stimulating factor (G, granulocyte; GM, granulocyte-monocyte; M, monocyte); Meg, megakaryocyte; IL, interleukin; Neut., neutrophil; NK, natural killer; PHSC, pluripotent hemopoietic stem cell.

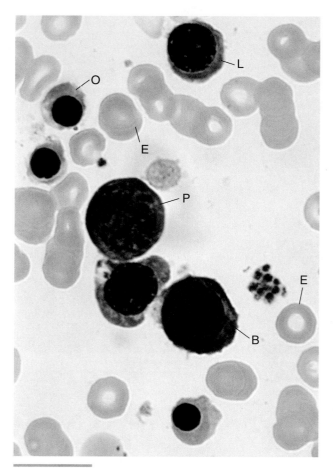

Figure 10–17 Light micrograph of bone marrow displaying all of the stages of red blood cell formation except for reticulocytes (×1325). B, basophilic erythroblast; E, erythrocyte; L, polychromatophilic erythroblast; O, orthochromatophilic erythroblast; P, proerythroblast.

CLINICAL CORRELATIONS

Iron-deficiency anemia, the most common form of anemia resulting from nutritional deficiency, affects about 10% of the U.S. population. Although the cause may be low dietary intake of iron, that is usually not the case in the United States; instead, it is caused by either malabsorption or chronic blood loss. The erythrocytes of an iron-deficient person are smaller than usual; the patient presents with a whitish pallor, and the nails appear spoon-shaped with accentuated longitudinal ridges. The patient complains of generalized weakness, constant tiredness, and lack of energy.

Granulocytopoiesis

Granulocytopoiesis, the formation of the granulocytes (neutrophils, eosinophils, and basophils), is under the influence of several cytokines, namely G-CSF and GM-CSF, as well as IL-1, IL-5, IL-6, TNF-α, and IL-5.

Although the granulocytic series usually is discussed under a single heading, as it is here, the three types of granulocytes are actually derived from their own unipotential (or bipotential, as with neutrophils) stem cells (see Table 10-5). Each of these stem cells is a descendant of the pluripotential stem cell CFU-GEMM. Thus, CFU-Eo, of the eosinophil lineage, and CFU-Ba, of the basophil lineage, each undergo cell division, giving rise to the precursor cell, or **myeloblast.** Neutrophils originate from the bipotential stem cell, **CFU-GM,** whose mitosis produces two unipotential stem cells, **CFU-G** (of the neutrophil line) and **CFU-M,** responsible for the monocyte lineage. Similar to CFU-Ba and CFU-Eo, CFU-G divides to give rise to myeloblasts.

The proliferation and differentiation of these stem cells are under the influence of G-CSF, GM-CSF, and IL-5. Therefore, these three factors facilitate the development of neutrophils, basophils, and eosinophils. In turn, IL-1, IL-6, and TNF-α are cofactors necessary for the synthesis and release of G-CSF and GM-CSF. In addition, IL-5 may also play a role in the activation of eosinophils.

Myeloblasts (Fig. 10-20; also see Fig. 10-16) are precursors of all three types of granulocytes, and they cannot be differentiated from one another. It is not known whether a single myeloblast can produce all three types of granulocytes or whether there is a specific myeloblast for each type of granulocyte. Myeloblasts undergo mitosis, giving rise to promyelocytes, which in turn divide to form myelocytes. It is at the myelocyte step that specific granules are present and the three granulocyte lines may be recognized. Each day, the average adult produces approximately 800,000 neutrophils, 170,000 eosinophils, and 60,000 basophils.

Table 10-8 details the neutrophil lineage. The eosinophil and basophil lineages appear to be identical to the neutrophil lineage except for the differences in their specific granules.

Newly formed neutrophils leave the hemopoietic cords by *piercing* the endothelial cells lining the sinusoids rather than by *migrating* between them. Once neutrophils enter the circulatory system, they **marginate;** that is, they adhere to the endothelial cells of the blood vessels and remain there until they are needed. The process of margination requires the sequential expression of various transmembrane adhesion molecules and integrins by the neutrophils as well as of specific surface receptor molecules by the endothelial cells, the description of which is beyond the scope of this textbook. Because of the process of margination, there are always many more neutrophils in the circulatory system than in the circulating blood.

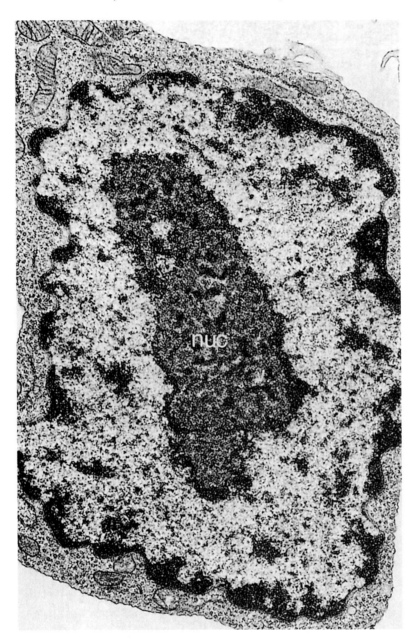

Figure 10–18 Electron micrograph of a proerythroblast, displaying its nucleolus (nuc) as well as the perinuclear cytoplasm (×14,000). Note that the nucleoplasm is relatively smooth in appearance and that the cytoplasm is rich in mitochondria and free ribosomes, indicating that the cell is active in protein synthesis. (From Hopkins CR: Structure and Function of Cells. Philadelphia, WB Saunders, 1978.)

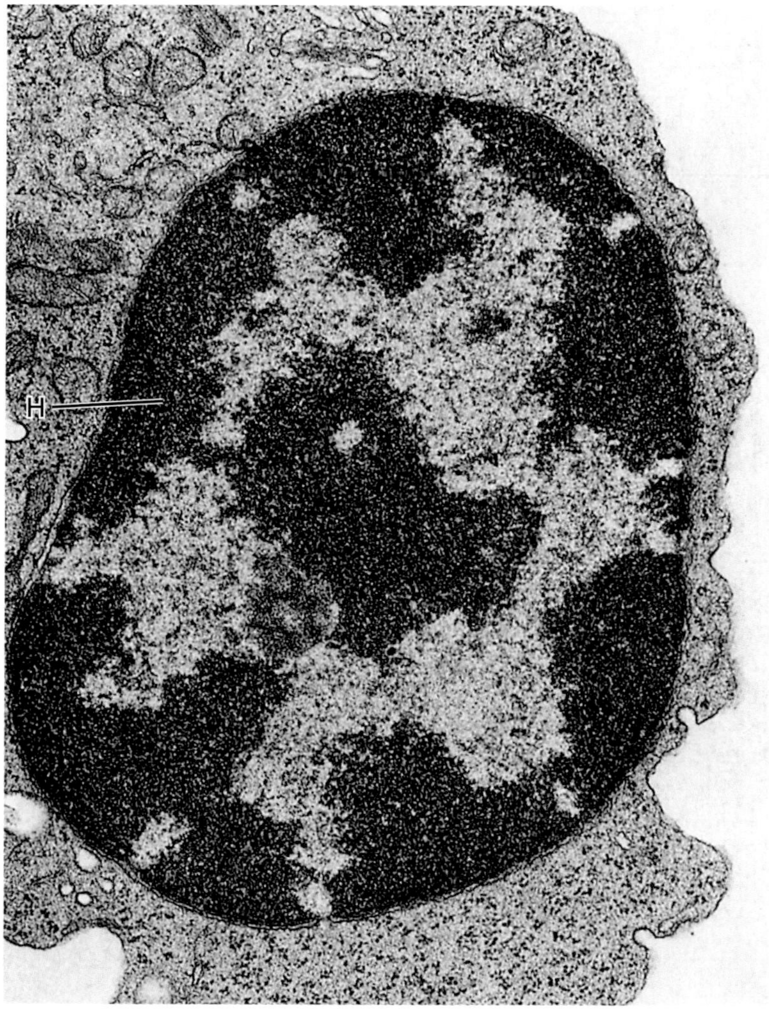

Figure 10–19 Electron micrograph of an orthochromatophilic erythroblast (×21,300). Observe that the nucleus possesses a large amount of heterochromatin (H). (From Hopkins CR: Structure and Function of Cells. Philadelphia, WB Saunders, 1978.)

TABLE 10–7 Cells of the Erythropoietic Series

Cell	Size (μm)	Nucleus* and Mitosis	Nucleoli	Cytoplasm*	Electron Micrographs
Proerythroblast	14-19	Round, burgundy-red; chromatin network: fine; mitosis	3-5	Gray-blue, peripheral clumping	Scant RER; many polysomes, few mitochondria; ferritin
Basophilic erythroblast		Same as above, but chromatin network is coarser; mitosis	1-2?	Similar to above, but slight pinkish background	Similar to above, but some hemoglobin is present
Polychromatophilic erythroblast	12-15	Round and densely staining; very coarse chromatin network; mitosis	None	Yellowish-pink in bluish background	Similar to above, but more hemoglobin is present
Orthochromatophilic erythroblast	8-12	Small, round, dense; excentric or is being extruded; no mitosis	None	Pink in a slight bluish background	Few mitochondria and polysomes; much hemoglobin
Reticulocyte	7-8	None	None	Like mature RBC, but when stained with cresyl blue; display bluish reticulum in pink cytoplasm	Clusters of ribosomes; cell is filled with hemoglobin
Erythrocyte	7.5	None	None	Pink cytoplasm	Only hemoglobin

*Colors as they appear using Romanovsky-type stains (or their modifications).
RBC, red blood cell; RER, rough endoplasmic reticulum.

CLINICAL CORRELATIONS

Acute myeloblastic leukemia results from uncontrolled mitosis of a transformed stem cell whose progeny do not differentiate into mature cells. The cells involved may be the CFU-GM, CFU-Eo, or CFU-Ba, whose differentiation stops at the myeloblast stage. The disease affects young adults between 15 and 40 years of age and is treated by intensive chemotherapy and, more recently, by bone marrow transplantation.

Monocytopoiesis

Monocytes share their bipotential cells with neutrophils. CFU-GM undergoes mitosis and gives rise to CFU-G and **CFU-M (monoblasts).** The progeny of CFU-M are **promonocytes,** large cells (16 to 18 μm in diameter) that have a kidney-shaped, acentrically located nucleus. The cytoplasm of promonocytes is bluish and houses numerous azurophilic granules.

Electron micrographs of promonocytes disclose a well-developed Golgi apparatus, abundant RER, and numerous mitochondria. The azurophilic granules are lysosomes, about 0.5 μm in diameter. Every day, the average adult forms more than 10^{10} monocytes, most of which enter the circulation. Within a day or two, the newly formed monocytes enter the connective tissue spaces of the body and differentiate into **macrophages.**

Platelet Formation

The formation of platelets is under the control of thrombopoietin, which induces the development and proliferation of giant cells known as megakaryoblasts.

The unipotential platelet progenitor, **CFU-Meg,** gives rise to a very large cell, the **megakaryoblast** (25 to 40 μm in diameter), whose single nucleus has several

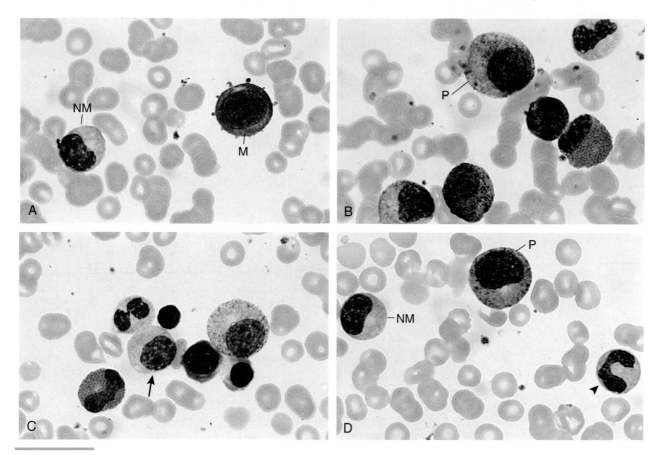

Figure 10–20 Light micrographs of granulocytopoiesis displaying the various intermediary cell types (×1234). **A,** Myeloblast (M) and neutrophilic metamyelocyte (NM). **B,** Promyelocyte (P). **C,** Neutrophilic myelocyte (*arrow*). **D,** Neutrophilic metamyelocyte (NM), promyelocyte (P), and neutrophilic stab cell (*arrowhead*).

lobes. These cells undergo **endomitosis,** whereby the cell does not divide; instead, it becomes larger and the nucleus becomes polyploid, as much as 64 N. The bluish cytoplasm accumulates azurophilic granules. These cells are stimulated to differentiate and proliferate by thrombopoietin.

Megakaryoblasts differentiate into **megakaryocytes** (see Fig. 10-14), which are large cells (40 to 100 μm in diameter), each with a single lobulated nucleus. Electron micrographs of megakaryocytes display a well-developed Golgi apparatus, numerous mitochondria, abundant RER, and many lysosomes (Fig. 10-21).

Megakaryocytes are located next to sinusoids, into which they protrude their cytoplasmic processes. These cytoplasmic processes fragment along complex, narrow invaginations of the plasmalemma, known as **demarcation channels,** into clusters of **proplatelets.** Shortly after the proplatelets are released, they disperse into individual platelets. Each megakaryocyte can form several thousand platelets. The remaining cytoplasm and nucleus of the megakaryocyte degenerate and are phagocytosed by macrophages.

Lymphopoiesis

Pluripotential hemopoietic stem cells give rise to the myeloid series of cells via CFU-GEMM cells as well as to the lymphoid series of cells via CFU-Ly cells.

The multipotential stem cell **CFU-Ly** divides in the bone marrow to form the two unipotential progenitor cells, CFU-LyB and CFU-LyT, neither of which is immunocompetent.

In birds, the **CFU-LyB** cell migrates to a diverticulum attached to the gut, known as the **bursa of Fabricius** (thus B cell). Here the CFU-LyB cell divides several times, giving rise to **immunocompetent** B lymphocytes expressing specific surface markers, including antibodies. A similar event occurs in mammals, but in the absence of a bursa this development of immunocompetence occurs in a bursa-equivalent location in the bone marrow.

CFU-LyT cells undergo mitosis, forming immunoincompetent T cells, which travel to the cortex of the thymus, where they proliferate, mature, and begin to

TABLE 10–8 Cells of the Neutrophilic Series

Cell	Size (μm)	Nucleus* and Mitosis	Nucleoli	Cytoplasm*	Granules	Electron Micrographs
Myeloblast	12-14	Round, reddish-blue; chromatin network: fine; mitosis	2-3	Blue clumps in a pale blue background; cytoplasmic blebs at cell periphery	None	RER, small Golgi, many mitochondria and polysomes
Promyelocyte	16-24	Round to oval, reddish blue; chromatin network: coarse; mitosis	1-2	Bluish cytoplasm; no cytoplasmic blebs at cell periphery	Azurophilic granules	RER, large Golgi, many mitochondria, numerous lysosomes (0.5 μm in diameter)
Neutrophilic myelocyte	10-12	Flattened, acentric; chromatin network: coarse; mitosis	0-1	Pale blue cytoplasm	Azurophilic and specific granules	RER, large Golgi, numerous mitochondria, lysosomes (0.5 μm) and specific granules (0.1 μm)
Neutrophilic metamyelocyte	10-12	Kidney-shaped, dense; chromatin network: coarse; no mitosis	None	Pale blue cytoplasm	Azurophilic and specific granules	Organelle population is reduced, but granules are as above
Neutrophilic band (stab; juvenile)	9-12	Horseshoe-shaped; chromatin network: very coarse; no mitosis	None	Pale blue cytoplasm	Azurophilic and specific granules	Same as above
Neutrophil	9-12	Multilobed; chromatin network: very coarse; no mitosis	None	Pale bluish-pink	Azurophilic and specific granules	Same as above

*Colors as appear using Romanovsky-type stains (or their modifications).
RER, rough endoplasmic reticulum.

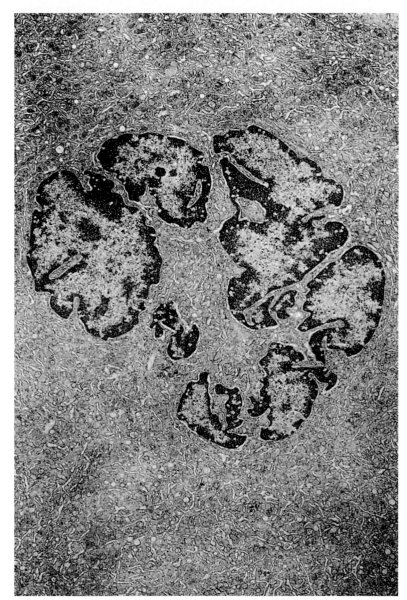

Figure 10–21 Electron micrograph of a mega-karyocyte displaying segmentation in the formation of platelets (×3166). Although this cell possesses a single nucleus, it is lobulated, which gives the appearance that the cell possesses several nuclei. (From Hopkins CR: Structure and Function of Cells. Philadelphia, WB Saunders, 1978.)

express cell surface markers. As these surface markers appear on the T-cell plasmalemma (such as T-cell receptors and clusters of differentiation markers), the cells become immunocompetent T lymphocytes. Most of these newly formed T cells are destroyed in the thymus and are phagocytosed by resident macrophages.

Both B lymphocytes and T lymphocytes proceed to lymphoid organs (such as the spleen and lymph nodes), where they form clones of immunocompetent T and B cells in well-defined regions of the organs. The lymphocytic series is discussed in more detail in Chapter 12.

11

Circulatory System

The circulatory system is composed of two separate but related components: the cardiovascular system and the lymphatic vascular system. The function of the **cardiovascular system** is to carry blood in both directions between the heart and the tissues. The function of the **lymphatic vascular system** is to collect **lymph,** the excess extracellular tissue fluid, and to deliver it back to the cardiovascular system. Thus, the lymphatic system provides one-way transport, whereas the cardiovascular system provides two-way circulation.

CARDIOVASCULAR SYSTEM

The cardiovascular system is composed of two circuits: the pulmonary circuit to the lungs and the systemic circuit to the tissues of the body.

The cardiovascular system comprises the **heart,** a muscular organ that pumps the blood into two separated circuits: the **pulmonary circuit,** which carries blood to and from the lungs, and the **systemic circuit,** which distributes blood to and from all of the organs and tissues of the body. These circuits consist of:

- **Arteries**—a series of vessels that transport blood away from the heart by branching into vessels of smaller and smaller diameter, eventually branching into capillaries to supply all regions of the body with blood
- **Capillaries**—thin-walled vessels with the smallest diameter, form capillary beds, where gases, nutrients, metabolic wastes, hormones, and signaling substances are interchanged or passed between the blood and the tissues of the body to sustain normal metabolic activities
- **Veins**—vessels that drain capillary beds and form larger and larger vessels returning blood to the heart

General Structure of Blood Vessels

Arteries generally have thicker walls and are smaller in diameter than their venous counterparts.

Most blood vessels have several features that are structurally similar, although dissimilarities exist and are the bases for classifying the vessels into different identifiable groups. For example, the walls of high-pressure vessels (e.g., subclavian arteries) are thicker than vessels conducting blood at low pressure (e.g., subclavian veins). However, arterial diameters continue to decrease at each branching, whereas vein diameters increase at each convergence, thus altering the respective layers of the walls of the vessels. Therefore, the descriptions used as distinguishing characteristics for a particular type of artery or vein are not always absolute. Indeed, the walls of the capillaries and venules are completely modified and less complex compared with those of larger vessels. Generally, arteries have thicker walls and are smaller in diameter than are the corresponding veins. Moreover, in histological sections, arteries are round and usually have no blood in their lumina.

Vessel Tunics

Walls of blood vessels are composed of three layers: the tunica intima, the tunica media, and the tunica adventitia.

Three separate concentric layers of tissue, or tunics, make up the wall of the typical blood vessel (Fig. 11-1). The innermost layer, the **tunica intima,** is composed of a single layer of flattened, squamous endothelial cells, which form a tube lining the lumen of the vessel, and the underlying subendothelial connective tissue. The intermediate layer, the **tunica media,** is composed mostly of smooth muscle cells oriented concentrically around the lumen. The outermost layer, the **tunica**

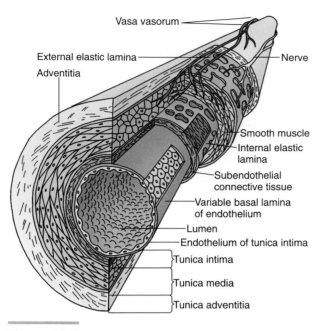

Figure 11–1 A typical artery.

adventitia, is composed mainly of fibroelastic connective tissue arranged longitudinally.

The tunica intima houses in its outermost layer the **internal elastic lamina,** a thin band of elastic fibers that is well developed in medium-sized arteries. The outermost layer of the tunica media houses another band of elastic fibers, the **external elastic lamina,** although it is not distinguishable in all arteries. The deeper cells of the tunica media and tunica adventitia are nourished by the **vasa vasorum.**

Tunica Intima

The tunica intima is composed of a simple squamous epithelium and the subendothelial connective tissue.

The endothelial cells (simple squamous epithelium) lining the lumen of the blood vessel rest on a basal lamina. These flattened cells are elongated into a sheet such that their long axis is more or less parallel to the long axis of the vessel, which permits each endothelial cell to nearly surround the lumen of a small-caliber vessel. In larger-bore vessels, several to many individual endothelial cells are required to line the circumference of the lumen. Endothelial cells not only provide an exceptionally smooth surface but also function in secreting types II, IV, and V collagens, lamin, endothelin, nitric oxide, and von Willebrand factor. Moreover, they possess membrane-bound enzymes, such as **angiotensin-converting enzyme (ACE),** which cleaves **angiotensin I** to generate **angiotensin II** (see

Regulation of Arterial Blood Pressure later), as well as enzymes that inactivate bradykinin, serotonin, prostaglandins, thrombin, and norepinephrine; moreover, they also bind lipoprotein lipase, the enzyme that degrades lipoproteins.

A **subendothelial layer** lies immediately beneath the endothelial cells. It is composed of loose connective tissue and a few scattered smooth muscle cells, both arranged longitudinally. Beneath the subendothelial layer is an **internal elastic lamina** that is especially well developed in muscular arteries. Separating the tunica intima from the tunica media, the internal elastic lamina is composed of **elastin,** which is a fenestrated sheet that permits the diffusion of substances into the deeper regions of the arterial wall to nourish the cells there.

Tunica Media

The tunica media, usually the thickest layer of the vessel wall, is composed of helically disposed layers of smooth muscle.

The tunica media is the thickest layer of the blood vessel. The **concentric cell layers** forming the tunica media comprise mostly helically arranged smooth muscle cells. Interspersed within the layers of smooth muscle are some elastic fibers, type III collagen, and proteoglycans. The fibrous elements form lamellae within the ground substance secreted by smooth muscle cells. Larger muscular arteries have an **external elastic lamina,** which is more delicate than the internal elastic lamina and separates the tunica media from the overlying tunica adventitia. Capillaries and postcapillary venules do not have a tunica media; in these small vessels, **pericytes** replace the tunica media (see Capillaries section).

Tunica Adventitia

The tunica adventitia, the outermost layer of the blood vessel wall, blends into the surrounding connective tissue.

Covering the vessels on their outside surface is the **tunica adventitia,** composed mostly of fibroblasts, type I collagen fibers, and longitudinally oriented elastic fibers. This layer becomes continuous with the connective tissue elements surrounding the vessel.

Vasa Vasorum

Vasa vasorum furnish the muscular walls of the larger blood vessels with a blood supply.

The thickness and muscularity of larger vessels—the tunica media and tunica adventitia—prevent the cells composing the tunics from being nourished by diffusion from the lumen of the vessel. These cells are nourished by the **vasa vasorum,** small arteries that enter the vessel walls and branch profusely to serve the cells located primarily in the tunica media and tunica adventitia. Compared with arteries, veins have more cells that cannot be supplied with oxygen and nutrients by diffusion, because venous blood contains less oxygen and nutrients than arterial blood. For this reason, the vasa vasorum are more prevalent in the walls of veins than arteries.

Nerve Supply to Blood Vessels

Sympathetic nerves supply vasomotor innervation to the smooth muscles of the tunica media.

A network of **vasomotor nerves** of the sympathetic component of the autonomic nervous system supplies smooth muscle cells of blood vessels. These unmyelinated, postganglionic sympathetic nerves are responsible for **vasoconstriction** of the vessel walls. Because the nerves seldom enter the tunica media of the vessel, they do not synapse directly on the smooth muscle cells. Instead, they release the neurotransmitter **norepinephrine,** which diffuses into the media and acts on smooth muscle cells nearby. These impulses are propagated throughout all of the smooth muscle cells via their gap junctions, thereby orchestrating contractions of the entire smooth muscle cell layer and thus reducing the diameter of the vessel lumen.

Arteries are more heavily endowed with vasomotor nerves than are veins, but veins also receive vasomotor nerve endings in the tunica adventitia. The arteries supplying skeletal muscles also receive cholinergic (parasympathetic) nerves to bring about vasodilation.

Arteries

Arteries are blood vessels that carry blood away from the heart.

Arteries are efferent vessels that transport blood away from the heart to the capillary beds. The two major arteries that arise from the right and left ventricles of the heart are the pulmonary trunk and the aorta, respectively.

The **pulmonary trunk** branches, shortly after exiting the heart, into right and left pulmonary arteries that enter the lungs for distribution. (Chapter 15 describes the branching and blood supply to the lungs.) The right and left coronary arteries, which supply the heart muscle, arise from the aorta as it exits the left ventricle.

The **aorta,** upon leaving the heart, courses in an obliquely posterior arch to descend in the thoracic cavity, where it sends branches to the body wall and the viscera; it then enters the abdominal cavity, where it sends branches to the body wall and viscera. The abdominal aorta terminates by bifurcating into the right and left common iliac arteries in the pelvis.

Three major arterial trunks—the right brachiocephalic artery, the left common carotid artery, and the left subclavian artery—arise from the arch of the aorta to supply the superior extremities and the head and neck. It is interesting to note that the right common carotid artery arises from the right brachiocephalic trunk, whereas the left common carotid artery arises directly from the aortic arch. Branching of all of these arteries into large numbers of smaller and smaller arteries continues until the vessel walls contain a single layer of endothelial cells. The resulting vessels, called **capillaries,** are the smallest functional vascular elements of the cardiovascular system.

Classification of Arteries

Arteries are of three types: elastic arteries (conducting arteries), muscular arteries (distributing arteries), and arterioles.

Arteries are classified into three major types based on their relative size, morphological characteristics, or both (Table 11-1). From largest to smallest, they are as follows:

- Elastic (conducting) arteries
- Muscular (distributing) arteries
- Arterioles

Because the vessels decrease in diameter in a continuous fashion, there are gradual changes in morphological characteristics as they morph from one type to another. Therefore, some vessels having characteristics of two categories cannot be assigned to a specific category with certainty.

Elastic Arteries

Concentric layers of elastic membranes, known as fenestrated membranes, occupy much of the tunica media.

The aorta and the branches originating from the aortic arch (the common carotid artery and the subclavian artery), the common iliac arteries, and the pulmonary trunk are elastic **(conducting)** arteries (Fig. 11-2). The walls of these vessels may be yellow in the fresh state because of the abundance of elastin.

The **tunica intima** of the elastic arteries is composed of an endothelium that is supported by a narrow layer of underlying connective tissue containing a few fibroblasts, occasional smooth muscle cells, and collagen fibers. Thin laminae of elastic fibers, the **internal elastic laminae,** are also present.

TABLE 11–1 Characteristics of Various Types of Arteries

Artery	Tunica Intima	Tunica Media	Tunica Adventitia
Elastic artery (*conducting*) (e.g., aorta)	Endothelium with Weibel-Palade bodies, basal lamina, subendothelial layer, incomplete internal elastic lamina	40 to 70 fenestrated elastic membranes; smooth muscle cells interspersed between elastic membranes; thin external elastic lamina; vasa vasorum in outer half	Thin layer of fibroelastic connective tissue, vasa vasorum, lymphatic vessels, nerve fibers
Muscular artery (*distributing*) (e.g., femoral artery)	Endothelium with Weibel-Palade bodies, basal lamina, subendothelial layer, thick internal elastic lamina	Up to 40 layers of smooth muscle cells; thick external elastic lamina	Thin layer of fibroelastic connective tissue; vasa vasorum not very prominent; lymphatic vessels, nerve fibers
Arteriole	Endothelium with Weibel-Palade bodies; basal lamina, subendothelial layer not very prominent; some elastic fibers instead of a defined internal elastic lamina	One or two layers of smooth muscle cells	Loose connective tissue, nerve fibers
Metarteriole	Endothelium, basal lamina	Smooth muscle cells form precapillary sphincter	Sparse, loose connective tissue

The endothelial cells of the elastic arteries are 10 to 15 μm wide and 25 to 50 μm long; their long axes are oriented parallel to the longitudinal axis of the vessel. These cells are connected to each other mostly by occluding junctions. Their plasma membranes contain small vesicles thought to be related to transport of water, macromolecules, and electrolytes. Occasional blunt processes may extend from the plasma membrane through the internal elastic lamina to form gap junctions with smooth muscle cells located in the tunica media. The endothelial cells contain **Weibel-Palade bodies,** membrane-bound inclusions 0.1 μm in diameter and 3 μm long, that have a dense matrix housing tubular elements containing the glycoprotein **von Willebrand factor.** This factor, which facilitates the coagulation of platelets during clot formation, is manufactured by most endothelial cells but is stored only in arteries.

CLINICAL CORRELATIONS

Patients with **von Willebrand disease,** an inherited disorder that results in impaired adhesion of platelets, have prolonged coagulation times and excessive bleeding at an injury site.

The **tunica media** of the elastic arteries consists of many fenestrated lamellae of elastin, known as **fenestrated membranes,** alternating with circularly oriented layers of smooth muscle cells. The number of lamellae of elastin increases with age; there are approximately 40 in newborns and 70 in adults. These fenestrated membranes also increase in thickness because of the continued deposition of elastin, which constitutes much of the tunica media; smooth muscles cells are less abundant in elastic arteries than in some of the muscular arteries. The extracellular matrix, secreted by the smooth muscle cells, is composed mostly of chondroitin sulfate, collagen, and reticular and elastin fibers. An **external elastic lamina** is also present in the tunica media.

The **tunica adventitia** of elastic arteries is relatively thin and is composed of loose fibroelastic connective tissue housing some fibroblasts. Vasa vasorum also are abundant throughout the adventitia. Capillary beds arise from the vasa vasorum and extend to the tissues of the tunica media, where they supply the connective tissue and smooth muscle cells with oxygen and nutrients. Fenestrations in the elastic laminae permit some diffusion of oxygen and nutrients to the cells in the tunica media from the blood flowing through the lumen, although most of the nourishment is derived from branches of the vasa vasorum.

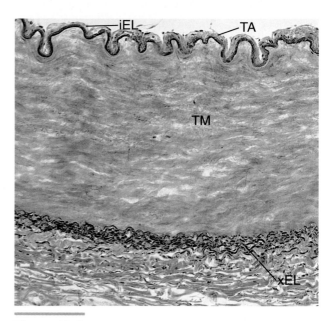

Figure 11–3 Light micrograph of a muscular artery (×132). Note the tunica adventitia (TA) and the internal (iEL) and external (xEL) elastic laminae within the thick tunica media (TM).

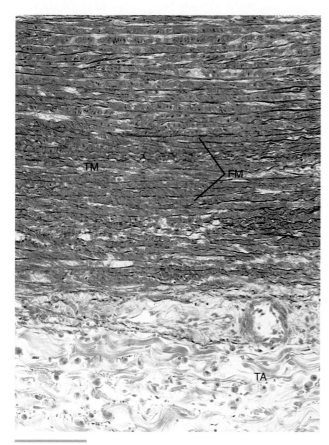

Figure 11–2 Light micrograph of an elastic artery (×132). Observe the fenestrated membranes (FM), tunica media (TM), and tunica adventitia (TA).

Muscular Arteries

Muscular arteries are characterized by a thick tunica media that is composed mostly of smooth muscle cells.

Muscular **(distributing)** arteries include most vessels arising from the aorta, except for the major trunks orginating from the arch of the aorta and the terminal bifurcation of the abdominal aorta, which are identified as elastic arteries. Indeed, most of the named arteries, even those with a diameter of only 0.1 mm, are classified as muscular arteries (e.g., brachial, ulnar, renal). The identifying characteristic of muscular arteries is a relatively thick tunica media composed mostly of smooth muscle cells (Fig. 11-3).

The **tunica intima** in the muscular arteries is thinner than that in the elastic arteries, but the subendothelial layer contains a few smooth muscle cells; also, in contrast with that of elastic arteries, the **internal elastic lamina** of the muscular arteries is prominent and displays an undulating surface to which the endothelium conforms. Occasionally the internal elastic lamina is duplicated; this is called **bifid internal elastic lamina.** As in elastic arteries, the endothelium has processes that pass through fenestrations within the internal elastic lamina and make gap junctions with smooth muscle cells of the tunica media that are near the interface with the tunica intima. It is believed that these gap junctions may couple metabolically the endothelium and the smooth muscle cells.

The **tunica media** of the muscular arteries is composed predominantly of smooth muscle cells, although these cells are considerably smaller than those located in the walls of the viscera. The orientation of most of the smooth muscle cells is circular where the tunica media interfaces with the tunica intima; however, a few bundles of smooth muscle fibers are arranged longitudinally in the tunica adventitia. Small muscular arteries have three or four layers of smooth muscle cells, whereas larger muscular arteries may have as many as 40 layers of circularly arranged smooth muscle cells. The number of cell layers decreases as the diameter of the artery diminishes.

Each smooth muscle cell is enveloped by an **external lamina** (similar to a **basal lamina**), although muscle cell processes extend through intervals in the basal lamina to form gap junctions with other muscle cells, ensuring coordinated contractions within the tunica media. Interspersed within the layers of smooth muscle cells are elastic fibers, type III collagen fibers, and chondroitin sulfate, all secreted by the smooth muscle cells. Type III collagen fibers (30 nm in diameter) are located in bundles within the intercellular spaces.

An **external elastic lamina** is identifiable in histological sections of larger muscular arteries as several layers of thin elastic sheets; in electron micrographs, these sheets display fenestrations.

The **tunica adventitia** of the muscular arteries consists of elastic fibers, collagen fibers (60 to 100 nm in diameter), and ground substance composed mostly of dermatan sulfate and heparan sulfate. This extracellular matrix is produced by fibroblasts in the adventitia. The collagen and elastic fibers are oriented longitudinally and blend into the surrounding connective tissues. Located at the outer regions of the adventitia are vasa vasorum and unmyelinated nerve endings. Neurotransmitters released at the nerve endings diffuse through fenestrations in the external elastic lamina into the tunica media to depolarize some of the superficial smooth muscle cells. Depolarization is propagated to all of the muscle cells of the tunica media via gap junctions.

CLINICAL CORRELATIONS

Aneurysm, a sac-like dilation of the wall of an artery (or less often of a vein), results from weakness in the vessel wall and is usually age related. The aneurysm occurs in regions of the vessel wall where, frequently as a result of atherosclerosis, Marfan syndrome, syphilis, and Ehlers-Danlos syndrome, elastic fibers are displaced by collagen fibers. The abdominal aorta is the most common vessel with this type of aneurysm. When discovered, the ballooned area can be repaired but if it is not discovered and it ruptures, there is rapid massive blood loss that may result in death of the individual.

Arterioles

Arteries with a diameter of less than 0.1 mm are considered to be arterioles.

Arterioles are the terminal arterial vessels that regulate blood flow into the capillary beds. In histological sections, the width of the wall of an arteriole is approximately equal to the diameter of its lumen (Fig. 11-4). The endothelium of the **tunica intima** is supported by a thin subendothelial connective tissue layer consisting of type III collagen and a few elastic fibers embedded in ground substance. A thin, fenestrated **internal elastic lamina** is absent in small and terminal arteri-

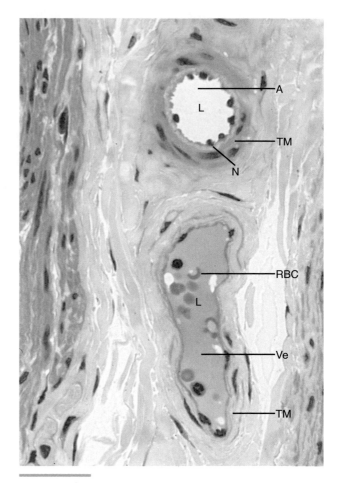

Figure 11–4 Light micrograph of an arteriole and a venule containing blood cells (×540). The arteriole (A) is well defined with a thick tunica media (TM). Nuclei of endothelial cells (N) bulge into the lumen (L). The venule (Ve) is poorly defined with a large poorly defined lumen containing red blood cells (RBC). The tunica media of the venule is not as robust as that in the arteriole.

oles but present in larger arterioles (Fig. 11-5). In small arterioles, the **tunica media** is composed of a single smooth muscle cell layer that completely encircles the endothelial cells (Fig. 11-6). In larger arterioles, the tunica media consists of two to three layers of smooth muscle cells. Arterioles do not have an external elastic lamina. The **tunica adventitia** of arterioles is scant and is represented by fibroelastic connective tissue housing a few fibroblasts.

Arteries that supply blood to capillary beds are called **metarterioles.** They differ structurally from arterioles in that the smooth muscle layer is not continuous; rather, the individual muscle cells are spaced apart, and each encircles the endothelium of a capillary arising from the metarteriole. It is believed that this arrangement permits these smooth muscle cells to function as

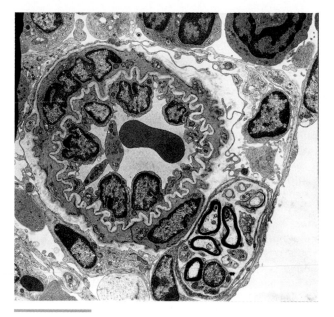

Figure 11–5 Electron micrograph of an arteriole. (From Yamazaki K, Allen TD: Ultrastructural morphometric study of efferent nerve terminals on murine bone marrow stromal cells, and the recognition of a novel anatomical unit: The "neuro-reticular complex." Am J Anat 187:261-276, 1990.)

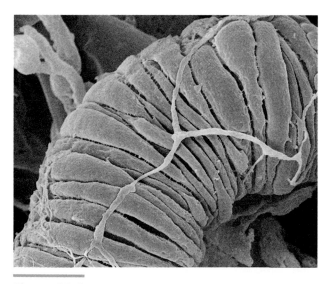

Figure 11–6 Scanning electron micrograph of an arteriole illustrating its compact layer of smooth muscle and its attendant nerve fibers (×4200). (From Fujiwara T, Uehara Y: The cytoarchitecture of the wall and innervation pattern of the microvessels in the rat mammary gland: A scanning electron microscopic observation. Am J Anat 170:39-54, 1984.)

a sphincter upon contraction, thus controlling blood flow into the capillary bed.

CLINICAL CORRELATIONS

Vessel walls that are weakened from embryological defects or damaged from diseases such as atherosclerosis, syphilis, and connective tissue disorders (e.g., **Marfan syndrome** and **Ehler-Danlos syndrome**) may balloon out at the affected site, forming an **aneurysm.** Further weakening may cause the aneurysm to rupture, a grave condition that may lead to death.

Specialized Sensory Structures in Arteries

Specialized sensory structures in the arteries include the carotid sinus, the carotid body, and aortic bodies.

Three types of specialized sensory structures are located in the major arteries of the body: **carotid sinuses, carotid bodies,** and **aortic bodies.** Nerve endings in these structures monitor blood pressure and blood composition, providing essential inputs to the brain for controlling heartbeat, respiration, and blood pressure.

Carotid Sinus

The carotid sinus is a baroreceptor located in the region of the internal carotid artery just distal to the bifurcation of the common carotid artery.

The carotid sinus is a baroreceptor; that is, it perceives changes in blood pressure. This structure is a specialization within the wall of the internal carotid artery just above the bifurcation of the common carotid artery. At this site, the adventitia of this vessel is relatively thicker and heavily endowed with sensory nerve endings from the glossopharyngeal nerve (cranial nerve IX). The tunica media at this site is relatively thinner, thus permitting it to be distended during increases in blood pressure; this distention stimulates the nerve endings. The afferent impulses, received at the vasomotor center in the brain, trigger adjustments in vasoconstriction, resulting in maintenance of proper blood pressure. Additional small baroreceptors are located in the aorta and in some of the larger vessels.

Carotid Body

The carotid body functions as a chemoreceptor, monitoring changes in oxygen and carbon dioxide levels as well as hydrogen ion concentration

Located at the bifurcation of the common carotid artery is a small, oval structure known as the carotid body. The carotid body possesses specialized chemoreceptor nerve endings responsible for monitoring changes in oxygen and carbon dioxide levels as well as blood H⁺ concentration. The carotid body, 3 to 5 mm in diameter, is composed of multiple clusters of pale-staining cells embedded in connective tissue. Two types of parenchymal cells are clearly distinguishable in electron micrographs: **glomus (type I) cells** and **sheath (type II) cells.**

Glomus cells have a large nucleus and the usual array of organelles. They are distinguished by the presence of dense-cored vesicles, 60 to 200 nm in diameter, that resemble vesicles located in the chromaffin cells of the suprarenal medulla. Cell processes also contain longitudinally oriented microtubules, dense-cored vesicles, and a few small electron-lucent vesicles. These processes contact other glomus cells and capillary endothelial cells.

Sheath cells are more complex and have long processes that almost completely ensheath the processes of the glomus cells. The nuclei of these cells are irregular and contain more heterochromatin compared with the nuclei of glomus cells; moreover, sheath cells contain no dense-cored vesicles. As nerve terminals enter clusters of glomus cells, they lose their Schwann cells and become covered by the sheath cells in much the same way as glial cells ensheath fibers in the central nervous system.

Carotid bodies contain catecholamines (as do the cells of the suprarenal medulla and paraganglia), but whether they produce hormones is unclear. The glossopharyngeal and vagus nerves supply the carotid body with numerous afferent fibers. In some of the synapses, the glomus cells appear to function as presynaptic cell bodies, but the specific relationships are as yet not understood.

Aortic Bodies

Aortic bodies are located on the arch of the aorta between the right subclavian and the right common carotid artery and between the left common carotid artery and the left subclavian artery. Their structure and function are similar to those of carotid bodies.

Regulation of Arterial Blood Pressure

Arterial blood pressure is regulated by the vasomotor center in the brain.

The heart, which serves as the cardiovascular pump, rests between each stroke, thus developing a pressur-

ized burst of blood that first enters into the elastic arteries, then moves into the muscular arteries and arterioles, and finally moves into capillaries, which serve the tissues. The **vasomotor center** in the brain responds to the continual monitoring of blood pressure by controlling **vasomotor tone,** the constant state of contraction of the vessel walls, which is modulated via vasoconstriction and vasodilation. **Vasoconstriction** is accomplished via **vasomotor nerves** of the sympathetic nervous system, whereas **vasodilation** is a function of the parasympathetic system. During vasodilation, acetylcholine from the nerve terminals in the vessel walls initiates release of **nitric oxide (NO)** from the endothelium to diffuse into the smooth muscle cells, which activates the cyclic guanosine monophosphate (cGMP) system, resulting in relaxation of the muscle cells, thus dilating the vessel lumen.

Smooth muscle cells of the arteries have receptors for substances besides the neurotransmitter norepinephrine. When the blood pressure is low, the kidneys secrete the enzyme **renin,** which cleaves **angiotensinogen** circulating in the blood, forming **angiotensin I.** This mild vasoconstrictor is converted to **angiotensin II** by ACE, which is located on the luminal plasmalemmae of capillary endothelia (especially capillaries of the lungs). Angiotensin II is a potent vasoconstrictor that initiates smooth muscle contraction, thereby reducing vessel lumen diameter, resulting in increased blood pressure. Severe hemorrhage induces pituitary secretion of **antidiuretic hormone (ADH),** or **vasopressin,** another powerful vasoconstrictor.

The structure of elastic arteries permits distention of their walls during **systole** (heart contraction), followed by recoil of their walls during **diastole** (heart relaxation), which assists in delivering a more constant blood pressure and flow of blood. Muscular arteries branching from the elastic arteries distribute blood to the body and are subject to constant changes in diameter resulting from vasoconstriction and vasodilation. To assist in accommodating for these events, the tunica adventitia blends loosely into the surrounding connective tissue, thus preventing restraint on the vessel during contractions and expansions for changes in blood pressure.

Artery location also dictates the thickness of the various tunics. For example, the thickness of the tunica media in the arteries of the leg is greater than that found in the arteries of the upper extremity. This is in response to the continued pressure resulting from gravitational forces. Moreover, the coronary arteries, serving the heart, are high-pressure arteries and, as such, have a thick tunica media. Conversely, arteries in the pulmonary circulation are under low pressure; thus, the tunica media in these vessels is thinner.

CLINICAL CORRELATIONS

Normal and Pathological Vascular Changes

The largest arteries continue to grow until about age 25 years, although there is progressive thickening of their walls and an increase in the number of elastic laminae. In the muscular arteries, from middle age on, deposits of collagen and proteoglycans increase in the walls, thus reducing their flexibility. The coronary vessels are the first to display the effects of aging, with the intima displaying the greatest age-related changes. These natural changes are not unlike the regressive changes observed in arteriosclerosis (hardening of the arteries).

Arteriosclerosis

Small arteries and arterioles, especially those of the kidneys, are prone to the most common type of arteriosclerosis, displaying a hyaline or concentric thickening which is often associated with hypertension and/or diabetes.

Atherosclerosis

The largest of the arteries—including the coronary arteries, carotid arteries, and the major arteries of the brain among others—are susceptible to atherosclerosis, a disease that is the forerunner of heart attack and stroke. Atherosclerosis is distinguished by infiltrations of soft, noncellular lipid material into the intima walls; these infiltrations can reduce the luminal diameter appreciably even by age 25. It is not clear whether these conditions are physiological or a manifestation of a disease process. The fibrous plaques that form in the intima of older persons, however, are pathological.

The smooth muscle cell layer in the tunica media of a healthy person undergoes renewal, but when the endothelium is injured, platelets that accumulate at the site release **platelet-derived growth factor (PDGF)**, stimulating proliferation of smooth muscle cells. As a consequence, these cells begin to be packed with cholesterol-rich lipids, which stimulate the muscle cells to manufacture additional collagen and proteoglycans, resulting in a cycle whereby the tunica intima becomes thickened. This further damage to the endothelium leads to necrosis, which attracts more platelets, and finally clotting, forming a thrombus that may occlude the vessel at that site or get into the general circulation and occlude a more dangerous vessel (e.g., a coronary vessel or a cerebral vessel).

The pathogenesis of cardiovascular heart diseases is still unclear, although current research theories point to the role of cholesterol, lipoproteins, and certain mitogens. A correlation between blood cholesterol levels and heart disease is established, but recently learned is that **C-reactive protein (CRP)**, synthesized by the liver, can be used as a marker for inflammation. Furthermore, CRP appears to be a far more accurate indicator of the risk for cardiovascular disease. Statins, which have been used extensively for reducing cholesterol levels in the blood and thereby reducing the risk of heart disease, have been shown to reduce CRP levels also. This fact is important because the response to inflammation is as critical in heart disease as are high levels of cholesterol. Thus there is a commonality between inflammation and cardiovascular disease.

Capillaries

Arising from the terminal ends of the arterioles are capillaries (Fig. 11-7), which form, by branching and anastomosing, a capillary bed (network) between the arterioles and the venules. Electron micrographs have revealed three types of capillaries: (1) **continuous** (Fig. 11-8), (2) **fenestrated,** and (3) **sinusoidal** (also see Fig. 11-12). The differences among them are discussed later.

General Structure of Capillaries

Capillaries, composed of a single layer of endothelial cells, are the smallest blood vessels.

Capillaries are the smallest of the vascular channels, on the average approximately 50 μm in length with a diameter of 8 to 10 μm. Capillaries are formed by a single layer of squamous endothelial cells rolled into a tube, with the long axis of these cells lying in the same direction as the blood flow. These endothelial cells are flattened, with the attenuated ends tapering to a thickness to 0.2 μm or less, although an elliptical nucleus bulges out into the lumen of the capillary. The cytoplasm contains a Golgi complex, a few mitochondria, some rough endoplasmic reticulum (RER), and free ribosomes (Fig. 11-9; also see Fig. 11-8). Intermediate filaments (9 to 11 nm in diameter), located around the perinuclear zone, vary in filament composition. For example, some cells contain filaments composed of **desmin,** others contain filaments composed of **vimentin,** and some endothelial cells contain both kinds of filaments. These filaments provide structural support to the endothelial cells, but the significance of their variation is unclear.

The large number of pinocytotic vesicles associated with the entire plasmalemma is an identifying charac-

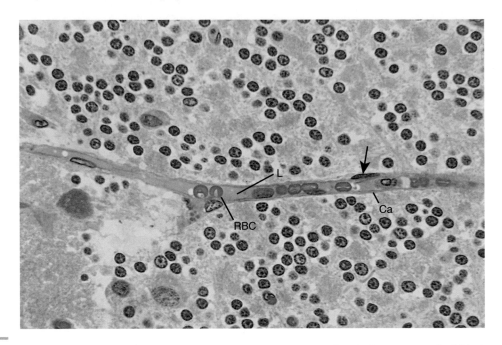

Figure 11–7   Light micrograph of a capillary in the monkey cerebellum (×270) A capillary (Ca) is present in the field of view, and red blood cells (RBC) are evident in its lumen (L). Note the nucleus (*arrow*) of an endothelial cell bulging into the lumen.

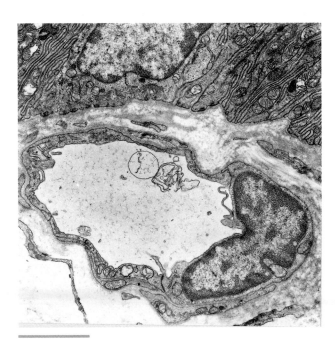

Figure 11–8   Electron micrograph of a continuous capillary in the rat submandibular gland (×13,000). The pericyte shares the endothelial cell's basal lamina. (From Sato A, Miyoshi S: Morphometric study of the microvasculature of the main excretory duct subepithelia of the rat parotid, submandibular, and sublingual salivary glands. Anat Rec 226:288-294, 1990.)

teristic of capillaries. These vesicles may be in singular array, two single vesicles may be fused together, or several vesicles may be fused, forming a transient channel. Where the endothelial cells are the thinnest, a single vesicle may span from the adluminal plasmalemma across the cytoplasm to the abluminal plasmalemma of the endothelial cell.

The endothelial cells of capillaries are rolled into a tube, giving the lumen a diameter that ranges from 8 to 10 mm but remains constant throughout the entire length of a capillary. This diameter is sufficient to permit individual cells of the blood to pass without being hindered. Although not all of the capillary beds are open at any one time, increased demand initiates the opening of more beds, thus increasing blood flow to meet physiological needs. The external surfaces of the endothelial cells are surrounded by a basal lamina secreted by the endothelial cells (see Fig. 11-9). When viewed in cross section, the endothelial walls making up small capillaries are formed by one endothelial cell, whereas portions of two or three endothelial cells contribute to forming the endothelial wall of larger capillaries. At these cellular junctions, the endothelial cells tend to overlap, forming a **marginal fold** that projects into the lumen. Endothelial cells are joined together by **fasciae occludentes,** or **tight junctions.**

Pericytes are located along the outside of the capillaries and small venules, and appear to be surrounding them (Figs. 11-10 and 11-11). These cells have long

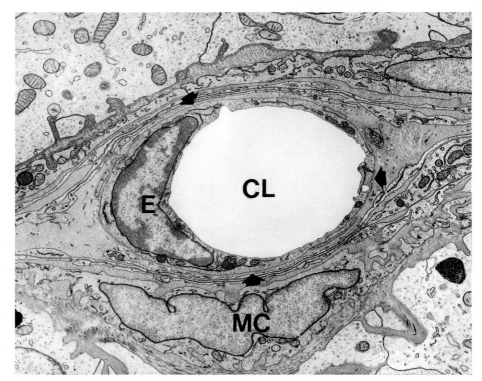

Figure 11–9 Electron micrograph of a testicular capillary. CL, capillary lumen; MC, myoid cell; E, nucleus of endothelial cell. *Arrows* represent the basal lamina. (From Meyerhofer A, Hikim APS, Bartke A, Russell LD: Changes in the testicular microvasculature during photoperiod-related seasonal transition from reproductive quiescence to reproductive activity in the adult golden hamster. Anat Rec 224:495-507, 1989.)

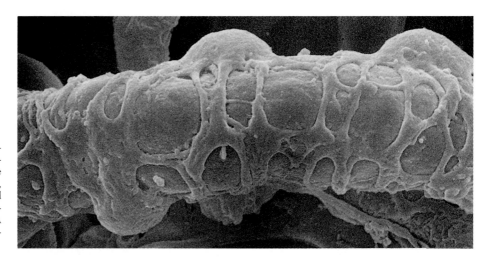

Figure 11–10 Scanning electron micrograph of a capillary displaying pericytes on its surface (×5000). (From Fujiwara T, Uehara, Y: The cytoarchitecture of the wall and innervation pattern of the microvessels in the rat mammary gland: A scanning electron microscopic observation. Am J Anat 170:39-54, 1984.)

primary processes that are located along the long axis of the capillary and from which secondary processes arise to wrap around the capillary, forming a few **gap junctions** with the endothelial cells. Pericytes share the basal lamina of the endothelial cells. Pericytes possess a small Golgi complex, mitochondria, RER, microtubules, and filaments extending into the processes. These cells also contain tropomyosin, isomyosin, and protein kinase, which are all related to the contractile process that regulates blood flow through the capillar-

ies. Further, as discussed in Chapter 6, after injury pericytes may undergo differentiation to become smooth muscle cells and endothelial cells in the walls of arterioles and venules.

Classification of Capillaries

Capillaries are of three types: (1) continuous, (2) fenestrated, and (3) sinusoidal (Fig. 11-12). They differ in their location and structure.

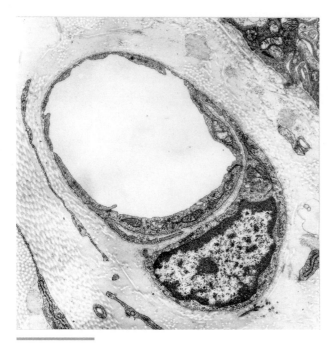

Figure 11–11 Electron micrograph of a fenestrated capillary and its pericyte in cross section. Note that the capillary endothelial cells and the pericyte share the same basal lamina. (From Sato A, Miyoshi S: Morphometric study of the microvasculature of the main excretory duct subepithelia of the rat parotid, submandibular, and sublingual salivary glands. Anat Rec 226:288-294, 1990.)

Continuous Capillaries

Continuous capillaries have no pores or fenestrae in their walls.

Continuous capillaries are present in muscle, nervous, and connective tissues; in the brain tissue they are classified as modified continuous capillaries. The intercellular junctions between their endothelial cells are a type of **fasciae occludentes,** which prevent passage of many molecules. Substances such as amino acids, glucose, nucleosides, and purines move across the capillary wall via carrier-mediated transport. The cells exhibit a polarity with the transport systems, such that Na^+,K^+-ATPase is located in the adluminal cell membrane only. There is evidence that barrier regulation resides within the endothelial cells but is influenced by products formed by the astrocytes associated with the capillaries.

Fenestrated Capillaries

Fenestrated capillaries possess pores (fenestrae) in their walls that are covered by pore diaphragms.

Fenestrated capillaries have **pores (fenestrae)** in their walls that are 60 to 80 nm in diameter and covered by

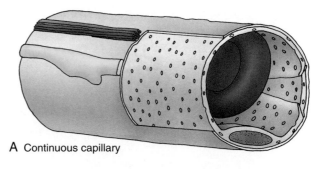

A Continuous capillary

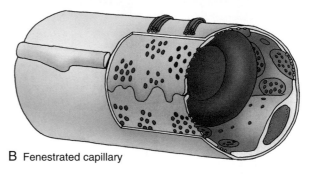

B Fenestrated capillary

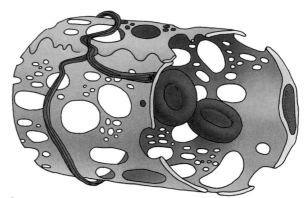

C Sinusoidal (discontinuous) capillary

Figure 11–12 The three types of capillaries: continuous, fenestrated, and sinosoidal (discontinuous).

a pore diaphragm. These capillaries are found in the pancreas, intestines, and endocrine glands.

The pores in fenestrated capillaries are bridged by an ultrathin diaphragm. When viewed after processing with platinum-carbon shadowing, the diaphragm displays eight fibrils radiating out from a central area and forming wedge-like channels, each with an opening of about 5.5 nm. These pore-diaphragm complexes are regularly spaced about 50 nm apart but are located in clusters; thus, most of the endothelial wall of the fenestrated capillary is without fenestrae (see Fig. 11-12B). An exception is the **renal glomerulus,** composed of fenestrated capillaries that lack diaphragms.

Sinusoidal Capillaries

> *Sinusoidal capillaries may possess discontinuous endothelial cells and basal lamina and contain many large fenestrae without diaphragms, enhancing exchange between blood and tissue.*

The vascular channels in certain organs of the body, including the bone marrow, liver, spleen, lymphoid organs, and certain of the endocrine glands, are called **sinusoids,** irregular blood pools or channels that conform to the shape of the structure in which they are located. The peculiar conformation of a sinusoid is determined by its being shaped between the parenchymal components of the organ during organogenesis.

Because of their location, sinusoidal capillaries have an enlarged diameter of 30 to 40 μm (Fig. 11-12C). They also contain many large fenestrae that lack diaphragms; the endothelial wall may be discontinuous, as is the basal lamina, permitting enhanced exchange between the blood and the tissues. Sinusoids are lined by endothelium. In certain organs, the endothelium is thin and continuous (as in some lymphoid organs); in others it may have continuous areas mixed with fenestrated areas (as in endocrine glands). Although the endothelial cells lack pinocytotic vesicles, macrophages may be located either in or along the outside of the endothelial wall.

Regulation of Blood Flow into a Capillary Bed

Arteriovenous Anastomoses

> *Arteriovenous anastomoses are direct vascular connections between arterioles and venules that bypass the capillary bed.*

Terminals of most arteries end in capillary beds, which deliver their blood to venules for the return back to the venous side of the cardiovascular system. In many parts of the body, however, the artery simply joins with a venous channel, forming an arteriovenous anastomosis (AVA). The structures of the arterial and venous ends of the AVA are similar to those of an artery and vein, respectively, whereas the intermediate segment has a thickened tunica media and its subendothelial layer is composed of plump polygonal cells that are modified, longitudinally arranged smooth muscle cells.

When the AVAs are closed, the blood passes through the capillary bed; when shunts are open, a large amount of blood bypasses the capillary bed and flows through the AVA. These shunts are useful in thermoregulation and are abundant in skin. The intermediate segments of the AVAs are richly innervated with adrenergic and cholinergic nerves. Whereas most peripheral nerves are controlled somewhat by local environmental stimuli, those nerves in the AVAs are controlled by the thermoregulatory system in the brain.

Glomera

Nail beds and the tips of the fingers and toes are vascularized by glomera (singular, glomus). The glomus is a small organ that receives an arteriole devoid of an elastic lamina and acquires a richly innervated smooth muscle cell layer that surrounds the vessel lumen, thus directly controlling blood flow to the region before emptying into a venous plexus. The entire glomera complex is not fully understood.

Central Channel

> *Metarterioles form the proximal portion of a central channel, and thoroughfare channels form the distal portion of a central channel.*

Blood flow from the arterial system is controlled either by **metarterioles** (with precapillary sphincters) or by **terminal arterioles.** Thus, metarterioles form the proximal portion of a central channel, whereas the channel's distal portion is formed by the **thoroughfare channel,** a structure so-named because it is without precapillary sphincters. The thoroughfare channels drain the capillary bed and empty the blood into **small venules** of the venous system (Fig. 11-13). When the precapillary sphincters are contracted, blood flows through the central channels, bypassing the capillary bed and entering directly into the venules.

Histophysiology of Capillaries

> *Capillaries are regions where blood flow is very slow, permitting exchange of material between the circulating blood and the extravascular connective tissue.*

The endothelial cells of capillaries may contain two distinct pore systems: **small pores** (~9 to 11 nm in diameter) and **large pores** (~50 to 70 nm in diameter). The smaller pores are believed to be discontinuities between endothelial cell junctions. The large pores are represented by fenestrae and transport vesicles. Oxygen, carbon dioxide, and glucose may diffuse or be transported across the plasmalemma and then diffuse through the cytoplasm and finally through the abluminal plasmalemma into the extravascular space. Water and hydrophilic molecules (~1.5 nm) simply diffuse through these intercellular junctions.

Water-soluble molecules greater than 11 nm in diameter are transported from the *adluminal* plasmalemma to the *abluminal* plasmalemma by the numerous pinocytotic vesicles adjacent to the cell membrane. This process is called **transcytosis** (Fig. 11-14) because the material traverses the entire cell instead of remaining

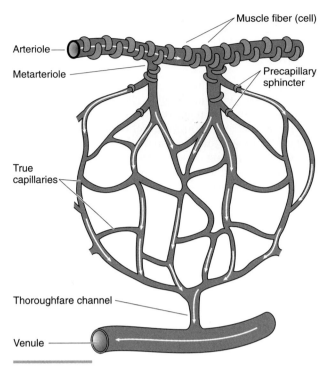

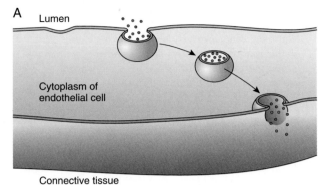

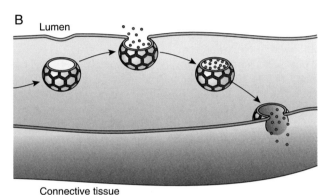

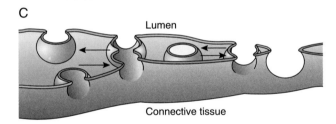

Figure 11–13 The control of blood flow through a capillary bed. The central channel, composed of the metarteriole on the arterial side and the thoroughfare channel on the venous side, can bypass the capillary bed by closure of the precapillary sphincters.

within the cell. In continuous capillaries, substances are taken up by open vesicles located on the *adluminal* plasmalemma. The vesicles are then transported across the cytoplasm to the *abluminal* plasmalemma, where the vesicles fuse with it to deliver their contents into the extravascular space. This is an efficient process because the number of vesicles in these endothelial cells may exceed 1000/mm². It appears that these vesicles are members of a stable population of vesicles arising from the Golgi complex via a fusion-fission mechanism of renewal.

Leukocytes leave the bloodstream to enter the extravascular space by passing through the junctions via a process called **diapedesis. Histamine** and **bradykinin,** whose levels are increased during the inflammatory process, increase capillary permeability, thus causing excessive fluid passage into the extravascular spaces. This excess extravascular fluid causes the tissues to swell, a condition known as **edema.**

The endothelial cells of capillaries also secrete a number of substances, including **fibronectin, laminin, and types II**, **IV, and V collagen,** all of which are released into and become part of the extracellular matrix. Additionally, endothelial cells produce several other important substances related to **clotting, vascu-**

Figure 11–14 The various methods of transport across capillary endothelia. **A,** Pinocytotic vesicles, which form on the luminal surface, traverse the endothelial cell, and their contents are released on the opposite surface into the connective tissue spaces. **B,** *Trans* Golgi network–derived vesicles possessing clathrin coats and receptor molecules fuse with the luminal surface of the endothelial cells and pick up specific ligands from the capillary lumen. They then detach and traverse the endothelial cell, fuse with the membrane of the opposite surface, and release their contents into the connective tissue spaces. **C,** In regions where the endothelial cells are highly attenuated, the pinocytotic (or *trans* Golgi network–derived) vesicles may fuse with each other to form transient fenestrations through the entire thickness of the endothelial cell, permitting material to travel between the lumen and the connective tissue spaces. (**A-C,** Adapted from Simionescu N, Simionescu M: In Ussing H, Bindslev, N, Sten-Knudsen O [eds]: Water Transport Across Epithelia. Copenhagen, Munksgaard, 1981.)

lar smooth muscle tone, lymphocyte circulation, and **neutrophil movement.**

A vasoconstrictor substance, **endothelin I,** secreted by the capillary endothelial cells, attaches to vascular smooth muscle cells. Endothelin I acts as a hypertensive agent, keeping the smooth muscle cells contracted for long periods and thus elevating blood pressure. Although endothelin I is much more effective than angiotensin II, it is unclear how widespread its effects really are.

Adhesion molecules (L-selectin and β₂-integrins) expressed on the plasma membranes of migrating leukocytes bind to receptors on the plasma membranes of capillary endothelial cells at sites of inflammation. The bound leukocytes then enter the connective tissue spaces, where they perform their functions in the inflammatory process. **Prostacyclin,** a potent vasodilator and inhibitor of platelet aggregation, is also released by capillaries.

In addition to these functions, capillaries also serve a maintenance role in converting such substances as serotonin, norepinephrine, bradykinin, prostaglandins, and thrombin into inactive compounds.

Enzymes on the luminal surface of endothelial cells of the capillaries in adipose tissue degrade lipoproteins into triglycerides and fatty acids for storage within adipocytes.

Veins

Veins are vessels that return blood to the heart.

At the discharging ends of capillaries are small venules, the beginning of the venous return, which conducts blood away from the organs and tissues and returns it to the heart. These venules empty their contents into larger veins, and the process continues as the vessels become larger and larger while going back to the heart.

Because veins not only outnumber arteries but also usually have larger luminal diameters, almost 70% of the total blood volume is in these vessels. In histological sections, veins parallel arteries; however, their walls are usually collapsed because they are thinner and less elastic than arterial walls because the venous return is a low-pressure system.

Classification of Veins

Veins are classified into three groups on the basis of their diameter and wall thickness: small, medium, and large.

The structure of veins is not necessarily uniform, even for veins of the same size or for the same vein along its entire length. Veins are described as having the same three layers (tunicae intima, media, and adventitia) as arteries (Table 11-2). Although the muscular and elastic layers are not as well developed, the connective tissue components in veins are more pronounced than in arteries. In certain areas of the body where the structures housing the veins protect them from pressure (retina, meninges, placenta, penis), the veins have little or no smooth muscle in their walls; moreover, the boundaries between the tunica intima and the tunica media of most veins are not clearly distinguishable.

Venules and Small Veins

Venules are similar to but larger than capillaries; larger venules possess smooth muscle cells instead of pericytes.

As the blood pools from the capillary bed, it is discharged into **postcapillary venules,** which are 15 to 20 μm in diameter. Their walls are similar to those of capillaries, with a thin endothelium surrounded by reticular fibers and pericytes (see Fig. 11-4). The peri-

---

TABLE 11–2 Characteristics of Veins

Type	Tunica Intima	Tunica Media	Tunica Adventitia
Large veins	Endothelium; basal lamina, valves in some; subendothelial connective tissue	Connective tissue; smooth muscle cells	Smooth muscle cells oriented in longitudinal bundles; cardiac muscle cells near their entry into the heart; collagen layers with fibroblasts
Medium and small veins	Endothelium, basal lamina; valves in some; subendothelial connective tissue	Reticular and elastic fibers, some smooth muscle cells	Collagen layers with fibroblasts
Venules	Endothelium, basal lamina (pericytes, postcapillary venules)	Sparse connective tissue and a few smooth muscle cells	Some collagen and a few fibroblasts

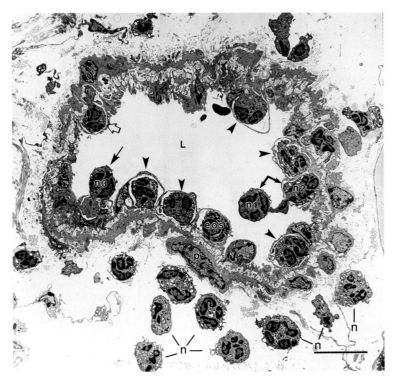

Figure 11–15 Large venule in guinea pig skin harvested 60 minutes after intradermal injection of 10^{-5} M of *N*-formyl-methionyl-leucyl-phenylalanine. Many neutrophils and a single eosinophil (eos) are captured at various stages of attachment to and extravasation across vascular endothelium and underlying *pericytes* (p). Two neutrophils (*joined arrows*), one in another lumen and another partway across the endothelium, are tethered together. Another neutrophil (*long arrow*) has projected a cytoplasmic process into an underlying endothelial cell. Other neutrophils (*arrowheads*) and the eosinophil have crossed the endothelial cell barrier but remain superficial to pericytes, forming dome-like structures that bulge into the vascular lumen (L). Still another neutrophil (*open arrow*) that has already crossed the endothelium has extended a process into the basal lamina and indents an underlying pericyte. Other neutrophils (n) have crossed both the endothelial cell and pericyte barriers and have entered the surrounding connective tissues. Bar, 10 mm. (Modified from Feng D, Nagy JA, Pyne K, et al: Neutrophils emigrate from venules by a transendothelial cell pathway in response to FMLP. J Exp Med 187:903-915, 1998.)

cytes of postcapillary venules form an intricate, loose network surrounding the endothelium. Pericytes are replaced by smooth muscle cells in larger venules (>1 mm in diameter), first as scattered smooth muscle cells; then, as venule diameter increases, the smooth muscle cells become more closely spaced, forming a continuous layer in the largest venules and small veins. Materials are exchanged between the connective tissue spaces and vessel lumina not only in the capillaries but also in the postcapillary venules, whose walls are even more permeable. Indeed, this is the preferred location for emigration of the leukocytes from the bloodstream into the tissue spaces (Fig. 11-15). These vessels respond to pharmacological agents such as histamine and serotonin.

The endothelial cells of venules located in certain lymphoid organs are cuboidal rather than squamous and are called **high-endothelial venules.** These function in lymphocyte recognition and segregation by type-specific receptors on their luminal surface, ensuring that specific lymphocytes migrate into the proper regions of the lymphoid parenchyma.

Medium Veins

Medium veins are less than 1 cm in diameter.

Medium veins are those draining most of the body, including most of the regions of the extremities. Their tunica intima includes the endothelium and its basal lamina and reticular fibers. Sometimes an elastic network surrounds the endothelium, but these elastic fibers do not form laminae characteristic of an internal elastic lamina. The smooth muscle cells of the tunica media are in a loosely organized layer interwoven with collagen fibers and fibroblasts. The tunica adventitia, the thickest of the tunicas, is composed of longitudinally arranged collagen bundles and elastic fibers, as well as a few scattered smooth muscle cells.

Large Veins

Large veins return venous blood directly to the heart from the extremities, head, liver, and body wall.

Large veins include the venae cavae and the pulmonary, portal, renal, internal jugular, iliac, and azygos veins. The tunica intima of the large veins is similar to that of the medium veins, except that large veins have a thick subendothelial connective tissue layer, containing fibroblasts and a network of elastic fibers. Although only a few major vessels (such as the pulmonary veins) have a well-developed smooth muscle layer, most large veins are without a tunica media; in its place is a well-developed tunica adventitia. An exception are the superficial veins of the legs, which have a well-defined muscular wall, perhaps to resist the distention caused by gravity.

The tunica adventitia of large veins contains many elastic fibers, abundant collagen fibers, and vasa vasorum, whereas the inferior vena cava has longitudinally arranged smooth muscle cells in its adventitia. As the pulmonary veins and the venae cavae approach the heart, their adventitia contains some cardiac muscle cells.

Valves of Veins

A venous valve is composed of two leaflets, each composed of a thin fold of the intima jutting out from the wall into the lumen.

Many medium veins have valves that function to prevent the backflow of blood. These valves are especially abundant in the veins of the legs, where they act against the force of gravity. A venous valve is composed of two leaflets, each having a thin fold of the intima jutting out from the wall into the lumen. The thin leaflets are structurally reinforced by collagen and elastic fibers that are continuous with those of the wall. As blood flows to the heart, the valve cusps are deflected in the direction of the blood flow toward the heart. Backward flow of blood forces the cusps to approximate each other, thus blocking backflow.

CLINICAL CORRELATIONS

Varicose veins are abnormally enlarged tortuous veins, usually the superficial veins in the legs of older persons. This condition results from loss of muscle tone, degeneration of vessel walls, and valvular incompetence. Varicose veins may also occur in the lower end of the esophagus (**esophageal varices**) or at the terminus of the anal canal (**hemorrhoids**).

Heart

The heart is a four-chambered pump of the cardiovascular system.

The muscular wall (**myocardium**) of the heart is composed of cardiac muscle (see Chapter 8). The heart consists of four chambers: two atria, which receive blood, and two ventricles, which discharge blood from the heart (Fig. 11-16). The **superior** and **inferior venae cavae** return systemic venous blood to the **right atrium** of the heart. From here, the blood passes through the **right atrioventricular valve (tricuspid valve)** into the **right ventricle.** As the ventricles contract, blood from the right ventricle is pumped out the

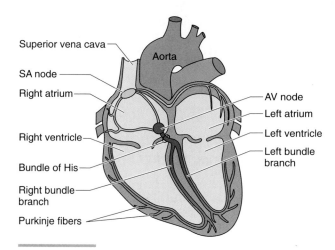

Figure 11–16 Diagram of the heart showing locations of the sinoatrial (SA) and atrioventricular (AV) nodes, Purkinje fibers, and bundle of His.

pulmonary trunk, a large vessel that bifurcates into the right and left pulmonary arteries to deliver deoxygenated blood to the lungs for gaseous exchange. Oxygenated blood from the lungs returns to the heart via the **pulmonary veins,** which empty into the **left atrium.** From here, the blood passes through the **left atrioventricular valve (bicuspid or mitral valve)** to enter the **left ventricle.** Again, ventricular contraction expels the blood from the left ventricle into the aorta, from which many branches emanate to deliver blood to the tissues of the body.

The atrioventricular valves prevent regurgitation of the ventricular blood back into the atria, whereas the **semilunar valves,** located in the pulmonary trunk and the aorta near their origins, prevent backflow from these vessels into the heart.

Layers of the Heart Wall

The three layers that constitute the heart wall are the **endocardium, myocardium,** and **epicardium,** homologous to the tunica intima, tunica media, and the tunica adventitia, respectively, of the blood vessels.

Endocardium

The endocardium, a simple squamous epithelium and underlying subendothelial connective tissue, lines the lumen of the heart.

The endocardium is continuous with the tunica intima of the blood vessels entering and leaving the heart. It is composed of an **endothelium,** consisting of a simple squamous epithelium and an underlying layer of fibroelastic connective tissue with scattered fibroblasts. Lying deeper is a layer of dense connective tissue, heavily endowed with elastic fibers interspersed with smooth muscle cells. Deep to the endocardium is a **subendocardial layer** of loose connective tissue that contains small blood vessels, nerves, and Purkinje fibers from the conduction system of the heart. The subendocardial layer forms the boundary of the endocardium as it attaches to the endomysium of the cardiac muscle.

CLINICAL CORRELATIONS

Children who have had **rheumatic fever** may later develop **rheumatic heart valve disease** as a result of scarring of the valves stemming from the rheumatic fever episode. This condition develops because the valves cannot properly close (incompetence) or open (stenosis) because of reduced elasticity as a result of rheumatic fever. The **bicuspid (mitral) valve,** followed by the **aortic valve**, is the valve most commonly affected.

Myocardium

The thick middle layer of the heart (the myocardium) is composed of cardiac muscle cells.

The myocardium, the middle and thickest of the three layers of the heart, contains cardiac muscle cells arranged in complex spirals around the orifices of the chambers. Certain cardiac muscle cells attach the myocardium to the fibrous cardiac skeleton, others are specialized for endocrine secretions, and still others are specialized for impulse generation or impulse conduction.

The heart rate (~70 beats per minute) is controlled by the **sinoatrial node (pacemaker)** located at the junction of the superior vena cava and the right atrium (see Fig. 11-16). These specialized nodal cardiac muscle cells can spontaneously depolarize 70 times per minute, creating an impulse that spreads over the atrial chamber walls by internodal pathways to the **atrioventricular node,** located in the septal wall just above the tricuspid valve. Modified cardiac muscle cells of the atrioventricular node, regulated by impulses arriving from the sinoatrial node, transmit signals to the myocardium of the atria via the **atrioventricular bundle (bundle of His).** Fibers from the atrioventricular bundle pass down the interventricular septum to conduct the impulse to the cardiac muscle, thus producing a rhythmic contraction. The atrioventricular bundle travels in the subendocardial connective tissue as large, modified cardiac muscle cells, forming **Purkinje fibers** (Fig. 11-17), which transmit impulses to the cardiac muscle cells located at the apex of the heart (Purkinje fibers are not

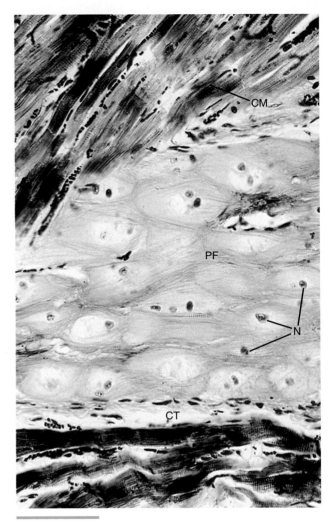

Figure 11–17 Light micrograph of Purkinje fibers. Cardiac muscle (CM) appears very dark, whereas Purkinje fibers (PF) with their solitary nuclei (N) appear light with this stain. Slender connective tissue elements (CT) surround the Purkinje fibers (×270).

be confused with the *Purkinje cells* in the cerebellar cortex). It should be noted that although the autonomic nervous system does not initiate the heartbeat, it does modulate the rate and stroke volume of the heartbeat. Stimulation of sympathetic nerves accelerates the heart rate, whereas stimulation of the parasympathetic nerves serving the heart slows the heart rate.

Specialized cardiac muscle cells, located primarily in the atrial wall and in the interventricular septum, produce an array of small secreted peptides (Fig. 11-18). These include **atriopeptin, atrial natriuretic polypeptide, cardiodilatin,** and **cardionatrin**, which are released into the surrounding capillaries. These hormones aid fluid maintenance and electrolyte balance and decrease blood pressure.

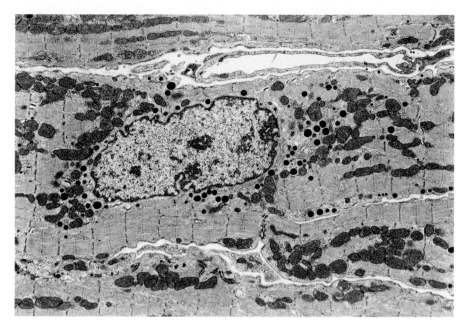

Figure 11–18 Electron micrograph of a cardiac muscle cell containing clusters of vesicles with atrial natriuretic peptide. (From Mifune H, Suzuki S, Honda J, et al: Atrial natriuretic peptide [ANP]: A study of ANP and its mRNA in cardiocytes, and of plasma ANP levels in non-obese diabetic mice. Cell Tissue Res 267:267-272, 1992.)

Epicardium

The epicardium represents the homologue of the tunica adventitia in blood vessels.

Epicardium, the outermost layer of the heart wall, is also called the **visceral layer of the pericardium** (composed of a simple squamous epithelium known as a **mesothelium**). The subepicardial layer of loose connective tissue contains the coronary vessels, nerves, and ganglia. It also is the region where fat is stored on the surface of the heart. At the roots of the vessels entering and leaving the heart, the visceral pericardium becomes continuous with the serous layer of the parietal pericardium. These two layers of the pericardium enclose the pericardial cavity, a space containing a small amount of serous fluid for lubricating the serous layer of the pericardium and the visceral pericardium.

CLINICAL CORRELATIONS

Infection in the pericardial cavity, called **pericarditis,** severely restricts the heart from beating properly because the space is obliterated by adhesions between the epicardium and the serous layer of the pericardium.

Cardiac Skeleton

The cardiac skeleton, composed of dense connective tissue, includes three main components:

- The **annuli fibrosi,** formed around the base of the aorta, pulmonary artery, and the atrioventricular orifices
- The **trigonum fibrosum,** formed primarily in the vicinity of the cuspal area of the aortic valve
- The **septum membranaceum,** constituting the upper portion of the interventricular septum

In addition to providing a structural framework for the heart and attachment sites for the cardiac muscle, the cardiac skeleton provides a discontinuity between the myocardia of the atria and ventricles, thus ensuring a rhythmic and cyclic beating of the heart, controlled by the conduction mechanism of the atrioventricular bundles.

CLINICAL CORRELATIONS

Ischemic (coronary) heart disease, especially prevalent in older persons, is related to **atherosclerosis of the coronary vessels** serving the myocardium. As atherosclerotic plaques reduce the lumina of the coronary vessels, the patient may experience referred pain and pressure, known as **angina pectoris,** as a result of lack of oxygen. Continued narrowing results in ischemia of the heart wall, which may be fatal if untreated. Angioplasty is the current mode of the initial invasive treatment for partially occluded arteries.

LYMPHATIC VASCULAR SYSTEM

The lymphatic vascular system consists of vessels that collect the excess interstitial fluid and return it to the cardiovascular system.

The lymphatic vascular system is composed of a series of vessels that remove excess extracellular fluid **(lymph)** from the interstitial tissue spaces and return it to the cardiovascular system. Lymphatic vessels are present throughout the body, except in the central nervous system and a few other areas, including the orbit, internal ear, epidermis, cartilage, and bone. Unlike the cardiovascular system, which contains a pump (the heart) and circulates blood in a *closed* system, the lymphatic vascular system is an *open* system in that there is no pump and no circulation of fluid.

The lymphatic vascular system begins in the tissues of the body as blind-ended **lymphatic capillaries** (Fig. 11-19), which simply act as drain fields for excess interstitial fluid. The lymphatic capillaries empty their contents into **lymphatic vessels,** which empty into successively larger vessels until one of the two **lym-**

phatic ducts is reached. From either of these ducts, the lymph is emptied into the venous portion of the cardiovascular system at the junctions of the internal jugular and the subclavian veins.

Lymph nodes are interposed along the paths of lymphatic vessels, and lymph must pass through them to be filtered. **Afferent lymphatic vessels** deliver lymph into the lymph nodes, where lymph is distributed into labyrinthine channels lined by an endothelium and abundant macrophages. Here the lymph is filtered and cleared of particulate matter. Lymphocytes are added to the lymph as it leaves by **efferent lymphatic vessels,** eventually reaching a lymphatic duct. Lymph nodes are discussed in Chapter 12.

Lymphatic Capillaries and Vessels

Lymphatic capillaries are composed of a single layer of attenuated endothelial cells with an incomplete basal lamina.

The blind-ended, thin-walled lymphatic capillaries are composed of a single layer of attenuated endothelial cells with an incomplete basal lamina (Fig. 11-20). The endothelial cells overlap each other in places but have intercellular clefts that permit easy access to the lumen of the vessel. These cells do not have fenestrae and do not make tight junctions with each other. Bundles of **lymphatic anchoring filaments** (5 to 10 nm in diameter) terminate on the abluminal plasma membrane. It is thought that these filaments may play a role in maintaining the luminal patency of these flimsy vessels.

Small and medium lymphatic vessels are characterized by closely spaced valves. Large lymphatic vessels resem-

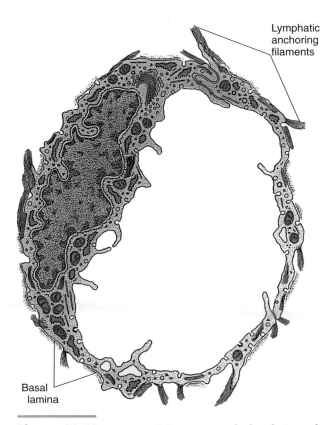

Figure 11–19 Diagram of ultrastructure of a lymphatic capillary. (From Lentz TL: Cell Fine Structure: An Atlas of Drawings of Whole-Cell Structure. Philadelphia, WB Saunders, 1971.)

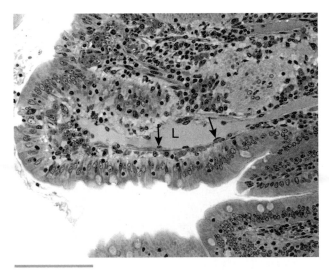

Figure 11–20 Light micrograph of a lymph vessel in the villus core of the small intestine is known as a lacteal (L) (×270). Observe endothelium lining the lacteal (*arrows*).

ble small veins structurally, except that their lumina are larger and their walls thinner. Large lymphatic vessels have a thin layer of elastic fibers beneath their endothelium and a thin layer of smooth muscle cells. This smooth muscle layer is then overlaid with elastic and collagen fibers that blend with the surrounding connective tissue, much like a tunica adventitia. Although some histologists describe tunics similar to those in blood vessels, most do not concur, because there are no clear boundaries between the layers and because the walls are so varied.

Lymphatic Ducts

Lymphatic ducts are similar to large veins; they empty their contents into the great veins of the neck.

The lymphatic ducts, which are similar in structure to large veins, are the final two collecting vessels of the lymphatic vascular system. The short **right lymphatic duct** empties its contents into the venous system at the junction of the right internal jugular and subclavian veins. The larger, the **thoracic duct,** begins in the abdomen as the **cisterna chyli** and ascends through the thorax and neck to empty its contents at the junction of the left internal jugular and subclavian veins. The right lymphatic duct collects lymph from the upper right quadrant of the body, whereas the thoracic duct collects lymph from the remainder of the body.

The tunica intima of lymphatic ducts is composed of an endothelium and several layers of elastic and collagen fibers. At the interface with the tunica media, there is a layer of condensed elastic fibers that resembles an internal elastic lamina. Both longitudinal and circular layers of smooth muscle are present in the media. The tunica adventitia contains longitudinally oriented smooth muscle cells and collagen fibers that blend into the surrounding connective tissue. Piercing the walls of the thoracic duct are small vessels homologous to the vasa vasorum of the arteries.

CLINICAL CORRELATIONS

Malignant tumor cells (especially carcinomas) are spread throughout the body by lymphatic vessels. When the malignant cells reach a lymph node, they are slowed and multiply there, eventually leaving to metastasize to a secondary site. Therefore, in surgical removal of a cancerous growth, examination of the lymph nodes and the removal of both enlarged lymph nodes in the pathway and associated lymphatic vessels are essential in preventing secondary growth of the tumor.

12

Lymphoid (Immune) System

The lymphoid system is responsible for the immunological defense of the body. Some of its component organs—**lymph nodes, thymus,** and **spleen**—are surrounded by connective tissue capsules, whereas its other components, members of the **diffuse lymphoid system,** are not encapsulated. The cells of the lymphoid system protect the body against foreign macromolecules, viruses, bacteria, and other invasive microorganisms, and they kill virally transformed cells.

OVERVIEW OF THE IMMUNE SYSTEM

The immune system has two components: the innate immune system and the adaptive immune system.

The immune system provides the second and the third lines of defense against invading pathogens. The first line of defense is the epithelial barrier, namely skin and mucosa, which forms a complete lining and covering of the body surfaces. Once this physical barrier is breached by a cut, tear, or abrasion, or even if foreign substances are able to penetrate, but have not yet penetrated, the intact barrier, the second and the third lines of defense may become activated; these are the innate and the adaptive immune systems.

The **innate immune system** (natural immune system) is nonspecific and is composed of (1) a system of blood-borne macromolecules known as **complement;** (2) groups of cells known as **macrophages** and **neutrophils,** which phagocytose invaders; and (3) another group of cells, **natural killer (NK) cells,** which kill tumor cells, virally infected cells, bacteria, and parasites.

The **adaptive immune system** (acquired immune system) is responsible for eliminating threats from spe-

cific invaders. Whereas a macrophage can phagocytose most bacteria, the adaptive immune system not only reacts against one specific antigenic component of a pathogen, but also its ability to react against that particular component improves with subsequent confrontations with it.

Although the two systems differ in their mode of responses, they are intimately related to one another, and each affects the other's activities.

The Innate Immune System

The innate immune system responds rapidly, has no immunological memory, and depends on Toll-like receptors for initiating inflammatory and immune responses.

Although the innate immune system is much older than the adaptive immune system, it responds rapidly, usually within a few hours, to an antigenic invasion; it responds in a nonspecific manner; and has no immunological memory. The critical components of the innate immune system are complement, antimicrobial peptides, cytokines, macrophages, neutrophils, NK cells, and Toll-like receptors (TLRs). (See Table 12-1 for acronyms and abbreviations used in this chapter).

Complement is a series of blood-borne proteins that attack microbes that found their way into the bloodstream. As they precipitate on the surface of these invading pathogens, they form a membrane attack complex (MAC) that damage the microbe's cell membrane. Phagocytic cells, such as neutrophils and macrophages, of the host have receptors for a specific moeity of complement (i.e., C3b) and the presence of C3b on the microbial surface facilitates phagocytosis of microbes by these host defense cells.

TABLE 12–1 Acronyms and Abbreviations Used in this Chapter

Acronym/Abbreviation	Definition
ADDC	Antibody-dependent cellular cytotoxicity
AIDS	Acquired immunodeficiency syndrome
APC	Antigen-presenting cell
BALT	Bronchus-associated lymphoid tissue
B lymphocyte	Bursa-derived lymphocyte (Bone marrow–derived lymphocyte)
C3b	Complement 3b
CD	Cluster of differentiation molecule (usually followed by an Arabic numeral)
CLIP	Class II–associated invariant protein
CSF	Colony-stimulating factor
CTL	Cytotoxic T lymphocyte (T killer cell)
Fab	Antigen-binding fragment of an antibody
Fas protein	CD95 (induces apoptosis)
Fc	Crystallized fragment (constant fragment of an antibody)
GALT	Gut-associated lymphoid tissue
G-CSF	Granulocyte colony-stimulating factor
GM-CSF	Granulocyte-monocyte colony-stimulating factor
HEVs	High endothelial venules
HIV	Human immunodeficiency virus
IFN-α	Interferon-alpha
IFN-γ	Interferon-gamma
Ig	Immunoglobulin (usually followed by a capital letter: A, D, E, G, or M)
IL	Interleukin (usually followed by an Arabic numeral)
M cell	Microfold cell
MAC	Membrane attack complex
MALT	Mucosa-associated lymphoid tissue
MHC	Major histocompatibility complex
MHC I and MHC II	MHC class I molecules and class II molecules
MIIC vesicle	MHC class II–enriched compartment
NK cell	Natural killer cell
PALS	Periarterial lymphatic sheath
RER	Rough endoplasmic reticulum
sIgs	Surface immunoglobulins
TAP	Transporter protein (1 and 2)
TCM	Central memory T cell
TCR	T-cell receptor
TEM	Effector T memory cell
TGF	Tumor growth factor
T_H cell	T-helper cell (usually followed by an Arabic numeral)
TLR	Toll-like receptor
T lymphocyte	Thymus-derived lymphocyte
TNF-α	Tumor necrosis factor-alpha
T reg cell	Regulatory T cell
TSH	Thyroid-stimulating hormone

Antimicrobial peptides, such as **defensins,** are synthesized and released by epithelial cells and not only defend the body against gram-negative bacteria but also are chemoattractants for immature dendritic cells and T lymphocytes.

Cytokines are signaling molecules that are released by various cells of the innate and adaptive immune systems to effect responses from their target cells. Cytokines that are released by lymphocytes are known as **interleukins (ILs),** whereas cytokines that possess chemoattractant capabilities are usually referred to as **chemokines.** Those cytokines that stimulate differentiation and mitotic activity of hemopoietic cells are known as **colony-stimulating factors (CSFs),** whereas cytokines displaying antiviral properties are referred to as **interferons.**

Macrophages possess receptors for the constant portions of antibodies (Fc receptors), complement receptors, and receptors that recognize carbohydrates that are not usually present on the surface of vertebrate cells. Macrophages are also antigen-presenting cells, presenting antigens to both T and B lymphocytes. They also release G-CSF and GM-CSF, which induce the formation of neutrophils and their release into the circulating blood.

Neutrophils leave the vascular system in the region of inflammation and enter the bacteria-laden connective tissue compartment where they phagocytose and destroy bacteria. Bacterial killing is effected either in an oxygen-dependent manner, by the formation of hydrogen peroxide, hydroxyl radicals, and singlet oxygen within the phagolysosomes, or via enzymatic digestion, utilizing cationic proteins as well as myeloperoxidase and lysozymes.

NK cells are similar to cytotoxic T cells (members of the adaptive immune system, as discussed later), but they do not have to enter the thymus gland to become mature killer cells. These are cells that use nonspecific markers to recognize their target cells, and they do so by the use of two different methods:

- NK cells possess Fc receptors that recognize the constant portion of the IgG antibody and act as a signal to kill the target cell. This is known as **antibody-dependent cellular cytotoxicity.**
- The NK cell surface also displays transmembrane proteins known as **killer-activating receptors** that bind to certain markers on the surface of nucleated cells. In order to control this killing process, NK cells also possess **killer-inhibitory receptors** that recognize MHC I molecules (major histocompatibility complex type I molecules) that are located on the plasma membranes of all cells. The presence of MHC I molecules prevents the killing of healthy cells by NK cells.

CLINICAL CORRELATIONS

MHC I molecules are required to be present on cell membranes of nucleated cells for cytotoxic T lymphocytes (CTLs) to recognize the cells as targets for destruction. However, tumor cells and cells that are infected by viruses suppress the production of MHC I molecules in order to prevent their recognition as targets for CTLs. This evasive maneuver allows tumor and virally infected cells to become targets of NK cells because their killer inhibitory receptors do not become activated.

Toll-like receptors (TLRs) are highly conserved integral proteins present in the membranes on cells of the innate immune system; humans have been shown to possess at least 12 different TLRs, each with different roles (Table 12-2). It appears that TLRs function in pairs, so that two TLR partners form a single active receptor. Some of the TLRs are present on cell membranes so that they have both intracellular and extracellular moieties, whereas other TLRs are located only intracellularly and possess no extracellular moieties. All TLRs (with the exception of TLR3) associate with and activate the nuclear factor NF-κB pathway that acts through several cytosolic proteins, including MyD88, that induces an intracellular cascade of TLR-specific responses. This sequence of events results not only in

---

TABLE 12–2 Toll-Like Receptors and Their Putative Functions

Domains	Toll-Like Receptor (TLR) Pair	Function
Intracellular and extracellular (on cell membrane)	TLR1-TLR2	Binds to bacterial lipoprotein; also binds to certain proteins of parasites
	TLR2-TLR6	Binds to lipoteichoic acid of gram-positive bacterial wall; also binds to zymosan, a fungus-derived polysaccharide
	TLR4-TLR4	Binds to lipoprotein saccharide of gram-negative bacteria
	TLR5-?*	Binds to flagellin of bacterial flagella
	TLR11-?*	Host recognition of *Toxoplasmosis gondii*
Intracellular only	TLR3-?*	Binds to double-stranded viral RNA
	TLR7-?*	Binds to single-stranded viral RNA
	TLR8-?*	Binds to single-stranded viral RNA
	TLR9-?*	Binds to bacterial and viral DNA
	TLR10-?*	Unknown
	TLR12-?*	Unknown

*Currently, TLR partner is unknown.

the release of cytokines appropriate to the pathogen being detected but also in the possible activation of B and T cells designed to mount a specific adaptive immune response. Therefore, TLRs have the ability to modulate the immune response, suggesting that the innate immune system is not a static, one-fits-all type of response but is dynamic in nature and is capable of regulating both the inflammatory and immune responses equally.

CLINICAL CORRELATIONS

Hypoactivity of TLRs can result in greater susceptibility to pathogens, whereas their hyperactivity may be responsible for some autoimmune diseases such as systemic lupus erythematosus, cardiovascular diseases, and rheumatoid arthritis.

The Adaptive Immune System

The adaptive immune system responds slower than the innate immune system, has immunological memory, and depends on B and T lymphocytes to mount an immune response.

The adaptive immune response exhibits four distinctive properties: **specificity, diversity, memory,** and **self/nonself recognition**—that is, the ability to distinguish between structures that belong to the organism, self, and those that are foreign, nonself. **T lymphocytes, B lymphocytes,** and specialized macrophages known as **antigen-presenting cells (APCs)** participate in the (adaptive) immune response. These cells communicate with members of the innate immune system as well as with each other by signaling molecules **(cytokines),** which are released in response to encounters with foreign substances called **antigens.**

Recognition of a substance as foreign by the immune system stimulates a complex sequence of reactions that result either in the production of **immunoglobulins** (also known as **antibodies**), which bind to the antigen, or in the induction of a group of cells that specialize in cytotoxicity, namely the killing of the foreign cell or altered self-cell (e.g., tumor cell). The immune response that depends on the formation of antibodies is called the **humoral immune response,** whereas the cytotoxic response is known as the **cell-mediated immune response.**

The cells that constitute the functional components of the innate and adaptive immune system (T cells, B cells, macrophages, and their subcategory, APCs) are all formed in the bone marrow. B cells become immunocompetent in the bone marrow, whereas T cells migrate to the thymus to become immunocompetent; therefore, bone marrow and the thymus are called the **primary (central) lymphoid organs**. After lymphocytes become immunocompetent in the bone marrow or in the thymus, they migrate to the **secondary (peripheral) lymphoid organs**—diffuse lymphoid tissue, lymph nodes, and spleen—where they come into contact with antigens.

Immunogens and Antigens

Immunogens are molecules that always elicit an immune response; antigens are molecules that bind to antibodies but do not necessarily elicit an immune response.

A foreign structure that can elicit an immune response in a particular host is known as an immunogen; an antigen is a molecule that can react with an antibody irrespective of its ability to elicit an immune response. Although not all antigens are immunogens, in this textbook the two terms are considered synonymous, and only the term *antigen* is used.

The region of the antigen that reacts with an antibody, or T-cell receptor, is known as its **epitope,** or antigenic determinant. Each epitope is a small portion of the antigen molecule and consists of only 8 to 12 or 15 to 22 hydrophilic amino acid or sugar residues that are accessible to the immune apparatus. Large foreign invaders such as bacteria have several epitopes, each capable of binding to a different antibody.

CLINICAL CORRELATIONS

The complexity of a foreign substance is also important in determining its antigenicity. Hence, large polymeric molecules that have relatively simple chemical compositions, such as certain man-made plastics, have minimal immunogenicity and are therefore used in the manufacture of artificial implants (as in hip replacement).

Clonal Selection and Expansion

During embryonic development, an extremely large number of small clusters (clones) of lymphocytes are formed. Each clone can recognize one specific foreign antigen.

The immune system can recognize and combat an astonishing number of different antigens. The explanation for this capability is that, during embryonic development, an enormous number (approximately 10^{15}) of lymphocyte clones are formed by rearrangement of the

400 or so genes encoding immunoglobulins or TCRs. All of the cells in a particular clone have identical surface markers and can react with a specific antigen, even though they have not yet been exposed to that antigen. The cell-surface proteins that enable lymphocytes to interact with antigens are **membrane-bound antibodies (B-cell receptors** or **surface immunoglobulins [sIgs])** in the case of B cells and **T-cell receptors (TCRs)** in the case of T cells. Although the molecular structures of antibodies and TCRs differ, they are functionally equivalent in their ability to recognize and interact with specific epitopes.

The first time the organism encounters an antigen, the adaptive immune response is slow to begin and not very robust; this response is called the **primary immune response.** Subsequent exposures to the same antigen elicit the **secondary immune response,** which begins rapidly and is much more intense than the primary response. The increased potency of the secondary reaction is due to the process of **immunological memory,** which is inherent to the immune system. Both B and T cells are said to be **virgin cells (naïve cells)** before exposure to antigens. Once a virgin cell comes in contact with an antigen, it proliferates to form activated cells and memory cells.

Activated cells, also known as **effector cells,** are responsible for carrying out an immune response. Effector cells derived from B cells are called **plasma cells** and produce and release antibodies. Effector cells derived from T cells either secrete cytokines or destroy foreign cells or altered self-cells.

Memory cells, similar to virgin lymphocytes, express either B-cell receptors (sIgs) or TCRs, which can interact with specific antigens. Memory cells are not directly involved in the immune response during which they are generated. However, these cells live for months or years and have a much greater affinity for antigens than do virgin lymphocytes. Moreover, formation of memory cells after first exposure to an antigen increases the size of the original clone, a process called **clonal expansion.** Because of the presence of an expanded population of memory cells with an increased affinity for the antigen, subsequent exposure to the same antigen induces a secondary response (**anamnestic response**) that is much faster, more potent, and longer in duration than the primary response.

Immunological Tolerance

Macromolecules of the self are not viewed as antigens and therefore do not elicit an immune response.

The immune system can recognize macromolecules that belong to the self and does not attempt to mount an immune response against them. This lack of action is due to immunological tolerance. The mechanism of immunological tolerance depends on killing or disabling cells that would react against the self. During embryonic development, if a lymphocyte encounters the substance to which it is designed to react, the cell is either killed (**clonal deletion**) so that this particular clone does not form, or the lymphocyte is disabled (**clonal anergy**) and cannot mount an immune response, even though it is present.

CLINICAL CORRELATIONS

Autoimmune diseases involve a malfunction of the immune system that results in the loss of immunological tolerance. One example is **Graves' disease,** in which the receptors for thyroid-stimulating hormone (TSH) on the follicular cells of the thyroid gland are perceived to be antigens. Antibodies formed against TSH receptors bind to these receptors and stimulate the cells to release an excess amount of thyroid hormone. Patients with Graves' disease have an enlarged thyroid gland and exophthalmos (protruding eyeballs).

Immunoglobulins

Immunoglobulins are antibodies that are manufactured by plasma cells. A typical immunoglobulin has one pair of heavy chains and one pair of light chains attached to each other by disulfide bonds.

Immunoglobulins (**antibodies**) are glycoproteins that inactivate antigens (including viruses) and elicit an extracellular response against invading microorganisms. The response may involve phagocytosis in the connective tissue spaces by macrophages (or neutrophils) or the activation of the blood-borne **complement system.**

CLINICAL CORRELATIONS

The complement system is composed of 20 plasma proteins that assemble in a specific sequence and fashion on the surface of invading microorganisms to form a **membrane attack complex (MAC)** that lyses the foreign cell. The key component of the complement system is **protein C3.** Deficiency of protein C3 predisposes a person to recurring bacterial infections.

Immunoglobulins are manufactured in large numbers by plasma cells, which release them into the

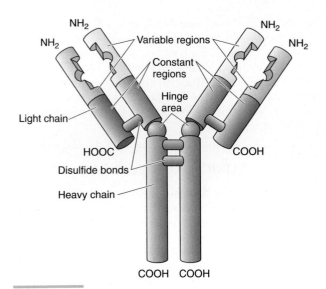

Figure 12–1 An antibody and its regions.

lymph or blood vascular system. The typical antibody is immunoglobulin G (IgG). Each IgG is a **Y**-shaped molecule, composed of two long, identical 55- to 70-kDa polypeptides, known as **heavy chains,** and two shorter, identical 25-kDa polypeptides, the **light chains.** The four chains are bound to each other by several disulfide bonds and noncovalent bonds in such a way that the stem of the **Y** is composed only of heavy chains and the diverging arms consist of both light and heavy chains (Fig. 12-1).

The region in the vicinity of the sulfide bonds between the two heavy chains—the **hinge region**—is flexible and permits the arms to move away from or toward each other. The distal regions on the tips of the arms (the four amino-terminal segments) are responsible for binding to the epitope; hence, each antibody molecule can bind two *identical* epitopes.

The enzyme papain cleaves the antibody molecule at its hinge regions (see Fig. 12-1), forming three fragments: one **Fc fragment** composed of the stem of the **Y** and containing equal parts of the two heavy chains, and two **Fab fragments,** each composed of the remaining part of one heavy chain and one entire light chain. Fc fragments are easily crystallized (hence the "c" designation), whereas the Fab fragment is the *a*ntigen-*b*inding region of the antibody (hence the "ab" designation).

The amino acid sequence of the Fc fragment is mostly constant in its class; thus the stem of an antibody binds to Fc receptors of many different cells. The amino acid sequence of the Fab region is variable, and it is the alterations of that sequence that determine the **specificity** of the antibody molecule for its specific antigen.

Each antibody is specific against a specific epitope; thus the Fab regions of all antibodies against that par-

ticular epitope are identical. It is believed that after the clones against the "self" are eliminated, there remain 10^6 to 10^9 different types of antibodies in a person, each specific against one particular antigen. Each type of antibody is manufactured by members of the same **clone.** Thus there are 10^6 to 10^9 clones whose members discern and react to a particular epitope (or a small number of similar epitopes).

As noted earlier, small amounts of immunoglobulins are made by B cells and inserted into their plasmalemma; these are known as sIgs or **B-cell receptors;** they function as antigen-receptor molecules. They are slightly different from antibodies in that they possess a membrane-binding component composed of two pairs of membrane-spanning chains, Igββ and Igβ, which bind the heavy chains of the antibody molecule to the cell membrane.

Classes of Immunoglobulins

Humans have five **isotypes** (classes) of immunoglobulins (Table 12-3):

IgM, which resembles five IgG molecules bound to each other (pentameric form of immunoglobulin)

IgA, which resembles two IgG molecules bound to each other (dimeric form of immunoglobulin)

IgG, the monomeric form of immunoglobulin described earlier

IgD, which is present in very low concentration in the blood, but is found on the B-cell surface as a monomeric form of immunoglobulin known as surface IgD (sIgD)

IgE, a monomeric form of immunoglobulin present on the surface of basophils and mast cells

The classes of immunoglobulins are also determined by the amino acid sequences of their heavy chains. The various heavy chains are designated by the Greek letters α, δ, γ, ε, and μ.

Cells of the Adaptive and Innate Immune Systems

The cells of the adaptive and innate immune system are B lymphocytes, T lymphocytes, macrophages, antigen-presenting cells, and natural killer cells.

B Lymphocytes

B lymphocytes originate and become immunocompetent in the bone marrow. They are responsible for the humorally mediated immune system.

B lymphocytes, also known as **B cells,** are small lymphocytes (see Chapter 10) that both originate and become **immunocompetent** in the bone marrow. However, in birds, in which B cells were first identified,

TABLE 12–3 Properties of Human Immunoglobulins

Class	Cytokines*	No. of Units†	Ig in Blood (%)	Crosses Placenta	Binds to Cells	Biological Characteristics
IgA	TGFβ	1 or 2	10-15	No	Epithelial cells (temporarily) during secretion	Also known as secretory antibody because it is secreted into tears, saliva the lumen of the gut, and the nasal cavity as **dimers**; individual units of the dimer are held together by **J protein** manufactured by plasma cells and protected from enzymatic degradation by a **secretory component** manufactured by the epithelial cell; combats antigens and microorganisms in the lumen of gut, nasal cavity, vagina, and conjunctival sac; secreted into milk, thus protecting neonate with passive immunity; **monomeric** form in bloodstream; assists eosinophils in recognizing and killing parasites
IgD		1	<1	No	B-cell plasma membrane	Surface immunoglobulin; assists B cells in recognizing antigens for which they are specific; functions in the activation of B cells subsequent to antigenic challenge to differentiate into plasma cells
IgE	IL-4, IL-5	1	<1	No	Mast cells and basophils	Reaginic antibody; when several membrane-bound antibodies are cross-linked by antigens, IgE facilitates degranulation of basophils and mast cells, with subsequent release of pharmacological agents, such as heparin, histamine, eosinophil and neutrophil chemotactic factors, and leukotrienes; elicits immediate hypersensitivity reactions; assists eosinophils in recognizing and killing parasites
IgG	IFN-γ, IL-4, IL-6	1	80	Yes	Macrophages and neutrophils	Crosses placenta—thus protects fetus with passive immunity; secreted in milk—thus protects neonate with passive immunity; fixes complement cascade; functions as **opsonins**—that is, by coating microorganisms; facilitates their phagocytosis by macrophages and neutrophils, cells that possess Fc receptors for the Fc region of these antibodies; also participates in **antibody-dependent cell-mediated cytotoxicity** by activating NK cells; produced in large quantities during secondary immune responses
IgM		1 or 5	5-10	No	B cells (in monometric form)	Pentameric form is maintained by J-protein links, which bind Fc regions of each unit; activates cascade of the complement system; is the first isotype to be formed in the primary immune response

*Cytokines responsible for switching to this isotype.
†A unit is a single immunoglobulin composed of two heavy and two light chains; thus, IgA exists both as a monomer and as a dimer.
Fc, crystallizable fragment; IFN, interferon; Ig, immunoglobulin; IL, interleukin; NK, natural killer; TGF, tumor growth factor.

they become immunocompetent in a diverticulum of the cloaca, known as the **bursa of Fabricius** (hence "B" cells). During the process of becoming immunocompetent, each cell manufactures 50,000 to 100,000 IgM and IgD immunoglobulins and inserts these in its plasma membrane so that the epitope-binding sites of the antibodies face the extracellular space. The Fc region of the antibody is embedded in the phospholipid bilayer with the assistance of two pairs of transmembrane proteins, Igβ and Igα, whose carboxyl termini are in contact with intracellular protein complexes. Every member of a particular clone of B cells has antibodies that bind to the same epitope.

When the surface immunoglobulin reacts with its epitope, the Igβ and Igα transduce (relay) the information to the intracellular protein complex with which they are in contact, initiating a chain of events that results in **activation** of the B cell. The activated B cell undergoes mitosis, forming antibody-producing **plasma cells** and **B memory cells,** as discussed earlier. Because the antibodies produced by plasma cells are released either into the blood or into the lymph circulation, B cells are responsible for the **humorally mediated immune response.**

As naïve B cells first become activated, they make IgM, which, when bound to the surface of an invading pathogen, is able to activate the complement system (complement fixation). IgM molecules can also bind to viruses, preventing them from contacting the cell surface, thus protecting the cells from viral invasion.

Once IgM is produced, the B cell can manufacture a different class of immunoglobulin. This capability is known as **class switching (isotype switching)** and is determined by the particular cytokines that are present in the B cell's microenvironment. These cytokines are released by T-helper (T_H) cells as a function of the type of pathogens present:

- During parasitic worm invasion, T-helper cells release IL-4 and IL-5, and B cells differentiate into plasma cells and after class switching form IgE to elicit mast cell degranulation on the surface of the parasites.
- During bacterial and viral invasions, T-helper cells release interferon-γ (IFN-γ) and IL-6, and B cells switch to forming IgG, which opsonizes bacteria, fixes complement, and stimulates NK cells to kill virally altered cells (antibody-dependent cell-mediated cytotoxicity [ADCC]).
- During viral or bacterial invasion of mucosal surfaces, T-helper cells release tumor growth factor-β (TGF-β), and B cells switch to IgA formation, which is secreted onto the mucosal surface.

Certain antigens (e.g., polysaccharides of microbial capsules) can elicit a humoral immune response without a T-cell intermediary. These are known as **thymic-independent antigens.** They cannot induce formation of B memory cells and can elicit only IgM-antibody formation. However, most antigens require participation of a T-cell intermediary before they can induce a humoral immune response (see below).

T Lymphocytes

T lymphocytes originate in the bone marrow and migrate to the thymus to become immunocompetent. They are responsible for the cellularly mediated immune response.

T lymphoctes (**T cells**) also are formed in the bone marrow, but they migrate to the thymic cortex, where they become immunocompetent by expressing specific molecules on their cell membranes that permit them to perform their functions. The process whereby T cells become immunocompetent is discussed later (see Thymus).

Although histologically T cells appear to be identical to B cells, there are important differences between them:

- T cells have TCRs rather than sIgs on their cell surface.
- T cells recognize only epitopes presented to them by other cells (APCs).
- T cells respond only to protein antigens.
- T cells perform their functions only at short distances.

Similar to sIgs on B cells, **TCRs** on the plasmalemma of T cells function as antigen receptors. The **constant regions** of the TCR are membrane-bound, whereas the variable **amino-terminal regions** containing the antigen-binding sites extend from the cell surface. In addition to TCR molecules, T cells express **clusters of differentiation proteins (CD molecules or CD markers)** on their plasmalemma. These accessory proteins bind to specific ligands on target cells. Although almost 200 CD molecules are known, Table 12-4 lists only those that are immediately pertinent to the subsequent discussion of cellular interactions in the immune process. The membrane-bound portion of the TCR associates with the membrane proteins, CD3, and either CD4 or CD8, forming the **TCR complex.** Several other membrane proteins play roles in signal transduction and in strengthening the interaction between the TCR and an epitope, thus facilitating antigen-stimulated T-cell activation.

A TCR can recognize an epitope only if the epitope is a polypeptide (composed of amino acids) and if the epitope is bound to a **major histocompatibility complex (MHC) molecule,** such as those in the plasmalemma of an APC. There are two classes of these glycoproteins: MHC class I and MHC class II. Most

TABLE 12–4 Selected Surface Markers Involved in the Immune Process

Protein	Cell Surface	Ligand and Target Cell	Function
CD3	All T cells	None	Transduces MHC-epitope complex binding into intracellular signal, activating T cell
CD4	T-helper cells	MHC II on APCs	Coreceptor for TCR binding to MHC II–epitope complex, activation of T-helper cell
CD8	Cytotoxic T cells and suppressor T cells	MHC I on most nucleated cells	Coreceptor for TCR binding to MHC I–epitope complex; activation of cytotoxic T cell
CD28 CD40	T-helper cells B cells	B7 on APCs CD40 receptor molecule expressed on activated T-helper cells	Assists in the activation of T-helper cells Binding of CD40 to CD40 receptor permits T-helper cell to activate B cell to proliferate into B memory cells and plasma cells

APC, antigen-presenting cell; CD, cluster of differentiation molecule; MHC, major histocompatibility complex; TCR, T-cell receptor.

nucleated cells express MHC I molecules on their surface, whereas APCs (discussed later) can express both MHC I and MHC II molecules on their plasmalemma. The MHC molecules are unique in each individual (except for identical twins), and to be activated, T cells must recognize not only the foreign epitope but also the MHC molecule as self. If a T cell recognizes the epitope but not the MHC molecule, it does not become stimulated; hence, the T cell's capacity to act against an epitope is **MHC-restricted.**

There are three types of T cells, some with two or more subtypes:

■ Naïve T cells
■ Memory T cells
■ Effector T cells

Naïve T Cells

Naïve T cells possess CD45RA molecules on their cell surface and they leave the thymus programmed as immunologically competent cells, but they are not as yet ready to function in that capacity until they become activated T cells. When a T lymphocyte becomes activated it undergoes cell division and forms both memory T cells and effector T cells.

Memory T Cells

There are two types of memory T cells: central memory T cells and effector memory T cells. They are responsible for the immunological memory of the adaptive immune system.

Memory T cells, unlike naïve T cells, express CD45R0 molecules on their cell membrane. They form the immunological memory of the adaptive immune system because they form a clone whose members are identical and have the capability of combating a particular antigen. These memory cells can become activated and express effector capabilities. There are two types of memory T cells: those that express CR7⁺ molecules on their surface, known as **central memory T cells (TCMs),** and CR7⁻ cells, known **as effector memory T cells (TEMs).** TCMs populate and remain in the T cell–rich area of lymph nodes, they are incapable of immediate effector function, and they interact with and stimulate antigen-presenting cells and cause them to release IL-12. This signaling molecule binds to IL-12 receptors of TCMs and stimulates TCMs to differentiate into effector memory T cells. TEMs express receptors that permit these cells to migrate to regions of inflammation, where they have immediate effector function by differentiating into effector T cells.

Effector T cells

There are three types of effector T cells: T_H cells, cytotoxic T lymphocytes, and regulatory T (T reg) cells. These are the cells that are able to respond to an immunological challenge.

Effector T cells are immunologically competent cells that are capable of responding to and mounting an immune response. There are three types of effector T cell: T_H cells, T killer cells (cytotoxic T lymphocytes

[CTLs]), and T reg cells; T_H and T reg cells have their own cell subtypes.

T-HELPER CELLS

The three subtypes of T_H cells display CD4 molecules on their cell membrane and are responsible for the recognition of foreign antigens as well as for mounting an immunological response against them.

T_H cells possess CD4 molecules as their cell membrane markers, are capable of interacting with other cells of the innate and adaptive immune systems, and can activate cells of the cell-mediated immune system to mount a response to invading pathogens and eliminate them. T_H cells also play a major role in stimulating the humorally mediated immune system by interacting with B cells and stimulating them to become antibody-producing plasma cells. There are three subtypes of Th cells: T_H0, T_H1, and T_H2; an additional subtype, Th3, has been reclassified as an inducible T reg cell.

T_H0 cells are precursor cells that have the capability of manufacturing and releasing a large number of cytokines. These cells can differentiate into either T_H1 or T_H2 cells, and then their repertoire of cytokine release becomes limited.

T_H1 cells secrete IL-2, IFN-γ, and TNF-β:

- IL-2 stimulates CD4 and CD8 T cell proliferation as well as cytotoxicity by CD8 T cells (CTLs)
- IFN-γ stimulates macrophages so that they can destroy pathogens, such as mycobacteria, protozoa, and fungi, that they have phagocytosed; this cytokine also activates NK cells of the innate immune system to become cytotoxic. Macrophages release IL-12, which induces the proliferation of T_H1 cells and inhibits the proliferation of T_H2 cells
- TNF-β stimulates neutrophils to facilitate the induction of acute inflammation
- T_H1 cells are crucial for the control of intracellular pathogens and are also responsible for the induction of the cell-mediated immune response, as in acute allograft rejection and in the cases of multiple sclerosis.

T_H2 cells secrete IL-4, IL-5, IL-6, IL-9, IL-10, and IL-13, and many of these interleukins facilitate the production of antibodies by plasma cells. T_H2 cells elicit a response against a parasitic (IgE) or mucosal (IgA) infection.

The secreted interleukins have varied effects, including the following functions:

- IL 4 stimulates B cells to switch to IgE synthesis; thus it plays an important role in allergic reactions
- IL 10, acting in concert with IL 4, suppresses the differentiation of T_H0 cells to T_H1 cells

- IL 5 induces the production of eosinophils
- IL-6 combats asthma and systemic lupus erythematosus

CYTOTOXIC T LYMPHOCYTES

Cytotoxic T lymphocytes (CTLs, T killer cells) display CD8 molecules on their cell membrane and are responsible for killing foreign cells, tumor cells, and virally altered cells.

CTLs possess CD8 molecules on their cell membrane. They recognize epitopes that are displayed on the cell membranes of foreign cells, tumor cells, as well as cells that have been altered by viruses and display viral epitopes on their plasmalemmae, and kill these cells. The killing of these cells is performed in one of two ways:

- CTLs place perforins into the cell membranes of the virally altered cell:
- Perforins stimulate the formation of pores in the plasmalemma.
- CTLs transfer granzymes into the cytoplasm of the virally altered cell.
- Granzymes stimulate capsases to induce apoptosis, thus killing the virally altered cell.
- CTLs express Fas L, also known as CD95L (the death ligand), on their cell membrane.
- Fas, also known as CD95 (death receptor), on the surface of the target cell is activated.
- Once Fas is activated, it stimulates an apoptotic cascade, resulting in the death of the target cell.

T REG CELLS

T reg cells possess CD 4 molecules on their cell membrane and function in suppressing the immune response.

T reg cells display CD4 molecules on their cell membrane and function in suppressing the immune response. Historically, the role of suppressing the immune response was ascribed to a theoretical T suppressor cell; however, many immunologists did not accept the existence of these cells. Recent investigations, however, showed that there are cells that suppress the immune function, and these cells were named regulatory T (T reg) cells. There are two types of T reg cells: natural (constitutive) and inducible (adaptive). Both express CD4 molecules on their plasma membrane.

- **Natural T reg cells** develop in the thymus; they leave the thymus and, when their TCRs bind to an APC, they suppress the immune response in a non–antigen-specific manner.

▪ **Inducible T reg cells** (also known as **T_H3 cells**) are derived from naïve T cells; they secrete cytokines, such as IL-10 and TGF-β, that inhibit the formation of **T_H1 cells.**

It is possible that the two types of T reg cells have overlapping functions and that they act in concert to suppress the autoimmune response to self-molecules.

NATURAL T KILLER CELLS

Natural T killer cells are effector T cells that resemble NK cells but must enter the thymic cortex to become immunocompetent effector cells. They release these cytokines: IFNγ, IL-4, and IL-10. Similar to NK cells, they can be activated almost immediately. These are very unusual cells because they are able to recognize *lipid antigens* that are presented to them on the surfaces of immature dendritic cells. In order for natural T killer cells to recognize antigenic lipids, the lipids must be presented to them in conjunction with **CD_I molecules.** There are four isoforms of CD_I molecules, and they are located either on the cell surface or are monitoring lysosomal and late endosomal compartments.

Major Histocompatibility Complex Molecules

> MHC molecules present epitopes of pathogens to T cells. There are two classes of MHC molecules: MHC I and MHC II.

The prime importance of MHC molecules is to permit APCs and cells under viral attack (or cells already virally transformed) to present the epitopes of the invading pathogen to the T cells. These epitopes are short polypeptides that fit into a groove on the surface of the MHC molecule.

There are two classes of MHC molecules:

▪ **MHC I molecules** function in presenting short polypeptide fragments (8 to 12 amino acids in length) derived from endogenous proteins (i.e., proteins manufactured by the cell).
▪ **MHC II molecules** function in presenting longer polypeptide fragments (13 to 25 amino acids in length) derived from exogenous proteins (i.e., proteins that were phagocytosed and cleaved by these cells from the extracellular space).

Almost every cell synthesizes and displays MHC I proteins, but only APCs synthesize and display MHC II proteins. In humans, MHC I and MHC II molecules exist in many forms, which permits T cells to recognize the MHC molecules of an individual as belonging to that particular individual—that is, T cells are capable of distinguishing "self."

Loading Epitopes on MHC I Molecules

> Epitopes derived from endogenous proteins are transported by specialized transporter proteins into the rough endoplasmic reticulum cisternae.

Proteins manufactured by a cell, whether they belong to the cell or to a virus or a parasite that has overtaken the protein synthetic machinery of the cell, are known as **endogenous proteins.** The quality of the proteins that the cell manufactures is controlled by **proteasomes,** which are modified to splice defective or foreign proteins into the proper-sized polypeptide fragments (8 to 12 amino acids in length). These fragments, known as **epitopes,** are transported by specialized transporter proteins (TAP1 and TAP2) into the cisternae of the rough endoplasmic reticulum (RER), where they are complexed to MHC I molecules that were manufactured on the RER surface. The MHC I–epitope complex is transported to the Golgi apparatus and is packaged, within the *trans* Golgi network, into clathrin-coated vesicles for transport to and insertion into the cell membrane. In this fashion, TCLs "look" at the cell surface and "see" whether the cell is producing self-proteins or nonself-proteins.

Loading Epitopes on MHC II Molecules

> Epitopes derived from proteins endocytosed by macrophages and APCs are loaded onto MHC II molecules within specialized intracellular compartments known as MHC II compartment (MIIC).

Macrophages and APCs endocytose proteins from their extracellular milieu by the formation of pinocytotic vesicles or phagosomes. The contents of these vesicles, known as **exogenous proteins,** are delivered to early endosomes, where they are enzymatically cleaved into polypeptide fragments. The polypeptide fragments are transported to late endosomes, where they are further cleaved to become the proper size (13 to 25 amino acids in length) so that they can fit into the groove of the MHC II molecule.

MHC II molecules are synthesized on the RER. As they are assembled in the RER cisternae, a protein known as **class II–associated invariant protein (CLIP)** is loaded into the groove of the MHC II molecule, preventing the accidental loading of the molecule with an endogenous epitope. The MHC II–CLIP complex is transported to the Golgi apparatus and is sorted into clathrin-coated vesicles within the *trans* Golgi network for delivery to MHC II–enriched compartments (MIIC vesicles), specialized vesicles that function in loading epitopes onto the MHC II molecule.

The MIIC vesicle receives not only the MHC II–CLIP complex but also the epitopes from the processed antigens from the late endosomes. Within the MIIC vesicle, the CLIP is enzymatically dissociated from the MHC II molecule and is replaced by an epitope. The MHC II–epitope complex is then transported to and inserted into the cell membrane. In this fashion, T_H cells can "look" at the cell surface and "see" whether the cell is encountering nonself-proteins.

Antigen-Presenting Cells (APCs)

APCs express both MHC I and MHC II on their plasmalemmae, and they phagocytose, catabolize, process, and present antigens.

APCs phagocytose, catabolize, and process antigens, attach their epitopes to MHC II molecules, and present this complex to T cells. Most APCs are derived from monocytes and therefore belong to the mononuclear phagocyte system. APCs include macrophages, dendritic cells (such as Langerhans cells of the epidermis and oral mucosa), and two types of non–monocyte-derived cells (B cells and epithelial reticular cells of the thymus).

Similar to T_H cells, APCs manufacture and release **cytokines.** These signaling molecules are needed to activate target cells to perform their specific functions, not only in the immune response but also in other processes. Table 12-5 lists some of these cytokines but includes only those properties that relate specifically to the immune response.

Interaction among the Lymphoid Cells

Cells of the lymphoid system interact with each other to effect an immune response. The process of interac-

TABLE 12–5 Origin and Selected Functions of Some Cytokines

Cytokine	Cell Origin	Target Cell	Function
IL-1a IL-1b	Macrophages and epithelial cells	T cells and macrophages	Activate T cells and macrophages
IL-2	T_H1 cells	Activated T cells and activated B cells	Promotes proliferation of activated T cells and activated B cells
IL-4	T_H2 cells	B cells	Promotes proliferation of B cells and their maturation to plasma cells; also facilitates switch from production of IgM to IgG and IgE
IL-5	T_H2 cells	B cells	Promotes B-cell proliferation and maturation; also facilitates switch from production of IgM to IgE
IL-6	APCs and T_H2 cells	T cells and activated B cells	Activates T cells; promotes B-cell maturation to IgG-producing plasma cells
IL-10	T_H2 cells	T_H1 cells	Inhibits development of T_H1 cells and inhibits them from secreting cytokines
IL-12	B cells and macrophages	NK cells and T cells	Activates NK cells and induces the formation of T_H1-like cells
TNF-α	Macrophage T_H1 cells	Macrophages Hyperactive macrophages	Self-activates macrophages to release IL-12 Stimulates hyperactive macrophages to produce oxygen radicals, thereby facilitating bacterial killing
IFN-α	Cells under viral attack	NK cells and macrophages	Activates macrophages and NK cell
IFN-β	Cells under viral attack	NK cells and macrophages	Activates macrophages and NK cells
IFN-γ	T_H1 cells	Macrophages and T cells	Promotes cell killing by cytotoxic T cells and phagocytosis by macrophages

APCs, antigent-presenting cells; Ig, immunoglobulin; IL, interleukin; IFN, interferon; NK, natural killer; T_H, T-helper; TNF, tumor necrosis factor.

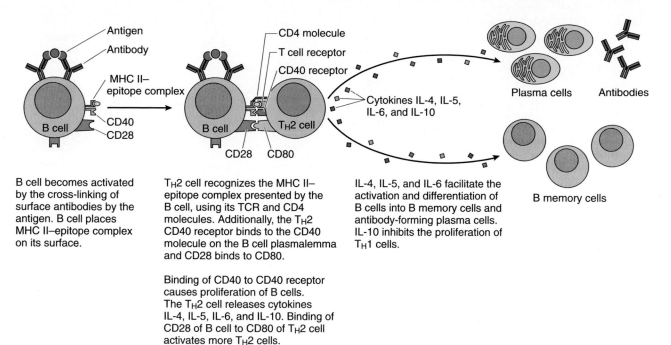

Figure 12–2 The interaction between B cells and a T-helper cell (T$_H$2 cell) in a thymus-dependent, antigen-induced, B memory, and plasma cell formation. CD, cluster of differentiation molecule; IL, interleukin; MHC, major histocompatibility complex; TCR, T-cell receptor.

tion is regulated by recognition of surface molecules; if the molecules are not recognized, the cell is eliminated to prevent an incorrect response. If the surface molecules are recognized, the lymphocytes proliferate and differentiate. The initiation of these two responses is called **activation.** At least two signals are required for activation:

■ Recognition of the antigen (or epitope)
■ Recognition of a second, costimulatory signal, which may be mediated by a cytokine or by a membrane-bound signaling molecule

T-Helper Cell–Mediated (T$_H$2 cells) Humoral Immune Response

Except for thymus-independent antigens, B cells can respond to an antigen only if instructed to do so by the T$_H$2 cell subtype (Fig. 12-2). When the B cell binds antigens on its sIgs, it internalizes the antigen-antibody complex, removes the epitope and attaches it to MHC II molecules, and places the epitope–MHC II complex on its surface and presents it to a T$_H$2 cell.

Signal 1. The T$_H$2 cell not only must recognize the epitope with its TCR but also must recognize the MHC II molecule with its CD4 molecule.
Signal 2. The T$_H$2 cell's CD40 receptor must bind to the B cell's CD40 molecule, and the T$_H$2 cell's CD28 has to contact the B cell's CD80 molecule.

If both signaling events are properly executed, the B cell becomes activated and rapidly proliferates. During proliferation, the T$_H$2 cell releases IL-4, IL-5, IL-6, and IL-10. The first three of these cytokines facilitate the differentiation of the newly formed B cells into **B memory cells** and antibody-secreting **plasma cells,** whereas IL-10 inhibits the proliferation of T$_H$1 cells. The interaction of CD40 with the CD40 ligand facilitates isotype switching from IgM to IgG, and the interaction between CD28 and CD80 enhances T$_H$2 cell activity. IL-4 facilitates the isotype switching to IgE.

T-Helper Cell–Mediated (T$_H$1 cells) Killing of Virally Transformed Cells

In most cases, CTLs need to receive a signal from a T$_H$1 cell to be capable of killing virally transformed cells. Before that signal can be given, however, the T$_H$1 cell must be activated by an APC that offers the proper epitope (Fig. 12-3).

Signal 1. The TCR and the CD4 molecule of the T$_H$1 cell must recognize the epitope–MHC II complex on the surface of an APC. If these events occur, the APC expresses a molecule called **B7** on its surface.
Signal 2. The CD28 molecule of the T$_H$1 cell binds to the B7 molecule of the APC.

The T$_H$1 cell is now activated and releases IL-2, IFN-γ, and TNF. **IFN-γ** causes activation and

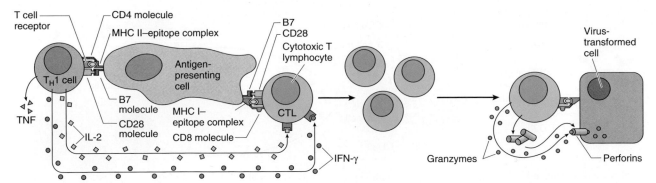

T$_H$1 cell TCR binds to MHC II–epitope complex of antigen-presenting cell. The CD4 molecule of the T$_H$1 cell recognizes MHC II. These two events cause the APC to express B7 molecules on its surface, which bind to CD28 of the T$_H$1 cell, causing it to release IL-2, IFN-γ, and TNF.

The same APC also has **MHC I–epitope** complex expressed on its surface that is bound by a CTL's CD8 molecule and T-cell receptor. Additionally, the CTL has CD28 molecules bound to the APC's B7 molecule. The CTL also possesses IL-2 receptors, which bind the IL-2 released by the T$_H$1 cell, causing the CTL to undergo proliferation, and IFN-γ causes its activation.

The newly formed CTLs attach to the MHC I–epitope complex via their TCR and CD8 molecules and secrete **perforins** and **granzymes**, killing the virus-transformed cells. Killing occurs when granzymes enter the cell through the pores established by perforins and act on the intracellular components to drive the cell into apoptosis.

Figure 12–3 T-helper cell (T$_H$1 cell) activation of cytotoxic T cells in killing virus-transformed cells. APC, antigen-presenting cell; CD, cluster of differentiation molecule; CTL, cytotoxic T lymphocyte; IFN-γ, interferon-gamma; MHC, major histocompatibility complex; TCR, T-cell receptor; TNF, tumor necrosis factor.

proliferation of the CTL if that CTL is bound to the same APC and if the following conditions are met:

Signal 1. The TCR and the **CD8 molecule** of the CTL must recognize the **epitope–MHC I complex** of the APC; also, the CD28 molecule of the CTL must bind with the B7 molecule of the APC.

Signal 2. IL-2 released by the T$_H$1 cell binds to the IL-2 receptors of the CTL.

The CTL is now activated and rapidly proliferates. The newly formed CTLs seek out virally transformed cells by binding with their TCR and CD8 to the transformed cell's epitope–MHC I complex. Target cell killing may occur in one of the following ways:

1 Binding (in the presence of calcium) causes release of **perforins,** a group of glycoproteins that are closely related to the C9 fraction of the complement membrane attack complex. Perforins embed themselves into the cell membranes of the transformed cells and, by aggregating, form hydrophilic pores. These pores may become so large and so abundant that the target cell cannot maintain its cytoplasmic integrity and the cells undergo necrosis. It is interesting to note that the CTL is protected from autodestruction by perforin because the proteoglycan chondroitin sulfate A is present in the vesicles that contain granzymes.

2 Binding (in the presence of calcium) causes the release of perforins and **granzymes.** Granzymes are released from the storage granules of the CTL; these

enzymes enter the transformed cells via the perforin-formed pores and drive the cells into apoptosis, killing them within a few minutes.

3 Binding can also bring the CTL's Fas ligand into contact with the target cell membrane's Fas protein (CD95). When a threshold number of these Fas ligands and Fas proteins bond, the clustering of the Fas proteins induces the intracellular protein cascade that leads to apoptosis.

Note that certain highly vigorous APCs can act as the first signal. In such an instance, the CTL does not require a T$_H$ cell intermediary but can release IL-2 and can activate itself.

T$_H$1 Cells Assist Macrophages in Killing Bacteria

Bacteria that are phagocytosed by macrophages can readily proliferate within the phagosome (becoming infected) because macrophages cannot destroy these microorganisms unless they are activated by T$_H$1 cells (Fig. 12-4).

Signal 1. The TCR and CD4 molecules of the T$_H$1 cell must recognize the epitope–MHC II complex of the macrophage that phagocytosed the bacteria.

Signal 2. The T$_H$1 cell expresses IL-2 receptors on its surface and releases IL-2, which binds to the receptors, thus activating itself.

T$_H$1 Cell Activation of Infected Macrophages

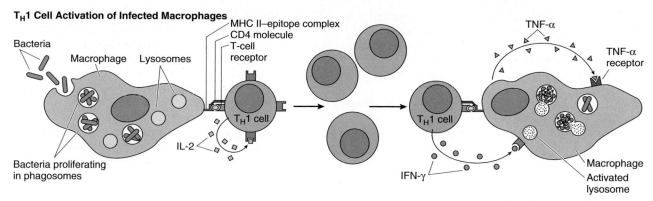

Figure 12–4 Macrophage activation by T cells. CD, cluster of differentiation molecule; IL, interleukin; IFN-γ, interferon-gamma; MHC, major histocompatibility complex; TCR, T-cell receptor; TNF-α, tumor necrosis factor-alpha.

The activated T$_H$1 cell rapidly proliferates, and the newly formed T$_H$1 cells contact macrophages that are infected with bacteria.

Signal 1. The TCR and CD4 molecules of the T$_H$1 cell must recognize the epitope–MHC II complex of the infected macrophage, and the T cell releases IFN-γ.

Signal 2. The IFN-γ activates the macrophage, which then expresses TNF-α receptors on its surface and releases the cytokine TNF-α.

When these two factors, IFN-γ and TNF-α, bind to their receptors on macrophages, they facilitate the production of oxygen radicals by the macrophage, resulting in killing of bacteria.

CLINICAL CORRELATIONS

Human immunodeficiency virus (HIV), the cause of **acquired immunodeficiency syndrome (AIDS),** binds to CD4 molecules of T$_H$ cells and injects its core into the cell. The virus incapacitates the cell, and as the virus spreads, it infects other T$_H$ cells, thereby reducing their numbers. As a result, infected persons eventually become incapable of mounting an immune response against bacterial or viral infections. Victims succumb to secondary infections due to opportunistic microorganisms or to malignancies.

LYMPHOID ORGANS

The lymphoid organs are classified into two categories:

1 **Primary (central) lymphoid organs** are responsible for the development and maturation of lymphocytes into mature, immunocompetent cells.
2 **Secondary (peripheral) lymphoid organs** are responsible for the proper environment in which immunocompetent cells can react with each other, as well as with antigens and other cells, to mount an immunological challenge against invading antigens or pathogens.

In humans, the fetal liver, prenatal and postnatal bone marrow, and thymus constitute the primary lymphoid organs. The lymph nodes, spleen, and mucosa-associated lymphoid tissues (as well as the postnatal bone marrow) constitute the secondary lymphoid organs.

Thymus

The thymus is a primary lymphoid organ that is the site of maturation of T lymphocytes.

The thymus, situated in the superior mediastinum and extending over the great vessels of the heart, is a small encapsulated organ composed of two **lobes.** Each lobe arises separately in the third (and possibly fourth) pharyngeal pouches of the embryo. The T lymphocytes that enter the thymus to become instructed to achieve immunological competence arise from mesoderm.

The thymus originates early in the embryo and continues to grow until puberty, when it may weigh as much as 35 to 40 g. After the first few years of life, the thymus begins to **involute** (atrophy) and becomes infiltrated by adipose cells. However, it may continue to function even in older adults.

The capsule of the thymus, composed of dense, irregular collagenous connective tissue, sends septa into the lobes, subdividing them into incomplete **lobules** (Fig. 12-5). Each lobule is composed of a cortex and a medulla, although the medullae of adjacent lobules are confluent with each other.

Thymic Cortex

Immunological competency of T cells, elimination of self-intolerant T lymphocytes, and MHC recognition occur in the thymic cortex.

The cortex of the thymus appears much darker histologically than does the medulla because of the presence of a large number of **T lymphocytes (thymocytes)** (Fig. 12-6; also see Fig. 12-5). Immunologically incompetent T cells leave the bone marrow and migrate to the periphery of the thymic cortex, where they undergo extensive proliferation and instruction to become immunocompetent T cells. In addition to the lymphocytes, the cortex houses macrophages and **epithelial reticular cells.** It is believed that in humans epithelial reticular cells are derived from the endoderm of the third (and possibly fourth) pharyngeal pouch. Three types of epithelial reticular cells are present in the thymic cortex:

■ **Type I cells** separate the cortex from the connective tissue capsule and trabeculae and surround vascular elements in the cortex. These cells form occluding junctions with each other, completely isolating the

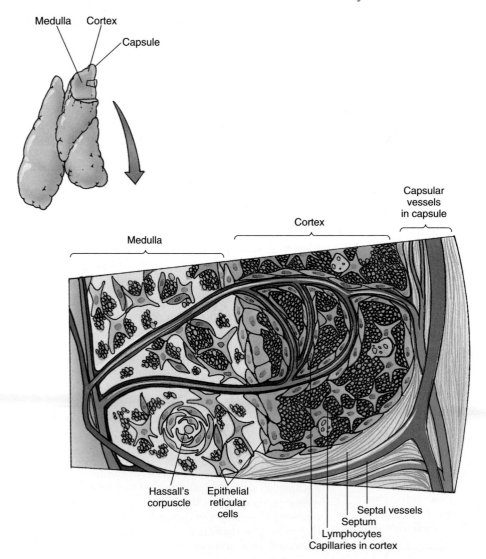

Figure 12–5 Diagram of the thymus demonstrating its blood supply and histological arrangement.

cells participate in the formation of occluding junctions with each other and with epithelial reticular cells of the medulla; this isolates the cortex from the medulla.

These three types of epithelial reticular cells completely isolate the thymic cortex and thus prevent developing T cells from contacting foreign antigens. Type II and III cells as well as bone marrow–derived interdigitating cells (APCs) also present **self-antigens, MHC I** molecules, and **MHC II** molecules to the developing T cells. Developing T lymphocytes whose TCRs recognize self-proteins, or whose CD4 or CD8 molecules cannot recognize the MHC I or MHC II molecules, undergo apoptosis before they can leave the cortex. It is interesting that 98% of developing T cells die in the cortex and are phagocytosed by resident macrophages, which are referred to as **tingible body macrophages.** The surviving cells enter the medulla of the thymus as naïve T lymphocytes, and from there (or from the corticomedullary junction) they are distributed to secondary lymphoid organs via the vascular system.

Medulla

The medulla is characterized by the presence of Hassall's corpuscles. All thymocytes of the medulla are immunocompetent T cells.

The thymic medulla stains much lighter than the cortex because its lymphocyte population is not nearly as profuse and because it houses a large number of endothelially derived epithelial reticular cells (see Figs. 12-5 and 12-6). There are three types of epithelial reticular cells in the medulla:

■ **Type IV cells** are found in close association with type III cells of the cortex and assist in the formation of the corticomedullary junction. The nuclei of these cells have a coarse chromatin network, and their cytoplasm is dark-staining and richly endowed with tonofilaments.
■ **Type V cells** form the cytoreticulum of the medulla. The nuclei of these cells are polymorphous, with a well-defined perinuclear chromatin network and a conspicuous nucleolus.
■ **Type VI cells** compose the most characteristic feature of the thymic medulla. These large, pale-staining cells coalesce around each other, forming whorl-shaped **thymic corpuscles (Hassall's corpuscles),** whose numbers increase with a person's age (see Figs. 12-5 and 12-6). Type VI cells may become highly cornified and even calcified. Unlike types IV and V, type VI epithelial reticular cells may be ectodermal in origin. The function of thymic corpuscles is not known, although they may be the site of T lymphocyte cell death in the medulla.

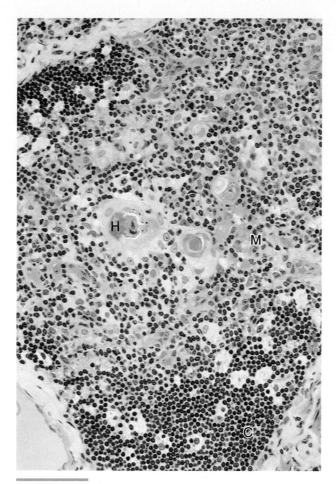

Figure 12–6 Light micrograph of a lobule of the thymus (×124). The peripheral cortex (C) stains darker than the central medulla (M) that is distinguished by the presence of Hassall's corpuscles (H).

thymic cortex from the remainder of the body. The nuclei of type I cells are polymorphous and have a well-defined nucleolus.
■ **Type II cells** are located in the midcortex. These cells have long, wide, sheath-like processes that form desmosomal junctions with each other. Their processes form a cytoreticulum that subdivides the thymic cortex into small, lymphocyte-filled compartments. The nuclei of type II cells are large, pale structures with little heterochromatin. The cytoplasm is also pale and is richly endowed with tonofilaments.
■ **Type III cells** are located in the deep cortex and at the corticomedullary junction. The cytoplasm and the nuclei of these cells are denser than those of type I and type II epithelial reticular cells. The RER of type III cells displays dilated cisternae, which is indicative of protein synthesis. Type III epithelial reticular cells also have wide, sheath-like processes that form lymphocyte-filled compartments. These

Vascular Supply

The cortical vascular supply forms a very powerful blood-thymus barrier to prevent developing T cells from contacting blood-borne macromolecules.

The thymus receives numerous small arteries, which enter the capsule and are distributed throughout the organ via the trabeculae between adjacent lobules. Branches of these vessels do not gain access to the cortex directly; instead, from the trabeculae they enter the corticomedullary junction, where they form capillary beds that penetrate the cortex.

The capillaries of the cortex are of the **continuous** type, possess a thick basal lamina, and are invested by a sheath of type I epithelial reticular cells that form a **blood-thymus barrier.** Thus, the developing T cells of the cortex are protected from contacting blood-borne macromolecules. However, self-macromolecules are permitted to cross the blood-thymus barrier (probably controlled by the epithelial reticular cells), possibly to eliminate those T cells that are programmed against self-antigens. The cortical capillary network drains into small venules in the medulla.

Newly formed, immunologically incompetent T cells arriving from the bone marrow leave the vascular supply at the corticomedullary junction and migrate to the periphery of the cortex. As these cells mature, they move deeper into the cortex and enter the medulla as naïve but immunocompetent cells. They leave the medulla via veins draining the thymus.

Histophysiology of the Thymus

The primary function of the thymus is to instruct immunoincompetent T cells to achieve immunocompetence.

The developing T cells proliferate extensively in the cortex, begin to express their surface markers, and are tested for their ability to recognize **self–MHC molecules** and **self-epitopes.** T cells that are unable to recognize self–MHC I and self–MHC II molecules are destroyed by being driven into apoptosis. Additionally, those T lymphocytes whose TCRs are programmed against self-macromolecules are also destroyed.

The process of testing for self-MHC molecules and self-epitopes is believed to be a function of type II and type III epithelial reticular cells and of bone marrow–derived dendritic cells, because these three cell types express both classes of the epitope–MHC molecule complex on their surface.

The epithelial reticular cells of the thymus produce at least four hormones that are necessary for the maturation of T cells. These are probably paracrine hormones, acting at short range, although some are believed to be released into the bloodstream. These hormones include **thymosin, thymopoietin, thymulin,** and **thymic humoral factor,** and they facilitate T-cell proliferation and the expression of their surface markers. Additionally, hormones from extrathymic sources, especially the gonads and the pituitary, thyroid, and suprarenal glands, influence T-cell maturation. The most potent effects are due to (1) **adrenocorticosteroids,** which decrease T-cell numbers in the thymic cortex; (2) **thyroxin,** which stimulates the cortical epithelial reticular cells to increase thymulin production; and (3) **somatotropin,** which promotes T-cell development in the thymic cortex.

CLINICAL CORRELATIONS

Congenital failure of the thymus to develop is called **DiGeorge's syndrome.** Patients with this disease cannot produce T cells. Therefore their cellularly mediated immune response is nonfunctional, and these patients die at an early age from infection. Because these patients also lack parathyroid glands, death also may be caused by **tetany.**

Lymph Nodes

Lymph nodes are small, encapsulated, oval structures that are interposed in the path of lymph vessels to serve as filters for the removal of bacteria and other foreign substances.

Lymph nodes are located in various regions of the body but are most prevalent in the neck, in the axilla, in the groin, along major vessels, and in the body cavities. Their parenchyma is composed of collections of T and B lymphocytes, APCs, and macrophages. These lymphoid cells react to the presence of antigens by mounting an immunological response in which macrophages phagocytose bacteria and other microorganisms that enter the lymph node by way of the lymph.

Each lymph node is a relatively small, soft structure that is less than 3 cm in diameter and that has a fibrous connective tissue capsule, usually surrounded by adipose tissue (Fig. 12-7). It has a convex surface that is perforated by **afferent lymph vessels** that have **valves,** which ensure that lymph from those vessels enters the substance of the node. The concave surface of the node, the **hilum,** is the site of arteries and veins entering and exiting the node. Additionally, lymph leaves the node via the **efferent lymph vessels,** which are also located at the hilum. The efferent lymph vessels have valves that prevent regurgitation of lymph back into the node.

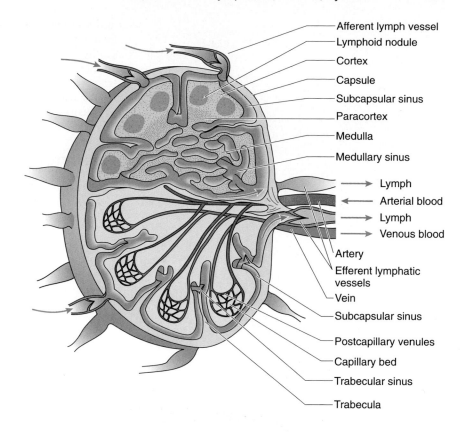

Afferent lymph vessel
Lymphoid nodule
Cortex
Capsule
Subcapsular sinus
Paracortex
Medulla
Medullary sinus
→ Lymph
← Arterial blood
→ Lymph
→ Venous blood
Artery
Efferent lymphatic vessels
Vein
Subcapsular sinus
Postcapillary venules
Capillary bed
Trabecular sinus
Trabecula

Figure 12–7 A typical lymph node.

CLINICAL CORRELATIONS

In the presence of antigens or bacteria, lymphocytes of the lymph node rapidly proliferate, and the node may increase to several times its normal size, becoming hard and palpable to the touch.

Histologically, a lymph node is subdivided into three regions: cortex, paracortex, and medulla. All three regions have a rich supply of sinusoids, enlarged endothelium-lined spaces through which lymph percolates.

Lymph Node Cortex

The cortex of the lymph node is subdivided into compartments that house B cell–rich primary and secondary lymphoid nodules.

The dense, irregular, collagenous connective tissue **capsule** sends **trabeculae** into the substance of the lymph node, subdividing the outer region of the **cortex** into incomplete compartments that extend to the vicinity of the hilum (Fig. 12-8; also see Fig. 12-7). The capsule is thickened at the hilum, and as vessels enter the substance of the node, they are surrounded by a connective tissue sheath derived from the capsule. Suspended from

the capsule and trabeculae is a three-dimensional network of reticular connective tissue that forms the architectural framework of the entire lymph node.

The afferent lymph vessels pierce the capsule on the convex surface of the node and empty their lymph into the **subcapsular sinus,** which is located just deep to the capsule. This sinus is continuous with the **cortical sinuses (paratrabecular sinuses)** that parallel the trabeculae and deliver the lymph into the **medullary sinuses,** eventually to enter the **efferent lymphatic vessels.** These sinuses have a network of stellate reticular cells whose processes contact those of other cells and the endothelium-like simple squamous epithelium. **Macrophages,** attached to the stellate reticular cells, avidly phagocytose foreign particulate matter. Additionally, lymphoid cells can enter or leave the sinusoids by passing between their squamous cell lining.

Lymphoid Nodules

There are two types of lymphoid nodules: primary and secondary. Secondary lymphoid nodules have a germinal center.

The incomplete compartments within the cortex house **primary lymphoid nodules,** which are spherical aggregates of B lymphocytes (both virgin B cells and B memory cells) that are in the process of entering or

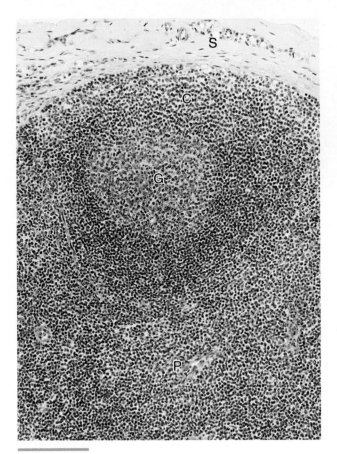

Figure 12–8 Light micrograph of the lymph node cortex (×132), displaying the subcapsular sinus (S), a secondary lymphoid nodule with its corona (C), germinal center (G), and the paracortex (P).

leaving the lymph node (see Figs. 12-7 and 12-8). Frequently, the centers of the lymphoid nodules are stained pale and house **germinal centers,** and these lymph nodes are then known as **secondary lymphoid nodules.** Secondary lymphoid nodules form only in response to an antigenic challenge; it is believed that they are the sites of B memory cell and plasma cell generation.

The region of the lymphoid nodule peripheral to the germinal center is composed of a dense accumulation of small lymphocytes that are migrating away from their site of origin within the germinal center. This peripheral region is called the **corona (mantle).**

Germinal centers display three zones: a dark zone, a basal light zone, and an apical light zone. The **dark zone** is the site of the intense proliferation of closely packed B cells (that do not possess sIgs). These cells, know as **centroblasts,** migrate into the **basal light zone,** express sIgs, switch immunoglobulin class, and are known as **centrocytes.** These cells are exposed to antigen-bearing **follicular dendritic cells** and

undergo hypermutation to become more proficient at forming antibodies against the antigen. Cells that do not synthesize the proper sIgs are forced into apoptosis and are destroyed by macrophages. The newly formed centrocytes that are permitted to survive enter the **apical light zone,** where they become either **B memory cells** or **plasma cells** and subsequently leave the secondary follicle.

Paracortex

The region of the lymph node between the cortex and the medulla is the paracortex. It houses mostly T cells and is the thymus-dependent zone of the lymph node.

APCs (e.g., Langerhans cells from skin or dendritic cells from the mucosa) migrate to the paracortex region of the lymph node to present their epitope–MHC II complex to T_H cells. If T_H cells become activated, they proliferate, increasing the width of the paracortex to such an extent that it may intrude deep into the medulla. Newly formed T cells then migrate to the medullary sinuses, leave the lymph node, and proceed to the area of antigenic activity.

High endothelial venules (HEVs) are located in the paracortex. Lymphocytes leave the vascular supply by migrating between the cuboidal cells of this unusual endothelium and enter the substance of the lymph node. B cells migrate to the outer cortex, whereas most T cells remain in the paracortex.

The lymphocyte plasma membrane expresses surface molecules, known as **selectins,** that aid the cell in recognizing the endothelial cells of HEVs and permit it to roll along the surface of these cells. When the lymphocyte contacts additional signaling molecules that are located on the endothelial cell plasmalemma, the selectins become activated, bind firmly to the endothelial cell, and stop the rolling action of the lymphocyte. Then, via **diapedesis,** the lymphocyte migrates between the cuboidal endothelial cells to leave the lumen of the postcapillary venule and enter the lymph node parenchyma.

Medulla

The medulla is composed of large, tortuous lymph sinuses surrounded by lymphoid cells that are organized in clusters known as medullary cords.

The cells of the medullary cords (lymphocytes, plasma cells, and macrophages) are enmeshed in a network of reticular fibers and reticular cells (Fig. 12-9; also see Fig. 12-7). The lymphocytes migrate from the cortex to enter the medullary sinuses, from which they enter the efferent lymphatic vessels to leave the lymph node. Histological sections of the medulla also display the presence of trabeculae arising from the thickened capsule

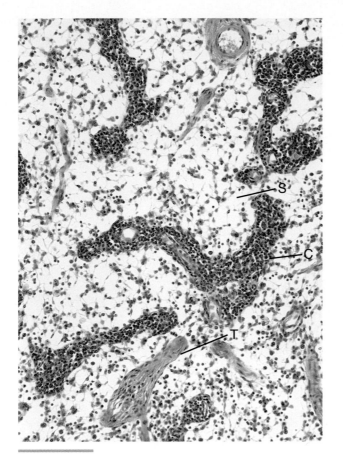

Figure 12–9 Light micrograph of the lymph node medulla (×132) with its medullary sinusoids (S), medullary cords (C), and trabecula (T).

of the hilum, conveying blood vessels into and out of the lymph node.

Vascularization of the Lymph Node

The arterial supply enters the substance of lymph nodes at the hilum. The vessels course through the medulla within trabeculae and become smaller as they repeatedly branch. Eventually, they lose their connective tissue sheath, travel within the substance of medullary cords, and contribute to the formation of the medullary capillary beds. The small branches of the arteries continue in the medullary cords until they reach the cortex. Here they form a cortical capillary bed, which is drained by **postcapillary venules.** Blood from postcapillary venules drains into larger veins, which exit the lymph node at the hilum.

Histophysiology of Lymph Nodes

Lymph nodes filter lymph and act as sites for antigen recognition.

As lymph enters the lymph node, the flow rate is reduced, which gives the macrophages that reside in (or have their processes intrude into) the sinuses more time to phagocytose foreign particulate matter. In this fashion, 99% of the impurities found in lymph are removed.

Lymph nodes also function as sites of antigen recognition, because APCs that contact antigens migrate to the nearest lymph node and present their epitope–MHC complex to lymphocytes. Additionally, antigens percolating through the lymph node are trapped by **follicular dendritic cells,** and lymphocytes that are in the lymph node or migrate into the lymph node recognize the antigen.

If an antigen is recognized and a B cell becomes activated, that B cell migrates to a **primary lymphoid nodule** and proliferates, forming a germinal center, and the primary lymphoid nodule becomes known as a **secondary lymphoid nodule.** The newly formed cells differentiate into B memory and plasma cells, leave the cortex, and form the medullary cords. About 10% of the newly formed plasma cells stay in the medulla and release antibodies into the medullary sinuses. The remainder of the plasma cells enter the sinuses and go to the bone marrow, where they continue to manufacture antibodies until they die. Some B memory cells stay in the primary lymphoid nodules of the cortex, but most leave the lymph node to take up residence in other secondary lymphatic organs of the body. Therefore, if there is a second exposure to the same antigen, a large number of memory cells are available so that the body can mount a prompt and potent secondary response.

CLINICAL CORRELATIONS

Lymph nodes are located along the paths of lymph vessels and form a chain of lymph nodes so that lymph flows from one node to the next. For this reason, infection can spread and malignant cells may metastasize through a chain of nodes to remote regions of the body.

Spleen

The spleen, the largest lymphoid organ in the body, is invested by a collagenous connective tissue capsule. It has a convex surface and a concave aspect known as the hilum.

The spleen, the largest lymphoid organ in the body, is located in the peritoneum in the upper left quadrant of the abdominal cavity. Its dense, irregular fibroelastic connective tissue capsule, occasionally housing **smooth muscle cells,** is surrounded by visceral peritoneum. The simple squamous epithelium of the peritoneum provides a smooth surface for the spleen. The spleen functions not only in the immunological capacity of antibody formation and T-cell and B-cell proliferation but also as a filter of the blood in destroying old erythrocytes. During fetal development, the spleen is a hemopoietic organ; if necessary, it can resume that function in the adult. Additionally, in some animals (but not in humans), the spleen acts as a reservoir of red blood cells, which may be released into circulation as the need arises.

The spleen has a convex surface as well as a concave aspect known as the **hilum.** The capsule of the spleen is thickened at the hilum, and it is here where arteries and their accompanying nerve fibers enter and veins and lymph vessels leave the spleen.

The trabeculae, arising from the capsule, carry blood vessels into and out of the parenchyma of the spleen (Fig. 12-10). Histologically, the spleen has a three-dimensional network of **reticular fibers** and

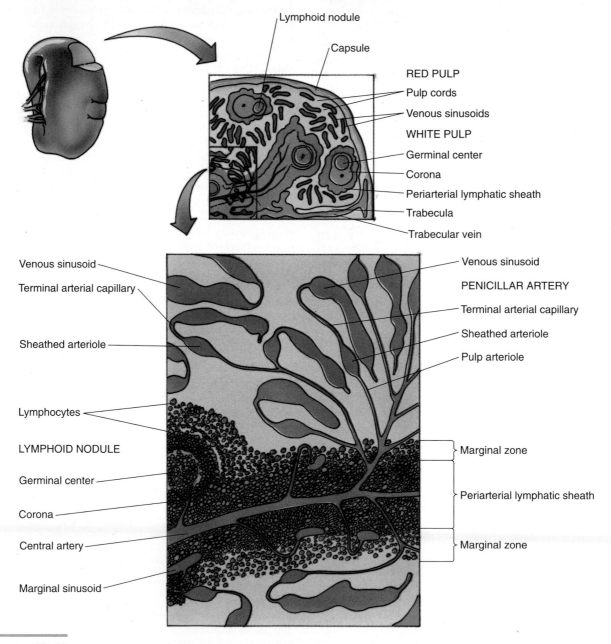

Figure 12–10
Schematic diagram of the spleen. *Top,* Low-magnification view of white pulp and red pulp. *Bottom,* Higher-magnification view of the central arteriole and its branches.

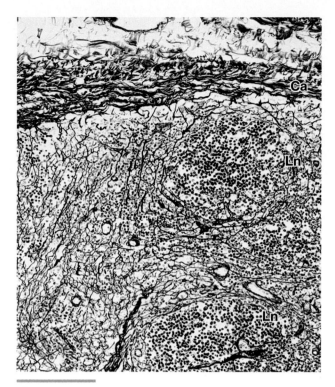

Figure 12–11 Silver-stained photomicrograph of the reticular fiber architecture of the spleen (×132). Note the capsule (Ca) and lymphoid nodule (Ln).

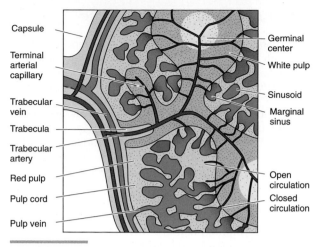

Figure 12–12 Open and closed circulation in the spleen.

associated reticular cells. The reticular fiber network is attached to the capsule as well as to the trabeculae and forms the architectural framework of this organ (Fig. 12-11).

The interstices of the reticular tissue network are occupied by **venous sinuses,** trabeculae conveying blood vessels, and the splenic parenchyma. The cut surface of a fresh spleen shows gray areas surrounded by red areas; the former are called **white pulp** and the latter are known as **red pulp.** Central to the appreciation of the organization and function of the spleen is an understanding of its blood supply.

Vascular Supply of the Spleen

The spleen is supplied by the splenic artery and is drained by the splenic vein; both vessels enter and leave the spleen at the hilum.

The splenic artery branches repeatedly as it pierces the connective tissue capsule at the hilum of the spleen. Branches of these vessels, **trabecular arteries,** are conveyed into the substance of the spleen by trabeculae of decreasing sizes (see Fig. 12-10). When the trabecular arteries are reduced to about 0.2 mm in diameter, they leave the trabeculae. The tunica adven-

titia of these vessels that left the trabeculae become loosely organized, and they become infiltrated by a sheath of lymphocytes, the **periarterial lymphatic sheath (PALS).** Because this vessel occupies the center of the PALS, it is called the **central artery.**

At its termination, the central splenic artery loses its lymphatic sheath and subdivides into several short, parallel branches, known as **penicillar arteries,** which enter the red pulp. The penicillar arteries have three regions: (1) the **pulp arteriole,** (2) the **sheathed arteriole** (a thickened region of the vessel surrounded by a sheath of macrophages termed the Schweigger-Seidel sheath), and (3) the **terminal arterial capillaries.**

Although it is known that the terminal arterial capillaries deliver their blood into the splenic sinuses, the method of delivery is not completely understood, which has prompted the formulation of three theories of spleen circulation: (1) closed circulation, (2) open circulation, and (3) a combination of the first two theories.

Proponents of the **closed circulation theory** believe that the endothelial lining of the terminal arterial capillaries is continuous with the sinus endothelium (Fig. 12-12). Investigators who subscribe to the **open circulation theory** believe that the terminal arterial capillaries terminate prior to reaching the sinusoids, and blood from these vessels percolates through the red pulp into the sinuses. Still other investigators believe that some vessels connect to the sinusoids and that other vessels terminate as open-ended channels in the red pulp, suggesting that the spleen has both **open and closed systems of circulation.**

Splenic sinuses are drained by small **veins of the pulp,** which are tributaries of larger and larger veins that merge to form the **splenic vein,** a tributary of the **portal vein.**

White Pulp and Marginal Zone

The white pulp is composed of the periarterial lymphatic sheath housing T cells, and lymphoid nodules housing B cells. The marginal zone houses B cells that are specialized to recognize thymic-independent antigens.

The structure of the white pulp is closely associated with the central arteriole. The PALS that surrounds the central arteriole is composed of T lymphocytes. Frequently, enclosed within the PALS are **lymphoid nodules,** which are composed of B cells and displace the central arteriole to a peripheral position. Lymphoid nodules may display **germinal centers,** indicative of antigenic challenge (Fig. 12-13; see Fig. 12-10). The PALS and lymphoid nodules constitute the white pulp, and as in the lymph node, the T and B cells are stationed in specific locations.

The white pulp is surrounded by a **marginal zone,** 100 μm in width, that separates the white pulp from the

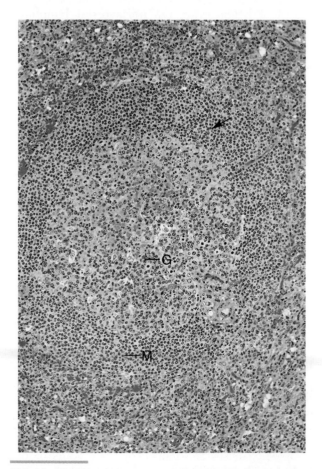

Figure 12–13 Light micrograph of the white pulp and marginal zone of the spleen (×116). G, germinal center; M, marginal zone. Note the central artery (*arrow*).

red pulp (Fig. 12-14; see Figs. 12-10 and 12-13). This zone is composed of plasma cells, T and B lymphocytes, macrophages, and **interdigitating dendritic cells** (APCs). Additionally, numerous small vascular channels, **marginal sinuses,** are present in the marginal zone, especially surrounding lymphoid nodules. Slender blood vessels, radiating from the central arteriole, pass into the red pulp, recur, and deliver their blood into the marginal sinuses.

Because the spaces between the endothelial cells of these sinuses may be as wide as 2 to 3 μm, it is here that blood-borne cells, antigens, and particulate matter have their first free access to the parenchyma of the spleen. Thus the following events occur at the marginal zone:

1 APCs sample the material traveling in blood, searching for antigens.
2 Macrophages attack microorganisms present in the blood.
3 The circulating pool of T and B lymphocytes leaves the bloodstream to enter its preferred locations within the white pulp.
4 Lymphocytes come into contact with the interdigitating dendritic cells; if they recognize their epitope-MHC complex, the lymphocytes initiate an immune response within the white pulp.
5 B cells recognize and react to thymus-independent antigens (such as polysaccharides of bacterial cell walls).

Red Pulp

The red pulp of the spleen is composed of splenic sinuses and splenic cords (of Billroth).

The red pulp resembles a sponge, in that the spaces within the sponge represent the sinuses and the sponge material among the spaces denotes the splenic cords (see Fig. 12-10).

The endothelial lining of **splenic sinuses** is unusual in that its cells are fusiform, resembling staves of a barrel (Fig. 12-15). Moreover, spaces (2 to 3 μm wide) between adjoining cells are common. The sinuses are surrounded by reticular fibers (continuous with those of the splenic cords) that wrap around the sinuses as individual, thin strands of thread. The reticular fibers are arranged perpendicular to the longitudinal axis of the sinuses and are coated by **basal lamina.** Thus, splenic sinuses have a discontinuous basal lamina.

The **splenic cords** are composed of a loose network of reticular fibers, whose interstices are permeated by extravasated blood. The reticular fibers are enveloped by **stellate reticular cells,** which isolate the type III collagen fibers from blood, preventing a platelet reaction to the collagen (coagulation). **Macrophages** are particularly numerous in the vicinity of the sinusoids.

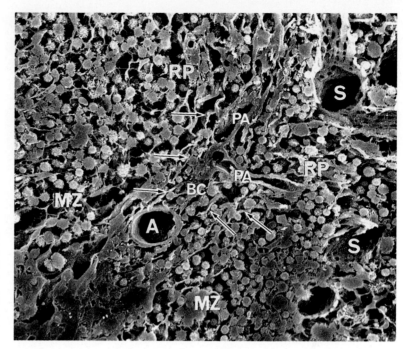

Figure 12–14 Scanning electron micrograph of the marginal zone and adjoining red pulp of the spleen (×680). Note the periarterial flat reticular cells (*arrows*). A, central artery; BC, marginal zone bridging channel; MZ, marginal zone; PA, penicillar artery; RP, red pulp; S, venous sinus. (From Sasou S, Sugai T: Periarterial lymphoid sheath in the rat spleen: A light, transmission, and scanning electron microscopic study. Anat Rec 232:15-24, 1992.)

Histophysiology of the Spleen

The spleen filters the blood, forms lymphoid cells, eliminates or inactivates blood-borne antigens, destroys aged platelets and erythrocytes, and participates in hemopoiesis.

As blood enters the marginal sinuses of the marginal zone, it flows past a macrophage-rich zone. These cells phagocytose blood-borne antigens, bacteria, and other foreign particulate matter. Material that is not eliminated in the marginal zone is cleared in the red pulp at the periphery of the splenic sinuses.

Lymphoid cells are formed in the white pulp in response to an antigenic challenge. B memory cells and plasma cells are formed in lymphoid nodules, whereas T cells of various subcategories are formed in the PALS. The newly formed B and T cells enter the marginal sinuses and migrate to the site of antigenic challenge or become part of the circulating pool of lymphocytes. Some plasma cells may stay in the marginal zone, manufacture antibodies, and release immunoglobulins into the marginal sinuses. Most plasma cells, however, migrate to the bone marrow to manufacture and release their antibodies into the bone marrow sinuses.

Soluble blood-borne antigens are inactivated by the antibodies formed against them, whereas bacteria become **opsonized** and are eliminated by macrophages or neutrophils. Virus-transformed cells are killed by CTLs formed in the PALS of the white pulp.

Macrophages kill aged platelets and monitor erythrocytes as they migrate from the splenic cords between the endothelial cells into the sinuses (Fig. 12-16). Because older erythrocytes lose their flexibility (as do erythrocytes infected by the malarial parasite), they cannot penetrate the spaces between the endothelial cells and are phagocytosed by macrophages. The phagocytes also monitor the surface coats of red blood cells, which are destroyed in the following manner:

1 Old erythrocytes lose sialic acid residues from their surface macromolecules, exposing galactose moieties.
2 Galactose moieties that are exposed on erythrocyte membranes induce their phagocytosis.
3 Erythrocytes phagocytosed by macrophages are destroyed within phagosomes.
4 Hemoglobin is catabolized into its heme and globin portions.
5 The globin moiety is disassembled into its constituent amino acids, which become part of the circulating amino-acid pool of the blood.
6 Iron molecules are conveyed to the bone marrow by **transferrin** and are used in the formation of new red blood cells.
7 Heme is converted to **bilirubin** and excreted by the liver in **bile.**
8 Macrophages also phagocytose damaged or defunct platelets and neutrophils.

During the second trimester of gestation, the spleen actively participates in **hemopoiesis;** after birth,

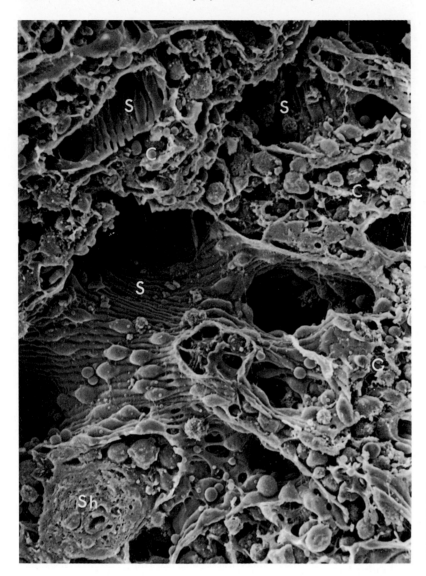

Figure 12–15 Scanning electron micrograph of sinusoidal lining cells bounded by splenic cords (×500). C, splenic cords; S, venous sinuses; Sh, sheathed arteriole. (From Leeson TS, Leeson CR, Paparo AA: Text-Atlas of Histology. Philadelphia, WB Saunders, 1988.)

however, blood cell formation occurs only in the bone marrow. If the necessity arises, the spleen can resume its hemopoietic function.

CLINICAL CORRELATIONS

Because the spleen is a friable (fragile) organ, major trauma to the upper left abdominal quadrant may cause rupture of the spleen. In severe cases, the spleen may be removed surgically, without compromising a person's life. Aged red blood cells are then phagocytosed by macrophages of the liver and bone marrow.

Mucosa-Associated Lymphoid Tissue

Mucosa-associated lymphoid tissue (MALT) is composed of a nonencapsulated, localized lymphocyte infiltration and lymphoid nodules in the mucosa of the gastrointestinal, respiratory, and urinary tracts. The best examples of these accumulations are those associated with the mucosa of the gut: **gut-associated lymphoid tissue (GALT), bronchus-associated lymphatic tissue (BALT),** and the **tonsils.**

Gut-Associated Lymphoid Tissue

The most prominent accumulation of GALT is located in the ileum and is known as Peyer's patches.

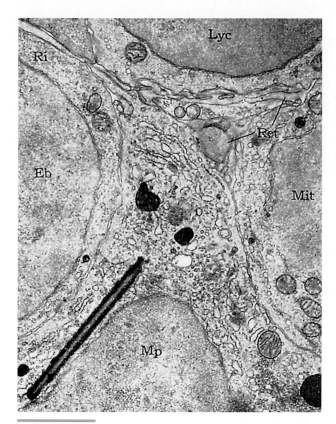

Figure 12–16 Electron micrograph of a macrophage containing phagocytosed materials, including a crystalloid body. Mp, macrophage; Mit, cell undergoing mitosis; Lyc, lymphocyte; Eb, erythroblast; Ret, reticular fibers in the interstitial spaces; Ri, ribosome. (From Rhodin JAG: An Atlas of Ultrastructure. Philadelphia, WB Saunders, 1963.)

GALT is composed of lymphoid follicles along the length of the gastrointestinal tract. Most of the lymphoid follicles are isolated from each other; in the ileum, however, they form lymphoid aggregates, known as **Peyer's patches** (Fig. 12-17). The lymphoid follicles of Peyer's patches are composed of B cells surrounded by a looser region of T cells and numerous APCs.

Although the ileum is lined by a simple columnar epithelium, the regions immediately adjacent to the lymphoid follicles are lined by squamous-like cells, known as **M cells (microfold cells).** It is believed that M cells capture antigens and transfer them (without first processing them into epitopes) to macrophages located in Peyer's patches (see Chapter 17).

Peyer's patches have no afferent lymphatic vessels, but they do have efferent lymph drainage. They receive small arterioles that form a capillary bed, drained by HEVs. Lymphocytes destined to enter Peyer's patches have homing receptors that are specific for the HEVs of GALT.

Bronchus-Associated Lymphoid Tissue

BALT is similar to Peyer's patches, except that it is located in the walls of bronchi, especially in regions where bronchi and bronchioles bifurcate. As in GALT, the epithelial cover over these lymphoid nodules changes from a pseudostratified ciliated columnar with goblet cells to **M cells.**

Afferent lymph vessels are absent, although lymph drainage has been demonstrated. The rich vascular supply of BALT indicates its possible systemic as well as localized role in the immune process. Most of the cells are B cells, although APCs and T cells are present. Lymphocytes destined to enter BALT have homing receptors that are specific for the HEVs of this lymphoid tissue.

The Tonsils

The tonsils (palatine, pharyngeal, and lingual) are incompletely encapsulated aggregates of lymphoid nodules that guard the entrance to the oral pharynx. Because of their locations, the tonsils are interposed into the path of airborne and ingested antigens. They react to these antigens by forming lymphocytes and mounting an immune response.

The bilateral **palatine tonsils** are located at the boundary of the oral cavity and the oral pharynx, between the palatoglossal and the palatopharyngeal folds. The deep aspect of each palatine tonsil is isolated from the surrounding connective tissue by a dense, fibrous **capsule.** The superficial aspect of the tonsils is covered by a stratified squamous nonkeratinized epithelium that dips into the 10 to 12 deep **crypts** that invaginate the tonsilar parenchyma. The crypts frequently contain food debris, desquamated epithelial cells, dead leukocytes, bacteria, and other antigenic substances.

The parenchyma of the tonsil is composed of numerous lymphoid nodules, many of which display germinal centers, indicative of B-cell formation.

The single **pharyngeal tonsil** is in the roof of the nasal pharynx. It is similar to the palatine tonsils, but its incomplete capsule is thinner. Instead of crypts, the pharyngeal tonsil has shallow, longitudinal infoldings called **pleats.** Ducts of seromucous glands open into the base of the pleats. Its superficial surface is covered by a pseudostratified ciliated columnar epithelium that is interspersed with patches of stratified squamous epithelium (Fig. 12-18).

The parenchyma of the pharyngeal tonsil is composed of lymphoid nodules, some of which have germinal centers. When this type of tonsil is inflamed, it is called the **adenoid.**

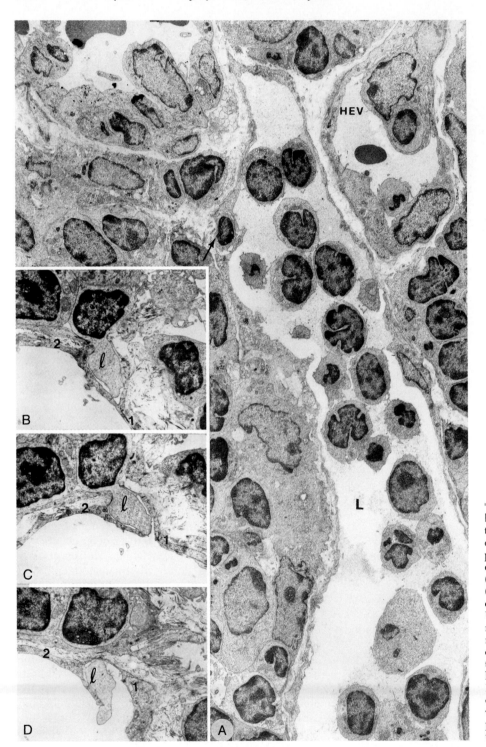

Figure 12–17 Transmission electron micrographs. **A,** ALPA vessel (L) of the interfollicular area full of lymphocytes that has an intraendothelial channel that includes lymphocytes (*arrow*) in the endothelial wall (×3000). Note the postcapillary high endothelium venula (HEV). **B-D,** Ultrathin serial sections that document various stages of lymphoctye migration through an intraendothelial channel composed of one (1) and two (2) endothelial cells (×9000). *ℓ,* lymphocyte. (From Azzali G, Arcari MA: Ultrastructural and three-dimensional aspects of the lymphatic vessels of the absorbing peripheral lymphatic apparatus in Peyer's patches of the rabbit. Anat Rec 258:76; 2000.)

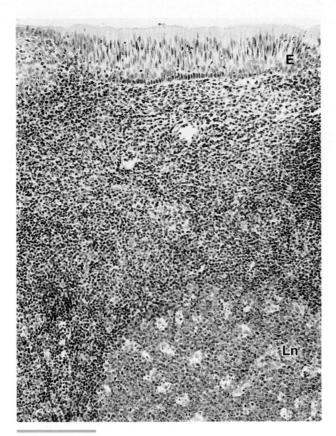

Figure 12–18 Light micrograph of a lymphoid nodule (Ln) of the pharyngeal tonsil, displaying its pseudostratified ciliated columnar epithelium (E) and a germinal center of the secondary nodule (×132).

The **lingual tonsil** is located on the dorsal surface of the posterior one third of the tongue and is covered, on its superficial aspect, by a stratified squamous nonkeratinized epithelium. The deep aspect of the lingual tonsil has a flimsy capsule that separates it from the underlying connective tissue. The tonsil has numerous crypts, whose bases receive the ducts of mucous minor salivary glands. The parenchyma of the lingual tonsil is composed of lymphoid nodules, which frequently have germinal centers.

Endocrine System

13

The endocrine system regulates metabolic activities in certain organs and tissues of the body, thereby helping to bring about homeostasis. The autonomic nervous system regulates certain organs and tissues via impulses that initiate the release of neurotransmitter substances, that produce rapid responses in the tissues that are affected. However, the endocrine system produces a slow and diffused effect via chemical substances called **hormones,** which are released into the bloodstream to influence target cells at remote sites. Although the nervous and endocrine systems function in different ways, the two systems interact to modulate and coordinate the metabolic activities of the body.

The **endocrine system** consists of **ductless glands,** distinct clusters of cells within certain organs of the body, and **endocrine cells,** isolated in the epithelial lining of the digestive tract and in the respiratory system. (The latter are discussed in Chapters 17 and 15, respectively.) The **endocrine glands,** the subject of this chapter, are abundantly and richly vascularized so that their secretory product may be released into slender connective tissue spaces between cells and the capillary beds from which they enter the bloodstream. The endocrine glands include the pineal body, the **pituitary gland,** the **thyroid gland,** the **parathyroid glands,** and the **suprarenal glands.** Unlike the endocrine glands, which are ductless, the various exocrine glands (discussed in other chapters) empty their secretions in a duct system and exert only local effects.

HORMONES

Hormones are chemical messengers that are produced by endocrine glands and delivered by the bloodstream to target cells or organs.

The chemical nature of a hormone dictates its mechanism of action. Most hormones elicit several effects on their target cells (e.g., short-term and long-term effects). Hormones are classified into three types based on their composition:

- **Proteins and polypeptides**—mostly water-soluble (e.g., insulin, glucagon, and follicle-stimulating hormone [FSH]).
- **Amino-acid derivatives**—mostly water-soluble (e.g., thyroxine and epinephrine).
- **Steroid and fatty acid derivatives**—mostly lipid-soluble (e.g., progesterone, estradiol, and testosterone).

Once a hormone has been released into the bloodstream and has arrived in the vicinity of its target cells, it first binds to specific receptors on (or in) the target cell. Receptors for certain hormones (mostly protein and peptide hormones) are located on the plasmalemma **(cell-surface receptors)** of the target cell, whereas other receptors are located in the cytoplasm and bind only to hormones that have diffused through the plasmalemma. The binding of a hormone to its receptor communicates a message to the target cell, initiating **signal transduction,** or translation of the signal into a biochemical reaction.

Thyroid and steroid hormones bind to cytoplasmic receptors. The resulting hormone-receptor complex translocates to the nucleus, where it binds directly to deoxyribonucleic acid (DNA) close to a promoter site, thereby stimulating gene transcription. However, at least some steroid hormones may bind to receptors that are located in the target cell plasma membrane, and thus the hormone's actions may be mediated directly without gene transcription or protein synthesis. Neither the hormone nor the receptor alone can initiate the target cell response.

Hormones that bind to cell-surface receptors located in the plasmalemma use several different mechanisms to elicit a response in their target cells. In each instance, the hormone-receptor complex is believed to induce a protein kinase to phosphorylate certain regulatory proteins, thereby generating a biological response to the hormone. For example, some hormone-receptor complexes stimulate adenylate cyclase to synthesize cyclic adenosine monophosphate (cAMP), which stimulates protein kinase A in the cytosol. In such an instance, cAMP acts as a **second messenger.** Several additional second messengers have been identified, including: (1) **cyclic guanosine 3′,5′-monophosphate (cGMP),** (2) **metabolites of phosphatidylinositol,** (3) **calcium ions,** and (4) **sodium ions** (in neurons).

Some hormone receptor complexes are associated with guanosine triphosphate-binding proteins (**G proteins),** which couple the receptor to the hormone-induced responses of the target cells. The receptors for epinephrine, thyroid-stimulating hormone (TSH), and serotonin, for example, use G proteins to activate a second messenger, which elicits a metabolic response. Other hormones, such as insulin and growth hormone, use **catalytic receptors** that activate protein kinases to phosphorylate target proteins.

Once a hormone activates its target cell, an inhibitory signal is generated and returned to the endocrine gland (**feedback mechanism),** either directly or indirectly, to halt hormone secretion. The feedback mechanism also operates in another way: When the hormone level is inadequate to elicit a sufficient metabolic response in the target, a positive feedback signal is released, travels to the endocrine gland, and initiates an increase in hormone secretion. Through the feedback mechanism, therefore, regulation of the endocrine glands maintains homeostasis.

Many of the hormones that circulate in the bloodstream are in oversupply. They are usually bound to plasma proteins, which makes them biologically inactive, but they can be released from their bound state quickly, thus becoming active. Hormones become permanently inactivated in their target tissue; additionally, they may be degraded and destroyed in the liver and kidneys.

PITUITARY GLAND (HYPOPHYSIS)

The pituitary gland, composed of portions derived from oral ectoderm and from neural ectoderm, produces hormones that regulate growth, metabolism, and reproduction.

The pituitary gland, or **hypophysis,** is an endocrine gland that produces several hormones that are responsible for regulating growth, reproduction, and metabolism. It has two subdivisions, which develop from different embryologic sources: (1) the **adenohypophysis** develops from an evagination of the oral ectoderm (**Rathke's pouch)** that lines the primitive oral cavity (stomadeum), and (2) the **neurohypophysis** develops

from neural ectoderm as a downgrowth of the diencephalon. Subsequently, both the adenohypophysis and the neurohypophysis are joined and encapsulated into a single gland. Because each subdivision has a distinctly different embryonic origin, however, the cellular constituents and the functions of each differ.

The pituitary gland lies below the hypothalamus of the brain, to which it is connected extending inferiorly from the diencephalon. It sits in the hypophyseal fossa, a bony depression in the sella turcica of the sphenoid bone that is lined by dura mater and covered over by a portion of the dura mater called the **diaphragma sellae.** The gland measures approximately 1 cm by 1 to 1.5 cm; it is 0.5 cm thick and weighs about 0.5 g in men and slightly more in women.

The pituitary is connected to the brain by neural pathways; it also has a rich vascular supply from vessels that supply the brain, attesting to the intercoordination of the two systems in maintaining a physiological balance. Indeed, secretion of nearly all of the hormones produced by the pituitary gland is controlled by either hormonal or nerve signals from the hypothalamus. In addition to controlling the pituitary, the hypothalamus also receives input from various areas of the central nervous system (i.e., information regarding plasma circulating levels of electrolytes and hormones) and controls the autonomic nervous system; therefore, the hypothalamus is the brain center for the maintenance of homeostasis.

Within each subdivision of the hypophysis are various regions having specialized cells that release different hormones (Figs. 13-1 and 13-2). The subdivisions of the hypophysis and the names of the regions are:

■ Adenohypophysis (anterior pituitary)
  ■ Pars distalis (pars anterior)
  ■ Pars intermedia
  ■ Pars tuberalis
■ Neurohypophysis (posterior pituitary)
  ■ Median eminence
  ■ Infundibulum
  ■ Pars nervosa

Interposed between the anterior and posterior lobes of the pituitary gland are remnants of Rathke's pouch (epithelial cells), which surround an amorphous colloid. The pars tuberalis forms a sleeve around the stem of the infundibulum.

Blood Supply and Control of Secretion

The hypophyseal portal system of veins delivers neurosecretory hormones from the primary capillary plexus of the median eminence to the secondary capillary plexus of the pars distalis.

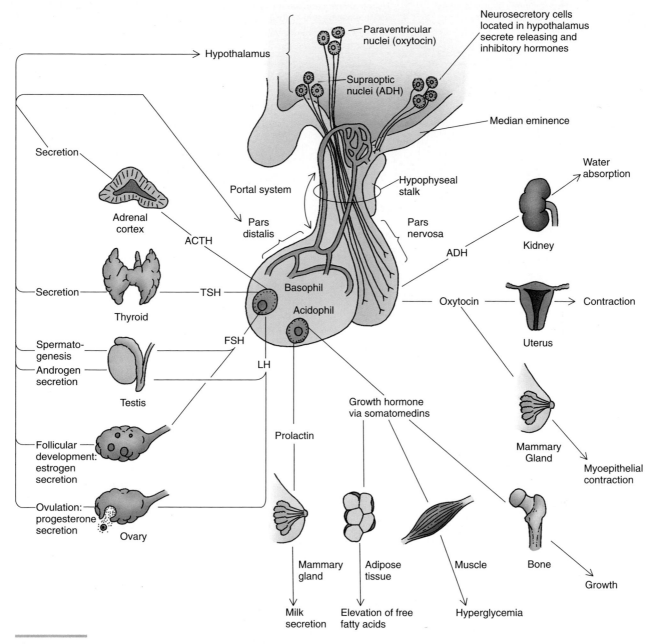

Figure 13–1 The pituitary gland and its target organs. ACTH, adrenocorticotropic hormone; ADH, antidiuretic hormone; FSH, follicle-stimulating hormone; LH, luteinizing hormone; TSH, thyroid-stimulating hormone.

The arterial supply for the pituitary gland is provided from two pairs of vessels that arise from the internal carotid artery (see Fig. 13-2). The **superior hypophyseal arteries** supply the pars tuberalis and the infundibulum. They also form an extensive capillary network, the **primary capillary plexus,** in the median eminence. **Inferior hypophyseal arteries** primarily supply the posterior lobe, although they also send a few branches to the anterior lobe.

Hypophyseal portal veins drain the primary capillary plexus of the median eminence, which delivers its blood into the **secondary capillary plexus,** located in the pars distalis (see Fig. 13-2). The capillaries of both plexuses axe fenestrated. **Hypothalamic**

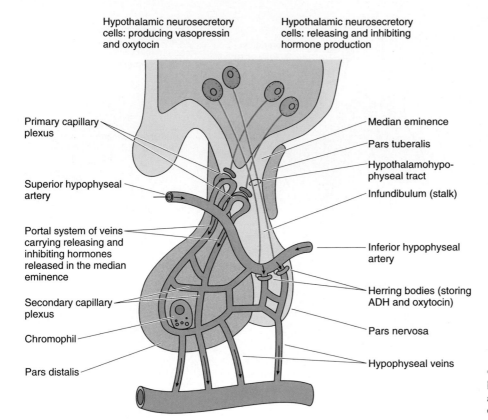

Hypothalamic neurosecretory cells: producing vasopressin and oxytocin

Hypothalamic neurosecretory cells: releasing and inhibiting hormone production

Primary capillary plexus

Superior hypophyseal artery

Portal system of veins carrying releasing and inhibiting hormones released in the median eminence

Secondary capillary plexus

Chromophil

Pars distalis

Median eminence

Pars tuberalis

Hypothalamohypo-physeal tract

Infundibulum (stalk)

Inferior hypophyseal artery

Herring bodies (storing ADH and oxytocin)

Pars nervosa

Hypophyseal veins

Figure 13–2 The pituitary gland and its circulatory system. ADH, anti-diuretic hormone.

neurosecretory hormones, manufactured in the hypothalamus and stored in the median eminence, enter the primary capillary plexus and are drained by the hypophyseal portal veins, which course through the infundibulum and connect to the secondary capillary plexus in the anterior lobe. Here the neurosecretory hormones leave the blood to stimulate or inhibit the parenchymal cells. Thus, the hypophyseal portal system is the vascular supply system that is used for hormonal regulation of the pars distalis by the hypothalamus.

Axons of neurons that originate in various portions of the hypothalamus terminate around these capillary plexuses. The endings of these axons differ from other axons of the body, because instead of delivering a signal to another cell, they liberate either **releasing** or **inhibiting hormones (factors)** directly into the primary capillary bed. These hormones are taken by the hypophyseal portal system and delivered to the secondary capillary bed of the pars distalis, where they regulate secretion of various anterior pituitary hormones. The following are the main releasing and inhibitory hormones (factors):

- **Thyroid-stimulating hormone–releasing hormone (thyrotropin-releasing hormone [TRH])** stimulates the release of TSH.

- **Corticotropin-releasing hormone (CRH)** stimulates the release of adrenocorticotropin.
- **Somatotropin-releasing hormone (SRH)** stimulates the release of somatotropin (growth hormone).
- **Luteinizing hormone–releasing hormone (LHRH)** stimulates the release of luteinizing hormone (LH) and FSH.
- **Prolactin-releasing hormone (PRH)** stimulates the release of prolactin.
- **Prolactin inhibitory factor (PIF)** inhibits prolactin secretion.

The physiological effects of pituitary hormones are summarized in Table 13-1.

Adenohypophysis

The anterior pituitary gland, the adenohypophysis, develops from Rathke's pouch, a diverticulum of the oral ectoderm. The adenohypophysis consists of the pars distalis, the pars intermedia, and the pars tuberalis.

Pars Distalis

The parenchymal cells of the pars distalis consist of the chromophils and chromophobes.

TABLE 13–1 Physiological Effects of Pituitary Hormones

Hormon	Releasing/Inhibiting	Function
Pars Distalis		
Somatotropin (growth hormone)	*Releasing:* SRH *Inhibiting:* Somatostatin	Generalized effect on most cells is to increase metabolic rates, stimulate liver cells to release somatomedins (insulin-like growth factors I and II), which increases proliferation of cartilage and assists in growth in long bones
Prolactin	*Releasing:* PRH *Inhibiting:* PIF	Promotes development of mammary glands during pregnancy; stimulates milk production after parturition (prolactin secretion is stimulated by suckling)
Adrenocorticotropic hormone (ACTH, corticotropin)	*Releasing:* CRH	Stimulates synthesis and release of hormones (cortisol and corticosterone) from suprarenal cortex
Follicle-stimulating hormone (FSH)	*Releasing:* LHRH *Inhibiting:* Inhibin (in males)	Stimulates secondary ovarian follicle growth and estrogen secretion; stimulates Sertoli cells in seminiferous tubules to produce androgen-binding protein
Luteinizing hormone (LH)	*Releasing:* LHRH	Assists FSH in promoting ovulation, formation of the corpus luteum, and secretion of progesterone and estrogen, forming a negative feedback to the hypothalamus to inhibit LHRH in women
Interstitial cell-stimulating hormone (ICSH) in men		Stimulates Leydig cells to secrete and release testosterone, which forms a negative feedback to the hypothalamus to inhibit LHRH in men
Thyroid-stimulating hormone (TSH) (thyrotropin)	*Releasing:* TRH *Inhibiting:* Negative feedback suppresses via the central nervous system	Stimulates synthesis and release of thyroid hormone, which increases metabolic rate
Pars Nervosa		
Oxytocin		Stimulates smooth muscle contractions of the uterus during orgasm; causes contractions of pregnant uterus at parturition (stimulation of cervix sends signal to hypothalamus to secrete more oxytocin); suckling sends signals to hypothalamus, resulting in more oxytocin, causing contractions of myoepithelial cells of the mammary glands, assisting in milk ejection
Vasopressin (antidiuretic hormone [ADH])		Conserves body water by increasing resorption of water by kidneys; thought to be regulated by osmotic pressure; causes contraction of smooth muscles in arteries, thus raising the blood pressure; may restore normal blood pressure after severe hemorrhage

CRH, corticotropin-releasing hormone; LHRH, luteinizing hormone–releasing hormone; PIF, prolactin inhibitory factor; PRH, prolactin-releasing hormone; SRH, somatotropin-releasing hormone; TRH, thyrotropin-releasing hormone.

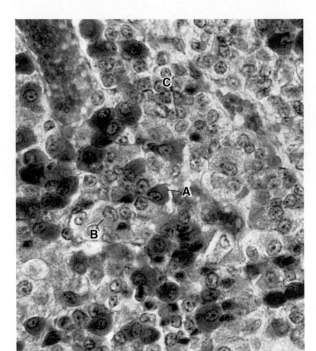

Figure 13–3   Light micrograph of the pituitary gland displaying chromophobes (C), acidophils (A), and basophils (B) (×470).

The pars distalis, or anterior lobe of the pituitary gland, is covered by a fibrous capsule and is composed of cords of parenchymal cells that are surrounded by reticular fibers; these fibers also surround the large sinusoidal capillaries of the secondary capillary plexus. Scant connective tissue is located primarily around the hypophyseal arteries and the portal veins. The endothelial lining of the sinusoids is fenestrated, which facilitates the diffusion of releasing factors to the parenchymal cells and provides entry sites for their released secretions. The parenchymal cells of the pars distalis that have an affinity for dyes are called **chromophils,** whereas those parenchymal cells that have no affinity for dyes are called **chromophobes.** Chromophils are further subdivided into **acidophils** (staining with acid dyes) and **basophils** (staining with basic dyes), which constitute the main secretory cells of the pars distalis (Fig. 13-3). However, it should be noted that these latter designations refer to the affinity of the secretory granules within the cells to the dyes, not to the parenchymal cell cytoplasm.

Chromophils

Secretory granules of chromophils have an affinity for histological dyes: those that stain orange-red with *acid* dyes and those that stain blue with *basic* dyes.

ACIDOPHILS

Acidophils, whose granules stain orange-red with eosin, are of two varieties: somatotrophs and mammotrophs.

The most abundant cells in the pars distalis are acidophils, whose granules are large enough to be seen by the light microscope and stain orange-to-red with eosin (Fig. 13-4).

Somatotrophs, one of the two varieties of the acidophils, have a centrally placed nucleus, a moderate Golgi complex, small rod-shaped mitochondria, abundant rough endoplasmic reticulum (RER), and numerous secretory granulesthat are 300 to 400 nm in diameter. These cells secrete **somatotropin (growth hormone);** thus, they are stimulated by **SRH** and inhibited by **somatostatin.** Somatotropin has a generalized effect of increasing cellular metabolic rates. This hormone also induces liver cells to produce **somatomedins (insulin-like growth factors I and II),** which stimulate mitotic rates of epiphyseal plate chondrocytes and thus promote elongation of long bones and, hence, growth.

Mammotrophs, the other variety of acidophils, are arranged as individual cells rather than as clumps or clusters. These small, polygonal acidophils have the usual unremarkable organelle population; during lactation, however, the organelles enlarge and the Golgi complex may become as large as the nucleus. These cells can be distinguished by their large secretory granules, formed by the fusion of smaller granules that are released by the *trans* Golgi network. These fused granules, which may be 600 nm in diameter, contain the hormone **prolactin,** which promotes mammary gland development during pregnancy as well as lactation after birth.

During pregnancy, circulating estrogen and progesterone inhibit secretion of prolactin. Following birth, estrogen and progesterone levels drop; thus their inhibitory effect is lost. The number of mammotrophs also increases at this time. At the conclusion of nursing, the granules are degraded and the excess mammotrophs regress. Release of prolactin from mammotrophs is stimulated by **prolactin-releasing factor (PRH)** and oxytocin, especially when nursing is taking place, and is inhibited by **PIF.**

BASOPHILS

Basophils, the granules of which stain blue with basic dyes, are of three varieties: corticotrophs, thyrotrophs, and gonadotrophs.

Basophils stain blue with basic dyes (especially with periodic acid–Schiff reagent) and are usually located at the periphery of the pars distalis (see Fig. 13-3).

Corticotrophs, which are scattered throughout the pars distalis, are round to ovoid cells, each with an

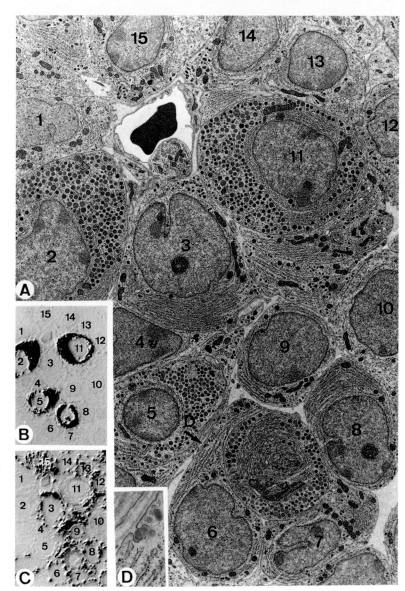

Figure 13–4 Light and electron micrographs of mouse adenohypophysis (×4000). Observe the mammotropes (cells 3, 6-9, 12-15) and somatotropes (cells 2, 5, 11), and note the secretory granules of these cells. (From Yamaji A, Sasaki, F, Iwama Y, Yamauchi S: Mammotropes and somatotropes in the adenophyophysis of androgenized female mice: Morphological and immunohistochemical studies by light microscopy correlated with routine electron microscopy. Anat Rec 233:103-110, 1992.)

eccentric nucleus and relatively few organelles. Their secretory granules are 250 to 400 nm in diameter. Corticotrophs secrete **adrenocorticotropic hormone (ACTH)** and **lipotropic hormone (LPH).** Secretion is stimulated by **CRH.** The hormone ACTH stimulates cells of the suprarenal cortex to release their secretory products.

Thyrotrophs are deeply embedded within cords of the parenchymal cells at a distance from sinusoids. These cells can be distinguished by their small secretory granules (150 nm in diameter), which contain **TSH,** also known as **thyrotropin.** Secretion is stimulated by **TRH** and inhibited by the presence of thyroxine (T_4) and triiodothyronine (T_3) (thyroid hormones) in the blood.

Gonadotrophs are round cells that have a well-developed Golgi complex and abundant RER and mitochondria. Their secretory granules vary in diameter from 200 to 400 nm. Gonadotrophs, situated near sinuses, secrete **FSH** and **LH;** sometimes LH is called **interstitial cell–stimulating hormone (ICSH),** because it stimulates steroid hormone production in interstitial cells of the testes. It remains unclear whether there are two subpopulations of gonadotrophs, one secreting FSH and the other LH, or whether both hormones are produced by one cell in different phases of the secretory cycle. Secretion is stimulated by **LHRH** and is inhibited by various hormones that are produced by the ovaries and testes.

Chromophobes

Chromophobes have very little cytoplasm; therefore, they do not take up stain readily.

Groups of small, weakly staining cells in the pars distalis are called chromophobes (see Fig. 13-3). These cells generally have less cytoplasm than chromophils do, and they may represent either nonspecific stem cells or partly degranulated chromophils, although some retain secretory granules. Because there is evidence for the cyclic nature of the secretory function of the chromophils, it is probable that chromophobes are degranulated chromophils.

Folliculostellate Cells

Nonsecretory folliculostellate cells constitute a large population of cells in the pars distalis. Although their function is not clear, they have long processes that form gap junctions with those of other folliculostellate cells. Whether they physically support parenchymal cells of the anterior pituitary or provide a network of intercommunication with each other is not known.

Pars Intermedia

The pars intermedia lies between the pars distalis and the pars nervosa and contains cysts that are remnants of Rathke's pouch.

The pars intermedia is characterized by many cuboidal, cell-lined, colloid-containing cysts (Rathke's cysts), which are remnants of the ectoderm of the evaginating Rathke's pouch. The pars intermedia, or more accurately in the adult human, the **zona intermedia,** sometimes houses cords of basophils along the networks of capillaries. These basophils synthesize the prohormone **pro-opiomelanocortin (POMC),** which undergoes post-translational cleavage to form **α-melanocyte-stimulating hormone (α-MSH),** corticotropin, β-lipotropin, and β-endorphin. However, it has been suggested that POMC is actually produced by corticotropin cells of the anterior lobe and that the intermediate lobe (or zone) is rudimentary in humans. Although α-MSH stimulates melanin production in lower animals, in humans it may stimulate the release of prolactin and is therefore referred to as **prolactin-releasing factor.**

Pars Tuberalis

The pars tuberalis surrounds the hypophyseal stalk and is composed of cuboidal to low-columnar basophilic cells.

The pars tuberalis surrounds the hypophyseal stalk but frequently is absent on its posterior aspect. Thin layers of pia arachnoid–like connective tissue separate the pars tuberalis from the infundibular stalk. The pars tuberalis is highly vascularized by arteries and the hypophyseal portal system, along which lie longitudinal cords of cuboidal to low-columnar epithelial cells. The cytoplasm of these basophilic cells contains small, dense granules, lipid droplets, interspersed colloid droplets, and glycogen. Although no specific hormones are known to be secreted by the pars tuberalis, some cells contain secretory granules that possibly contain **FSH** and **LH.**

Neurohypophysis

The posterior pituitary gland, the neurohypophysis, develops from a downgrowth of the hypothalamus. The neurohypophysis is divided into the median eminence, the infundibulum (continuation of the hypothalamus), and the pars nervosa (see Fig. 13-1).

Hypothalamohypophyseal Tract

Axons of neurosecretory cells of supraoptic and paraventricular nuclei extend into the posterior pituitary as the hypothalamohypophyseal tract.

Unmyelinated axons of neurosecretory cells, the cell bodies of which lie in the **supraoptic** and **paraventricular nuclei** of the hypothalamus, enter the posterior pituitary to terminate in the vicinity of the capillaries. These axons form the hypothalamohypophyseal tract and constitute the bulk of the posterior pituitary gland. Neurosecretory cells of the supraoptic and paraventricular nuclei synthesize two hormones: **vasopressin (antidiuretic hormone [ADH])** and **oxytocin.** A carrier protein, **neurophysin,** also produced by the cells of these nuclei, binds to each of these hormones as they travel down the axons to the posterior pituitary, where they are released into the bloodstream from the axon terminals.

Pars Nervosa

The pars nervosa of the posterior pituitary gland receives terminals of the neurosecretory hypothalamohypophyseal tract.

Technically, the pars nervosa of the posterior pituitary gland is not an endocrine gland. The distal terminals of the axons of the hypothalamohypophyseal tract (Fig. 13-5) end in the pars nervosa and store the neurosecretions that are produced by their cell bodies, which are located in the hypothalamus. These axons are supported by glia-like cells known as pituicytes. Although only the nuclei of the pituicytes stain well enough to be evident by light microscopy, electron micrographs reveal that one population of axons contains membrane-bound granules of

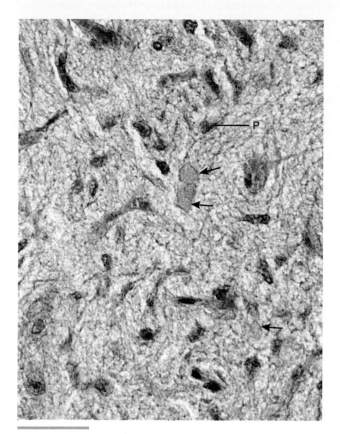

Figure 13–5 Light micrograph of the pars nervosa of the pituitary gland displaying pituicytes (P) and Herring bodies *(arrows)* (×132). Herring bodies are the expanded terminals of the nerve fibers where the neurosecretory products, vasopressin (antidiuretic hormone) and oxytocin are stored.

vasopressin and that another population contains **oxytocin.** Cell bodies of neurons that secrete vasopressin are located chiefly in the supraoptic nucleus of the hypothalamus, whereas cell bodies of neurons that secrete oxytocin are located mostly in the paraventricular nucleus of the hypothalamus. Each of these peptide hormones travel down the axons of their respective neurons in association with a precursor protein known as a **neurophysin.** By the time that they reach the pars nervosa of the hypophysis, the hormones have matured and cleaved from their precursors Chrome-alum hematoxylin staining reveals blue-black distentions of the axons by light microscopy; these are called **Herring bodies,** which represent accumulations of neurosecretory granules (see Fig. 13-5) not only at the termini but also along the length of the axons. In response to nerve stimulation, the contents of these granules are released into the perivascular space near the fenestrated capillaries of the capillary plexus.

The target for vasopressin (ADH) are the collecting ducts of the kidney, where it modulates plasma membrane permeability, which has the effect of lowering urine volume but increasing its concentration (see Chapter 19). The target for oxytocin is the myometrium of the uterus, where it is released in the late phases of pregnancy. During labor, oxytocin is believed to play a role in parturition by stimulating contraction of the smooth muscles of the uterus. Additionally, oxytocin functions in milk ejection from the mammary gland by stimulating contraction of the myoepithelial cells surrounding the glandular alveoli and the ducts of the mammary gland (see Chapter 20).

Pituicytes occupy about 25% of the volume of the pars nervosa. They are similar to neuroglial cells and help support the axons of the pars nervosa by ensheathing them as well as their dilations. Pituicytes contain lipid droplets, lipochrome pigment, and intermediate filaments; they have numerous cytoplasmic processes that contact and form gap junctions with each other. Beyond supporting the neural elements in the pars nervosa, additional functions of pituicytes have not been elucidated. However, it is believed that they may contribute a trophic function to the normal operation of the neurosecretory axon terminals and neurohypophysis.

CLINICAL CORRELATIONS

Pituitary adenomas are common tumors of the anterior pituitary gland. Their growth and enlargement may suppress hormonal production in other secretory cells of the pars distalis. When left unattended, these adenomas may erode surrounding bone and other neural tissues.

Diabetes insipidus may be caused by lesions in the hypothalmus or pars nervosa that reduce the production of ADH by neurosecretory cells whose axon terminals are located in the neurohypophysis. This condition leads to renal dysfunction, which leads to inadequate water resorption by the kidneys, resulting in polyuria (high urinary output) and dehydration.

THYROID GLAND

The thyroid gland, located in the anterior portion of the neck, secretes the hormones thyroxine, triiodothyronine, and calcitonin.

The hormones T_4 and T_3, the secretions of which are under the control of **TSH** secreted by the anterior pituitary gland, stimulate the rate of metabolism. Another hormone, **calcitonin,** aids in decreasing blood calcium levels and facilitates the storage of calcium in bones (Table 13-2).

TABLE 13–2   Hormones and Functions of the Thyroid, Parathyroid, Adrenal, and Pineal Glands

Hormone	Cell Source	Regulating Hormone	Function
Thyroid Gland			
Thyroxine (T_4) and triiodothyronine (T_3)	Follicular cells	Thyroid-stimulating hormone (TSH)	Facilitate nuclear transcription of genes responsible for protein synthesis; increase cellular metabolism, growth rates; facilitate mental processes; increase endocrine gland activity; stimulate carbohydrate and fat metabolism; decrease cholesterol, phospholipids, and triglycerides; increase fatty acids; decrease body weight; increase heart rate, respiration, muscle action
Calcitonin (thyrocalcitonin)	Parafollicular cells	Feedback mechanism with parathyroid hormone	Lowers plasma calcium concentration by suppressing bone resorption
Parathyroid Gland			
Parathyroid hormone (PTH)	Chief cells	Feedback mechanism with calcitonin	Increases calcium concentration in body fluids
Suprarenal (Adrenal) Glands Suprarenal Cortex			
Mineralocorticoids: aldosterone and deoxycorticosterone	Cells of the zona glomerulosa	Angiotensin II and adrenocorticotropic hormone (ACTH)	Control body fluid volume and electrolyte concentrations by acting on distal tubules of the kidney, causing excretion of potassium and resorption of sodium
Glucocorticoids: cortisol and corticosterone	Cells of the zona fasciculata (spongiocytes)	ACTH	Regulate metabolism of carbohydrates, fats, and proteins; decrease protein synthesis, increasing amino acids in blood; stimulate gluconeogenesis by activating liver to convert amino acids to glucose; release fatty acid and glycerol; act as anti-inflammatory agents; reduce capillary permeability; suppress immune response
Androgens: dehydroepiandrosterone and androstenedione	Cells of the zona reticularis	ACTH	Provides weak masculinizing characteristics
Suprarenal Medulla			
Catecholamines: epinephrine and norepinephrine	Chromaffin cells	Preganglionic, sympathetic, and splanchnic nerves	*Epinephrine:* Operates the "fight or flight" mechanism preparing the body for severe fear or stress; increases cardiac heart rate and output, augmenting blood flow to the organs and release of glucose from the liver for energy; *Norepinephrine:* Causes an elevation in blood pressure by vasoconstriction
Pineal Gland			
Melatonin	Pinealocytes	Norepinephrine	May influence cyclic gonadal activity

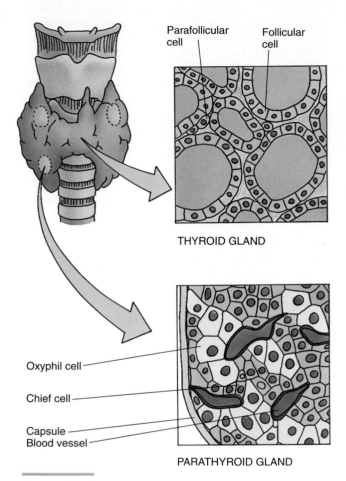

THYROID GLAND

PARATHYROID GLAND

Figure 13–6 The thyroid and parathyroid glands.

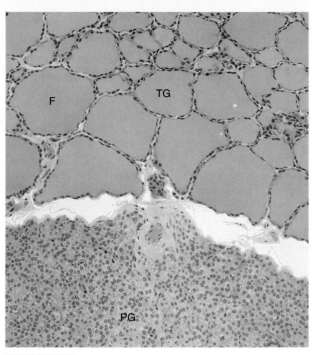

Figure 13–7 Light micrograph of the thyroid and parathyroid glands (×132). Observe the colloid-filled follicles (F) of the thyroid gland (TG) in the upper portion of the figure. At bottom is the parathyroid gland (PG), as evidenced by the presence of chief and oxyphil cells.

The thyroid gland lies just inferior to the larynx, anterior to the junction of the thyroid and cricoid cartilages (Fig. 13-6). It is composed of a **right lobe** and a **left lobe,** which are connected across the midline by an **isthmus.** In some people, the gland has an additional lobe, called the **pyramidal lobe,** that ascends from the left side of the isthmus. The pyramidal lobe is an embryological remnant of the path of descent of the thyroid primordium from its origin in the forming tongue by way of the thyroglossal duct.

The thyroid gland is surrounded by a slender, dense, irregular collagenous connective tissue capsule, a derivative of the deep cervical fascia. Septa derived from the capsule subdivide the gland into lobules. Embedded within the capsule, on the posterior aspect of the gland, are the parathyroid glands.

Cellular Organization

The thyroid follicle is the structural and functional unit of the thyroid gland.

Unlike most of the endocrine glands, which store their secretory substances within the parenchymal cells, the thyroid gland stores its secretory substances in the lumina of **follicles** (Fig. 13-7). These cyst-like structures, ranging from 0.2 to 0.9 mm in diameter, are composed of a simple cuboidal epithelium surrounding a central colloid-filled lumen. Each follicle can store several weeks' supply of hormone within the **colloid.** The hormones T_4 and T_3 are stored in the colloid, which is bound to a large (660,000 Da) secretory glycoprotein called **thyroglobulin.** When the hormones are to be released, the hormone-bound thyroglobulin is endocytosed and the hormones are cleaved from it by lysosomal proteases.

Connective tissue septa derived from the capsule invade the parenchyma and provide a conduit for blood vessels, lymphatic vessels, and nerve fibers. Slender connective tissue elements, composed mostly of reticular fibers and housing a rich capillary plexus, surround each follicle but are separated from the **follicular** and **parafollicular** cells by a thin **basal lamina.** Occasionally, follicular cells of neighboring follicles may come into contact with each other and disrupt the continuity of the basal lamina.

Follicular Cells (Principal Cells)

Follicular (principal) cells are squamous to low-columnar in shape and are tallest when stimulated.

Follicular cells have a round to ovoid nucleus with two nucleoli and basophilic cytoplasm. Frequently, their RER is distended and displays zones that are ribosome-free. These cells also have numerous apically located lysosomes, rod-shaped mitochondria, a supranuclear Golgi complex, and numerous short villi that extend into the colloid (Fig. 13-8). Numerous small vesicles, dispersed throughout the cytoplasm, are believed to contain thyroglobulin that was packaged in the Golgi complex and is destined for exocytosis into the follicle lumen. **Iodide** is essential for the synthesis of the thyroid hormones (T_3 and T_4); iodination of tyrosine residues occurs in the follicles at the colloid-follicular cell interface. Thus follicular cells secrete triiodothyronine (T_3) and thyroxine (T_4), which increases basal metabolic rates.

During great demand for thyroid hormone, follicular cells extend pseudopods into the follicles to envelop and absorb the colloid. When demand for the hormone declines, the amount of colloid in the follicle lumen increases.

Synthesis of Thyroid Hormones (T_3 and T_4)

Thyroid hormone synthesis is regulated by iodide levels and by TSH binding to TSH receptors of follicular cells.

The synthesis of thyroid hormone is regulated by the iodide levels in the follicular cell as well as by the binding of TSH to TSH receptors of the follicular cells. The occupation of TSH receptors triggers cAMP production, resulting in protein kinase A activity and synthesis of T_3 and T_4. Figure 13-9 outlines the pathway for the synthesis and release of thyroid hormones.

Thyroglobulin is synthesized in the RER and subsequently glycosylated in both the RER and the Golgi apparatus. The modified protein is packaged in the *trans* Golgi network. The vesicles containing thyroglobulin are transported to the apical plasmalemma, where their contents are released into the colloid and stored in the lumen of the follicle.

Iodine is reduced to iodide (I^-) within the alimentary canal and is preferentially absorbed and transported by the bloodstream to the thyroid gland. Iodide is actively transported via sodium/iodide symporters, which are located in the basal plasmalemma of the follicular cells, so that the intracellular iodide concentration is 20-fold to 40-fold that of plasma. Once in the cytosol, iodide is transferred to the colloid-cell membrane interface, where iodide oxidation occurs by the enzyme **thyroid peroxidase,** a process that requires the presence of hydrogen peroxide (H_2O_2). The activated iodide enters the colloid and iodinates tyrosine residues of thyroglobulin at the interface of the colloid and the apical plasmalemma of the thyroid follicular cell. Tyrosine residues of thyroglobulin are iodinated, forming **monoiodinated tyrosine (MIT)** and **diiodinated tyrosine** (DIT). Triiodinated and tetraiodinated

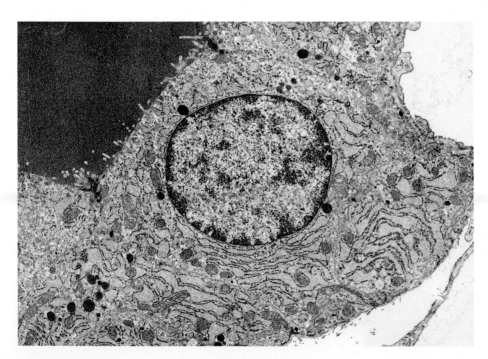

Figure 13–8 Electron micrograph of a thyroid follicular cell bordering the colloid (*dark area, upper left corner*) (×10,700). (From Mestdagh C, Many MC, Haalpern S, et al: Correlated autoradiographic and ion-microscopic study of the role of iodine in the formation of "cold" follicles in young and old mice. Cell Tissue Res 260:449-457, 1990.)

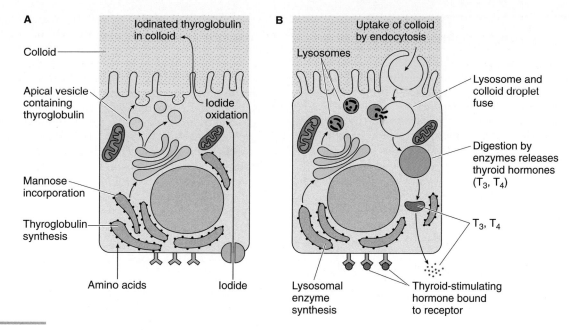

Figure 13–9 The synthesis and iodination of thyroglobulin (**A**) and release of thyroid hormone (**B**).

tyrosines are then formed by the coupling of an MIT and a DIT or of two DITs, respectively. Each thyroglobulin molecule has fewer than four T_4 molecules and fewer than 0.3 T_3 residues. The iodinated thyroglobulin is released by the follicular cells to be stored in the colloid.

Release of Thyroid Hormones (T_3 and T_4)

> *TSH stimulates follicular cells of the thyroid gland to release T_3 and T_4 into the bloodstream.*

TSH, released from the basophils of the anterior pituitary, binds to TSH receptors on the basal plasmalemma of the follicular cells. Binding of TSH facilitates formation of filopodia at the apical cell membrane, resulting in endocytosis of aliquots of the colloid. Cytoplasmic vesicles containing colloid fuse with early (or late) endosomes. Within the endosomes, iodinated residues are cleaved from thyroglobulin by proteases and are transferred into the cytosol as free MIT, DIT, T_3, and T_4.

MIT and DIT are stripped of their iodine by the enzyme **iodotyrosine dehalogenase,** and both the iodine and the amino acid tyrosine become part of their respective pools within the cytosol, to be used later.

T_3 and T_4 are released at the basal plasmalemma of the follicular cells, entering the connective tissue spaces of the thyroid for distribution by the bloodstream. T_4 constitutes about 90% of the released hormone, although it is not as effective as T_3.

Physiological Effects of Triiodothyronine and Thyroxine

Once they enter the bloodstream, **T_3 and T_4** bind to plasma-binding proteins and are slowly released to the tissues and contact cells. As they enter the cytoplasm, they are bound to intracellular proteins and slowly used over a period of several days to weeks. Because only the free hormone has the ability to enter the cell and because T_3 is bound less avidly, more of it gains entry into the cytoplasm than does T_4. Moreover, both T_3 and T_4 bind to **nuclear thyroid hormone receptor proteins,** but T_3 binds with a much greater affinity than does T_4, which also accounts for the greater biological activity of T_3.

These hormones stimulate transcription of many genes that encode various types of proteins (see Table 13-2), resulting in a generalized increase in cellular metabolism that may be as great as twice the resting rate. T_3 and T_4 also increase the growth rate in the young, facilitate mental processes, and stimulate endocrine gland activity.

Generally, thyroid hormones stimulate carbohydrate metabolism. They decrease synthesis of cholesterol, phospholipids, and triglycerides but increase synthesis of fatty acids and the uptake of various vitamins. Increased thyroid hormone production also decreases body weight and increases heart rate, metabolism, respiration, muscle function, and appetite. Excessive amounts of thyroid hormone cause muscle tremor, tiredness, impotence in men, and reduced or absence of menstrual bleeding in women.

Graves' disease is characterized by hyperplasia of the follicular cells, increasing the size of the thyroid gland two to three times above normal. Thyroid hormone production is also greatly increased, from 5 to 15 times normal **(hyperthyroidism)**. Other symptoms include **exophthalmos,** protrusion of the eyeballs. Although Graves' disease may develop from several causes, the most common agent is the binding of autoimmune immunoglobulin G (IgG) antibodies to TSH receptors, which stimulates thyroid follicular cells.

Insufficient dietary intake of iodine causes the thyroid gland to enlarge, a condition called **simple goiter.** Goiter usually is not associated with hyperthyroidism or hypothyroidism. This condition can be treated with supplementation of iodine in the diet.

Hypothyroidism is characterized by such conditions as fatigue, sleeping for up to 14 to 16 hours a day, muscular sluggishness, slowed heart rate, decreased cardiac output and blood volume, mental sluggishness, failure of body functions, constipation, and loss of hair growth. Patients with severe hypothyroidism may develop **myxedema,** which is characterized by bagginess under the eyes and a swollen face that is due to nonpitting edema of the skin, infiltration of excess glycosaminoglycans, and proteoglycans into the extracellular matrix. **Cretinism** is an extreme form of hypothyroidism occurring in fetal life through childhood that is characterized by failure of growth and mental retardation owing to a congenitally missing thyroid gland.

The nerves supplying the laryngeal musculature (i.e., external laryngeal nerves and recurrent laryngeal nerves) are closely applied to the thyroid gland and must be isolated and protected during **thyroidectomy.** Damage to either of these two nerves results in hoarseness and, possibly, loss of speech.

Parafollicular Cells (Clear Cells, C Cells)

Parafollicular cells secrete calcitonin. They are found individually or may form small clusters of cells at the periphery of the follicle.

The pale-staining parafollicular cells lie singly or in clusters among the follicular cells, but they do not reach the lumen of the follicle. Although these cells are two to three times larger than follicular cells, they account for only about 0.1% of the epithelium. Electron micrographs display a round nucleus, moderate amounts of RER, elongated mitochondria, a well-developed Golgi complex, and small, dense secretory granules (0.1 to 0.4 μm in diameter) located in the basal cytoplasm. These secretory granules contain **calcitonin (thyrocalcitonin),** a peptide hormone that inhibits bone resorption by osteoclasts, thereby lowering calcium concentrations in blood. When the circulating level of calcium is high, release of calcitonin is stimulated (see Chapter 7).

PARATHYROID GLANDS

The absence of parathyroid glands is incompatible with life because parathyroid hormone (PTH) regulates blood calcium levels.

The parathyroid glands, usually four in number, are located on the posterior surface of the thyroid gland; each gland is enveloped in its own thin, collagenous connective tissue capsule (see Fig. 13-6). The glands function in producing **PTH,** which acts on bone, kidneys, and the intestines in maintaining the optimal concentrations of calcium within blood and interstitial tissue fluid.

Normally, one parathyroid gland is located on both poles (superior and inferior) of the right and left lobes of the thyroid gland. Because of their embryological origin and descent in the neck with the primordium of the thymus and thyroid tissues, the parathyroid glands may be located anywhere along the pathway of descent, even in the thorax, and there may also be supernumerary parathyroid glands.

The parathyroid glands develop from the third and fourth pharyngeal pouches during embryogenesis. The parathyroid glands that develop in the third pharyngeal pouches descend with the thymus (also developing in the third pouches) to become the **inferior parathyroid glands.** The parathyroid glands that develop in the fourth pharyngeal pouches descend only a short distance to become the **superior parathyroid glands.** The glands grow slowly, reaching the adult size at about 20 years of age.

Parathyroid Cellular Organization

The parenchyma of the parathyroid glands consists of two cell types: chief cells and oxyphil cells.

Each parathyroid gland is a small, ovoid structure about 5 mm in length, 4 mm wide, and 2 mm in thickness and weighs about 25 to 50 mg. Extensions of the connective tissue capsule enter the gland as septa, accompanied by blood vessels, lymphatics, and nerves. The septa serve mainly to support the parenchyma and consist of cords or clusters of epithelial cells surrounded by reticular fibers, which also support the parenchyma and a rich capillary network. The connective tissue stroma in older adults often contains several to many adipose cells, which may occupy up to 60% of the gland. The parenchyma of the parathyroid glands is composed of two cell types: **chief cells** and **oxyphil cells** (see Fig. 13-7).

Chief Cells

Chief cells synthesize parathyroid hormone.

The major functional parenchymal cells of the parathyroid glands are the slightly eosinophilic-staining chief cells (5 to 8 μm in diameter), which contain granules of lipofuscin pigment that is scattered throughout the cytoplasm. Smaller, dense granules, 200 to 400 nm in diameter, arising from the Golgi complex and moving to the cell periphery, represent the secretory granules and contain **parathyroid hormone (PTH).** Electron micrographs also reveal a juxtanuclear Golgi complex, elongated mitochondria, and abundant RER. Occasionally, desmosomes join adjacent chief cells. A single cilium may extend into the intercellular space. Some chief cells have a smaller Golgi complex, scant secretory granules, and large amounts of glycogen; these cells are thought to be in an inactive phase.

The precursor, **preproparathyroid hormone,** is synthesized on ribosomes of the RER and rapidly cleaved as it is transported to the lumen of the RER to form **proparathyroid hormone** and a polypeptide. On reaching the Golgi complex, the proparathyroid hormone is cleaved again into PTH and a small polypeptide. The hormone is packaged into secretory granules and is released from the cell surface by exocytosis.

Oxyphil Cells

Oxyphil cells are believed to be the inactive phase of chief cells.

The second cell type located in the parathyroid glands is the oxyphil cell. Its function is unknown, although it is believed that oxyphil cells and a third cell, described as an **intermediate cell,** probably represent inactive phases of a single cell type, with chief cells being the actively secreting phase.

Oxyphil cells are less numerous, larger (6 to 10 μm in diameter), and stain more deeply with eosin than

chief cells do. Oxyphils appear in groups and as isolated cells. They have more abundant mitochondria than do chief cells, but their Golgi apparatus is small and there is little RER. Glycogen is also located in the cytosol and is surrounded by mitochondria.

Physiological Effect of Parathyroid Hormone

PTH, produced by chief cells of the parathyroid glands, helps to maintain the extracellular fluid as well as the plasma concentration of calcium ions (8.5 to 10.5 mg/dL). This hormone acts on cells of the bones, the kidneys, and, indirectly, the intestines, leading to an increased calcium ion concentration in body fluids (see Table 13-2). When calcium ion concentration in body fluids falls below normal, the chief cells increase their production and release of PTH, quickly increasing their normal secretion rate 10-fold. This rapid response is especially important because of the many functions of calcium in homeostasis, including its role in stabilizing ion gradients across the plasmalemmae of muscle and nerve cells and its role in the release of neurotransmitter at axon terminals.

The interplay of PTH and calcitonin represents a dual mechanism for regulating calcium levels in the blood: PTH acts to increase serum calcium levels, whereas calcitonin has the opposite effect.

In bone, PTH binds to receptors on osteoblasts, signaling the cells to increase their secretion of **osteoclast-stimulating factor.** This factor induces activation of osteoclasts, thereby increasing bone resorption and the ultimate release of calcium ions into the blood (see Chapter 7). In the kidneys, PTH prevents loss of calcium in the urine. Finally, PTH controls the rate of calcium uptake in the gastrointestinal tract by indirectly regulating the production of vitamin D in the kidneys; vitamin D is necessary for intestinal uptake of calcium. Vitamin D functions to stimulate the intestinal mucosa to reabsorb calcium by inducing epithelial cells of the intestinal villus to form calcium-binding protein that becomes localized on the microvilli that facilitates the transport of calcium into the epithelial cells.

SUPRARENAL (ADRENAL) GLANDS

Suprarenal glands produce two different groups of hormones: steroids and catecholamines.

The suprarenal glands are located at the superior poles of the kidneys and are embedded in adipose tissue. The right and left suprarenal glands are not mirror images of each other; rather, the right suprarenal gland is

---

CLINICAL CORRELATIONS

A condition called **primary hyperparathyroidism,** which may be caused by a tumor in one of the parathyroid glands, is marked by high blood calcium levels, low blood phosphate levels, loss of bone mineral, and sometimes kidney stones. **Secondary hyperparathyroidism** may develop in patients with **rickets,** because calcium cannot be absorbed from the intestines owing to vitamin D deficiency; therefore, calcium ion concentrations in the blood are low.

Hypoparathyroidism results from deficiency in secretion of PTH, commonly caused by injury of the parathyroid glands or by their removal during thyroid gland surgery. Hypoparathyroidism is marked by low blood calcium levels, retention of bone calcium, and increased phosphate resorption in the kidney. The main symptoms are numbness, tingling, **carpopedal spasms** (muscle cramps) in the hands and feet, **muscle tetany** (tremors) in the facial and laryngeal muscles, mental confusion, and memory loss. The only treatment for survival is large intravenous doses of calcium gluconate, vitamin D, and oral calcium.

---

pyramid-shaped and sits directly on top of the right kidney, whereas the left suprarenal gland is more crescent-shaped and lies along the medial border of the left kidney from the hilus to its superior pole.

Both glands are about 1 cm in thickness, 2 cm in width at the apex, and up to 5 cm at the base; each weighs 7 to 10 g. The parenchyma of the gland is divided into two histologically and functionally different regions: an outer yellowish portion, accounting for about 80% to 90% of the organ, called the **suprarenal cortex,** and a small, dark, inner portion called the **suprarenal medulla** (Fig. 13-10). Although both entities are endocrine in function, each develops from a different embryological origin and performs a different role. The suprarenal cortex, arising from mesoderm, produces a group of hormones called **corticosteroids,** which are synthesized from **cholesterol.** Secretion of these hormones, including **cortisol** and **corticosterone,** is regulated by **ACTH,** a hormone secreted by the anterior pituitary gland. The suprarenal medulla, arising from neural crest, is functionally related to and regulated by the sympathetic nervous system; it produces the hormones **epinephrine** and **norepinephrine** (see Table 13-2).

The suprarenal glands are retroperitoneal, located behind the peritoneum, and surrounded by a connective tissue capsule that contains large amounts of adipose tissue. Each gland has a thick capsule of connective tissue that sends septa into the parenchyma of the gland, accompanied by blood vessels and nerves.

Blood Supply to the Suprarenal Glands

Arteries from three separate sources provide the suprarenal glands with an abundant blood supply:

The suprarenal glands have one of the richest blood supplies in the body (Fig. 13-11). Each suprarenal gland is served by three separate arteries that arise from three separate sources:

■ The **inferior phrenic arteries,** from which the superior suprarenal arteries originate.
■ The **aorta,** from which the **middle suprarenal arteries** originate.
■ The **renal arteries,** from which the inferior suprarenal arteries originate.

These branches pass over the capsule, penetrate it, and form a **subcapsular plexus.**

Arising from the plexus are **short cortical arteries,** which, in the cortical parenchyma, form a network of sinusoidal fenestrated capillaries (with diaphragms). The pore diameters of the fenestrated endothelial walls of the capillaries increase from 100 nm at the outer cortex to 250 nm in the deep cortex, where the sinusoidal capillaries become confluent with a venous plexus. Small venules arising from this area pass through the suprarenal medulla and drain into a suprarenal vein, emerging from the hilus. The right suprarenal vein joins the inferior vena cava, and the left suprarenal vein drains into the left renal vein.

Additional **long cortical arteries** pass unbranched through the cortex and into the medulla, where they form networks of capillaries. Thus, the medulla receives a dual blood supply: (1) an arterial supply from the long cortical arteries and (2) numerous vessels from the cortical capillary beds.

Suprarenal Cortex

The suprarenal cortex is subdivided into three zones that produce three classes of steroids.

The suprarenal cortex contains parenchymal cells that synthesize and secrete several steroid hormones without storing them. The cortex is subdivided histologically into three concentric zones named, from the capsule inward, the **zona glomerulosa,** the **zona fasciculata,** and the **zona reticularis** (Fig. 13-12; also see Fig. 13-10). Although each of the three identified zones

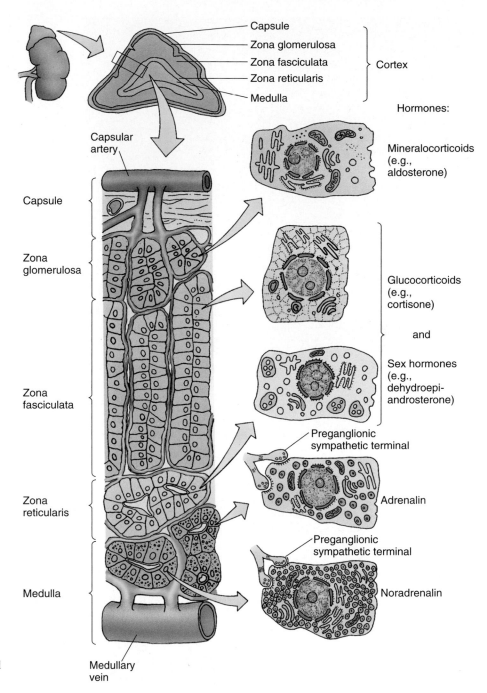

Figure 13–10 The suprarenal gland and its cell types.

of the suprarenal cortex is said to secrete specific hormones, it should be remembered that the boundaries between these zone overlap; thus it is better to remember the cortex as a secreting unit for the three classes of adrenocortical hormones (of course, the student's instructor may deem otherwise, in which case it is in the student's best interest to follow the instructor's point of view).

The three classes of adrenocortical hormones—**mineralocorticoids, glucocorticoids,** and **androgens**—are all synthesized from **cholesterol,** the major component of **low-density lipoprotein.** Cholesterol is taken up from the blood and stored esterified in lipid droplets within the cytoplasm of the cortical cells. When these cells are stimulated, cholesterol is freed and used in hormone synthesis in the **smooth endoplasmic**

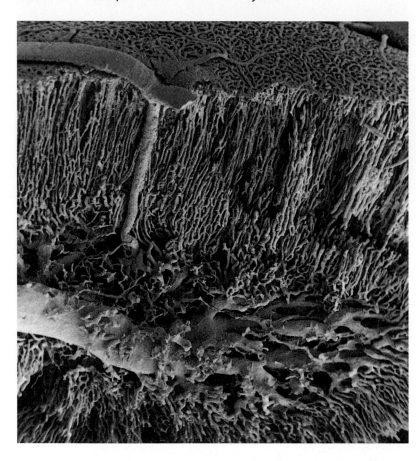

Figure 13–11 Scanning electron micrograph of the rat adrenal gland demonstrating microcirculation in the cortex and medulla (×80). (From Kikuta A, Murakami T: Microcirculation of the rat adrenal gland: A scanning electron microscope study of vascular casts. Am J Anat 164:19-28, 1982.)

reticulum (SER) by enzymes that are located there and in the mitochondria. The intermediate products of the hormone that is being synthesized are transferred between the SER and the mitochondria until the final hormone is produced.

Zona Glomerulosa

Parenchymal cells of the zona glomerulosa, when stimulated by angiotensin II and ACTH, synthesize and release the hormones aldosterone and deoxycorticosterone.

The outer concentric ring of capsular parenchymal cells, located just beneath the suprarenal capsule, is the zona glomerulosa, which constitutes approximately 13% of the total adrenal volume (see Fig. 13-10). The small columnar cells composing this zone are arranged in cords and clusters. Their small, dark-staining nuclei contain one or two nucleoli, and their acidophilic cytoplasm contains an abundant and extensive SER, short mitochondria with shelf-like cristae, a well-developed Golgi complex, abundant RER, and free ribosomes. Some lipid droplets also are dispersed in the cytoplasm. Occasional desmosomes and small gap junctions join cells to each other, and some cells have short microvilli.

The parenchymal cells of the zona glomerulosa synthesize and secrete the **mineralocorticoid hormones,** principally **aldosterone** and some **deoxycorticosterone**. Synthesis of these hormones is stimulated by **angiotensin II** and **ACTH,** both required for normal existence of glomerulosa cells. The mineralocorticoid hormones function in controlling fluid and electrolyte balance in the body by affecting the function of the renal tubules, specifically the distal convoluted tubules (see Chapter 19).

Zona Fasciculata

Parenchymal cells of the zona fasciculata (spongiocytes), when stimulated by ACTH, synthesize and release the hormones cortisol and corticosterone.

The intermediate concentric layer of cells in the suprarenal cortex is the zona fasciculata, the largest layer of the cortex, which accounts for up to 80% of the total volume of the gland. This zone contains sinusoidal capillaries that are arranged longitudinally between the columns of parenchymal cells. The polyhedral cells in

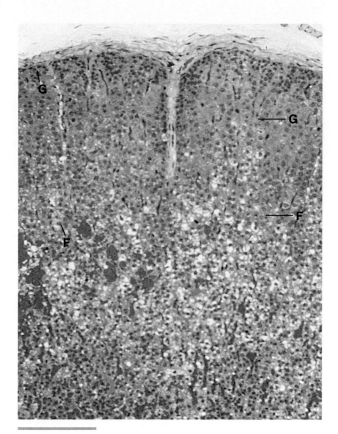

Figure 13–12 Light micrograph of the cortex of the suprarenal gland (×132). Observe the zona glomerulosa (G) and the zona fasciculata (F).

this layer are larger than the cells of the zona glomerulosa and are arranged in radial columns, one to two layers thick, and stain lightly acidophilic. Because they have many lipid droplets in their cytoplasm, which are extracted during histological processing, these cells appear vacuolated and are called **spongiocytes.** Spongiocytes have spherical mitochondria with tubular and vesicular cristae, extensive networks of SER, some RER, lysosomes, and granules of lipofuscin pigment.

Cells of the zona fasciculata synthesize and secrete the **glucocorticoid hormones cortisol** and **corticosterone.** The synthesis of these hormones is stimulated by ACTH. Glucocorticoids function in the control of carbohydrate, fat, and protein metabolism.

Zona Reticularis

The cells of the zona reticularis, when stimulated by ACTH, synthesize and release dehydroepiandrosterone, androstenedione, and some glucocorticoids.

The innermost layer of the suprarenal cortex is the zona reticularis, constituting about 7% of gland volume.

The darkly staining acidophilic cells in this layer are arranged in anastomosing cords. They are similar to the spongiocytes of the zona fasciculata but are smaller with fewer lipid droplets. They frequently contain large amounts of lipofuscin pigment granules. Several cells near the suprarenal medulla are dark with electron-dense cytoplasm and pyknotic nuclei, which suggests that this zone contains degenerating parenchymal cells.

Cells of the zona reticularis synthesize and secrete **androgens,** principally **dehydroepiandrosterone** and some **androstenedione.** Additionally, these cells may synthesize and secrete small amounts of glucocorticoids. The secretion of these hormones is stimulated by ACTH. Both dehydroepiandrosterone and androstenedione are weak, masculinizing hormones with negligible effects under normal conditions.

Histophysiology of the Suprarenal Cortex

The three classes of hormones that are secreted by the suprarenal cortex are steroids: (1) mineralocorticoids, (2) glucocorticoids, and (3) weak androgens. ACTH from the pars distalis of the pituitary is the trophic hormone that stimulates secretion of the suprarenal cortex hormones.

Mineralocorticoids

The mineralocorticoids secreted by the zona glomerulosa include **aldosterone** predominantly and some deoxycorticosterone. The targets of these hormones include the gastric mucosa, salivary glands, and sweat glands, where they stimulate absorption of sodium. However, their main target are the cells of the distal convoluted tubules of the kidney, where they function to stimulate the regulation of water balance and the homeostasis of sodium and potassium by absorbing sodium and excreting potassium.

Glucocorticoids

Glucocorticoids, secreted by the zona fasciculata, include **hydrocortisone (cortisol)** and **corticosterone.** These steroid hormones have a wide range of functions that affect most tissues of the body as well as control general metabolism. Glucocorticoids exert an **anabolic** effect in the liver that promotes the uptake of fatty acids, amino acids, and carbohydrates for glucose synthesis and glycogen polymerization; in other tissues, however, the effect is **catabolic.** For example, in adipocytes glucocorticoids stimulate **lipolysis,** and in muscle these hormones stimulate **proteolysis.** Glucocorticoids, when circulating at above normal levels, also influence anti-inflammatory responses by inhibiting macrophage and leukocyte infiltration at sites of inflammation. These hormones also suppress the immune response by inducing atrophy of the lymphatic system, thereby reducing the circulating lymphocyte population.

The **negative feedback** mechanism for the glucocorticoids is partly controlled by their plasma concentration. When blood glucocorticoid levels are high, **corticotropin-releasing hormone (CRH)** cells of the hypothalamus are inhibited, which in turn inhibits **corticotrophs** of the pars distalis of the pituitary gland from releasing ACTH.

Weak Androgens

Androgens secreted by the zona reticularis include **dehydroepiandrosterone** and androstenedione, both weak, masculinizing sex hormones that are only a small fraction as effective as the androgens that are produced in the testes. Under normal conditions, the influence of these hormones is insignificant.

CLINICAL CORRELATIONS

Addison's disease is characterized by decreased secretion of the adrenocortical hormones as a result of destruction of the suprarenal cortex. This disease is most often caused by an autoimmune process; it also can develop as a sequela of tuberculosis or of some other infectious diseases. Death occurs if steroid treatment is not provided.

Cushing's disease (hyperadrenocorticism) is caused by small tumors in the basophils of the anterior pituitary gland that lead to an increase in the output of **ACTH.** The excess ACTH causes enlargement of the suprarenal glands and hypertrophy of the suprarenal cortex, resulting in overproduction of cortisol. Patients are obese, predominantly in the face, neck, and trunk, and exhibit osteoporosis and muscle wasting. Males become impotent, and females have amenorrhea.

Suprarenal Medulla

Chromaffin cells of the suprarenal medulla are modified postganglionic neurons that have a secretory function.

The central portion of the suprarenal gland, the suprarenal medulla, is completely invested by the suprarenal cortex. The suprarenal medulla, which develops from ectodermal neural crest cells, comprises two populations of parenchymal cells: **chromaffin cells** (Fig. 13-13), which produce the **catecholamines (epinephrine** and **norepinephrine),** and **sympathetic**

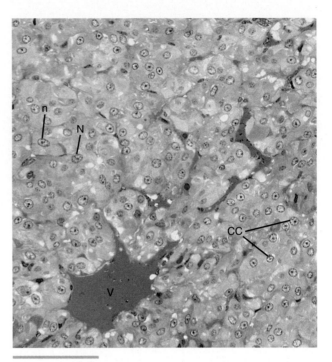

Figure 13–13 Light micrograph of the medulla of the suprarenal gland (×270). Note the chromaffin cells (CC) whose nucleus (N) houses a single nucleolus (n). Observe the rich arterial supply and venous drainage (V) of the suprarenal medulla.

ganglion cells, which are scattered throughout the connective tissue.

Chromaffin Cells

The suprarenal medulla functions as a modified sympathetic ganglion, housing postganglionic sympathetic cells that lack dendrites and axons.

Chromaffin cells of the suprarenal medulla are large epithelioid cells, arranged in clusters or short cords; they contain granules that stain intensely with chromaffin salts. The reaction of the granules, which turn deep brown when exposed to chromaffin salts, indicates that the cells contain **catecholamines,** transmitters produced by postganglionic cells of the sympathetic nervous system. Thus, the suprarenal medulla functions as a modified sympathetic ganglion, housing postganglionic sympathetic cells that lack dendrites and axons. The catecholamines synthesized by the chromaffin cells are the sympathetic transmitters **epinephrine** and **norepinephrine** (Fig. 13-14). These transmitters are secreted by the chromaffin cells in response to stimulation by **preganglionic sympathetic (cholinergic) splanchnic nerves.** Each chromaffin cell of primates, including the human, has the capability of producing both epinephrine and norepinephrine and storing them

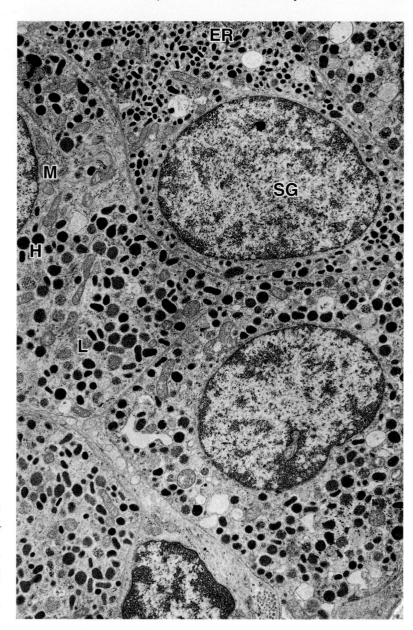

Figure 13–14 Electron micrograph of baboon adrenal medulla (×14,000). The different osmiophilic densities of the vesicles may be a reflection of their maturational phases. ER, endoplasmic reticulum; H, high-electron-density vesicle; L, low-electron-density vesicle; M, mitochondrion; SG, small granule cell. (From Al-Lami F, Carmichael SW: Microscopic anatomy of the baboon [*Papio hamadryas*] adrenal medulla. J Anat 178:213-221, 1991.)

in secretory vesicles. Although in electron micrographs two types of secretory vesicles, high-electron-density and low-electron-density, are evident, the density differential may be one of the maturational state of epinephrine and not necessarily indicative of the presence of two types of catecholamines.

In some animals, but not in primates including humans, two types of chromaffin cells have been identified by histochemical staining: those producing and storing norepinephrine and those producing and storing epinephrine. The granules of the norepinephrine-storing cells have an eccentric, electron-dense core within the limiting membrane of the granule, whereas the granules of chromaffin cells storing epinephrine are more homogeneous and less dense. Primate chromaffin cells have a well-developed juxtanuclear Golgi complex, some RER, and numerous mitochondria. The identifying characteristic of the chromaffin cells is the 30,000 or so small, membrane-bound, dense granules in the cytoplasm; approximately 20% of these granules contain either epinephrine or norepinephrine. The remaining granules are composed of **adenosine triphosphate, enkephalins,** and soluble proteins called **chromagranins.** Chromagranins are proteins that are believed to bind epinephrine and norepinephrine.

Histophysiology of the Suprarenal Medulla

The secretory activity of the suprarenal medulla is controlled by the splanchnic nerves. Release of the aggregated **catecholamines** from chromaffin cells is induced by stimulation of the sympathetic ganglion cells in the suprarenal medulla. Release of **acetylcholine** from these preganglionic sympathetic nerve endings depolarizes the chromaffin cell membranes, leading to an influx of calcium ions. The rise in intracellular calcium then induces release of **epinephrine** or **norepinephrine** via exocytosis.

When the stimulus is derived from an emotional source, secretion of norepinephrine predominates; when the stimulus is physiological (e.g., pain), secretion of epinephrine predominates. Catecholamines released by the suprarenal medulla exhibit a more generalized overall effect than do the catecholamines released by sympathetic neurons. However, these effects are not uniform for all tissues. Generally, they increase oxygen consumption, increase heat production, and mobilize fat for energy; in the cardiovascular system, they function in controlling the heart rate and the arterial smooth muscles, thus increasing blood pressure. Additionally, catecholamines regulate muscle contractions in some tissues (e.g., bladder sphincters); in other organs, they influence muscle relaxation (e.g., intestinal smooth muscle).

In severe fear or stress, increased epinephrine is released to prepare the body for "fight or flight." The resulting plasma levels of epinephrine, up to 300 times the normal level, increase alertness, cardiac output, and heart rate, as well as increase the release of glucose from the liver.

Epinephrine is most effective in controlling cardiac output, heart rate, and increasing blood flow through organs. Norepinephrine has little effect on these but brings about an elevation in blood pressure by vasoconstriction.

Norepinephrine is also produced in the brain and in peripheral nerves, functioning as a neurotransmitter; however, norepinephrine produced in the suprarenal medulla has a short half-life because it is destroyed in the liver shortly after its release.

PINEAL GLAND

The pineal gland is responsive to diurnal light and dark periods and is thought to influence gonadal activity.

The pineal gland (or **pineal body**) is an endocrine gland whose secretions are influenced by the light and dark periods of the day. It is a cone-shaped, midline projection from the roof of the diencephalon, within a recess of the third ventricle extending into the stalk that is attached to it. It is 5 to 8 mm long and 3 to 5 mm wide; it weighs approximately 120 mg. The gland is covered by pia mater, forming a capsule from which septa extend, dividing the pineal gland into incomplete lobules. Blood vessels enter the gland via the connective tissue septa. The parenchymal cells of the gland are composed primarily of **pinealocytes** and **interstitial cells** (Fig. 13-15).

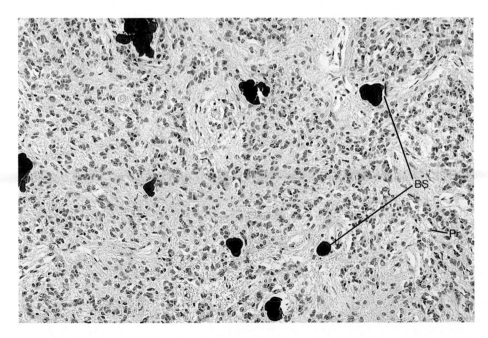

Figure 13–15 Pineal gland (×132). The large, darkly staining structures are brain sand (BS) scattered among the pinealocytes (Pi). Neuroglial cells are present but difficult to distinguish at this magnification.

Pinealocytes

Pinealocytes are the parenchymal cells of the pineal gland that are responsible for secreting melatonin.

Pinealocytes are slightly basophilic cells with one or two long processes whose terminal dilations approximate capillaries and, occasionally, other parenchymal cells. Their spherical nuclei have a single prominent nucleolus. The cytoplasm contains SER and RER, a small Golgi apparatus, numerous mitochondria, and small secretory vesicles, some with electron-dense cores. Pinealocytes also contain a well-developed cytoskeleton composed of microtubules, microfilaments, and dense tubular structures invested by spherical vesicular elements. These unusual structures, known as **synaptic ribbons** (also observed in the retina and inner ear), increase in number during the dark period of the diurnal cycle, but their function is not understood.

Melatonin, synthesized from tryptophan by pinealocytes and released at night, inhibits the release of growth hormone and gonadotropin by the hypophysis and hypothalamus, respectively. It has been suggested that melatonin induces the feeling of sleepiness and, therefore, some individuals use it as a supplement to combat sleep disorders, mood disorders, and depression.

CLINICAL CORRELATIONS

It has been suggested that **melatonin** may act to protect the central nervous system by its ability to scavenge and eliminate free radicals that are produced during oxidative stress. Additional theory suggest that melatonin may alter human moods, causing depression during shortened daylight hours of winter months. It has been reported that exposure to bright artificial light may reduce the secretion of melatonin and may result in alleviation of depression.

Interstitial Cells

Interstitial cells of the pineal gland are believed to be astroglia-like cells.

Interstitial cells, believed to be astrocyte-like neuroglial cells, are scattered throughout the pinealocytes and are particularly abundant in the pineal stalk that leads to the diencephalon. These cells have deeply staining, elongated nuclei and well-developed RER; some have deposits of glycogen. Their long cellular processes are rich in intermediate filaments, microtubules, and microfilaments.

The pineal gland also contains concretions of calcium phosphates and carbonates, which are deposited in concentric rings around an organic matrix. These structures, called **corpora arenacea ("brain sand"),** appear in early childhood and increase in size throughout life. Although it is unclear how they are formed or function, they increase during short photoperiods and are reduced when the pineal gland is actively secreting.

Histophysiology of the Pineal Gland

Although the pineal gland is connected to the midline of the brain as a projection of the roof of the diencephalon, no brain-derived, afferent or efferent nerve fibers enter the gland. Instead, the pineal body is innervated by **postganglionic sympathetic nerves** from the superior cervical ganglion. As the axons enter the gland, their myelin is lost and they synapse on the pinealocytes. **Norepinephrine,** released at the pinealocytes, controls production of **melatonin** (see Table 13-2). Synthesis of pineal hormones exhibits a diurnal rhythm, in that it is increased during dark periods and is inhibited during light periods. Melatonin is released into the connective tissue spaces to be distributed by blood vessels, whereas serotonin is taken up by presynaptic axon terminals. Continued research on the pineal gland is focused on the pineal hormones and their functions.

14

Integument

The integument, composed of **skin** and its appendages—the **sweat glands, sebaceous glands, hair,** and **nails**—is the largest organ of the body, constituting 16% of body weight. It invests the entire body, becoming continuous with the mucous membranes of the digestive system at the lips and the anus, the respiratory system in the nose, and the urogenital systems where they surface. Additionally, the skin of the eyelids becomes continuous with the conjunctiva lining the anterior portion of the orb. Skin also lines the external auditory meatus and covers the external surface of the tympanic membrane.

SKIN

Skin, the largest organ of the body, is composed of an epidermis and the underlying dermis.

Besides providing a cover for the underlying soft tissues, skin performs many additional functions, including (1) **protection** against injury, bacterial invasion, and desiccation; (2) **regulation of body temperature;** (3) **reception** of continual sensations from the environment (e.g., touch, temperature, and pain); (4) **excretion** from sweat glands; and (5) **absorption** of ultraviolet radiation from the sun for the synthesis of vitamin D.

Skin consists of two layers: an outer epidermis and a deeper connective tissue layer, the dermis (Fig. 14-1). The **epidermis** is composed of an **ectodermally** derived stratified squamous keratinized epithelium. Lying directly below and interdigitating with the epidermis is the **dermis,** derived from **mesoderm** and composed of dense, irregular collagenous connective tissue. The interface between the epidermis and dermis is formed by raised ridges of the dermis, the **dermal ridges (papillae),** which interdigitate with invaginations of the epidermis called **epidermal ridges.** Collectively, the two types of ridges are known as the **rete apparatus.** Additional downgrowths of the epidermal derivatives (i.e., hair follicles, sweat glands, and sebaceous glands) that come to lie in the dermis cause the interface to have an irregular contour.

The **hypodermis,** a loose connective tissue containing varying amounts of fat, underlies the skin. The hypodermis is not part of the skin but is the **superficial fascia** of gross anatomical dissection that covers the entire body, immediately deep to the skin. Individuals who are overnourished or who live in cold climates possess a large amount of fat deposited in the superficial fascia (hypodermis), named **panniculus adiposus.**

In certain regions of the body, the skin displays different textures and thicknesses. For example, skin of the eyelid is soft, fine, and thin and has fine hairs, whereas only a short distance away, on the eyebrow, the skin is thicker and manifests coarse hair. Skin of the forehead produces oily secretions; the skin on the chin lacks oily secretions but develops much hair.

The palms of the hands and soles of the feet are thick and do not produce hair but contain many sweat glands. Finger and toe pad surfaces have well-defined, alternating ridges and grooves that form patterns of loops, curves, arches, and whorls called **dermatoglyphs** (fingerprints), which develop in the fetus and remain unchanged throughout life. Dermatoglyphs are so individualized that they are used for identification purposes in forensic medicine and in criminal investigations. Although fingerprints are determined genetically, perhaps by multiple genes, other grooves and flexure lines about the knees, elbows, and hands are, for the most part, related to habitual use and physical stresses in a person's environment.

Epidermis

Epidermis, the surface layer of skin, is derived from ectoderm and is composed of stratified squamous keratinized epithelium.

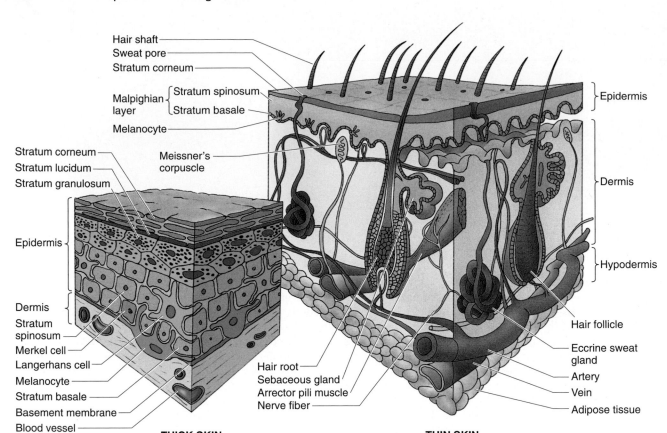

Figure 14–1 Comparison of thick skin and thin skin.

The epidermis is 0.07 to 0.12 mm in thickness over most of the body, with increased localized thickening on the palms of the hands and the soles of the feet (where it may be as much as 0.8 mm and 1.4 mm in thickness, respectively). Thicker skin on the palms and soles is evident in the fetus, but use, applied pressure, and friction result in continued increases in skin thickness in these areas over time.

The stratified squamous keratinized epithelium of skin is composed of four populations of cells:

▪ Keratinocytes
▪ Langerhans cells
▪ Melanocytes
▪ Merkel cells

Keratinocytes

Keratinocytes, which form the largest population of cells, are arranged in five recognizable layers; the remaining three cell types are interspersed among keratinocytes in specific locations (see later). Because keratinocytes are continually being sloughed from the surface of the epidermis, this cell population must be constantly renewed. Renewal is accomplished through mitotic activity of the keratinocytes in the basal layers of the epidermis. Keratinocytes undergo mitosis at night, and as the new cells are forming, the cells above continue to be pushed toward the surface. Along their way to the surface, the cells differentiate and begin to accumulate **keratin filaments** in their cytoplasm. Eventually, as they near the surface, the cells die and are sloughed off, a process that takes 20 to 30 days.

Because of the **cytomorphosis** of keratinocytes during their migration from the basal layer of the epidermis to its surface, five morphologically distinct zones of the epidermis can be identified. From the inner to the outer layer, they are (1) **stratum basale (germinativum),** (2) **stratum spinosum,** (3) **stratum granulosum,** (4) **stratum lucidum,** and (5) **stratum corneum.** Skin is classified as thick or thin according to the thickness of the epidermis (see Fig. 14-1). However, these two classifications are also are distinguished by the presence or absence of certain epidermal layers and the presence or absence of hair.

Thick skin covers the the palms and soles (Table 14-1). The epidermis of thick skin (see Fig. 14-2), which

TABLE 14–1 Strata and Histological Features of Thick Skin

Layer	Histological Features
Epidermis	Derived from ectoderm; composed of stratified squamous keratinized epithelium (keratinocytes)
Stratum corneum	Numerous layers of dead flattened keratinized cells, keratinocytes, without nuclei and organelles (squames, or horny cells) that will be sloughed off
Stratum lucidum°	Lightly stained thin layer of keratinocytes without nuclei and organelles; cells contain densely packed keratin filaments and eleidin
Stratum granulosum°	A layer three to five cell layers thick; these keratinocytes still retain nuclei; cells contain large, coarse keratohyalin granules as well as membrane-coating granules
Stratum spinosum	Thickest layer of epidermis, whose keratinocytes, known as prickle cells, interdigitate with one another by forming intercellular bridges and a large number of desmosomes; prickle cells have numerous tonofilaments and membrane-coating granules and are mitotically active; this layer also houses Langerhans cells
Stratum basale (germinativum)	This single layer of cuboidal to low columnar, mitotically active cells is separated from the papillary layer of the dermis by a well-developed basement membrane; Merkel cells and melanocytes are also present in this layer
Dermis	Derived from mesoderm; composed mostly of type I collagen and elastic fibers, the dermis is subdivided into two regions: the papillary layer and the reticular layer, a dense, irregular collagenous connective tissue
Papillary layer	Interdigitates with epidermis, forming the dermal papilla component of the rete apparatus; type III collagen and elastic fibers in loose arrangement and anchoring fibrils (type VII collagen); abundant capillary beds, connective tissue cells, and mechanoreceptors are located in this layer; occasionally, melanocytes are also present in the papillary layer
Reticular layer	Deepest layer of skin; type I collagen, thick elastic fibers, and connective tissue cells; contains sweat glands and their ducts, hair follicles and arrector pili muscles, and sebaceous glands as well as mechanoreceptors (such as pacinian corpuscles)

°Present only in thick skin. All layers are usually thinner in thin skin.

is 400 to 600 mm thick, is characterized by the presence of all five layers. Thick skin lacks hair follicles, arrector pili muscles, and sebaceous glands but does possess sweat glands.

Thin skin covers most of the remainder of the body. The epidermis of thin skin, which ranges from 75 to 150 mm in thickness, has a thin stratum corneum and lacks a definite stratum lucidum and stratum granulosum, although individual cells of these layers are present in their proper locations. Thin skin has **hair follicles, arrector pili muscles**, **sebaceous glands,** and **sweat glands.**

Stratum Basale (Stratum Germinativum)

Stratum basale, the germinal layer that undergoes mitosis, forms interdigitations with the dermis and is separated from it by a basement membrane.

The deepest layer of the epidermis, the stratum basale, is supported by a **basement membrane** and sits on the dermis, forming an irregular interface. The stratum basale consists of a single layer of mitotically active, cuboidal to low columnar cells containing basophilic cytoplasm and a large nucleus (Fig. 14-3). Many desmosomes are located on the lateral cell membrane attaching stratum basale cells to each other and to cells of the stratum spinosum. Basally located hemidesmosomes attach the cells to the basal lamina. Electron micrographs reveal a few mitochondria, a small Golgi complex, a few rough endoplasmic reticulum (RER) profiles, and abundant free ribosomes. Numerous bundles and single (10-nm) **intermediate filaments (tonofilaments)** course through the plaques of the laterally placed desmosomes and end in plaques of hemidesmosomes.

Mitotic figures should be common in the stratum basale because this layer is partially responsible for cell

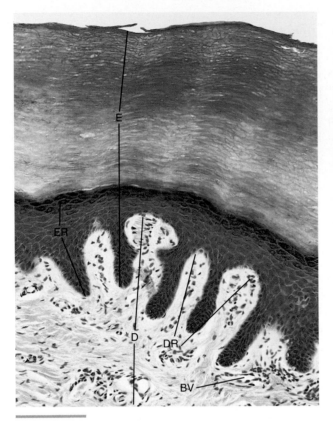

Figure 14–2 Light micrograph of thick skin (×132). Observe the epidermis (E) and dermis (D) as well as the dermal ridges (DR) that are interdigitating with epidermal ridges (ER). Several blood vessels (BV) are present.

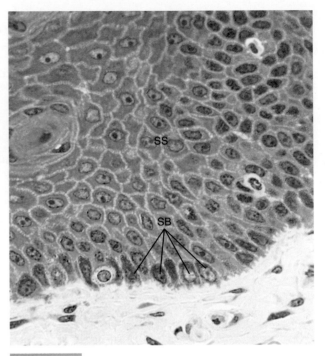

Figure 14–3 Light micrograph of thick skin demonstrating the stratum basale (SB) and stratum spinosum (SS) (×540).

renewal in the epithelium. However, mitosis occurs mostly during the night, and histological specimens are procured during the day; thus, mitotic figures are rarely seen in histological slides of skin. When new cells are formed via mitosis, the previous layer of cells is pushed surfaceward to join the next layer of the epidermis, the stratum spinosum.

Stratum Spinosum

The stratum spinosum is composed of several layers of mitotically active polymorphous cells whose numerous processes give this layer a prickly appearance.

The thickest layer of the epidermis is the stratum spinosum, composed of polyhedral to flattened cells. The basally located keratinocytes in the stratum spinosum also are mitotically active, and the two strata together, frequently referred to as the **malpighian layer,** are responsible for the turnover of epidermal keratinocytes. Keratinocytes of the stratum spinosum have the same organelle population as described for the stratum basale. However, the cells in the stratum spinosum are richer in bundles of intermediate filaments **(tonofilaments),** representing **cytokeratin,** than cells in the stratum basale. In the stratum spinosum cells, these bundles radiate outward from the perinuclear region toward highly interdigitated cellular processes, which attach adjacent cells to each other by desmosomes. These processes, called "intercellular bridges" by early histologists, give cells of the stratum spinosum a "prickle cell" appearance (see Fig. 14-3). As keratinocytes move toward the surface through the stratum spinosum, they continue to produce tonofilaments, which become grouped in bundles called **tonofibrils,** causing the cytoplasm to become eosinophilic (Fig. 14-4). Cells of the stratum spinosum also contain cytoplasmic secretory granules (0.1 to 0.4 μm in diameter) called **membrane-coating granules (lamellar granules).** These flattened vesicles house lipid substance arranged in a closely packed, lamellar configuration.

Stratum Granulosum

The stratum granulosum is composed of three to five layers of cells housing keratohyalin granules.

The stratum granulosum, consisting of three to five layers of flattened keratinocytes, is the most superficial layer of the epidermis in which cells still possess nuclei. The cytoplasm of these keratinocytes contains large,

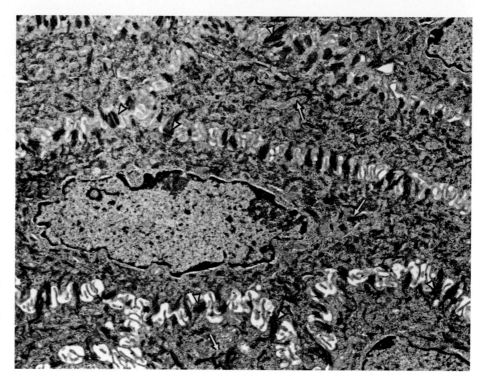

Figure 14–4 Electron micrograph of the stratum spinosum (×6800). The tonofibrils (*arrows*) and the cytoplasmic processes are bridging the intercellular spaces. (From Leeson TS, Leeson CR, and Paparo AA: Text-Atlas of Histology. Philadelphia, WB Saunders, 1988.)

irregularly shaped, coarse, basophilic **keratohyalin granules,** which are not membrane-bound. Bundles of keratin filaments pass through these granules.

Cells of the stratum granulosum also contain membrane-coating granules. The contents of these granules are released by exocytosis into the extracellular space, forming sheets of lipid-rich substance that acts as a waterproof barrier, one of the functions of skin. This impermeable layer prevents cells lying superficial to this region from being bathed in the nutrient-filled aqueous extracellular fluid, thus hastening their death.

Stratum Lucidum

> Present only in thick skin, cells of the stratum lucidum are devoid of nuclei and organelles but contain eleidin.

The clear, homogeneous, lightly staining, thin layer of cells immediately superficial to the stratum granulosum is the stratum lucidum. This layer is present only in thick skin (i.e., palms of the hands and soles of the feet). Although the flattened cells of the stratum lucidum lack organelles and nuclei, they contain densely packed keratin filaments oriented parallel to the skin surface and **eleidin,** a transformation product of keratohyalin. The cytoplasmic aspect of the plasma membrane of these cells has a thickened appearance because of the deposition of a nonkeratin protein, known as **involucrin,** whose function is not known.

Stratum Corneum

> The stratum corneum is composed of several layers of flattened, keratin-containing dead cells known as squames.

The most superficial layer of skin, the stratum corneum, is composed of numerous layers of flattened, keratinized cells with a thickened plasmalemma. These cells lack nuclei and organelles but are filled with keratin filaments embedded in an amorphous matrix. Those cells farther away from the skin surface display desmosomes, whereas cells near the surface of the skin, called **squames,** or **horny cells,** lose their desmosomes and become **desquamated** (sloughed off).

Nonkeratinocytes in the Epidermis

In addition to keratinocytes, the epidermis contains three other cell types: Largerhans cells, merkel cells, and melanocytes.

Langerhans Cells

> Langerhans cells are antigen-presenting cells located among the cells of the stratum spinosum.

Although they are scattered throughout the epidermis where they normally represent 2% to 4% of the epidermal cell population, Langerhans cells, sometimes called **dendritic cells** because of their numerous long processes, are located primarily in the stratum spinosum. These cells also may be found in the dermis as well as in the stratified squamous epithelia of the oral cavity, esophagus, and vagina. However, they are most prevalent in the epidermis, where their numbers may reach 800 per mm^2.

Viewed with light microscopy, Langerhans cells display a dense nucleus, pale cytoplasm, and long slender processes that radiate out from the cell body into the intercellular spaces between keratinocytes. Electron micrographs reveal the nucleus to be polymorphous; the electron-lucent cytoplasm houses a few mitochondria, sparse RER, and no intermediate filaments but contains lysosomes, multivesicular bodies, and small vesicles. Although the irregularly contoured nucleus and the absence of tonofilaments distinguish Langerhans cells from surrounding keratinocytes, the most unique feature of Langerhans cells are the membrane-bound **Birbeck granules (vermiform granules),** which in section resemble Ping-Pong paddles (15 to 50 nm in length and 4 nm thick). These granules form as a result of clathrin-assisted endocytosis; however, their function is not known.

Langerhans cells, once thought to be derived from neural crest cells, are now known to originate from precursors in the bone marrow and are a part of the mononuclear phagocyte system. Although they are capable of mitosis, this activity is restricted; thus, they are continually replaced by precursor cells leaving the bloodstream to migrate into the epidermis and differentiate into Langerhans cells. These cells function in the immune response. and have cell-surface Fc (antibody) and C3 (complement) as well as other receptors, and they phagocytose and process foreign antigens, after which they migrate to lymph nodes in the vicinity, where they present epitopes of processed foreign antigens to T lymphocytes; thus, Langerhans cells are **antigen-presenting cells.**

Merkel Cells

Merkel cells, scattered among cells of the stratum basale, may serve as mechanoreceptors.

Merkel cells, which are interspersed among the keratinocytes of the stratum basale of the epidermis, are especially abundant in the fingertips and oral mucosa and at the base of hair follicles. These cells are derived from the neural crest and are usually found as single cells oriented parallel to the basal lamina; however, they may extend their processes between keratinocytes, to which they are attached by desmosomes (Fig. 14-5). Merkel cell nuclei are deeply indented, and three types of cytokeratins within the cytoplasm make up the cytoskeletal filaments. Dense-cored granules located in the perinuclear zone

and in the processes, whose function is unclear, are the distinguishing feature of Merkel cells.

Myelinated sensory nerves traverse the basal lamina to approximate the Merkel cells, thus forming **Merkel cell–neurite complexes.** These complexes may function as **mechanoreceptors.** These cells exhibit a synaptophysin-like immunoreactivity, indicating that Merkel cells may release neurocrine-like substances, suggesting that the cells display diffuse neuroendocrine system–related activity.

Melanocytes

Melanocytes, derived from neural crest cells, produce melanin pigment that imparts a brown coloration to skin.

Melanocytes, derived from the neural crest, are located among the cells of the stratum basale, although they may also reside in the superficial portions of the dermis (Fig. 14-6).

Melanocytes are round to columnar cells whose long, undulating processes extend from the superficial surfaces of the cells and penetrate the intercellular spaces of the stratum spinosum (see Fig. 14-6). Tyrosinase produced by the RER of the melanocyte is packaged by its Golgi apparatus into oval granules known as **melanosomes** (although the melanosomes of red-haired individuals are round instead of oval). The amino acid tyrosine is preferentially transported into melanosomes, where tyrosinase converts it into **melanin** by means of a series of reactions progressing through 3,4-dihydroxyphenylalanine (dopa, methyldopa) and dopaquinone. It is interesting that the enzyme tyrosinase is activated by ultraviolet light.

CLINICAL CORRELATIONS

Ultraviolet light darkens the melanin and speeds tyrosinase synthesis, thus increasing melanin production. Also, pituitary ACTH influences pigmentation. In **Addison's disease** there is insufficient production of cortisol by the adrenal cortex so excess ACTH is produced, which leads to hyperpigmentation.

Albinism is the absence of melanin production resulting from a genetic defect in tyrosinase synthesis. Melanosomes are present but the melanocytes fail to produce tyrosinase.

Melanosomes leave the cell body of the melanocytes and travel to the tips of their long processes. Once there, the tips of the melanocyte processes penetrate the cytoplasm of the stratum spinosum cells and become

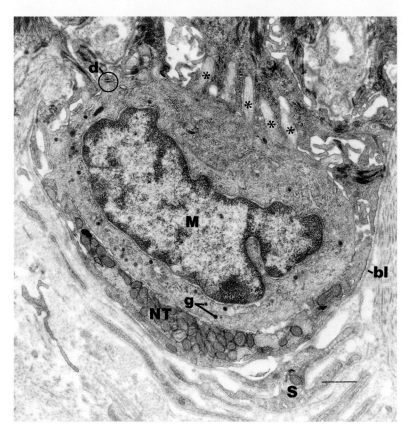

Figure 14–5 Electron micrograph of a Merkel cell (M) and its nerve terminal (NT) in an adult rat. (Scale bar = 0.5 μm). Note the spine-like processes (*asterisks*) that project into the intercellular spaces of the stratum spinosum. Merkel cells form desmosomes (d) with cells of the stratum spinosum and share the basal lamina (bl) of cells of the stratum basale. (From English KB, Wang ZZ, Stayner N, et al: Serotonin-like immunoreactivity in Merkel's cells and their afferent neurons in touch domes from hairy skin of rats. Anat Rec 232:112-120, 1991.)

pinched off via a special secretory process called **cytocrine secretion.** Each truncated melanocyte process elongates and receives more melanosomes, and the cycle is repeated. A particular melanocyte serves a number of keratinocytes with which it is associated, constituting an **epidermal melanin unit.** Within the cells of the stratum intermedium, the melanosomes are transported to the supranuclear region (that is, between the nucleus and the surfacemost region of the cell) so that the melanosomes form a protective barrier between the nucleus and the impinging ultraviolet rays from the sun. Eventually, the melanin pigment is attacked and degraded by lysosomes of the keratinocyte. This process occurs over a period of several days.

The number of melanocytes per square millimeter varies in different regions of skin of an individual, ranging from 800 to 2300. For example, there are much fewer melanocytes on the insides of the arms and thighs than on the face. The difference in skin pigmentation is related more to location of the melanin than to the total number of melanocytes in the skin, which is nearly the same for all races. For instance, there are more melanocytes in the skin on the dorsum than on the palmar surface of the hand; however, these numbers are very similar among the various races. The reason for the darker pigmentation is due not to the effective number of melanocytes but to an increase in their tyrosinase activity.

Although limited exposure to ultraviolet radiation increases the size and functional activity of melanocytes, their population remains the same. After continued exposure to ultraviolet radiation, however, there is also an increase in the melanocyte population. In Blacks, melanosomes are large, numerous, and dispersed throughout the cytoplasm of the keratinocytes, whereas in Caucasians, melanosomes are smaller and fewer and congregate in the vicinity of the nucleus. Also, melanosomes are degraded and removed more rapidly in the Caucasian population than in the Black population.

CLINICAL CORRELATIONS

Ultraviolet rays exist as two types. Ultraviolet B (UVB) is the component in sunlight that produces sunburn, whereas ultraviolet A (UVA) is responsible for tanning. Until recently, it was believed that UVA was relatively safe but it appears that UVA radiation penetrates the skin and damages the deep layers, producing mutations that are implicated in tumor progression.

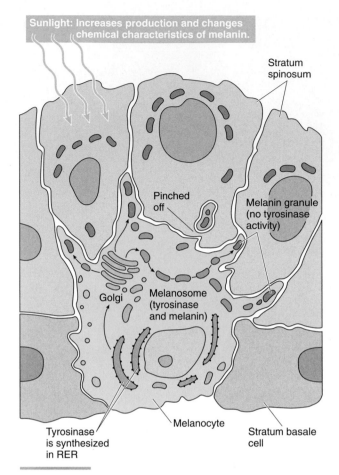

Figure 14–6 Melanocytes and their function. RER, rough endoplasmic reticulum.

Dermis (Corium)

The dermis, the layer of skin immediately deep to the epidermis, is derived from mesoderm and comprises a loose papillary layer and a deeper, denser reticular layer.

The region of the skin lying directly beneath the epidermis, called the dermis, is derived from the mesoderm and is divided into two layers: the superficial, loosely woven **papillary layer** and the deeper, much denser **reticular layer.** The dermis is composed of dense, irregular collagenous connective tissue, containing mostly type I collagen fibers and networks of elastic fibers, which support the epidermis and bind the skin to the underlying **hypodermis** (superficial fascia). The dermis ranges in thickness from 0.6 mm in the eyelids to 3 mm or so on the palm of the hand and the sole of the foot. However, there is not a sharp line of demarcation at its interface with the underlying connective tissue of the superficial fascia. Normally, the dermis is thicker in men than in women and on the dorsal rather than on the ventral surfaces of the body.

Papillary Layer of the Dermis

The most superficial layer of the dermis, the papillary layer, interdigitates directly with the epidermis but is separated from it by the basement membrane.

The superficial papillary layer of the dermis is uneven where it interdigitates with the epidermis, forming the dermal ridges **(papillae)** (see Fig. 14-2). It is composed of a loose connective tissue whose thin, **type III collagen fibers** (reticular fibers) and **elastic fibers** are arranged in loose networks. **Anchoring fibrils,** composed of type VII collagen, extend from the basal lamina into the papillary layer, binding the epidermis to the dermis (see Chapter 4, Figs. 4-13 and 4-14). The papillary layer contains fibroblasts, macrophages, plasma cells, mast cells, and other cells common to connective tissue.

The papillary layer also possesses many capillary loops, which extend to the epidermis-dermis interface. These capillaries regulate body temperature and nourish the cells of the avascular epidermis. Located in some dermal papillae are pear-shaped encapsulated **Meissner corpuscles,** mechanoreceptors specialized to respond to slight deformations of the epidermis. These receptors are most common in areas of the skin that are especially sensitive to tactile stimulation (e.g., lips, external genitalia, and nipples). Another encapsulated mechanoreceptor present in the papillary layer is the **Krause end bulb.** Although this receptor was once thought to respond to cold, its function is currently unclear.

Reticular Layer of the Dermis

The reticular layer of the dermis also contains epidermally derived structures, including sweat glands, hair follicles, and sebaceous glands.

The interface between the papillary layer and reticular layer of the dermis is indistinguishable because the two layers are continuous with each other. Characteristically, the reticular layer is composed of dense, irregular collagenous connective tissue, displaying thick **type I collagen fibers,** which are closely packed into large bundles lying mostly parallel to the skin surface. Networks of **thick elastic fibers** are intermingled with the collagen fibers, appearing especially abundant near sebaceous and sweat glands. Proteoglycans, rich in **dermatan sulfate,** fill the interstices of the reticular layer. Cells are more sparse in this layer than in the papillary layer. They include fibroblasts, mast cells, lymphocytes, macrophages, and, frequently, fat cells in the deeper aspects of the reticular layer.

Sweat glands, sebaceous glands, and **hair follicles,** all derived from the epidermis, invade the dermis and hypodermis during embryogenesis, where they remain permanently (see Fig. 14-1). Groups of **smooth muscle cells** are located in the deeper regions of the reticular layer at particular sites such as the skin of the penis and scrotum and the areola around the nipples; contractions of these muscle groups wrinkle the skin in these regions. Other smooth muscle fibers, called **arrector pili muscles,** are inserted into the hair follicles; contractions of these muscles erect the hairs when the body is cold or suddenly exposed to a cold environment, giving the skin "goose bumps." Additionally, a particular group of striated muscles located in the face, parts of the anterior neck, and scalp **(muscles of facial expression)** originate in the superficial fascia and insert into the dermis.

At least two types of encapsulated mechanoreceptors are located in the deeper portions of the dermis: (1) **pacinian corpuscles,** which respond to pressure and vibrations, and (2) **Ruffini corpuscles,** which respond to tensile forces. The latter are most abundant in the dermis of the soles of the feet.

Epidermis-Dermis Interface

The interdigitation of the epidermal ridges with the dermal ridges is known as the rete apparatus.

The interdigitations of the epidermal and dermal layers are translated through the epidermis and are apparent on the surface of the skin, especially of the palms and soles, where they are represented by whorls, arches, and loops (dermatoglyphs or fingerprints). Because these interdigitations are not easily visualized from two-dimensional histological sections, ethylenediaminetetraacetic acid (EDTA) can be used to chelate calcium ions (Ca^{2+}) of hemidesmosomes, permitting the dissociation of the epidermis from the dermis. Once the epidermis and dermis are dissociated, the three-dimensional surface of the papillary layer of the dermis may be examined with scanning electron microscopy.

The papillary layer presents parallel **primary dermal ridges** on its surface separated by **primary grooves,** which house projections of the epidermis (see

---

CLINICAL CORRELATIONS

Freckles are hyperpigmented spots located on sun-exposed areas of the skin, especially in fair-skinned individuals who sunburn easily. Freckles are usually exhibited by 3 years of age and are the result of increased melanin production and accumulation in the basal area of the epidermis without an increase in melanocytes. They tend to fade in the winter and darken with exposure to ultraviolet light.

Psoriasis is a disease characterized by patchy lesions caused by greater keratinocyte proliferation in the stratum basale and stratum spinosum and an accelerated cell cycle (turnover is increased as much as seven times), resulting in accumulations of keratinocytes and stratum corneum. The lesions are common on the scalp, elbows, and knees, but they may occur almost anywhere on the body. In some cases, the nails may also be involved. Psoriasis is an incurable but manageable chronic condition whose symptoms periodically escalate and then diminish with no apparent cause.

Warts are benign epidermal growths caused by infection of the keratinocytes with **papillomaviruses.** The resulting epidermal hyperplasia thickens the epidermis with scaling. Deeper ingrowth of the dermis brings capillaries closer to the surface. Warts are common in children, young adults, and immunosuppressed patients.

Basal cell carcinoma, the most common human malignancy, arises in the **stratum basale cells** of the epidermis and usually is caused by exposure to ultraviolet radiation. Although basal cell carcinomas do not usually metastasize, they are destructive to local tissue. Of the several types of lesions that occur, the most common is the nodular variety, characterized by a papule or nodule with a central depressed "crater" that eventually ulcerates and crusts. These lesions are most common on the face, especially the nose. Surgery is the usual treatment, and up to 90% of patients recover with no additional sequelae.

Squamous cell carcinoma, the second most common skin cancer, arises in the keratinocytes of the epidermis. It is locally invasive and may metastasize. It is characterized by a hyperkeratotic scaly plaque or nodule that often bleeds or ulcerates. It invades deeply, resulting in fixation to the underlying tissues. Several factors may cause this disease, including ultraviolet radiation, x-irradiation, soot, chemical carcinogens, and arsenic. The lesions are most common on the head and neck. Surgery is the usual treatment of choice.

Malignant melanoma, a skin cancer, is most prevalent in fair-skinned individuals and is increasing in incidence. It is usually associated with excessive exposure to the sun. Malignant melanoma is very invasive because the malignant cells originate from transformed melanocytes; the melanocytes penetrate the dermis and enter lymphatic vessels as well as the bloodstream to gain wide distribution throughout the body.

Fig. 14-2). In the center of each primary dermal ridge is a **secondary groove,** which receives a downgrowth of the epidermis known as an interpapillary peg. Along this and other adjacent ridges are rows of round-topped **dermal papillae** that project into concavities in the epidermis, thus firmly interlocking the epidermis and dermis at the interface. The epidermis-dermis interface in thin skin is much less complex, lacking such deep and widespread interlocking.

Histophysiology of Skin

The structural protein produced by the keratinocytes is **keratin,** which forms 10-nm filaments within the cytoplasm of keratinocytes. Approximately 10 different species of keratin have been identified, and four of these are present within the epidermis.

Stratum basale cells synthesize two of the four keratins, whereas the cells of the stratum spinosum synthesize the other two, which tend to form coarser bundles of filaments. Cells of the stratum spinosum also produce and deposit the protein **involucrin** on the cytoplasmic aspect of their plasmalemma. Moreover, cells of the stratum spinosum also form the **membrane-coating granules,** which later release their lipid-rich contents into the intercellular spaces, forming a permeability barrier.

The keratin-synthesizing machinery shuts down after keratinocytes enter the stratum granulosum. The cells in this layer produce **filaggrin,** a protein thought to help assemble keratin filaments into still coarser bundles. Once keratinocytes reach this stratum they also become permeable to calcium ions, which assist in cross-linking involucrin with other proteins, thereby forming a tough layer beneath the plasmalemma. As keratinocytes move through the stratum granulosum into the stratum lucidum, enzymes released from lysosomes digest the organelles and the nucleus. When the cells finally enter the stratum corneum, they are nonliving, organelle-free, tough shells filled with bundles of keratin filaments.

Epidermal growth factor (EGF) and **interleukin (IL-1α)** influence the growth and development of keratinocytes, at least in tissue culture. In contrast, **transforming growth factor (TGF)** suppresses keratinocyte proliferation and differentiation.

Glands of the Skin

The glands of the skin include eccrine glands, apocrine sweat glands, sebaceous glands, and the mammary gland (a modified and highly specialized type of sweat gland). The mammary gland is described in Chapter 20.

Eccrine Sweat Glands

Eccrine sweat glands are abundant throughout the skin. They release their secretory product, sweat, via the merocrine method of secretion.

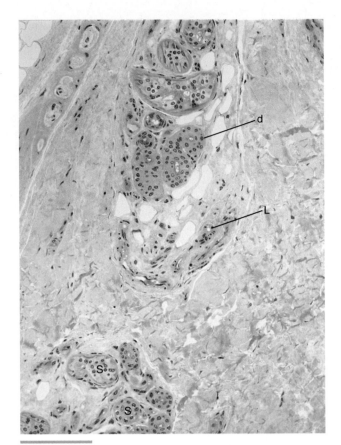

Figure 14–7   Light micrograph of sweat gland showing secretory units (S) and ducts (d), some displaying a lumen (L) (×132).

Eccrine sweat glands are about 0.4 mm in diameter and are located in the skin throughout most of the body. Numbering as many as 3 to 4 million, they are important organs of thermoregulation. Eccrine sweat glands develop as invaginations of the epithelium of the dermal ridge that grows down into the dermis, with its deep aspect becoming the glandular portion of the sweat gland. These glands, which begin to function soon after birth, excrete sweat and may secrete as much as 10 L of sweat a day under extreme conditions in highly active people engaged in vigorous exercise.

Eccrine sweat glands are **simple coiled tubular glands** located deep in the dermis or in the underlying hypodermis (Figs. 14-7 and 14-8). Passing from the secretory portion of each gland is a slender, coiled **duct** that traverses the dermis and epidermis to open on the surface of the skin at a **sweat pore.** Eccrine sweat glands are merocrine in their method of releasing their secretory product. The eccrine glands are innervated by postganglionic fibers of the sympathetic nervous system.

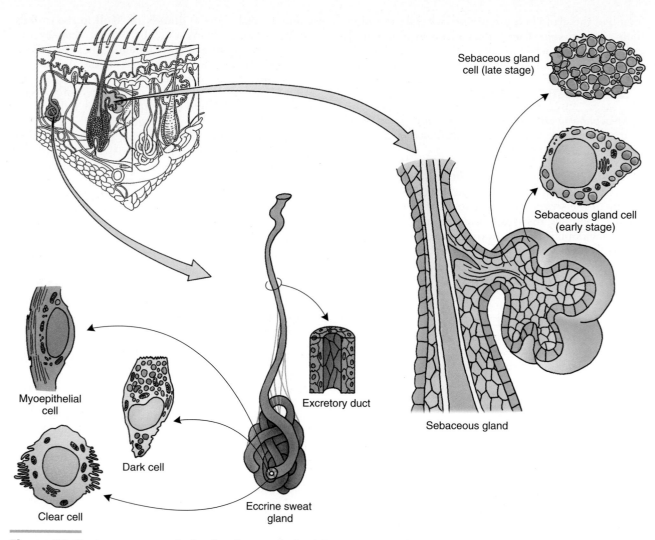

Figure 14–8 An eccrine sweat gland and a sebaceous gland and their constituent cells.

Secretory Unit

The secretory portion of the gland is said to be a simple cuboidal to low columnar epithelium composed of dark cells and clear cells; however, some investigators consider the secretory portion to be pseudostratified.

DARK CELLS (MUCOID CELLS)

Dark cells line the lumen of the secretory unit and secrete a mucus-rich substance.

Dark cells resemble an inverted cone, with the broad ends lining the lumen. The narrowed ends, which seldom reach the basal lamina, conform to fit between adjacent clear cells. Electron micrographs reveal some RER, numerous free ribosomes, elongated mitochondria, and a well-developed Golgi complex. Moderately dense glycoprotein-containing secretory granules are located in the apical cytoplasm of the dark cells, and the secretion released by these cells is **mucous** in nature.

CLEAR CELLS

Clear cells do not possess secretory granules; they release a watery secretion.

Clear cells have a narrow apical area and a broader base that extends to the basal lamina. Unlike dark cells, clear cells do not contain secretory granules but do contain accumulations of **glycogen;** their organelles are similar to those of dark cells, except that they have little RER. The bases of the clear cells are tortuously infolded, similar to those of other cell types involved in transepithelial transport. Clear cells have limited access to the lumen of the gland because of the dark cells; therefore, their **watery secretion** enters **intercellular canali-culi** interposed between adjacent clear cells, where it mixes with the mucous secretion of the dark cells.

MYOEPITHELIAL CELLS

Myoepithelial cells surrounding the secretory portion of the gland contain actin and myosin, imparting a contractile ability to these cells.

Myoepithelial cells surrounding the secretory portion of the eccrine sweat glands are enveloped by the basal lamina of the secretory cells. The cytoplasm of myoep-ithelial cells has **myosin filaments** as well as many deeply acidophil-staining **actin filaments,** which give the cell contractile capability. Contractions of the myoepithelial cells assist in expressing the fluid from the gland.

Duct

The duct of eccrine sweat glands, composed of basal and luminal cells, is highly coiled and traverses the dermis and epidermis on its way to opening on the skin surface.

The duct of an eccrine sweat gland is continuous with the secretory unit at its base but narrows as it passes through the dermis on its way to the epidermal surface. The duct is composed of a stratified cuboidal epithe-lium made up of two layers (see Figs. 14-7 and 14-8). The **cells of the basal layer** have a large, heterochro-matic nucleus and abundant mitochondria. The **cells of the luminal layer** have an irregularly shaped nucleus, little cytoplasm, only a few organelles, and a terminal web immediately deep to the apical plasma membrane.

The ducts follow a helical path through the dermis. As a duct reaches the epidermis, keratinocytes envelop the duct on its way to the sweat pore. The fluid secreted by the secretory portion of the gland is similar to blood plasma in regard to electrolyte balance, including potas-sium and sodium chloride as well as ammonia and urea. However, most of the potassium, sodium, and chloride ions are reabsorbed by cells of the duct as the secretion travels through its lumen. Duct cells excrete ions, urea, lactic acid, and some drugs into the lumen.

Apocrine Sweat Glands

Apocrine sweat glands are found only in the axilla, areola of the nipple, and anal region and may represent vestigial scent glands.

Apocrine sweat glands are found only in certain loca-tions: the axilla (arm pit), the areola of the nipple, and the anal region. Modified apocrine sweat glands consti-tute the **ceruminous (wax) glands** of the external

auditory canal and the **glands of Moll** in the eyelids. Apocrine sweat glands are much larger than eccrine sweat glands, up to 3 mm in diameter. These glands are embedded in the deeper portions of the dermis and hypodermis. Unlike the ducts of eccrine sweat glands, which open onto the skin surface, the ducts of apocrine sweat glands open into canals of the hair follicles just superficial to the entry of the sebaceous gland ducts.

The secretory cells of apocrine glands are simple cuboidal to low columnar in profile. When the lumen of the gland is filled with secretory product, these cells may become squamous. The lumina of these glands are much larger than those of eccrine glands, and the secre-tory cells contain granules that are isolated from the apical membrane by a prominent terminal web. The viscous secretory product of apocrine glands is odorless upon secretion, but when metabolized by bacteria, it presents a distinctive odor. Myoepithelial cells surround the secretory portion of the apocrine sweat glands and assist in expressing the secretory product into the duct of the gland.

An apocrine sweat gland arises from the epithelium of the hair follicles as an epithelial bud that develops into a gland. Secretion by apocrine glands is under the influence of hormones and does not begin until puberty. Their innervation is provided by fibers of the postgan-glionic sympathetic nervous system. Because of the sim-ilarity of their location, their histology, and the fact that the odor is most likely due to the bacterial metabolism of 3-methyl-1,2-hexanoic acid (a volatile acid similar to pheromone signals), it is speculated that apocrine sweat glands evolved from glands that secrete sex attractants in lower animals. As an interesting note, apocrine sweat glands in women undergo cyclical changes that seem to be related to the menstrual cycle—that is, the secretory cells and lumina enlarge before the premenstrual period and diminish during menstruation.

The term *apocrine* given to these special sweat glands implies that the secretion contains a portion of the cytoplasm of the secreting cells. Although some researchers suggest that these cells release their secre-tion via the apocrine method, most investigators report that, despite their name, apocrine sweat glands release their secretory product via the merocrine mode of secretion.

Sebaceous Glands

Sebaceous glands secrete an oily substance known as sebum, which maintains the suppleness of the skin.

Except for the palms of the hands, soles of the feet, and sides of the feet inferior to the hairline, sebaceous glands are found throughout the body, embedded in the dermis and hypodermis. These glands are most abun-dant on the face, scalp, and the forehead. The secretory product of the sebaceous glands, **sebum,** is a wax-like, oily mixture of cholesterol, triglycerides, and secretory cellular debris. Sebum is believed to facilitate the maintenance of proper skin texture and hair flexibility.

Like apocrine sweat glands, sebaceous glands are appendages of hair follicles. The ducts of the sebaceous glands open into the upper third of the follicular canal, where they discharge their secretory product to coat the hair shaft and, eventually, the skin surface (see Fig. 14-8). The ducts of sebaceous glands in certain regions of the body lacking hair follicles (i.e., the lips, glans penis, areola of the nipples, labia minora, and mucous surface of the prepuce) open onto the surface of the skin to empty their secretions. Sebaceous glands are under the influence of sex hormones and increase their activity greatly after puberty.

Sebaceous glands are lobular with clusters of acini opening into single short ducts. Each acinus is composed of peripherally located small basal cells (resting on the basal lamina), which surround larger round cells that fill the remainder of the acinus (Fig. 14-9). The basal cells have a spherical nucleus, both smooth endoplasmic reticulum (SER) and RER, glycogen, and lipid droplets. These cells undergo cell division to form more

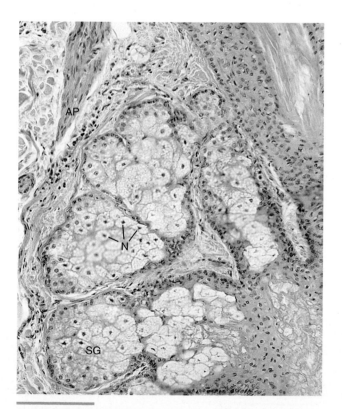

Figure 14–9 Light micrograph showing human sebaceous glands (SG) and the nuclei (N) of their cells (×132). AP, arrector pili muscle.

basal cells and larger round cells. The larger cells have abundant SER and cytoplasm filled with lipid droplets. The central region of the acinus is filled with cells in different stages of degeneration. These pale-staining cells display only strands of cytoplasm, deeply staining pyknotic nuclei, ruptured plasmalemmae, and coalescing lipid droplets. Lipid synthesis continues for a short time, followed by necrosis of the cells and the ultimate release of lipid and cellular debris, which form the secretory product (holocrine secretion). The secretory product is released into a duct lined with a stratified squamous epithelium that is continuous with the follicular canal at the hair follicle.

CLINICAL CORRELATIONS

Acne, the most common disease seen by dermatologists, is a chronic inflammatory disease involving the sebaceous glands and hair follicles. Obstructions resulting from impaction of sebum and keratinous debris within hair follicles is one cause of acne lesions. Anaerobic bacteria near these obstructions may contribute to development of acne, although the role of bacteria is not clear. However, the efficacy of antibiotic treatment for acne supports the idea of bacterial involvement in its pathogenesis. The disease is most severe in boys, with onset commonly from age 9 to 11 years, when increasing levels of sex hormones begin to stimulate the sebaceous glands. Acne usually subsides through the later teen years, but it may not resolve until the fourth decade of life. In some people, acne does not begin until adulthood.

Hair

Hairs are filamentous, keratinized structures that project from the epidermal surface of the skin (see Fig. 14-1). Hair grows over most of the body except on the vermilion zone of the lips, palms and sides of the palms, soles and sides of the feet, dorsum of the distal phalanges of the fingers and toes, glans penis, glans clitoris, labia minora, and vestibular aspect of the labia majora.

Two types of hairs are present on the human body. Hairs that are soft, fine, short, and pale (e.g., those covering the eyelids) are called **vellus hairs;** those that are hard, large, coarse, long, and dark (e.g., those of the scalp and eyebrows) are called **terminal hairs.** Additionally, very fine hair, called **lanugo,** is present on the fetus.

The number of hairs on humans is essentially the same as on other primates, but most human hair is of the vellus type, whereas terminal hairs predominate on other primates. Human hair does not provide thermal insulation, as does the fur of animals. Instead, human hairs serve in tactile sensation, such that any stimulus that deforms a hair is translated down the shaft to sensory nerves that surround the hair follicle.

Hair growth is optimal from about 16 to 46 years of age; after age 50, hair growth begins to diminish. During pregnancy, hair growth is normal; after parturition, the cycle of hair growth subsides and hair loss is temporarily increased.

Hair Follicles

Hair follicles develop from the epidermis and invade the dermis and hypodermis.

Hair follicles, the organs from which hairs develop, arise from invaginations of the epidermis that invade the dermis, hypodermis, or both. Hair follicles are surrounded by dense accumulations of fibrous connective tissue belonging to the dermis (Fig. 14-10). A thickened basement membrane, the **glassy membrane,** separates the dermis from the epithelium of the hair follicle (Fig. 14-11). The expanded terminus of the hair follicle, the **hair root,** is indented, and the concavity conforms to the shape of the **dermal papilla** occupying it. The hair root and the dermal papilla together are known as the **hair bulb.** The dermal papilla contains a rich supply of capillaries that provide nutrients and oxygen for the cells of the hair follicle. The dermal papilla also acts as an inductive force controlling the physiological activities of the hair follicle.

The bulk of the cells composing the hair root is called the **matrix.** Proliferation of these matrix cells accounts for the growth of hair; thus, they are homologous to the stratum basale of the epidermis. The outer layers of follicular epithelium form the **external root sheath,** which is composed of a single layer of cells at the hair bulb and several layers of cells near the surface of the skin (Fig. 14-12).

The external root sheath surrounds several layers of epidermally derived cells, the **internal root sheath,** which consists of three components: (1) an outer single row of cuboidal cells, **Henle's layer,** which contacts the innermost layer of cells of the external root sheath; (2) one or two layers of flattened cells forming **Huxley's layer;** and (3) the **cuticle of the internal root sheath,** formed by overlapping scale-like cells whose free ends project toward the base of the hair follicle. The internal root sheath ends where the duct of the sebaceous gland attaches to the hair follicle (see Fig. 14-12).

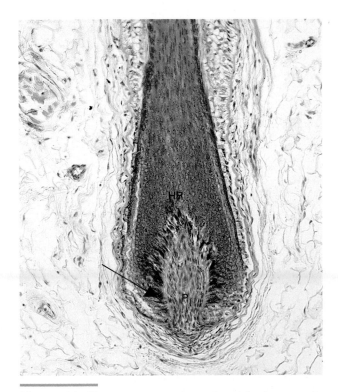

Figure 14–10 Light micrograph of a longitudinal section of a hair follicle with its hair root (HR) and papilla (P) (×132). The dark areas (*arrow*) are pigment.

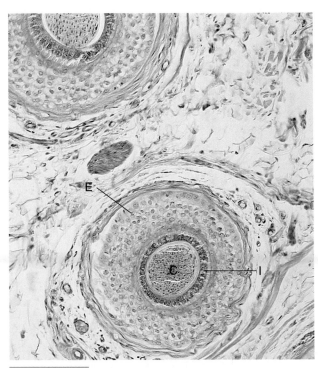

Figure 14–11 Light micrograph of hair follicles in cross section (×132). Observe the external root sheath (E), the internal root sheath (I), and the cortex (C).

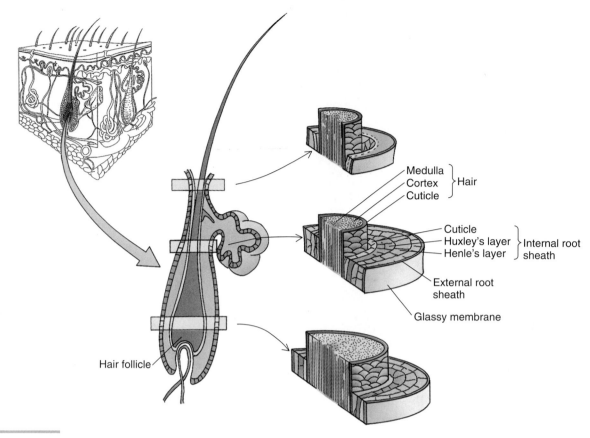

Figure 14–12 The hair follicle.

The hair shaft is a long slender filament that extends to and through the surface of the epidermis (Fig. 14-13). It consists of three regions: **medulla, cortex,** and the **cuticle of the hair.** As the cells of the matrix within the hair root proliferate and differentiate, they move toward the surface of the skin, eventually developing into the hair shaft. The cells in the center of the matrix are closest to the underlying dermal papilla and thus are most influenced by it; cells lying more and more peripheral to the matrix center are progressively less influenced by the dermal papilla. The distinctive layers of the follicle develop from different matrix cells as follows:

- The *most central* matrix cells give rise to large vacuolated cells that form the core of the hair shaft (the **medulla**). This layer is present only in thick hair.
- Matrix cells *slightly peripheral* to the center become the **cortex** of the hair shaft.
- *More peripheral* matrix cells become the **cuticle** of the hair.
- The *most peripheral* matrix cells develop into the cells of the **internal root sheath.**

As the cells of the cortex are displaced surfaceward, they synthesize abundant **keratin filaments** and **tri-** **chohyalin granules** (resembling keratohyalin granules of the epidermis). These granules coalesce, forming an amorphous substance in which the keratin filaments are embedded. Scattered among the cells of the matrix nearest to the dermal papilla are large **melanocytes,** with long dendritic processes that transfer **melanosomes** to the cells of the cortex. The melanosomes remain in these cells, imparting to the hair a color based on the amount of melanin present. With age, the melanocytes gradually lose their ability to produce **tyrosinase,** which is essential for the production of melanin, and the hair becomes gray.

Arrector Pili Muscles

Arrector pili muscles are smooth muscle cells extending from midshaft of the hair follicle to the papillary layer of the dermis.

Attached to the connective tissue sheath surrounding the hair follicles and to the papillary layer of the dermis are the arrector pili muscles (see Fig. 14-1). These smooth muscles attach to the hair follicle above its middle at an oblique angle. Contractions of these

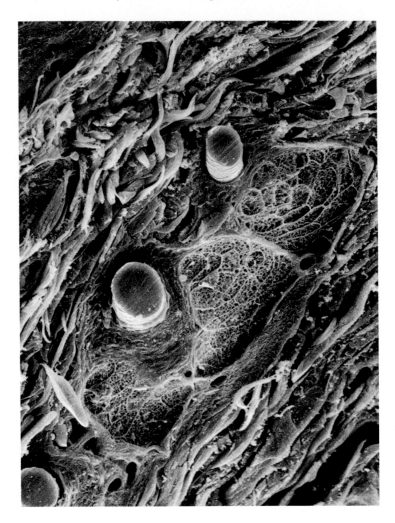

Figure 14–13 Scanning electron micrograph of monkey scalp that shows three hair shafts and their sebaceous glands surrounded by the dense, irregular, collagenous connective tissue of the dermis (×235). (From Leeson TS, Leeson, CR, and Paparo AA: Text/Atlas of Histology. Philadelphia, WB Saunders, 1998.)

muscles depress the skin over their attachment and elevate the hair shaft and the skin around the hair shaft, forming tiny "goose bumps" on the surface of the skin. These are easily observed when a person is chilled or suddenly frightened.

Histophysiology of Hair

Hair grows at an average rate of about 1 cm/month, but hair growth is not continuous. The hair growth cycle consists of three successive phases: (1) the growth period, the **anagen phase;** (2) a brief period of involution, the **catagen phase**; and (3) the final phase of rest, the **telogen phase,** in which the mature, aged hair is shed (falls out or is pulled out). Hairs shed in this fashion are called **club hairs** because they retain their club-shaped root. Soon afterward, a new hair is formed by the hair follicle and the hair growth cycle begins again.

The duration of the hair growth cycle varies in different areas of the body. For example, the life span of an axillary hair is roughly 4 months, whereas scalp hair may remain in the anagen phase for as long as 6 years and in the telogen phase for 4 months.

Hair follicles in certain regions of the body respond to male sex hormones. For this reason, men begin to develop more dark-pigmented terminal hairs about the chin, cheeks, and upper lip at puberty. Although women possess the same number of hair follicles in these regions, these hairs remain the fine, pale, vellus type. In both sexes at puberty, however, heavily pigmented, coarse terminal hairs begin to grow in the axillary and pubic regions.

The keratinization processes in hair and in skin, although generally similar, differ in some respects. The superficial cell layers of the epidermis of the skin form a **soft keratin,** consisting of keratin filaments embedded in filaggrin; the keratinized cells are sloughed continuously. In contrast, not only does keratinization of hair form a **hard keratin,** consisting of keratin filaments embedded in trichohyalin, but the keratinizing

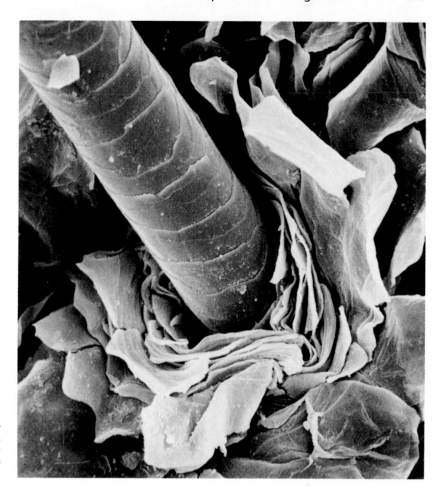

Figure 14–14 Scanning electron micrograph of a hair from a monkey's scalp (×1115). (From Leeson TS, Leeson CR, Paparo AA: Text/Atlas of Histology. Philadelphia, WB Saunders, 1988.)

cells are not shed; instead they accumulate, becoming compressed and hard.

The arrangement of cells composing the cuticle of the hair and cuticle of the internal root sheath interlocks the apposing free edges of these cells, making it difficult to pull the hair shaft out of its follicle (Fig. 14-14).

Nails

Nails represent keratinized epithelial cells arranged in plates of hard keratin.

Nails, located on the distal phalanx of each finger and toe, are composed of plates of heavily compacted, highly keratinized epithelial cells that form the **nail plate,** lying on the epidermis, known as the **nail bed** (Figs. 14-15 and 14-16). The nails develop from cells of the **nail matrix** that proliferate and become keratinized. The nail matrix, a region of the **nail root,** is located beneath the **proximal nail fold.** The stratum corneum of the proximal nail fold forms the **eponychium (cuticle),** which extends from the proximal end up

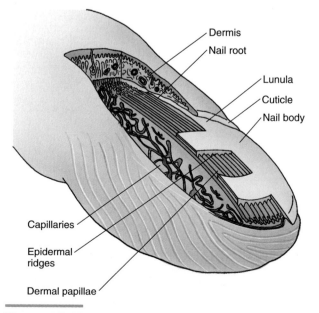

Figure 14–15 Structure of the thumbnail.

Dermis
Nail root
Lunula
Cuticle
Nail body
Capillaries
Epidermal ridges
Dermal papillae

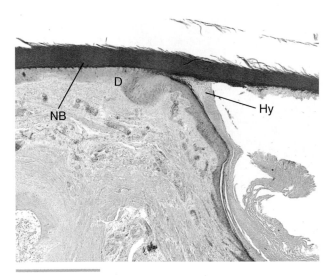

Figure 14–16 Light micrograph of a longitudinal section through a fingernail (×14). Observes the dermis (D), hyponychium (Hy) and the nail bed (NB).

on the nail for about 0.5 to 1 mm. Laterally, the skin turns under as **lateral nail folds,** forming the **lateral nail grooves;** the epidermis continues beneath the nail plate as the nail bed, and the nail plate occupies the position (and function) of the stratum corneum.

The white crescent observed at the proximal end of the nail is called the **lunula.** The distal end of the nail plate is not attached to the nail bed, which becomes continuous with the skin of the fingertip (or end of the toe). Near this junction is an accumulation of stratum corneum called the **hyponychium.**

Fingernails grow continuously at the rate of about 0.5 mm/week; toenails grow somewhat more slowly. The translucency of the fingernails provides a quick indication of the health of an individual; pinkness indicates a well-oxygenated blood supply.

Respiratory System

15

The respiratory system, comprising the lungs and a sequence of airways leading to the external environment, functions in providing oxygen (O_2) to and eliminating carbon dioxide (CO_2) from the cells of the body. The realization of this goal requires the fulfillment of the following four discrete events, collectively known as respiration:

- Movement of air in and out of the lungs (**breathing** or **ventilation**)
- Exchange of O_2 in the inspired air for carbon dioxide in the blood (**external respiration**)
- Conveyance of O_2 and CO_2 to and from the cells (**transport of gases**)
- Exchange of CO_2 for O_2 in the vicinity of the cells (**internal respiration**)

The first two of these events, ventilation and external respiration, occur within the confines of the respiratory system, whereas the transport of gases is performed by the circulatory system and internal respiration occurs in the tissues throughout the body.

The respiratory system is subdivided into two major components: the conducting portion and the respiratory portion (Table 15-1). The **conducting portion,** situated both outside and within the lungs, conveys air from the external milieu to the lungs. The **respiratory portion,** located strictly within the lungs, functions in the actual exchange of oxygen for carbon dioxide (external respiration).

CONDUCTING PORTION OF THE RESPIRATORY SYSTEM

The conducting portion of the respiratory system conveys air to and from the respiratory portion of the respiratory system.

The conducting portion of the respiratory system, listed in order from the exterior to the inside of the lung, is composed of the nasal cavity, mouth, nasopharynx, pharynx, larynx, trachea, primary bronchi, secondary bronchi (lobar bronchi), tertiary bronchi (segmental bronchi), bronchioles, and terminal bronchioles. These structures not only transport but also filter, moisten, and warm the inspired air before it reaches the respiratory portion of the lungs.

The patency of the conducting airways is maintained by a combination of bone, cartilage, and fibrous elements. As the air progresses along the airway during inspiration, it encounters a branching system of tubules. Although the luminal diameter of each succeeding tubule continues to decrease, the *total* cross-sectional diameter of the various branches increases at each level of branching. As a result, the velocity of air flow for a given volume of inhaled air decreases as the air proceeds toward the respiratory portion.

Nasal Cavity

The nasal cavity is divided into right and left halves by the cartilaginous and bony nasal septum. Each half of the nasal cavity is bounded laterally by a bony wall and a cartilaginous ala (wing) of the nose; it communicates with the outside, anteriorly, via the **naris** (nostril) and with the nasopharynx by way of the **choana.** Projecting from the bony lateral wall are three thin scroll-like bony shelves, situated one above the other: the superior, middle, and inferior **nasal conchae.**

Anterior Portion of the Nasal Cavity

The anterior portion of the nasal cavity, in the vicinity of the nares, is dilated and is known as the **vestibule.** This region is lined with thin skin and has **vibrissae—** short, stiff hairs that prevent larger dust particles from entering the nasal cavity. The dermis of the vestibule houses numerous sebaceous and sweat glands. The

TABLE 15–1 Divisions and Characteristic Features of the Respiratory System

Region	Support	Glands	Epithelium	Cell Types	Additional Features
Extrapulmonary Conducting Division					
Nasal vestibule	Hyaline cartilage	Sebaceous and sweat glands	Stratified squamous keratinized	Epidermal	Vibrissae
Nasal cavity: respiratory	Hyaline cartilage and bone	Seromucous glands	Respiratory	Basal, goblet, ciliated, brush, serous, and DNES	Erectile-like tissue
Nasal cavity: olfactory	Bone	Bowman's glands (serous)	Olfactory	Olfactory, sustentacular, and basal	Olfactory vesicle
Nasopharynx	Skeletal muscle	Seromucous glands	Respiratory	Basal, goblet, ciliated, brush, serous, and DNES	Pharyngeal tonsils and eustachian tubes
Larynx	Hyaline and elastic cartilages	Mucous and seromucous glands	Respiratory stratified squamous nonkeratinized	Basal, goblet, ciliated, brush, serous, and DNES	Epiglottis, vocal folds, and vestibular folds
Trachea and primary bronchi	Hyaline cartilage and dense, irregular, collagenous, connective tissue	Mucous and seromucous glands	Respiratory	Basal, goblet, ciliated, brush, serous, and DNES	C-rings and trachealis muscle (smooth muscle) in adventitia
Intrapulmonary Conducting Division					
Secondary (intrapulmonary) bronchi	Hyaline cartilage and smooth muscle	Seromucous glands	Respiratory	Basal, goblet, ciliated, brush, serous, and DNES	Plates of hyaline cartilage and two ribbons of helically oriented smooth muscle
(Primary) bronchioles	Smooth muscle	No glands	Simple columnar to simple cuboidal	Ciliated cells and Clara cells (and occasional goblet cells in larger bronchioles)	Less than 1 mm in diameter; supply air to lobules; two ribbons of helically oriented smooth muscle
Terminal bronchioles	Smooth muscle	No glands	Simple cuboidal	Some ciliated cells and many Clara cells (no goblet cells)	Less than 0.5 mm in diameter; supply air to lung acini; some smooth muscle
Respiratory Division					
Respiratory bronchioles	Some smooth muscle and collagen fibers	No glands	Simple cuboidal and highly attenuated simple squamous	Some ciliated cuboidal cells, Clara cells, and types I and II pneumocytes	Alveoli in walls; alveoli have smooth muscle sphincters in their openings
Alveolar ducts	Type III collagen (reticular) fibers and smooth muscle sphincters of alveoli	No glands	Highly attenuated simple squamous	Type I and type II pneumocytes of alveoli	No walls of their own; only a linear sequence of alveoli

TABLE 15–1 Divisions and Characteristic Features of the Respiratory System—cont'd

Region	Support	Glands	Epithlium	Cell Types	Additional Features
Alveolar sacs	Type III collagen and elastic fibers	No glands	Highly attenuated simple squamous	Type I and type II pneumocytes	Clusters of alveoli
Alveoli	Type III collagen and elastic fibers	No glands	Highly attenuated simple squamous	Type I and type II pneumocytes	200 μm in diameter; have alveolar macrophages

DNES, diffuse neuroendocrine system.

dermis is anchored by numerous collagen bundles to the perichondria of the hyaline cartilage segments that form the supporting skeleton of the ala.

Posterior Aspect of the Nasal Cavity

Except for the vestibule and the olfactory region, the nasal cavity is lined by pseudostratified ciliated columnar epithelium, frequently called the **respiratory epithelium** (see discussion of the trachea later), which is well endowed with goblet cells in the more posterior regions of the nasal cavity. The subepithelial connective tissue (**lamina propria**) is richly vascularized, especially in the region of the conchae and the anterior aspect of the nasal septum, housing large arterial plexuses and venous sinuses. The lamina propria has many seromucous glands and abundant lymphoid elements, including occasional lymphoid nodules, mast cells, and plasma cells. Antibodies produced by plasma cells (immunoglobulins IgA, IgE, and IgG) protect the nasal mucosa against inhaled antigens as well as against microbial invasion.

CLINICAL CORRELATIONS

Nasal bleeding usually occurs from **Kiesselbach's area,** the anteroinferior region of the nasal septum, which is the site of anastomosis of the arterial supply of the nasal mucosa. The bleeding may be arrested by applying pressure on the region or by packing the nasal cavity with cotton.

Olfactory Region of the Nasal Cavity

The olfactory region comprises the olfactory epithelium and the underlying lamina propria that houses Bowman's glands and a rich vascular plexus.

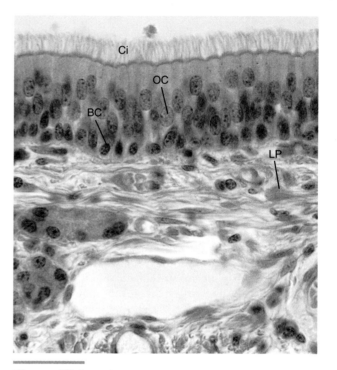

Figure 15–1 Light micrograph of the human olfactory mucosa (×540). Observe that the olfactory cilia (Ci) are well represented and that the connective tissue displays the presence of Bowman's glands. BC, basal cell; OC, olfactory cell; LP, lamina propria.

The roof of the nasal cavity, the superior aspect of the nasal septum, and the superior concha are covered by an olfactory epithelium 60 μm thick. The underlying lamina propria houses serous fluid–secreting Bowman's glands, a rich vascular plexus, and collections of axons that arise from the olfactory cells of the **olfactory epithelium.** The olfactory epithelium, which is yellow in the living person, is composed of three types of cells: olfactory, sustentacular, and basal (Fig. 15-1).

OLFACTORY CELLS

Olfactory cells are bipolar neurons whose apical aspect, the distal terminus of its slender dendrite, is modified

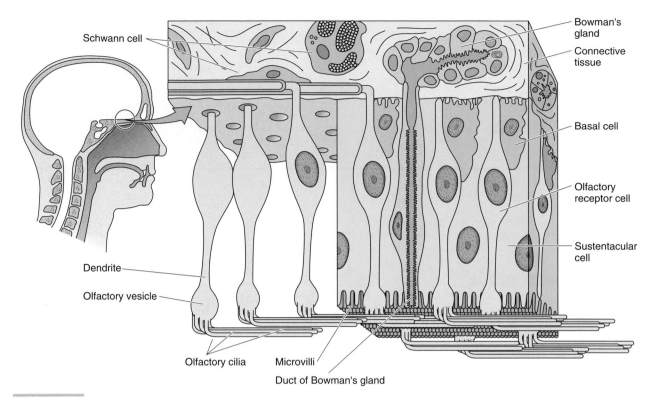

Figure 15–2   The olfactory epithelium, displaying basal, olfactory, and sustentacular cells. (Compare with Fig. 15-1.)

to form a bulb, the **olfactory vesicle,** which projects above the surface of the sustentacular cells (Figs. 15-2 and 15-3). The nucleus of the cell is spherical and is closer to the basal lamina than to the olfactory vesicle. Most of the organelles of the cell are in the vicinity of the nucleus.

Scanning electron micrographs demonstrate that six to eight long, nonmotile olfactory cilia extend from the olfactory vesicle and lie on the free surface of the epithelium. Transmission electron micrographs of these cilia display an unusual axoneme pattern that begins as a typical peripheral ring of nine **doublet** microtubules surrounding two central **singlets** (9 + 2 configuration) but without the characteristic dynein arms. The axoneme changes distally so that it is composed of nine **singlets** surrounding the two central singlets, and near the end of the cilium only the central singlets are present.

The basal region of the olfactory cell is its **axon,** which penetrates the basal lamina and joins similar axons to form bundles of nerve fibers. Each axon, although unmyelinated, has a sheath composed of Schwann cell–like olfactory ensheathing (glial) cells. The nerve fibers pass through the cribriform plate in the roof of the nasal cavity to synapse with secondary neurons in the olfactory bulb.

SUSTENTACULAR AND BASAL CELLS

Sustentacular cells are columnar cells, 50 to 60 μm tall, whose apical aspects have a striated border composed of microvilli. Their oval nuclei are in the apical third of the cell, somewhat superficial to the location of the olfactory cell nuclei. The apical cytoplasm of these cells has secretory granules housing a yellow pigment whose color is characteristic of the olfactory mucosa. Electron micrographs of sustentacular cells demonstrate that they form junctional complexes with the olfactory vesicle regions of olfactory cells as well as with contiguous sustentacular cells. The morphology of sustentacular cells is not remarkable, although they do display a prominent terminal web of actin microfilaments. These cells are believed to provide physical support, nourishment, and electrical insulation for the olfactory cells.

Basal cells are of two types, horizontal and globose. Horizontal cells are flat and lie against the basement membrane, whereas globose cells are short, basophilic, pyramid-shaped cells whose apical aspects do not reach the epithelial surface. Their nuclei are centrally located, but because these are short cells, the nuclei occupy the basal third of the epithelium. The globose type of basal cells have considerable proliferative capacity and can

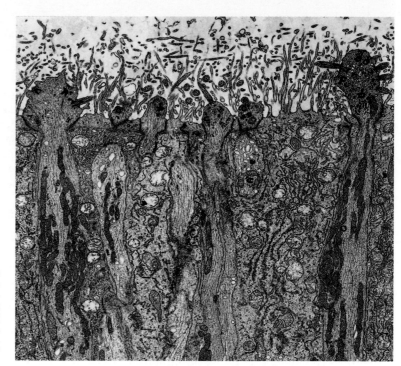

Figure 15–3 Transmission electron micrograph of the apical region of the rat olfactory epithelium (×8260). Note the olfactory vesicles and the cilia projecting from them. (Compare with the Figs. 15-1 and 15-2.) (From Mendoza AS, Kühnel W: Postnatal changes in the ultrastructure of the rat olfactory epithelium: The supranuclear region of supporting cells. Cell Tissue Res 265:193-196, 1991.)

replace both sustentacular and olfactory cells. In a healthy person, the olfactory cells live for less than three months and sustentacular cells have a life span of less than a year. The horizontal basal cells replicate to replace the globose basal cells.

LAMINA PROPRIA

The lamina propria of the olfactory mucosa is composed of a richly vascularized, loose to dense, irregular collagenous connective tissue that is firmly attached to the underlying periosteum. It houses numerous lymphoid elements as well as the collection of axons of the olfactory cells, which form fascicles of unmyelinated nerve fibers. **Bowman's glands (olfactory glands),** which produce a serous secretory product, are also present and are indicative of the olfactory mucosa. These glands release IgA, lactoferrin, lysozyme, and odorant-binding protein, a molecule that prevents the odorant from leaving the region of the olfactory epithelium, thus enhancing a person's ability to detect odors.

Histophysiology of the Nasal Cavity

The nasal mucosa filters, warms, and humidifies the inhaled air and also is responsible for the perception of odors.

The moist nasal mucosa filters inhaled air. Particulate matter, such as dust, is trapped by the mucus produced by the goblet cells of the epithelium and the seromu-cous glands of the lamina propria. The serous fluid, produced by the seromucous glands, is situated between the mucus and the apical plasmalemmae of the respiratory epithelial cells. Because the cilia of the ciliated columnar cells do not reach the mucous layer, their movement is restricted to the serous fluid layer. As the cilia move within that watery fluid, the mucus is swept along ("hydroplaned") at the interface of the two fluids. The particulate matter trapped in mucus is thus delivered, by ciliary action, to the pharynx to be swallowed or expectorated.

In addition to being filtered, the air is also warmed and humidified by being passed over the mucosa, which is kept warm and moist by its rich blood supply. Warming of the inspired air is facilitated by the presence of an extensive network of rows of arched vessels grouped in an anteroposterior arrangement. Capillary beds arising from these vessels lie just beneath the epithelium and the flow of blood into this vascular network is directed from posterior to anterior, opposite to the flow of air; thus, heat is continuously being transferred to the inspired air by a countercurrent mechanism.

Antigens and allergens carried by the air are combated by lymphoid elements of the lamina propria. Secretory immunoglobulin (IgA), produced by plasma cells, is transported across the epithelium into the nasal cavity by ciliated columnar cells and by the acinar cells of the seromucous glands. IgE, which is also produced by plasma cells, binds to IgE receptors (FcεRI receptors) of mast cell and basophil plasmalemmae. Subsequent binding of a specific antigen or allergen to the bound IgE causes the mast cell (and basophil) to release various mediators of inflammation. These, in turn, act on the nasal mucosa, inducing the symptoms associated with colds and hay fever.

CLINICAL CORRELATIONS

The nasal mucosa is protected from dehydration by alternating blood flow to the venous sinuses of the lamina propria overlying the conchae of the right and left nasal cavities. The erectile tissue-like region (**swell bodies**) of one side expands when its venous sinuses become engorged with blood, reducing the flow of air through that side. Seepage of plasma from the sinuses and seromucous secretions from the glands thus rehydrate the mucosa approximately every half hour.

Chemical irritants and particulate matter are removed from the nasal cavity by the **sneeze reflex.** The sudden explosive expulsion of air usually clears the nasal passage of the irritant.

The olfactory epithelium is responsible for the perception of odors, which also makes a major contribution to the sense of taste discrimination. The mechanism of odor discernment is poorly understood, although it is known that the plasmalemma of the olfactory cilia of a particular olfactory cell has numerous copies of one particular **odor receptor molecule.** Molecules of an odoriferous substance dissolved in the serous fluid bind to its specific receptor. When a threshold number of odor receptors are occupied, the olfactory cell becomes stimulated, an action potential is generated, and the information is transmitted via its axon to the olfactory bulb, a projection of the central nervous system, for processing. Axons of olfactory cells synapse with the dendrites of 1 of 30 mitral cells within small spherical regions of the olfactory bulb known as **glomeruli.** If a threshold level of impulses reaches a mitral cell, it becomes depolarized and relays the signal to the olfactory cortex for further processing.

Each glomerulus receives input (information) from approximately 2000 olfactory neurons, each specific for the same odoriferous substance. Similar to antigens, which may have several epitopes, each of which binds a specific antibody, odoriferous substances possess several small regions, each of which binds to a specific odor receptor molecule. Thus, a particular odoriferous substance may bind to several odor receptor molecules, activating a number of olfactory neurons and providing input to several glomeruli. Although there are only about 1000 glomeruli, each receiving information concerning a single odor receptor molecule, the olfactory cortex has the ability to distinguish about 10,000 different scents. It does so by recognizing information arising from a particular combination of glomeruli as a single scent. Thus, a particular glomerulus may be active in the recognition of several scents.

To ensure that a single stimulus does not produce repeated responses, the continuous flow of serous fluid from Bowman's glands provides a constant refreshment of the olfactory cilia.

Paranasal Sinuses

The ethmoid, sphenoid, frontal, and maxilla bones of the skull house large, mucoperiosteum-lined spaces, the paranasal sinuses (named after their location), which communicate with the nasal cavity. The mucosa of each sinus comprises a vascular connective tissue lamina propria fused with the periosteum. The thin lamina propria resembles that of the nasal cavity, in that it houses seromucous glands as well as lymphoid elements. The respiratory epithelial lining of the paranasal sinuses, similar to that of the nasal cavity, has numerous ciliated columnar cells whose cilia sweep the mucus layer toward the nasal cavity.

Nasopharynx

The pharynx begins at the choana and extends to the opening of the larynx. This continuous cavity is subdivided into three regions: (1) the superior nasopharynx, (2) the middle oral pharynx, and (3) the inferior laryngeal pharynx. The nasopharynx is lined by a respiratory epithelium, whereas the oral and laryngeal regions are lined by a stratified squamous epithelium. The lamina propria is composed of a loose to dense, irregular type of vascularized connective tissue housing seromucous glands and lymphoid elements. It is fused with the epimysium of the skeletal muscle components of the pharynx. The lamina propria of the posterior aspect of the nasopharynx houses the **pharyngeal tonsil,** an unencapsulated collection of lymphoid tissue described in Chapter 12.

Larynx

The larynx, or voice box, is responsible for phonation and for preventing the entry of food and fluids into the respiratory system.

The larynx, situated between the pharynx and the trachea, is a rigid, short, cylindrical tube 4 cm in length and approximately 4 cm in diameter. It is responsible for phonation and prevents the entry of solids or liquids into the respiratory system during swallowing. The wall of the larynx is reinforced by several hyaline cartilages (the unpaired thyroid and cricoid cartilages and the inferior aspect of the paired arytenoids) and elastic cartilages (the unpaired epiglottis, the paired corniculate and cuneiform cartilages, and the superior aspect of the arytenoids). These cartilages are connected to one another by ligaments, and their movements with respect to one another are controlled by **intrinsic and extrinsic skeletal muscles.**

The thyroid and cricoid cartilages form the cylindrical support for the larynx, whereas the epiglottis provides a cover over the laryngeal **aditus** (opening). During respiration, the epiglottis is in the vertical position, permitting the flow of air. During swallowing of food, fluids, or saliva, however, it is positioned horizontally, closing the laryngeal aditus; yet normally, even in the absence of an epiglottis, swallowed material bypasses the laryngeal opening. The arytenoid and corniculate cartilages are occasionally fused to each other, and most of the intrinsic muscles of the larynx move the two arytenoids with respect to each other and to the cricoid cartilage.

The lumen of the larynx is characterized by two pairs of shelf-like folds, the superiorly positioned vestibular folds and the inferiorly placed vocal folds. The **vestibular folds** are immovable. Their lamina propria, composed of loose connective tissue, houses seromucous glands, adipose cells, and lymphoid elements. The free edge of each **vocal fold** is reinforced by dense, regular elastic connective tissue, the **vocal ligament.** The vocalis muscle, attached to the vocal ligament, assists the other intrinsic muscles of the larynx in altering the tension on the vocal folds. These muscles also regulate the width of the space between the vocal folds (the **rima glottidis**), thus permitting precisely regulated vibrations of their free edges by the exhaled air.

During silent respiration, the vocal folds are partly *abducted* (pulled apart), and during forced inspiration, they are fully abducted. During phonation, however, the vocal folds are strongly *adducted* (drawn together), forming a narrow interval between them. The movement of air against the edges of the strongly adducted vocal folds produces and modulates sound (but not speech, which is formed by movements of the pharynx, soft palate, tongue, and lips). The longer and more relaxed the vocal folds, the deeper the **pitch** of the sound. Because the larynx of a postpubescent male is larger than that of a female, men tend to have deeper voices than women.

The larynx is lined by **pseudostratified ciliated columnar epithelium,** except on the superior surfaces of the epiglottis and vocal folds, which are covered by stratified squamous nonkeratinized epithelium. The cilia of the larynx beat toward the pharynx, transporting mucus and trapped particulate matter toward the mouth to be expectorated or swallowed.

CLINICAL CORRELATIONS

Laryngitis (inflammation of the laryngeal tissues, including the vocal folds) prevents the vocal folds from vibrating freely. Persons suffering from laryngitis sound hoarse or can only whisper.

The presence of chemical irritants or particulate matter in the upper air passages, including the trachea or bronchi, elicits the **cough reflex,** producing an explosive rush of air in an effort to remove the irritant. The cough reflex begins with the inhalation of a large volume of air and the closure of the epiglottis and glottis (abduction of the vocal folds), followed by powerful contraction of the muscles responsible for forced expiration (intercostal and abdominal muscles). Sudden opening of the glottis and epiglottis generates a rush of air whose velocity can exceed 100 miles per hour, removing the irritant with an enormous force.

Trachea

The trachea has three layers: mucosa, submucosa, and adventitia. C-rings are located in the adventitia.

The trachea is a tube, 12 cm in length and 2 cm in diameter, that begins at the cricoid cartilage of the larynx and ends when it bifurcates to form the primary bronchi. The wall of the trachea is reinforced by 10 to 12 horseshoe-shaped hyaline cartilage rings (**C-rings).** The open ends of these rings face posteriorly and are connected to each other by smooth muscle, the trachealis muscle. Because of this arrangement of the C-rings, the trachea is rounded anteriorly but flattened posteriorly. The perichondrium of each C-ring is connected to the perichondria lying directly above and below it by fibroelastic connective tissue, which provides flexibility to the trachea and permits its elongation during inspiration. Contraction of the trachealis muscle decreases the diameter of the tracheal lumen, resulting in faster air flow, which assists in the dislodging of foreign material (or mucus or other irritants) from the larynx by coughing.

The trachea has three layers: mucosa, submucosa, and adventitia (Fig. 15-4).

Mucosa

The mucosal lining of the trachea is composed of pseudostratified ciliated columnar (respiratory) epithelium, the subepithelial connective tissue (lamina propria), and

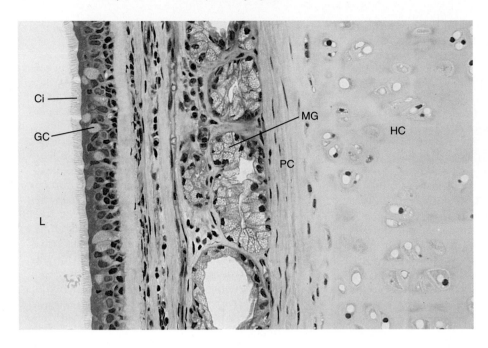

Figure 15–4 Light photomicrograph of the trachea in a monkey (×270). There are numerous cilia (Ci) as well as goblet cells (GC) in the epithelium. Also observe the mucous glands (MG) in the subepithelial connective tissue and the hyaline C-ring (HC) in the adventitia. L, lumen; PC, perichondrium.

a relatively thick bundle of elastic fibers separating the mucosa from the submucosa.

Respiratory Epithelium

The respiratory epithelium is a pseudostratified ciliated columnar epithelium composed of six cell types; goblet cells, ciliated columnar cells, and basal cells constitute 90% of the cell population.

The respiratory epithelium, a pseudostratified ciliated columnar epithelium, is separated from the lamina propria by a thick basement membrane. The epithelium is composed of six cell types: goblet cells, ciliated columnar cells, basal cells, brush cells, serous cells, and cells of the diffuse neuroendocrine system (DNES). All of these cells come into contact with the basement membrane, but they do not all reach the lumen (Fig. 15-5).

Goblet cells constitute about 30% of the total cell population of the respiratory epithelium. They produce mucinogen, which becomes hydrated and is known as **mucin** when released into an aqueous environment. Like goblet cells elsewhere, goblet cells in the respiratory epithelium have a narrow, basally positioned **stem** and an expanded **theca** containing secretory granules. Electron micrography demonstrates that the nucleus and most organelles are located in the stem. This region displays a rich network of rough endoplasmic reticulum (RER), a well-developed Golgi complex, numerous mitochondria, and an abundance of ribosomes. The theca is filled with numerous mucinogen-containing secretory granules of varied diameters. The apical

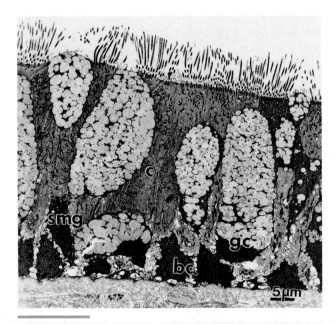

Figure 15–5 Transmission electron micrograph of monkey respiratory epithelium from the anterior nasal septum. Note the presence of goblet cells (gc), ciliated cells (c), basal cells (bc), and small granule mucous cells (smg). (From Harkema JR, Plopper CG, Hyde DM, et al: Nonolfactory surface epithelium of the nasal cavity of the bonnet monkey: A morphologic and morphometric study of the transitional and respiratory epithelium. Am J Anat 180:266-279, 1987.)

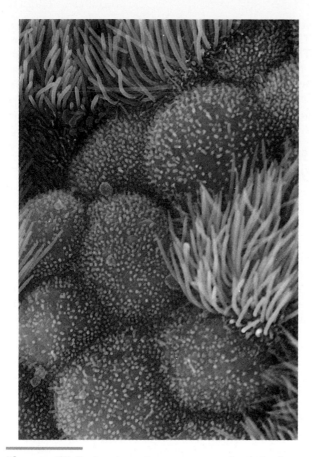

Figure 15–6 Scanning electron micrograph of the human fetal trachea displaying ciliated and nonciliated cells (×5500). (From Montgomery PQ, Stafford ND, Stolinski C: Ultrastructure of the human fetal trachea: A morphologic study of the luminal and glandular epithelia at the mid-trimester. J Anat 173:43-59, 1990.)

plasmalemma has a few short, blunt microvilli (see Fig. 15-5).

Ciliated columnar cells constitute approximately 30% of the total cell population. These tall, slender cells have a basally located nucleus and possess cilia and microvilli on their apical cell membrane (Fig. 15-6). The cytoplasm just below these structures is rich in mitochondria and has a Golgi complex. The remainder of the cytoplasm possesses some RER and a few ribosomes. These cells move the mucus and its trapped particulate matter, via ciliary action, toward the nasopharynx for elimination.

The short **basal cells** constitute about 30% of the total cell population. They are located on the basement membrane, but their apical surfaces do not reach the lumen (see Fig. 15-5). These relatively undifferentiated cells are considered to be stem cells that proliferate to replace defunct goblet, ciliated columnar, and brush cells.

Brush cells (small-granule mucous cells) constitute about 3% of the total cell population. They are narrow,

columnar cells with tall microvilli. Their function is unknown, but they have been associated with nerve endings; thus, some investigators suggest that they may have a sensory role. Other investigators believe that brush cells are merely goblet cells that have released their mucinogen.

Serous cells, which make up about 3% of the total cell population of the respiratory epithelium, are columnar cells. They have apical microvilli and apical granules containing an electron-dense secretory product, a serous fluid of unknown composition.

DNES cells, also known as small-granule cells or Kulchitsky cells, constitute about 3% to 4% of the total cell population. Many of these cells possess long, slender processes that extend into the lumen, and it is believed that they have the ability to monitor the oxygen and carbon dioxide levels in the lumen of the airway. These cells are closely associated with naked sensory nerve endings with which they make synaptic contact, and together with these nerve fibers they are referred to as **pulmonary neuroepithelial bodies.** DNES cells contain numerous granules in their basal cytoplasm that house pharmacological agents such as amines, peptides, acetylcholine, and adenosine triphosphate. Under hypoxic conditions, these agents are released not only into the synaptic clefts but also into the connective tissue spaces of the lamina propria, where they act as paracrine hormones or may enter the vascular supply to act as hormones. Therefore, it has been suggested that these pulmonary neuroepithelial bodies can exert local effects to alleviate localized hypoxic conditions by regulating perfusion and ventilation in their vicinity or they may have generalized effects via the efferent nerve fibers that relay information about hypoxic conditions to the **respiratory regulators** located in the medulla oblongata.

Lamina Propria and Elastic Fibers

The lamina propria of the trachea is composed of a loose, fibroelastic connective tissue. It contains lymphoid elements (e.g., lymphoid nodules, lymphocytes, and neutrophils) as well as mucous and seromucous glands, whose ducts open onto the epithelial surface. A dense layer of elastic fibers, the elastic lamina, separates the lamina propria from the underlying submucosa.

Submucosa

The tracheal submucosa is composed of a dense, irregular fibroelastic connective tissue housing numerous mucous and seromucous glands. The short ducts of these glands pierce the elastic lamina and the lamina propria to open onto the epithelial surface. Lymphoid elements are also present in the submucosa. Moreover, this region has a rich blood and lymph supply, the smaller branches of which reach the lamina propria.

Adventitia

The adventitia of the trachea is composed of a fibro-elastic connective tissue (see Fig. 15-4). The most prominent features of the adventitia are the hyaline cartilage C-rings and the intervening fibrous connective tissue. The adventitia also is responsible for anchoring the trachea to the adjacent structures (i.e., esophagus and connective tissues of the neck).

CLINICAL CORRELATIONS

The respiratory epithelium of people chronically exposed to irritants such as cigarette smoke and coal dust undergoes reversible alterations known as **metaplasia,** associated with an increase in the number of goblet cells relative to ciliated cells. The increased number of goblet cells produces a thicker layer of mucus to remove the irritants, but the reduced number of cilia retards the rate of mucus elimination, resulting in congestion. Moreover, the seromucous glands of the lamina propria and submucosa increase in size, forming a more copious secretion. A few months after elimination of the pollutants, the cell ratio returns to normal (1:1) and the seromucous glands revert to their previous size.

Bronchial Tree

The bronchial tree begins at the bifurcation of the trachea, as the right and left primary bronchi, which *arborize* (form branches that gradually decrease in size). The bronchial tree is composed of airways located outside the lungs (primary bronchi, extrapulmonary bronchi) and airways located inside the lungs: intrapulmonary bronchi (secondary and tertiary bronchi), bronchioles, terminal bronchioles, and respiratory bronchioles (Fig. 15-7). The bronchial tree divides 15 to 20 times before reaching the level of the terminal bronchioles. As the airways progressively decrease in size, several trends are observed, including a *decrease* in the amount of cartilage, the numbers of glands and goblet cells, and the height of epithelial cells and an *increase* in smooth muscle and elastic tissue (with respect to the thickness of the wall).

Primary (Extrapulmonary) Bronchi

The structure of the primary bronchi is identical to that of the trachea, except that primary bronchi are smaller in diameter and their walls are thinner. Each primary bronchus, accompanied by the pulmonary arteries, veins, and lymph vessels, pierces the root of the lung. The right bronchus is straighter than the left bronchus. The right bronchus trifurcates to lead to the three lobes of the right lung, and the left bronchus bifurcates, sending branches to the two lobes of the left lung. These branches then enter the substance of the lungs as intrapulmonary bronchi.

Secondary and Tertiary (Intrapulmonary) Bronchi

Each intrapulmonary bronchus serves a lobe of the lung; tertiary bronchi serve bronchopulmonary segments.

Each intrapulmonary bronchus is the airway to a lobe of the lung. These airways are similar to primary bronchi, with the following exceptions. The cartilage C-rings are replaced by irregular plates of hyaline cartilage that completely surround the lumina of the intrapulmonary bronchi; thus, these airways do not have a flattened region but are completely round. The smooth muscle is located at the interface of the fibro-elastic lamina propria and submucosa as two distinct smooth muscle layers spiraling in opposite directions. Elastic fibers, which radiate from the adventitia, connect to elastic fibers arising from the adventitia of other parts of the bronchial tree.

As in the primary bronchi and in the trachea, seromucous glands and lymphoid elements are present in the lamina propria and the submucosa of the intrapulmonary bronchi. Ducts of these glands deliver their secretory products onto the surface of the pseudostratified, ciliated epithelial lining of the lumen. Lymphoid nodules are particularly evident where these airways branch to form increasingly smaller intrapulmonary bronchi. The smaller intrapulmonary bronchi have thinner walls, decreasing amounts of hyaline cartilage plates, and shorter epithelium-lining cells.

Secondary bronchi, direct branches of the primary bronchi leading to the lobes of the lung, are also known as **lobar bronchi.** The left lung has two lobes and thus has two secondary bronchi; the right lung has three lobes and thus has three secondary bronchi.

As secondary bronchi enter the lobes of the lung, they subdivide into smaller branches, tertiary (segmental) bronchi. Each tertiary bronchus arborizes but leads to a discrete section of lung tissue known as a **bronchopulmonary segment.** Each lung has 10 bronchopulmonary segments that are completely separated from one another by connective tissue elements and are clinically important in surgical procedures involving the lungs.

As the arborized branches of intrapulmonary bronchi decrease in diameter, they eventually lead to bronchioles.

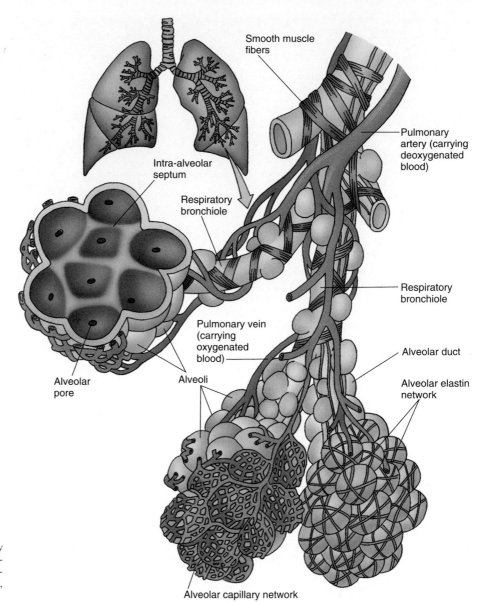

Figure 15–7 The respiratory system, displaying bronchioles, terminal bronchioles, respiratory bronchioles, alveolar ducts, alveolar pores, and alveoli.

Bronchioles

Bronchioles possess no cartilage in their walls, are less than 1 mm in diameter, and have Clara cells in their epithelial lining.

Each bronchiole (or **primary bronchiole**) supplies air to a pulmonary lobule. Bronchioles are considered the 10th to 15th generation of dichotomous branching of the bronchial tree. Their diameter commonly is described as less than 1 mm, although this number varies among authors from 5 mm to 0.3 mm. This disagreement concerning the diameter of bronchioles may lead to confusion in the descriptions of their structure

(but should not be regarded as a reason to complicate the life of the student).

The epithelial lining of bronchioles ranges from ciliated simple columnar with occasional goblet cells in larger bronchioles to simple cuboidal (many with cilia) with occasional Clara cells and no goblet cells in smaller bronchioles.

Clara cells are columnar cells with dome-shaped apices that have short, blunt microvilli (Fig. 15-8). Their apical cytoplasm houses numerous secretory granules containing glycoproteins manufactured on their abundant RER. Clara cells are believed to protect the bronchiolar epithelium by lining it with their secretory product. Additionally, these cells degrade toxins in the

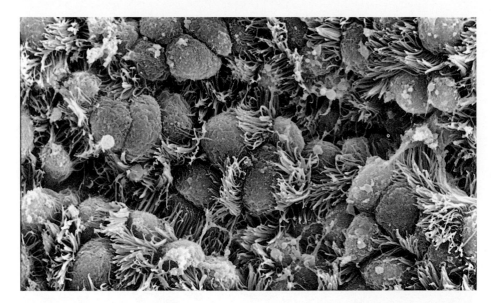

Figure 15-8 Scanning electron micrograph of Clara cells and ciliated cuboidal cells of rat terminal bronchioles (×1817). (From Peao MND, Aguas AP, De Sa CM, Grande NR: Anatomy of Clara cell secretion: Surface changes observed by scanning electron microscopy. J Anat 183:377-388, 1993.)

inhaled air via cytochrome P-450 enzymes in their smooth endoplasmic reticulum. Some investigators suggest that Clara cells produce a surfactant-like material that reduces the surface tension of bronchioles and facilitates the maintenance of their patency. Moreover, Clara cells divide to regenerate the bronchiolar epithelium.

The lamina propria of bronchioles has no glands; it is surrounded by a loose meshwork of helically oriented smooth muscle layers (Fig. 15-9). The walls of bronchioles and their branches have no cartilage. Elastic fibers radiate from the fibroelastic connective tissue that surrounds the smooth muscle coats of bronchioles. These elastic fibers connect to elastic fibers ramifying from other branches of the bronchial tree. During inhalation, as the lung expands in volume, the elastic fibers exert tension on the bronchiolar walls; by pulling uniformly in all directions, the elastic fibers help maintain the patency of the bronchioles.

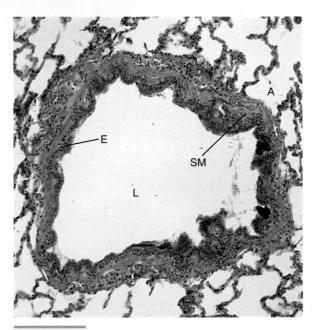

Figure 15-9 Light photomicrograph of a bronchiole (×117). Note the presence of smooth muscle (SM) and the absence of cartilage in its wall. Observe that the entire structure is intrapulmonary and is surrounded by lung tissue. A, alveolus; E, epithelium; L, lumen.

CLINICAL CORRELATIONS

The smooth muscle layers of bronchioles are controlled by the parasympathetic nervous system. Normally, the smooth muscle coats contract at the *end of* expiration and relax during inspiration. In persons with **asthma,** however, the smooth muscle coat undergoes prolonged contraction *during* expiration; thus, these individuals have difficulty in expelling air from their lungs. Steroids and β_2-agonists relax bronchiolar smooth muscle and are frequently used to relieve asthmatic attacks.

Terminal Bronchioles

Terminal bronchioles form the smallest and most distal region of the conducting portion of the respiratory system.

Each bronchiole subdivides to form several smaller terminal bronchioles, which are less than 0.5 mm in diameter and constitute the terminus of the conducting portion of the respiratory system. These structures supply air to lung acini, subdivisions of the lung lobule. The epithelium of terminal bronchioles is composed of Clara cells and cuboidal cells, some with cilia. The narrow lamina propria consists of fibroelastic connective tissue and is surrounded by one or two layers of smooth muscle cells. Elastic fibers radiate from the adventitia and, as with bronchioles, bind to elastic fibers radiating from other members of the bronchial tree. Terminal bronchioles branch to give rise to respiratory bronchioles.

RESPIRATORY PORTION OF THE RESPIRATORY SYSTEM

The respiratory portion of the respiratory system is composed of respiratory bronchioles, alveolar ducts, alveolar sacs, and alveoli.

Respiratory Bronchioles

Respiratory bronchioles are the first region of the respiratory system where exchange of gases can occur.

Respiratory bronchioles are similar in structure to terminal bronchioles, but their wall is interrupted by the presence of thin-walled, pouch-like structures known as **alveoli,** where gaseous exchange (O_2 for CO_2) can occur. As respiratory bronchioles branch, they become narrower in diameter and their population of alveoli increases. Subsequent to several branchings, each respiratory bronchiole terminates in an alveolar duct (Fig. 15-10).

Alveolar Duct, Atrium, and Alveolar Sac

Alveolar ducts, atria, and alveoli are supplied by a rich capillary network.

Alveolar ducts do not have walls of their own; they are merely linear arrangements of alveoli (Figs. 15-11 and 15-12). An alveolar duct that arises from a respiratory bronchiole branches, and each of the resultant alveolar ducts usually ends as a blind outpouching composed of two or more small clusters of alveoli, in which each cluster is known as an **alveolar sac.** These alveolar sacs thus open into a common space, which some investigators call the **atrium.**

Slender connective tissue elements between alveoli, the **interalveolar septa,** reinforce the alveolar duct, stabilizing it somewhat. Additionally, the opening of each alveolus to the alveolar duct is controlled by a single smooth muscle cell (smooth muscle "knob"), embedded in type III collagen, which forms a delicate sphincter regulating the diameter of the opening.

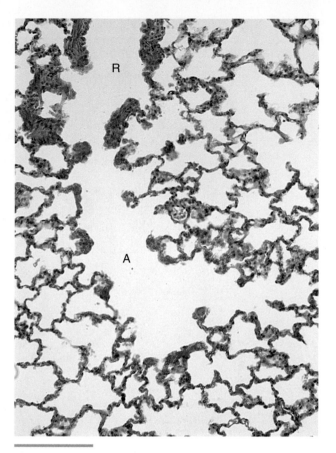

Figure 15–10 Light micrograph of a human respiratory bronchiole (R) giving rise to an alveolar duct (A). Respiratory bronchioles have definite walls with alveoli interjected. Alveolar ducts have no walls of their own; the ducts are created by neighboring alveoli.

Fine elastic fibers ramify from the periphery of alveolar ducts and sacs to intermingle with elastic fibers radiating from other intrapulmonary elements. This network of elastic fibers not only maintains the patency of these delicate structures during inhalation but also protects them against damage during distention and is responsible for nonforced exhalation.

Alveoli

Alveoli are small air sacs composed of highly attenuated type I pneumocytes and larger type II pneumocytes.

Each **alveolus** is a small outpouching, about 200 µm in diameter, of respiratory bronchioles, alveolar ducts, and alveolar sacs (Fig. 15-13; also see Figs. 15-11A and B and 15-12). Alveoli form the primary structural and functional unit of the respiratory system, because their thin walls permit exchange of CO_2 for O_2 between the air in their lumina and blood in adjacent capillaries. Although each alveolus is a small structure, about

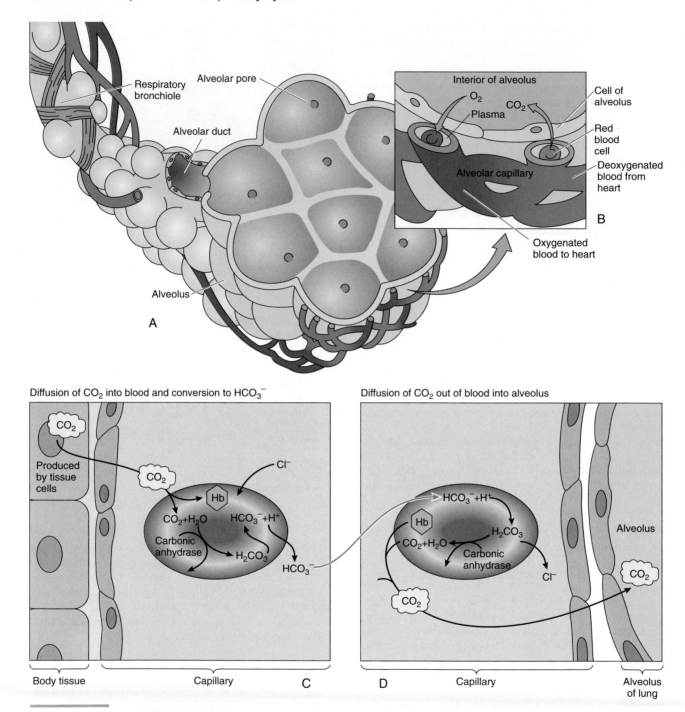

Figure 15–11 **A,** A respiratory bronchiole, alveolar sac, alveolar pore, and alveoli. **B,** Interalveolar septum. **C,** Carbon dioxide uptake from body tissues by erythrocytes and plasma. **D,** Carbon dioxide release by erythrocytes and plasma in the lung. (Compare **A** with the alveolar duct shown in Fig. 15-10.)

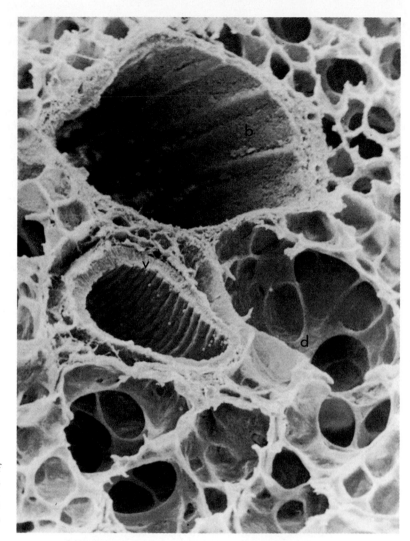

Figure 15–12 Scanning electron micrograph of a rat lung displaying a bronchiole (b), small artery (v), and alveoli (d), some of which present alveolar pores. (From Leeson TS, Leeson CR, and Paparo AA: Text/Atlas of Histology. Philadelphia, WB Saunders, 1988.)

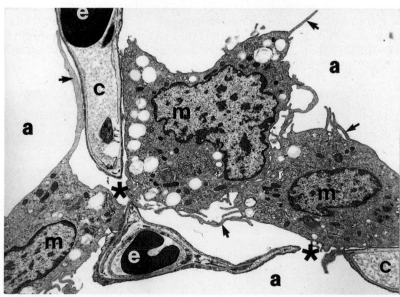

Figure 15–13 Transmission electron micrograph of the interalveolar septum in a monkey. Note the presence of alveoli (a), erythrocytes (e) within capillaries (c), and alveolar macrophages (m). Filopodia (*arrows*) and alveolar pores (*asterisks*) are evident. (From Maina JN: Morphology and morphometry of the normal lung of the adult vervet monkey (*Cercopithecus aethiops*). Am J Anat 183:258-267, 1988.)

0.002 mm³, their total number approximates 300 million, conferring on the lung its sponge-like consistency. It has been estimated that the total surface area of all the alveoli available for gas exchange exceeds 140 m² (the approximate floor space of an average-sized two-bedroom apartment or the size of a singles tennis court).

Because of their large number, alveoli are frequently pressed against each other, eliminating the connective tissue interstitium between them. In such areas of contact, the air spaces of the two alveoli may communicate with each other through an **alveolar pore (pore of Kohn),** whose diameter varies from 8 to 60 μm (see Fig. 15-12). These pores presumably function to equilibrate air pressure within pulmonary segments. The region between adjacent alveoli is known as the **interalveolar septum.** It is occupied by an extensive capillary bed composed of **continuous capillaries,** supplied by the pulmonary artery and drained by the pulmonary vein. The connective tissue of the interalveolar septum is rich in elastic fibers and type III collagen (reticular) fibers.

Because alveoli and capillaries are composed of epithelial cells, they are invested by a prominent basal lamina. The openings of alveoli associated with alveolar sacs, unlike those of respiratory bronchioles and alveolar ducts, *are devoid of smooth muscle cells.* Instead, their orifices are circumscribed by elastic and, especially, reticular fibers. Walls of alveoli are composed of two types of cells: type I pneumocytes and type II pneumocytes.

Type I Pneumocytes

Approximately 95% of the alveolar surface is composed of simple squamous epithelium, whose cells are known as **type I pneumocytes** (also called **type I alveolar cells** and **squamous alveolar cells**). Because the cells of this epithelium are highly attenuated, their cytoplasm may be as thin as 80 nm in width (Fig. 15-14; also see Fig. 15-12). The region of the nucleus is, as expected, wider, and it houses much of the cell's organelle population, composed of a small number of mitochondria, a few profiles of RER, and a modest Golgi apparatus.

Type I pneumocytes form occluding junctions with each other, thus preventing the seepage of extracellular fluid (tissue fluid) into the alveolar lumen. The adluminal aspect of these cells is covered by a well-developed basal lamina, which extends almost to the rim of the alveolar pores. The rim of each alveolar pore is formed by the fusion of the cell membranes of two closely apposed type I pneumocytes that belong to two discrete alveoli. The luminal aspect of type I pneumocytes is lined by surfactant as detailed below.

Type II Pneumocytes

Although **type II pneumocytes** (also known as **great alveolar cells, septal cells,** and **type II alveolar cells**) are more numerous than type I pneumocytes, they occupy only about 5% of the alveolar surface. These cuboidal cells are interspersed among, and form occluding junctions with, type I pneumocytes. Their dome-shaped apical surface juts into the lumen of the alveolus (Figs. 15-15 and 15-16). Type II pneumocytes are usually located in regions where adjacent alveoli are separated from each other by a septum (hence the name septal cells), and their adluminal surface is covered by basal lamina.

Electron micrographs of type II pneumocytes display short, apical microvilli. They have a centrally placed nucleus, an abundance of RER profiles, a well-developed Golgi apparatus, and mitochondria. The most distinguishing feature of these cells is the presence of membrane-bound **lamellar bodies** that contain **pulmonary surfactant,** the secretory product of these cells.

Pulmonary surfactant, synthesized on the RER of type II pneumocytes, is composed primarily of two phospholipids, **dipalmitoyl phosphatidylcholine** and **phosphatidylglycerol;** neutral lipid; and four unique proteins, **surfactant apoproteins SP-A, SP-B, SP-C,**

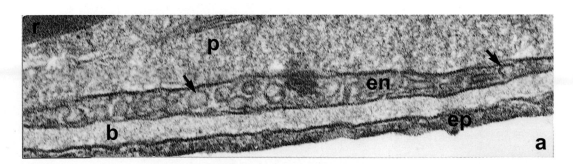

Figure 15–14 Transmission electron micrograph of the blood-gas barrier (×71,250). Note the presence of the alveolus (a), attenuated type I pneumocytes (ep), fused basal laminae (b), attenuated endothelial cell of the capillary (en) with pinocytotic vesicles (*arrows*), plasma (p), and an erythrocyte (r) within the capillary lumen. (From Maina JN: Morphology and morphometry of the normal lung of the adult vervet monkey (*Cercopithecus aethiops*). Am J Anat 183:258-267, 1988.)

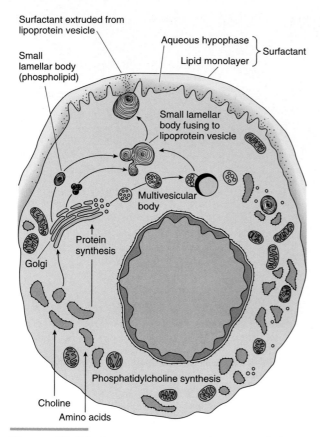

Surfactant extruded from lipoprotein vesicle

Small lamellar body (phospholipid)

Aqueous hypophase

Lipid monolayer ⎱ Surfactant

Small lamellar body fusing to lipoprotein vesicle

Multivesicular body

Protein synthesis

Golgi

Phosphatidylcholine synthesis

Choline

Amino acids

Figure 15–15 A type II pneumocyte. (Compare with the type II pneumocyte shown in Fig. 15-16.)

The surfactant is released by exocytosis into the lumen of the alveolus. Here it forms a broad, lattice-like network known as **tubular myelin,** which becomes separated into lipid and protein portions. The lipid is inserted into a monomolecular phospholipid film, forming an interface with air, and the protein enters an aqueous layer between the pneumocytes and the phospholipid film. The surfactant decreases surface tension, thus preventing atelectasis, namely the collapse of the alveolus. It is continuously manufactured by type II pneumocytes and is phagocytosed and recycled by type II pneumocytes and, less frequently, by alveolar macrophages.

In addition to producing and phagocytosing surfactant, type II pneumocytes undergo mito-sis to regenerate themselves as well as type I pneumocytes.

Alveolar Macrophages (Dust Cells)

Alveolar macrophages phagocytose particulate matter in the lumen of the alveolus as well as in the interalveolar spaces.

Monocytes gain access to the pulmonary interstitium, become alveolar macrophages (dust cells), migrate between type I pneumocytes, and enter the lumen of the alveolus. These cells phagocytose particulate matter, such as dust and bacteria, and thus maintain a sterile environment within the lungs (Fig. 15-17; also see Fig. 15-13). Dust cells also assist type II pneumocytes in the uptake of surfactant. Approximately 100 million macrophages migrate to the bronchi each day and are transported from there by ciliary action to the pharynx to be eliminated by being swallowed or expectorated. Some alveolar macrophages, however, reenter the pulmonary interstitium and migrate into lymph vessels to exit the lungs.

and **SP-D.** The surfactant is modified in the Golgi apparatus and is then released from the *trans* Golgi network into secretory vesicles, known as **composite bodies,** the immediate precursors of lamellar bodies.

CLINICAL CORRELATIONS

At birth, the infant's lungs expand upon the first intake of breath, and the presence of pulmonary surfactant permits the alveoli to remain patent. Immature infants (those born before 7 months of gestation) who have not as yet produced surfactant (or who have produced an inadequate supply of surfactant) suffer from the potentially fatal **respiratory distress of the newborn.** These newborns are treated with a combination of synthetic surfactant and glucocorticoid therapy. The synthetic surfactant acts immediately to reduce surface tension, and the glucocorticoids stimulate type II pneumocytes to produce surfactant.

CLINICAL CORRELATIONS

Alveolar macrophages of patients with pulmonary congestion and congestive heart failure contain phagocytosed, extravasated red blood cells. These macrophages are frequently called **heart failure cells.**

Emphysema is a disease usually associated with the sequelae of long-term exposure to cigarette smoke and other inhibitors of the protein α_1-antitrypsin. This protein safeguards the lungs against the destruction of elastic fibers by elastase synthesized by dust cells. In such patients, elasticity of the lung tissue is reduced and large, fluid-filled sacs are present that decrease the gas-exchange capability of the respiratory portion of the respiratory system.

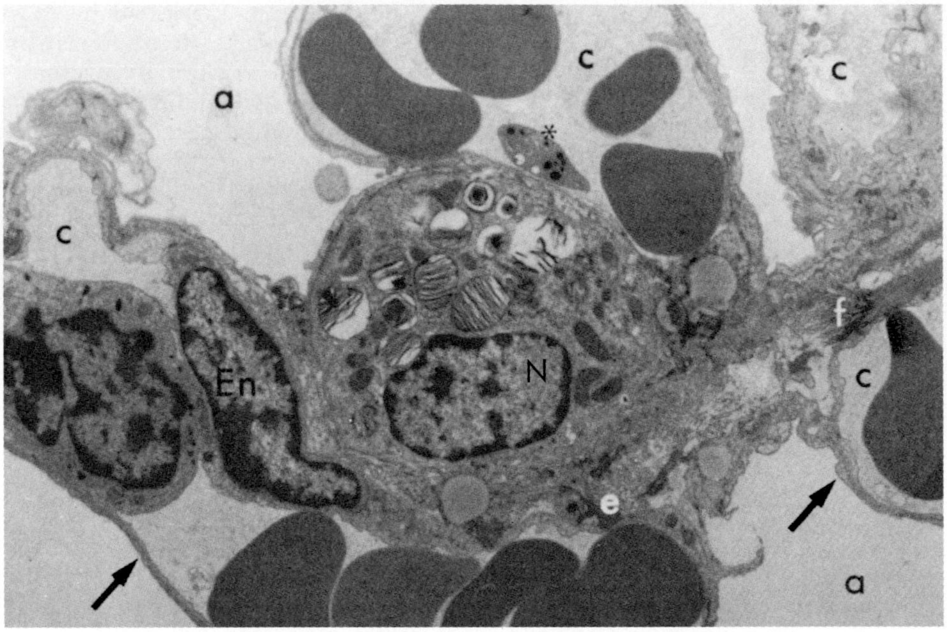

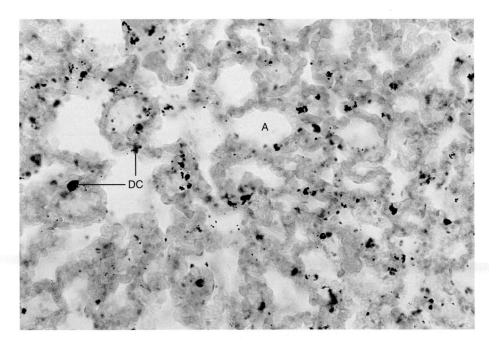

Figure 15–16 Transmission electron micrograph of a type II pneumocyte. Observe the centrally placed nucleus (N) flanked by several lamellar bodies. a, alveolus; c, capillaries; e, elastic fibers; En, nucleus of endothelial cell; f, collagen fibers. *Arrows* mark the blood-gas barrier; *asterisk* indicates a platelet. (From Leeson TS, Leeson CR, and Paparo AA: Text/Atlas of Histology. Philadelphia, WB Saunders, 1988.)

Figure 15–17 Alveolar macrophages (dust cells) in the human lung (×270). Dust cells (DC) appear as black spots on the image because they have phagocytosed dust particles that were present in the air spaces of the lung. A, alveolus.

Interalveolar Septum

The region between two adjacent alveoli, known as an interalveolar septum, is lined on both sides by alveolar epithelium (see Fig. 15-13). The interalveolar septum may be extremely narrow, housing only a **continuous capillary** and its basal lamina, or it may be somewhat wider, including connective tissue elements, such as type III collagen and elastic fibers, macrophages, fibroblasts (and myofibroblasts), mast cells, and lymphoid elements.

Blood-Gas Barrier

The blood-gas barrier is that region of the interalveolar septum that is traversed by O_2 and CO_2 as these gases go from the lumen of the blood vessel to the lumen of the alveolus, and vice versa.

The thinnest regions of the interalveolar septum where gases can be exchanged are called the blood-gas barriers (see Fig. 15-14). The narrowest blood-gas barrier, where type I pneumocytes are in intimate contact with the endothelial lining of the capillary and where the basal laminae of the two epithelia become fused, is most efficient for the exchange of O_2 (in the alveolar lumen) for CO_2 (in the blood). These regions are composed of the following structures:

- Surfactant and type I pneumocytes
- Fused basal laminae of type I pneumocytes and endothelial cells of the capillary
- Endothelial cells of the continuous capillary

Exchange of Gases between the Tissues and Lungs

In the lungs, O_2 is exchanged for CO_2 carried by blood; in the tissues of the body, CO_2 is exchanged for O_2 carried by blood.

During inspiration, oxygen-containing air enters the alveolar spaces of the lung. Because the total surface area of all the alveoli exceeds 140 m^2 and the total blood volume in all of the capillaries in the lungs at any one time is no more than 140 mL, the space available for diffusion of gases is enormous. Moreover, the diameter of the capillaries is small enough so that red blood cells may travel only in single file; thus, oxygen can reach each erythrocyte from all around, utilizing all the surface area of the red blood cells available for gas exchange. Oxygen diffuses through the blood-gas barrier to enter the lumina of the capillaries and binds to the **heme** portion of the erythrocyte hemoglobin, forming **oxyhemoglobin.** CO_2 leaves the blood, diffuses through the blood-gas barrier into the lumina of the alveolus, and exits the alveolar spaces as the CO_2-

rich air is exhaled. The passage of O_2 and CO_2 across the blood-gas barrier is due to passive diffusion in response to the partial pressures of these gases within the blood and alveolar lumina.

Approximately 200 mL of CO_2 is formed by the cells of the body per minute. CO_2 enters the bloodstream and is transported in three forms: (1) as a dissolved gas in plasma (20 mL), (2) bound to hemoglobin (40 mL), and (3) as plasma bicarbonate ion (140 mL). The following sequence of events occurs (see Fig. 15-11C):

1 Most of the CO_2 dissolved in the plasma diffuses into the cytosol of the erythrocytes.
2 Some of the CO_2 binds to the globin moiety of hemoglobin. Although CO_2 is carried in a different region of the hemoglobin molecule, its binding capacity is greater in the absence than in the presence of O_2 in the heme portion.
3 Within the cytosol of the erythrocyte, most of the CO_2 combines with water, a reaction catalyzed by the enzyme **carbonic anhydrase,** to form carbonic acid, which dissociates into hydrogen ion (H^+) and bicarbonate ion (HCO_3^-). The hydrogen ion binds to hemoglobin and the bicarbonate ion leaves the erythrocyte to enter the plasma. To maintain ionic equilibrium, chloride ion (Cl^-) enters the erythrocyte from the plasma; this exchange of bicarbonate for chloride ions is known as the **chloride shift.**

The bicarbonate-rich blood is delivered to the lungs by the pulmonary arteries. Because the level of CO_2 is greater in the blood than in the lumina of the alveoli, CO_2 is released (following the concentration gradient). The mechanism of release is the reverse of the previous reactions. The following sequence of events occurs (see Fig. 15-11D):

1 Bicarbonate ions enter the erythrocytes (with a consequent release of Cl^- from the red blood cells into the plasma, known as the chloride shift).
2 Bicarbonate ions and hydrogen ions within the erythrocyte cytosol combine to form carbonic acid.
3 In the lung, the combining of O_2 with hemoglobin makes the hemoglobin more acidic and reduces its ability to bind CO_2. Additionally, the excess hydrogen ions released because of the greater acidity of hemoglobin become bound to bicarbonate ions, forming carbonic acid.
4 **Carbonic anhydrase** catalyzes the cleavage of carbonic acid to form water and CO_2.
5 CO_2 dissolved in the plasma, bound to hemoglobin, and cleaved from carbonic acid follows the concentration gradient to diffuse across the blood-gas barrier to enter the lumina of the alveoli.

Hemoglobin also has two types of binding sites for **nitric oxide (NO),** a neurotransmitter substance that, when released by endothelial cells of blood vessels, causes relaxation of the vascular smooth muscle cells with a resultant dilation of the blood vessels. Hemoglobin, S-nitrosylated (binding site 1) by nitric oxide manufactured by blood vessels of the lung, ferries bound nitric oxide to arterioles and metarterioles of the tissues, where NO is released and causes vasodilation. In this fashion, hemoglobin not only contributes to the modulation of blood pressure but also facilitates the more efficient exchange of O_2 for CO_2. Moreover, once O_2 leaves the heme portion of hemoglobin to oxygenate the tissues, NO takes its place on the iron atoms (binding site 2) and is transported into the lungs, where it is released into the alveoli to be exhaled along with CO_2.

Pleural Cavities and the Mechanism of Ventilation

Alteration of the volume of the pleural cavities by muscle action is responsible for the movement of gases into and out of the respiratory system.

The thoracic cage is separated into three regions: the left and right thoracic cavities and the centrally located mediastinum. Each thoracic cavity is lined by a serous membrane, the **pleura,** composed of simple squamous epithelium and subserous connective tissue. The pleura may be imagined as an inflated balloon; as the lung develops, it pushes against the serous membrane, as if a fist were pushing against the outer surface of a balloon. In this fashion, a portion of the pleura, the **visceral pleura,** covers and adheres to the lung, and the remainder of the pleura, the **parietal pleura,** lines and adheres to the walls of the thoracic cavity.

The space between the visceral and parietal pleura (inside the balloon) is known as the **pleural cavity.** This space contains a slight amount of serous fluid (produced by the serous membranes) that permits a nearly frictionless movement of the lungs during **ventilation** (breathing), which involves air moving into the lungs (inhalation) and out of the lungs (exhalation).

Inhalation is an energy-requiring process because it involves contraction of the diaphragm, intercostal, and scalenus muscles, as well as accessory respiratory muscles. As these muscles contract, the volume of the thoracic cage expands. Because the parietal pleura is firmly attached to the walls of the thoracic cage, the pleural cavities also increase in volume, and consequently, the pressure within the pleural cavities decreases. The pressure differential between the atmospheric pressure outside the body and the pressure within the pleural cavities drives air into the lungs. With the influx of air the lungs expand, stretching the elastic fiber network of the pleural interstitium, and the visceral pleura is brought closer to the parietal pleura, reducing the volume of the pleural cavities and thus increasing the pressure inside the pleural cavities.

For **exhalation** to occur, the respiratory (and accessory respiratory) muscles relax, decreasing the volume of the pleural cavities, with a consequent increase in the pressure within the pleural cavities. Additionally, the stretched elastic fibers return to their resting length, driving air out of the lungs. Thus, normal expiration does not require energy. In forced expiration, the internal intercostal and abdominal muscles also contract, further decreasing the volume of the pleural cavity, forcing additional air to leave the lungs.

CLINICAL CORRELATIONS

In persons afflicted with **poliomyelitis,** the muscles of respiration may become so weakened that the accessory muscles hypertrophy because they become responsible for the elevation of the thoracic cage. In other diseases, such as **myasthenia gravis** and **Guillain-Barré syndrome,** the weakness of the respiratory and accessory respiratory muscles may lead to respiratory failure and consequent death even though the lungs function normally.

Gross Structure of the Lungs

The left lung has two lobes; the right lung has three lobes.

Each lung has a medial indentation, the **hilum,** where the primary bronchi, bronchiolar arteries, and pulmonary arteries enter and the bronchiolar veins, pulmonary veins, and lymph vessels leave the lung. This group of vessels and the airway that enter the hilum make up the **root** of the lung.

Each lobe is subdivided into several **bronchopulmonary segments** supplied by a tertiary intrapulmonary (segmental) bronchus. In turn, bronchopulmonary segments are subdivided into many **lobules,** each served by a bronchiole. Lobules are separated from one another by connective tissue septa, in which lymph vessels and tributaries of pulmonary veins travel. Branches of bronchial and pulmonary arteries follow bronchioles in their passage through the center of the lobule.

Pulmonary Vascular and Lymphatic Supply

The pulmonary arteries supply deoxygenated blood to the lungs from the right side of the heart at a rate of 5 L per minute. Branches of these vessels follow the bronchial tubes into the lobules of the lung (see Fig. 15-7). When they reach the respiratory bronchioles, these vessels form an extensive pulmonary capillary network composed strictly of **continuous capillaries.** Because these capillaries are only 8 μm in diameter, erythrocytes, as indicated above, follow each other in single file through them, reducing the space that gases have to traverse and maximally exposing the erythrocytes to oxygen.

The blood in the capillary bed becomes oxygenated and then drains into veins of increasing diameter. These tributaries of the pulmonary vein carry oxygenated blood and travel in the septa between lobules of the lung. Thus, the veins follow a path that is different from that of the arteries, until they reach the apex of the lobule, where they accompany the bronchial tubes to the hilum of the lung to deliver oxygenated blood to the left side of the heart.

Bronchial arteries, which are branches of the thoracic aorta, bring nutrient-laden and oxygen-laden blood to the bronchial tree, interlobular septa, and pleura of the lungs. Many of the small branches anastomose with those of the pulmonary system. Others are drained by tributaries of the **bronchial veins,** which return the blood to the azygos system of veins.

The lung has dual-lymph drainage, a superficial system of vessels in the visceral pleura and a deep network of vessels in the pulmonary interstitium, but these systems have numerous interconnections. The superficial system of lymph vessels forms several larger vessels, which drain into the hilar (bronchopulmonary) lymph nodes at the root of each lung. The deep network is organized into three groups following the pulmonary arteries, pulmonary veins, and bronchial tree down to the levels of the respiratory bronchioles. All of these networks drain into the hilar lymph nodes at the root of each lung. Efferent lymph vessels from these lymph nodes deliver their lymph to the thoracic duct or the right lymphatic duct, which returns the lymph to the junction of the internal jugular and subclavian veins of the left or right side, respectively.

Pulmonary Nerve Supply

The thoracic sympathetic chain ganglia provide sympathetic fibers and the vagus nerve supplies parasympathetic fibers to the smooth muscles of the bronchial tree. **Sympathetic fibers** (β-adrenergic) cause *relaxation* of bronchial smooth muscles and thus bronchodilation (while causing constriction of pulmonary blood vessels: "paradoxical response"); **parasympathetic fibers** are cholinergic; they elicit *contraction* of bronchial smooth muscles, causing bronchoconstriction. Additionally, nonadrenergic, noncholinergic fibers, also traveling with the vagus nerve, cause bronchodilation by releasing NO near bronchial smooth muscle, effecting their relaxation.

Synapses occasionally involve type II pneumocytes, suggesting the possibility of some neural control over the production of pulmonary surfactant.

16

Digestive System: Oral Cavity

The digestive system, composed of the oral cavity, alimentary tract, and associated glands, functions in the ingestion, mastication, deglutition (swallowing), digestion, and absorption of food as well as in the elimination of its indigestible remnants. Regions of the digestive system are modified and have specialized structures to be able to perform these varied tasks.

This and the following two chapters detail the histology and function of the component parts of the digestive system. The current chapter discusses the oral cavity; Chapter 17 describes the alimentary tract (esophagus, stomach, small and large intestines, rectum, and anus); and Chapter 18 considers the glands of the digestive system (major salivary glands, pancreas, liver, and gallbladder).

ORAL MUCOSA: OVERVIEW

The oral mucosa, composed of a wet stratified squamous epithelium (nonkeratinized, parakeratinized, or orthokeratinized) and an underlying dense irregular collagenous connective tissue, may be divided into three classifications: lining mucosa, masticatory mucosa, and specialized mucosa.

The oral cavity is lined by the oral mucosa, composed of a wet **stratified squamous keratinized, nonkeratinized,** or **parakeratinized epithelium** and an underlying connective tissue. Regions of the oral cavity that are exposed to considerable frictional and shearing forces (gingiva, dorsal surface of the tongue, and hard palate) are lined or covered by a **masticatory mucosa** composed of parakeratinized to completely keratinized stratified squamous epithelium with an underlying dense irregular collagenous connective tissue. The

remainder of the oral cavity is lined or covered by a **lining mucosa,** composed of a nonkeratinized stratified squamous epithelium overlying a looser type of dense irregular collagenous connective tissue. Moreover, the aspects of the oral mucosa that bear taste buds (dorsal surface of the tongue and patches of the soft palate and pharynx) are covered by **specialized mucosa** (specialized to perceive taste).

Ducts of the three pairs of major salivary glands (parotid, submandibular, and sublingual) open into the oral cavity, delivering saliva to moisten the mouth. These glands also manufacture and release the enzyme **salivary amylase** to break down carbohydrates, **lactoferrin** and **lysozymes,** antibacterial agents, and **secretory immunoglobulin (IgA).** In addition, minor salivary glands, located in the connective tissue elements of the oral mucosa, add to the flow of saliva into the oral cavity. It is in the oral cavity that food is moistened with saliva, chewed, and isolated by the tongue, ultimately forming spherical masses about 2 cm in diameter. These spherical masses, each known as a **bolus,** are forced by the tongue into the pharynx to be swallowed.

The lips form the anterior boundary, and the palatoglossal folds form the posterior boundary of the oral cavity. The structures of interest in and about the oral cavity are the lips, the teeth and their associated structures, the palate, and the tongue.

Lips

The lip has three regions: the skin aspect, the vermilion zone, and the mucous (internal) aspect.

The upper and lower lips are usually in contact with one another and thus resemble a drawstring, in that they guard the entrance into the oral cavity. The core of the lips is composed of skeletal muscle fibers that are responsible for lip mobility. Each lip may be subdivided into three regions: the external aspect, the vermilion zone, and the mucous (internal, wet) aspect.

The **external aspect** of the lip is covered with thin skin and is associated with sweat glands, hair follicles, and sebaceous glands. This region is continuous with the **vermilion zone,** the pink region of the lip, which is also covered by thin skin. However, the vermilion zone is devoid of sweat glands and hair follicles, although occasional, nonfunctional sebaceous glands are present there. The interdigitation between the epithelial and connective tissue components of the oral mucosa (the **rete apparatus**) is highly developed, so that the capillary loops of the dermal papillae are close to the surface of the skin, imparting a pink color to the vermilion zone. The absence of functional glands in this region necessitates the occasional moistening of the vermilion zone by the tongue.

The **mucous (internal) aspect** of the lip is always wet and is lined by stratified squamous nonkeratinized epithelium. The subepithelial connective tissue is of the dense, irregular collagenous type and houses numerous, mostly mucous, minor salivary glands.

Teeth

Each tooth, whether deciduous or permanent, has a crown, a cervix, and a root.

Humans have two sets of teeth: 20 **deciduous (milk) teeth,** which are replaced by 32 permanent (adult) teeth composed of 20 **succedaneous teeth** and 12 **molars** (accessional teeth). Both the deciduous and permanent dentitions are evenly distributed between the maxillary and mandibular arches.

The various teeth have different morphologic features, numbers of roots, and functions, such as seizing prey, cutting smaller pieces from large chunks, and macerating the chunks to form a bolus. Only the general structure of teeth is discussed here.

Each tooth is suspended in its bony socket, the **alveolus,** by a dense, irregular collagenous connective tissue, the **periodontal ligament.** The gingiva also supports the tooth, and its epithelium seals the oral cavity from the subepithelial connective tissue spaces (Fig. 16-1).

The portion of the tooth that is visible in the oral cavity is called the **clinical crown,** whereas the region housed within the alveolus is known as the **root.** The portion between the crown and the root is the **cervix.** The entire tooth is composed of three mineralized substances, which enclose a soft, gelatinous connective tissue known as the **pulp,** located in a continuous space

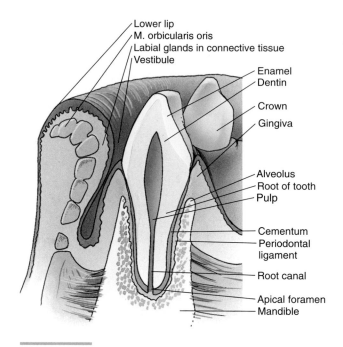

Figure 16–1 A tooth in the oral cavity. Note the location of the vestibule between the lip and the labial aspect of the tooth enamel and the gingiva, as well as the oral cavity on the buccal aspect of the teeth and gingiva.

subdivided into the pulp chamber and root canal. The root canal communicates with the periodontal ligament space via a small opening, the apical foramen, at the tip of each root. It is through this opening that blood and lymph vessels as well as nerves enter and leave the pulp (Fig. 16-2).

Mineralized Components

The mineralized structures of the tooth are enamel, dentin, and cementum. Dentin surrounds the pulp chamber and root canal and is covered on the crown by enamel and on the root by cementum. Thus, the bulk of the hard substance of the tooth is composed of dentin. Enamel and cementum meet each other at the **cervix** of the tooth.

Enamel

Enamel overlies dentin of the crown; it is composed of 96% calcium hydroxyapatite and is the hardest substance in the body.

Enamel is the hardest substance in the body. It is translucent, and its coloration is due to the color of the underlying dentin. Enamel consists of 96% calcium hydroxyapatite and 4% organic material and water. The

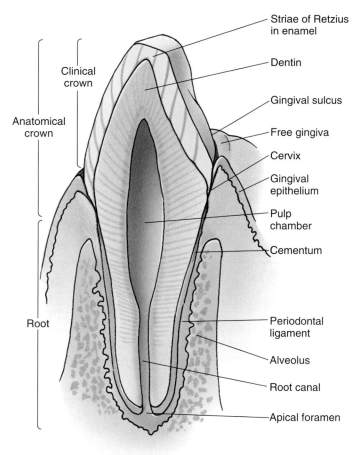

Striae of Retzius in enamel

Clinical crown

Anatomical crown

Dentin

Gingival sulcus

Free gingiva

Cervix

Gingival epithelium

Pulp chamber

Cementum

Root

Periodontal ligament

Alveolus

Root canal

Apical foramen

Figure 16–2 A tooth and its surrounding structures. Note that the clinical crown is that portion of the crown that is visible in the oral cavity, whereas the anatomical crown extends from the cemento-enamel junction to the occlusal surface of the tooth.

calcified portion of enamel is composed of large crystals coated with a thin layer of organic matrix. The organic constituents of enamel are the keratin-like, high molecular weight glycoproteins, tyrosine-rich **enamelins** as well as a related protein, **tuftleins.**

Enamel is produced by cells known as **ameloblasts,** which elaborate enamel daily in 4- to 8-μm segments known as **rod segments.** Successive rod segments adhere to one another, forming keyhole-shaped **enamel rods (prisms),** which extend over the complete width of the enamel from the dentinoenamel junction to the enamel surface. The calcium hydroxyapatite crystal orientation within rods varies, permitting a subdivision of the enamel rod into a cylindrical head to which a tail (interrod enamel), in the shape of a rectangular solid, is attached. Enamel is a nonvital substance; because the

ameloblasts die before the tooth erupts into the oral cavity, the body cannot repair enamel.

CLINICAL CORRELATIONS

Caries (cavities) usually result from the accumulation of microorganisms in and on slight defects of the enamel surface. As these bacteria metabolize nutrients in the saliva and on the tooth surface, they produce acids that begin to decalcify the enamel. As the bacteria proliferate in the cavity that they have "excavated," they and the toxins that they release enlarge the caries.

Fluoride increases the hardness of enamel, especially in young individuals, making the enamel more resistant to caries. The incidence of cavities has been greatly reduced by the addition of fluoride to the public water supply and to toothpastes and by its topical application in the dental office. As an individual ages, the enamel crystals enlarge in size and there is less space available for the exchange of hydroxyl ions for fluoride ions. Therefore, the use of fluoride treatments in adults is not nearly as effective as for young children.

During its formation, enamel is elaborated in daily segments; because of this, the quality of the enamel produced varies with the health of the mother during prenatal stages and with the health of the child after birth. The **enamel rod** then reflects the metabolic state of the person during the time of enamel formation, resulting in successive rod segment sequences of hypocalcified and normally calcified enamel. These alternating sequences, analogous to growth rings in a tree trunk, are evident histologically and are called **striae of Retzius.**

The free surface of a newly erupted tooth is covered by a basal lamina-like substance, the **primary enamel cuticle,** manufactured by the same cells that elaborated enamel. This cuticle wears away shortly after the tooth's emergence into the oral cavity.

Dentin

Dentin forms the bulk of the tooth; it is composed of 70% calcium hydroxyapatite and is the second hardest substance in the body.

Dentin is the second hardest tissue in the body (Fig. 16-3; also see Fig. 16-2). It is yellowish in color, and its high degree of elasticity protects the overlying brittle enamel

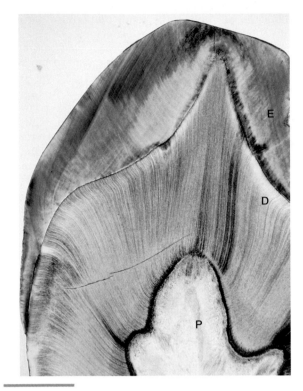

Figure 16–3 Light micrograph of the crown and neck of a tooth (×14). Observe that this is a ground section (nondecalcified) and that the enamel (*E*) appears brown and the dentin (*D*) appears grayish in this preparation. The pulp (*P*) cavity occupies the center of the tooth.

from becoming fractured. Dentin is composed of 65% to 70% calcium hydroxyapatite, 20% to 25% organic materials, and about 10% bound water. Most of the organic substance is **type I collagen** associated with proteoglycans and glycoproteins.

The cells that produce dentin are known as **odontoblasts.** Unlike ameloblasts, they maintain their association with dentin for the life of the tooth. These cells are located at the periphery of the pulp, and their cytoplasmic extensions, **odontoblastic processes,** occupy tunnel-like spaces within dentin. These extracellular fluid–filled spaces, known as **dentinal tubules,** extend from the pulp to the dentinoenamel (in the crown) and to the dentinocemental (in the root) junctions.

During dentinogenesis, odontoblasts manufacture about 4 to 8 μm of dentin every day. The quality of dentin, as of enamel, varies with the health of the mother prenatally and of the child postnatally. Thus, along the length of the dentinal tubule, dentin displays alternating regions of normal calcification and hypocalcification. These are recognizable histologically as **lines of Owen,** analogous to the striae of Retzius in enamel.

Because odontoblasts remain functional, dentin has the capability of self-repair, and **reparative dentin** is elaborated on the surface of preexisting dentin within the pulp chamber, thus reducing the size of the pulp chamber with age.

CLINICAL CORRELATIONS

Dentin sensitivity is mediated by sensory nerve fibers that are closely associated with odontoblasts, their processes, and the dentinal tubules. Disturbance of the tissue fluid within dentinal tubules is thought to depolarize the nerve fibers somehow, sending a signal to the brain, where the signal is interpreted as pain.

Cementum

Cementum overlies dentin of the roots. It is composed of about 50% calcium hydroxyapatite and 50% organic matrix and bound water; therefore, it is approximately as hard as bone.

The third mineralized tissue of the tooth is cementum, a substance that is restricted to the root (see Figs. 16-2 and 16-3). Cementum is composed of 45% to 50% calcium hydroxyapatite and 50% to 55% organic material and bound water. Most of the organic material is composed of **type I collagen** with associated proteoglycans and glycoproteins.

The apical region of cementum is similar to bone in that it houses cells, **cementocytes** within lenticular spaces, known as lacunae. Processes of cementocytes extend from lacunae within narrow **canaliculi** that extend toward the vascular periodontal ligament. Because of the presence of cementocytes, this type of cementum is called **cellular cementum.** The coronal region of cementum is without cementocytes, and thus this type of cementum is called **acellular cementum.** Both cellular cementum and acellular cementum have **cementoblasts.** These cells, which are responsible for the formation of cementum, cover cementum at its interface with the periodontal ligament and continue to elaborate cementum for the life of the tooth.

Collagen fibers of the periodontal ligament, known as **Sharpey's fibers,** are embedded in cementum and in the alveolus, and in this fashion the ligament suspends the tooth in its bony socket.

Cementum can be resorbed by osteoclast-like cells known as **odontoclasts.** During exfoliation, the replacement of deciduous teeth by their succedaneous counterparts, odontoclasts resorb cementum (and dentin) of the root.

Pulp

Pulp, a richly vascularized and innervated loose connective tissue, is surrounded by dentin and communicates with the periodontal ligament via the apical foramen.

The pulp of the tooth is composed of a loose, gelatinous connective tissue that is rich in proteoglycans and glycosaminoglycans, has an extensive vascular and nerve supply, and has some lymph circulatory elements (Fig. 16-4; also see Fig. 16-2). The pulp communicates with the periodontal ligament through the apical foramen, a small opening at the tip of each root. Vessels and nerves enter and leave the pulp through these openings.

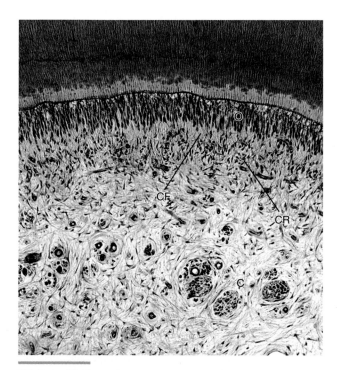

Figure 16–4 Light micrograph of the pulp of a tooth (×132). Note the three layers-odontoblastic zone (*O*), cell-poor (cell-free) zone (*CF*), cell-rich zone (*CR*)-and the core of the pulp (*C*).

It is customary to subdivide the pulp into three concentric zones around a central **core:**

- The outermost **odontoblastic zone** of the pulp is composed of a single layer of **odontoblasts,** whose processes extend into the adjacent dentinal tubules of dentin.
- The **cell-free zone** forms the layer deep to the odontoblastic zone, and as its name implies, it is devoid of cells.
- The **cell-rich zone,** consisting of fibroblasts and mesenchymal cells, is the deepest zone of the pulp, immediately surrounding the pulp core.

The **core of the pulp** resembles most other loose connective tissues but lacks adipose cells. Another notable difference is that the pulp core is highly vascularized and occasionally houses calcified elements called **pulp stones (denticles).**

The nerve fibers of the pulp are of two types: (1) **sympathetic** (vasomotor) fibers control the luminal diameters of blood vessels, and (2) **sensory** fibers are responsible for the transmission of pain sensation. **Pain fibers** are thin myelinated fibers that form the **Raschkow plexus,** just deep to the cell-rich zone. As nerve fibers continue through this plexus, they lose their myelin sheath, pass through the cell-free zone, and penetrate the space between odontoblasts to enter the dentinal tubule. Some nerve fibers synapse on the odontoblasts or their processes instead of entering the dentinal tubules.

Odontogenesis

Odontogenesis begins with the appearance of the dental lamina.

The first sign of odontogenesis **(tooth development)** occurs between the 6th and 7th weeks of gestation, when the ectodermally derived **oral epithelium** proliferates (Fig. 16-5). The result of this mitotic activity is the formation of a horseshoe-shaped band of epithelial cells, the **dental lamina,** surrounded by **neural crest**–derived **ectomesenchyme** of the mandibular and maxillary arches. The dental lamina is separated from the ectomesenchyme by a well-defined basal lamina.

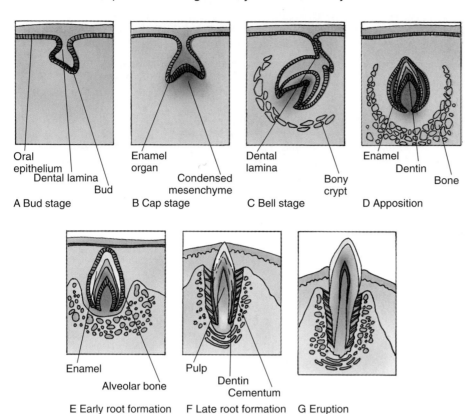

Oral
epithelium
Dental lamina
Bud
A Bud stage

Enamel
organ
Condensed
mesenchyme
B Cap stage

Dental
lamina
Bony
crypt
C Bell stage

Enamel
Dentin
Bone
D Apposition

Enamel
Alveolar bone
E Early root formation

Pulp
Dentin
Cementum
F Late root formation

G Eruption

Figure 16–5 Odontogenesis.

Bud Stage

Shortly after the appearance of the dental lamina, mitotic activity increases on the inferior aspect of this epithelial band of each arch. This activity is responsible for the formation of 10 discrete epithelial structures, known as buds, initiating the bud stage of tooth development. These buds presage the 10 deciduous teeth of both the maxillary and the mandibular arches. At the inferior tip of each bud, ectomesenchymal cells congregate to form the presumptive **dental papilla.** Further development, although similar for each bud, is asynchronous, corresponding to the order of emergence of the various teeth of the child.

Cap Stage

The cap stage of tooth development is recognized by the three-layered enamel organ. The three layers are: outer enamel epithelium, stellate reticulum, and inner enamel epithelium.

As cells of the bud proliferate, this structure not only increases in size but also alters its shape to form a three-layered configuration, known as the cap, initiating the cap stage of tooth development. Two of the three

layers—the convex simple squamous **outer enamel epithelium** and the concave simple squamous **inner enamel epithelium**—are continuous with each other at a rim-like region, the **cervical loop.** They enclose a third layer, the **stellate reticulum,** whose cells have numerous processes that are in contact with one another. These epithelially derived layers, constituting the "plump" **enamel organ,** are separated from the surrounding ectomesenchyme by a basal lamina. The concavity of the cap is occupied by a congregation of ectomesenchymal cells, the **dental papilla.** The dental papilla becomes vascularized and innervated during the cap stage of tooth development.

The process of morphodifferentiation is responsible for the establishment of the template of the presumptive tooth; that is, the enamel organ assumes the shape of an incisiform, caniniform, or molariform tooth. This event is controlled by the **enamel knot,** a dense clump of cells located adjacent to the inner enamel epithelium within the substance of the enamel organ. It appears that the ectomesenchymal cells of the dental papilla induce the cells of the enamel knot to begin to express signalling molecules, thus transforming the enamel knot into one of the principal signaling centers of tooth morphogenesis.

Cells of the enamel knot synthesize and release **bone morphogenic proteins BMP-2, BMP-4, BMP-7, sonic hedgehog,** and **fibroblast growth factor-4 (FGF-4)** at specific time intervals, thus establishing a pattern of inductive events resulting in the formation of teeth with cusps. However, the cells of the enamel knot require the presence of **epidermal growth factor (EGF)** and **FGF-4;** otherwise, the cells undergo apoptosis and die. Therefore, the enamel knot is responsible for cusp formation; however, once the cusp pattern is established, EGF and FGF-4 are removed, the cells of the enamel knot die, and that structure can no longer exert any influence on odontogenesis. Moreover, the enamel knot of presumptive teeth, such as incisors that do not develop cusps, never becomes a principal signaling center; instead, its cells undergo apoptosis and die during the cap stage.

The **dental papilla** and the enamel organ are collectively called the **tooth germ.** The dental papilla, whose most peripheral layer of cells is separated from the inner enamel epithelium by the basal lamina, is responsible for the formation of the pulp and dentin of the tooth. Ectomesenchymal cells surrounding the tooth germ form a vascularized membranous capsule, the **dental sac,** which gives rise to the cementum, periodontal ligament, connective tissue of the gingiva, and alveolus. Cells of the inner enamel epithelium differentiate into preameloblasts, which mature into ameloblasts to form enamel. Therefore, except for enamel, the tooth and its associated structures are derived from cells of neural crest origin.

During the cap stage of tooth development, a solid cord of epithelial cells, the **succedaneous lamina,** derived from the dental lamina, grows deep into the ectomesenchyme. The cells at the tip of the succedaneous lamina proliferate to form a bud, the precursor of the **succedaneous tooth** that eventually replaces the **deciduous tooth** being developed. Because there are only 20 deciduous teeth, only the same number of succedaneous teeth are formed. The remaining 12 permanent teeth, known as **accessional teeth** (three permanent molars in each quadrant) because they do not replace existing deciduous dentition, arise from the posterior extensions of the maxillary and mandibular dental laminae. The formation of the posteriorly directed extension of the original dental laminae begins in the 5th month of gestation.

Bell Stage and Appositional Stage

The bell stage is recognized by the four-layered enamel organ. The four layers are the outer enamel epithelium, stellate reticulum, stratum intermedium, and inner enamel epithelium.

Proliferation of the cells of the tooth germ increases its size, and the accumulation of fluid within the enamel organ increases its plump appearance. In addition, its concavity deepens and another layer of cells develops between the stellate reticulum and inner enamel epithelium of the enamel organ. This new layer of cells is the **stratum intermedium,** and its appearance characterizes the bell stage of tooth development. Because of changes in the morphology of the enamel organ and changes in the shape of certain cells of the tooth germ, this stage of odontogenesis is also called the **stage of morphodifferentiation and histodifferentiation.**

As most of the fluid within the enamel organ is resorbed, much of the outer enamel epithelium collapses over the stratum intermedium, bringing the vascularized dental sac close to that new layer. The proximity of blood vessels apparently causes the stratum intermedium to induce the simple squamous cells of the inner enamel epithelium to differentiate into preameloblasts that will mature into enamel-producing columnar cells, known as **ameloblasts** (Fig. 16-6). In response to the histodifferentiation of the inner enamel

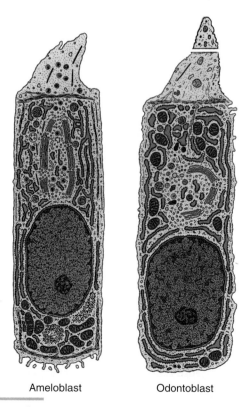

Ameloblast   Odontoblast

Figure 16–6 An ameloblast and an odontoblast. Note that the odontoblastic process is very long and a large section of it has been cut out (*white space*). (From Lentz TL: Cell Fine Structure: An Atlas of Drawings of Whole-Cell Structure. Philadelphia, WB Saunders, 1971.)

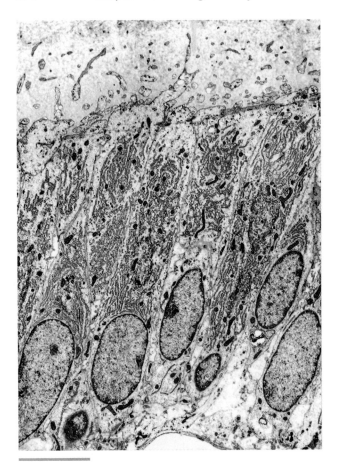

Figure 16–7 Electron micrograph of rat incisor odontoblasts (×3416). (From Ohshima H, Yoshida S: The relationship between odontoblasts and pulp capillaries in the process of enamel-related cementum-related dentin formation in rat incisors. Cell Tissue Res 268:51-63, 1992.)

epithelial cells, the most peripheral cells of the dental papilla, those in contact with the basal lamina, also differentiate to become preodontoblasts that will mature into dentin-producing columnar cells, known as **odontoblasts** (Fig. 16-7; also see Fig. 16-6).

Shortly after the odontoblasts begin to elaborate the matrix of dentin into the basal lamina, the ameloblasts also begin to manufacture the matrix of enamel. The dentin and enamel adjoin each other, and the junction between them is called the **dentinoenamel junction (DEJ)** (see Fig. 16-3). The tooth germ is now said to be in the **appositional stage** of odontogenesis.

During the formation of dentin, as the odontoblasts move away from the DEJ, the distal tip of their process remains at that junction and the process continues to elongate. This cytoplasmic extension, known as the **odontoblastic process,** is surrounded by dentin. The space occupied by the odontoblastic process is the dentinal tubule.

As the ameloblasts secrete the enamel matrix, their apical region becomes constricted by the matrix, forming **Tomes' process.** The ameloblasts then move away from the newly elaborated enamel, and the constricted region expands to its previous size, and ameloblasts secrete more enamel matrix to fill the space that the Tomes' process previously occupied. This block of new enamel matrix is known as a **rod segment.** The cyclic nature of the Tomes' process formation continues until enamel formation ceases. As dentin matrix becomes calcified to form dentin, the process of calcification spreads into the enamel matrix, which becomes known as **enamel.**

Root Formation

Root formation begins after the completion of the crown and is organized by the Hertwig epithelial root sheath.

When all of the enamel and coronal dentin (dentin of the crown) have been manufactured, the tooth germ enters the next stage of odontogenesis, root formation. The outer and inner enamel epithelia of the cervical loop elongate, forming a sleeve-like structure known as the **Hertwig epithelial root sheath (HERS),** which encompasses ectomesenchymal cells located deep to the developing crown, forming an elongation of the dental papilla.

The absence of the stratum intermedium prevents the cells of the inner enamel epithelium from differentiating into ameloblasts; thus, enamel is not formed on the developing root surface. However, the most peripheral cells of the root dental papilla differentiate into odontoblasts and begin to elaborate root dentin. As the HERS elongates, more and more of the root continues to be manufactured and the region of HERS closer to the cervical loop begins to disintegrate, forming perforations in this sleeve-like structure. Ectomesenchymal cells from the dental sac migrate through the openings in the HERS, approximate the newly formed dentin, and differentiate into **cementoblasts.** These newly differentiated cells manufacture cementum matrix, which subsequently calcifies and is referred to as **cementum.**

The elongation of the root is a consequence of the lengthening of the HERS. As the root becomes longer, the crown approaches and eventually erupts into the oral cavity. Although the two processes are simultaneous, the root is not "pushing" on the tissue apical to it; instead, it is believed that specialized fibroblasts, **myofibroblasts,** of the dental sac pull the forming tooth into the proper position.

Structures Associated with Teeth

The structures associated with teeth are the periodontal ligament, alveolus, and gingiva.

Periodontal Ligament

The periodontal ligament is a dense, irregular collagenous connective tissue whose principal fiber groups, composed of type I collagen, suspend the tooth in its alveolus.

The periodontal ligament (PDL) is located in the PDL space, defined as the region between the cementum of the root and the bony alveolus (see Figs. 16-1 and 16-2). The PDL space is less than 0.5 mm wide. Although this richly vascularized connective tissue is classified as dense irregular collagenous connective tissue, it has **principal fiber groups,** composed of **type I collagen fibers,** that are arranged in specific, predetermined patterns to absorb and counteract masticatory forces. The ends of the principal fiber groups are embedded in the alveolus and cementum as **Sharpey's fibers,** which permit the periodontal ligament to suspend the tooth in its socket (Fig. 16-8).

Fibroblasts are the most populous cells of the periodontal ligament. These cells not only manufacture the collagen and amorphous intercellular components of the PDL but also help to **resorb** collagen fibers, thus being responsible for the **high turnover of collagen** in the PDL. In addition, mast cells, macrophages, plasma cells, and leukocytes are also present in the PDL.

Nerves of the PDL include: (1) **autonomic fibers,** which regulate the luminal diameter of the arterioles; (2) **pain fibers,** which mediate pain sensation; and (3) **proprioceptive fibers,** which are responsible for the perception of spatial orientation.

CLINICAL CORRELATIONS

Proprioceptive fibers in the periodontal ligament are responsible for the **jaw-jerk reflex,** an involuntary opening of the jaw when one unexpectedly bites down on something hard. This reflex causes relaxation of the muscles of mastication and contraction of muscles responsible for opening the jaw, thus protecting the teeth from fracture.

Alveolus

The alveolus is the bony socket in which the tooth is suspended by fibers of the periodontal ligament.

The alveolar process, a bony continuation of the mandible and maxilla, is divided into compartments, each known as an alveolus, that house the root or, in the case of multirooted teeth, roots of a tooth. Adjacent alveoli are separated from each other by a bony interalveolar septum. The alveolus has three regions (see Figs. 16-1 and 16-2). The **cortical plates,** disposed lingually and labially, form a firm supporting ledge of compact bone, lined by cancellous bone, the **spongiosa.** The spongiosa surrounds a thin layer of compact bone, the **alveolar bone proper,** whose shape mirrors that of the root suspended in it.

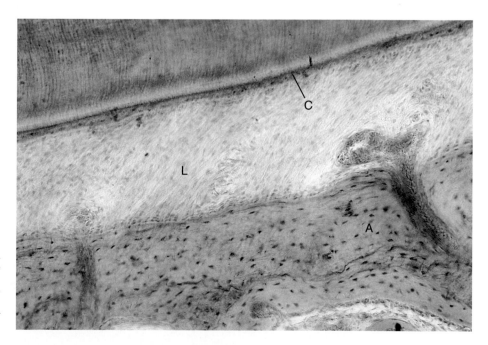

Figure 16–8 Light micrograph of tooth socket (bony alveolus). The periodontal ligament (*L*) is a dense, irregular, collagenous connective tissue located between the cementum (*C*) of the root and the bony alveolus (*A*) (×132).

Nutrient arteries travel in canals (referred to as nutrient canals) within the spongiosa, supplying the bony alveolus. The alveolar bone proper, said to be supported by the cortical plate and the spongiosa, has numerous perforations. Branches of the nutrient artery, named perforating arteries, pass from the spongiosa into the periodontal ligament, contributing to its vascularization.

Gingiva (Gums)

The gingiva is attached to the enamel surface by a thin, wedge-shaped, stratified squamous nonkeratinized epithelium, known as the junctional epithelium.

Since the gingiva is exposed to strenuous frictional forces, its stratified squamous epithelium is either fully keratinized (**orthokeratinized**) or partially keratinized (**parakeratinized**) (see Figs. 16-1 and 16-2). Deep to the epithelium is a dense, irregular collagenous connective tissue whose type I collagen fibers form principal fiber groups that resemble those of the periodontal ligament.

As the epithelium of the gingiva approaches the tooth, it forms a hairpin turn, proceeds apically (toward the root tip) for 1 to 2 mm, and then attaches to the enamel surface by the formation of hemidesmosomes. The 1- to 2-mm-deep space between the gingiva and the tooth is the gingival sulcus.

The region of the gingival epithelium that attaches to the enamel surface is known as the **junctional epithelium,** which forms a collar around the neck of the tooth. The junctional epithelium forms a robust barrier between the bacteria-laden oral cavity and the sterile environment of the gingival connective tissue. The principal fiber groups of the gingiva assist in the adherence of the junctional epithelium to the tooth surface, maintaining the integrity of the epithelial barrier. This barrier is a wedge-shaped structure, about 1 mm long, and is only about 35 to 50 cells wide coronally and 5 to 7 cells wide apically.

Palate

The palate, comprising the hard palate, the soft palate, and the uvula, separates the oral cavity from the nasal cavity.

The oral and nasal cavities are separated from each other by the hard palate and the soft palate. The hard palate, positioned anteriorly, is immovable and receives its name from the bony shelf contained within it. In contrast, the soft palate is movable, and its core is occupied by skeletal muscle responsible for its movements.

The **masticatory mucosa** on the oral aspect of the **hard palate** is composed of a wet stratified squamous keratinized (or parakeratinized) epithelium underlain by dense, irregular collagenous connective tissue. The connective tissue of the anterior lateral region of the hard palate displays clusters of adipose tissue, whereas its posterior lateral aspect exhibits acini of mucous minor salivary glands. The nasal aspect of the hard palate is covered by respiratory epithelium with occasional patches of stratified squamous nonkeratinized epithelium.

The oral surface of the **soft palate** is covered by a **lining mucosa,** composed of a wet stratified squamous nonkeratinized epithelium and a subjacent dense, irregular collagenous connective tissue housing mucous minor salivary glands that are continuous with those of the hard palate. The epithelium of its nasal aspect, like that of the hard palate, is of the pseudostratified ciliated columnar type. The most posterior extension of the soft palate is the uvula, whose histological appearance is similar to that of the soft palate, but its epithelium is composed solely of stratified squamous nonkeratinized epithelium. The connective tissue of the uvula is also a dense irregular collagenous type and possesses mucous minor salivary glands and its core is composed of skeletal muscle that is responsible for its movement.

Tongue

The tongue has three regions: the anterior two-thirds, the posterior one-third, and a root.

The tongue is the largest structure in the oral cavity. Its extreme mobility is due to the large intertwined mass of skeletal muscle fibers that compose its bulk (Fig. 16-9). The muscle fibers may be classified into two groups: those that originate outside the tongue, the **extrinsic muscles,** and those that originate within and insert into the tongue, the **intrinsic muscles.** The extrinsic muscles are responsible for moving the tongue in and out of the mouth as well as from side to side, whereas the intrinsic muscles alter the shape of the tongue. The intrinsic muscles are arranged in four groups: superior and inferior longitudinal, vertical, and transverse.

The tongue has a dorsal surface, a ventral surface, and two lateral surfaces. The dorsal surface is observed to have two unequal regions, the larger **anterior two-thirds** and the smaller **posterior one-third.** The two regions are separated from one another by a shallow, V-shaped groove, the **sulcus terminalis,** whose apex

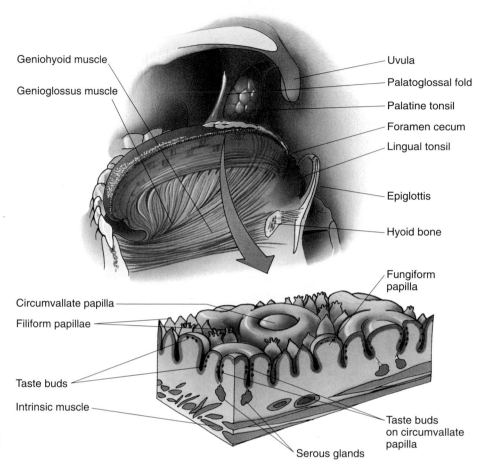

Geniohyoid muscle
Genioglossus muscle

Uvula
Palatoglossal fold
Palatine tonsil
Foramen cecum
Lingual tonsil
Epiglottis
Hyoid bone

Fungiform papilla
Circumvallate papilla
Filiform papillae
Taste buds
Intrinsic muscle
Taste buds on circumvallate papilla
Serous glands

Figure 16–9 The tongue and its lingual papillae.

points posteriorly and contains a deep concavity, the **foramen cecum.**

The dorsal surface of the posterior one third of the tongue is uneven because of the presence of the lingual tonsil (see Chapter 12). The most posterior portion of the tongue is known as the **root of the tongue.** Lingual papillae, most of which project above the surface, cover the anterior two thirds of the tongue's dorsal surface.

Lingual Papillae

There are four types of lingual papillae: filiform, fungiform, foliate, and circumvallate.

On the basis of their structure and function, the lingual papillae are of four types: filiform, fungiform, foliate, and circumvallate (Fig. 16-10; also see Fig. 16-9). They are all located anterior to the sulcus terminalis on the dorsal or lateral aspect of the tongue.

The numerous **filiform papillae** are slender structures that impart a velvety appearance to the dorsal surface (see Figs. 16-9 and 16-10). These papillae are covered by stratified squamous keratinized epithelium and help to scrape food off a surface. The high degree of keratinization is especially apparent in the sandpaper-like quality of the cat tongue. Filiform papillae do not have taste buds.

Each **fungiform papilla** resembles a mushroom whose slender stalk connects a broad cap to the tongue surface (see Figs. 16-9 and 16-10). The epithelial covering of these papillae is stratified squamous nonkeratinized; thus, the blood coursing through the subepithelial capillary loops is evident as red dots distributed randomly among the filiform papillae on the dorsum of the tongue. Fungiform papillae have taste buds on the dorsal aspect of their cap.

Foliate papillae are located along the posterolateral aspect of the tongue. They appear as vertical furrows, reminiscent of pages of a book. These papillae have functional taste buds in the neonate, but these taste

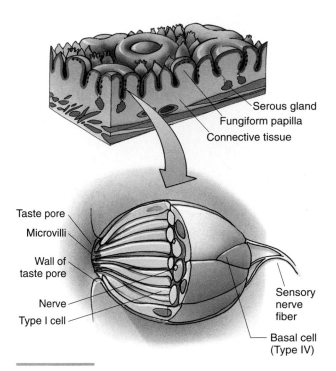

Figure 16–10 Lingual papillae and a taste bud.

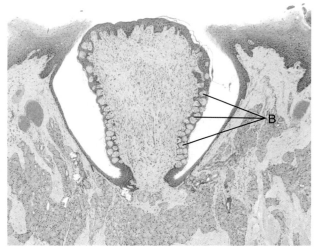

Figure 16–11 Light micrograph of monkey taste buds (×497). The taste bud (*B*) is completely within the epithelium and appears to be composed of several types of cells; however, these are the same cells at various times of their life cycle.

buds degenerate by the second or third year of life. Slender ducts of serous minor salivary **glands of von Ebner,** located in the core of the tongue, empty into the base of the furrows.

There are 8 to 12 large **circumvallate papillae** in a V-shaped arrangement just anterior to the sulcus terminalis. These papillae are submerged into the surface of the tongue so that they are surrounded by an epithelially lined groove, whose base is pierced by slender ducts of glands of von Ebner (see Figs. 16-9 and 16-10). The epithelial lining of the groove and the side (but not the dorsum) of these papillae have taste buds.

TASTE BUDS

Taste buds are intraepithelial sensory organs that function in the perception of taste. The surface of the tongue and the posterior aspect of the oral cavity have approximately 3000 taste buds. Each taste bud, composed of 60 to 80 spindle-shaped cells, is an oval structure, 70 to 80 μm long and 30 to 40 μm wide, and is distinctly paler than the epithelium surrounding it (Figs. 16-11 and 16-12; see Fig. 16-10). The narrow end of the taste bud, located at the free surface of the epithelium, projects into an opening, the **taste pore,** formed by the squamous epithelial cells that overlie the taste bud (see Fig. 16-12).

Four types of cells constitute the taste bud:

■ Basal cells (type IV cells)
■ Dark cells (type I cells)
■ Light cells (type II cells)
■ Intermediate cells (type III cells)

The relationship among the various cell types is not clear, although researchers agree that basal cells function as reserve cells and regenerate the cells of the taste buds, which have an average life span of 10 days. Most investigators believe in the following progression: Basal cells give rise to dark cells, which mature into light cells, which become intermediate cells and die.

Nerve fibers enter the taste bud and form synaptic junctions with type I, type II, and type III cells, indicating that all three cell types probably function in the discernment of taste. Each of these cell types has long, slender microvilli that protrude from the taste pore (see Fig. 16-12). In the past, these microvilli were noted with the light microscope and were called **taste hairs.**

Tastants, chemicals from food dissolved in saliva, interact either with ion channels or with receptors located on the microvilli of the taste cells, effecting electrical alterations in the resting potentials of these cells resulting in depolarization of the cell and initiating an action potential that is transmitted to the brain where the signals are interpreted as specific taste sensations. There are five primary taste sensations: salty, sweet, sour, bitter, and umami (a savory taste sensed via glutamate receptors). It is believed that although every taste bud can discern each of the five sensations, each taste bud specializes in two of the five tastes. The reaction to

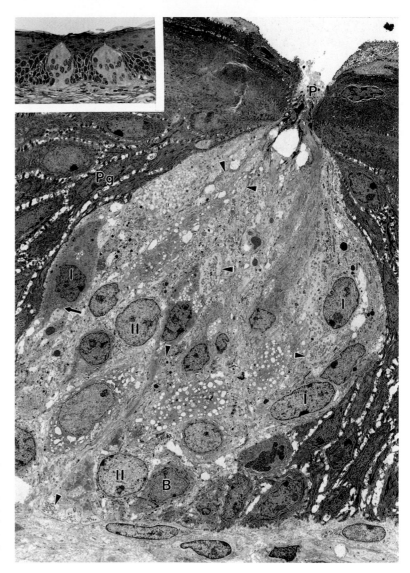

Figure 16–12 Low-power electron micrograph of a taste bud from the lamb epiglottis (×2353). B, basal cell; I, type I cell; II, type II cell; P, taste pore; Pg, perigemmal cell. *Arrowheads* represent nerve fibers; *arrow* represents synapse-like structure between a type I cell and a nerve fiber. (From Sweazy RD, Edwards CA, Kapp BM: Fine structure of taste buds located on the lamb epiglottis. Anat Rec 238:517-527, 1994.)

these taste modalities is due to the presence of specific ion channels (salty and sour) and G protein-coupled membrane receptors (bitter, sweet, and umami) in the plasmalemma of the cells of the taste bud. Recently, another receptor was localized on taste buds, CD36, a fatty acid transporter, that has the ability to detect fat and some individuals prefer foods that are fatty.

The process of complex taste perception is due more to the olfactory apparatus than to the taste buds, as evidenced by the decreased taste ability of people with nasal congestion from colds.

17

Digestive System: Alimentary Canal

The alimentary canal, the continuation of the oral cavity, is the tubular portion of the digestive tract. It is here that food is churned, liquefied, and digested; its nutritional elements and water are absorbed; and its indigestible components are eliminated. The alimentary canal, which is about 9 meters long, is subdivided into morphologically recognizable regions: the esophagus, stomach, small intestine (duodenum, jejunum, and ileum), and large intestine (cecum, colon, rectum, anal canal, and appendix).

Before a discussion of the individual regions of the alimentary canal is presented, it is reasonable and preferable to describe the general plan of the digestive tract. Once the conceptual design of the alimentary canal is understood, variations on that common theme are easier to assimilate.

GENERAL PLAN OF THE ALIMENTARY CANAL

The alimentary canal comprises four concentric layers: mucosa, submucosa, muscularis externa, and serosa (or adventitia).

The alimentary canal is composed of several histological layers (Fig. 17-1). These layers are innervated by the enteric nervous system and modulated by parasympathetic and sympathetic nerves; they are also served by sensory fibers.

Alimentary Canal Histology

The histology of the alimentary canal often is discussed in terms of four broad layers: the mucosa, submucosa, muscularis externa, and serosa (or adventitia). These layers are similar throughout the length of the digestive tract but display regional modifications and specializations.

Mucosa

The lumen of the alimentary canal is lined by an **epithelium,** deep to which is a loose connective tissue known as the **lamina propria.** This richly vascularized connective tissue houses glands as well as lymph vessels and occasional lymphoid nodules, members of the mucosa-associated lymphoid tissue (MALT) system. Certain cells of the lamina propria are responsible for the synthesis and release of growth factors that control the cell cycle of the overlying epithelium. Surrounding this connective tissue coat is the **muscularis mucosae,** composed of an inner circular layer and an outer longitudinal layer of smooth muscle. The epithelium, lamina propria, and muscularis mucosae are collectively called the mucosa.

Submucosa

The mucosa is surrounded by a dense, irregular fibroelastic connective tissue layer, the submucosa (see Fig. 17-1); this layer houses no glands except in the esophagus and duodenum. The submucosa also contains blood and lymph vessels as well as a component of the **enteric nervous system** known as **Meissner's submucosal plexus.** This plexus, which also houses postganglionic parasympathetic nerve cell bodies, controls the motility of the mucosa (and, to a limited extent, motility of the submucosa) and the secretory activities of its glands.

Muscularis Externa

The muscularis externa is usually composed of inner circular and outer longitudinal smooth muscle layers.

The submucosa is invested by a thick muscular layer, the muscularis externa, responsible for **peristaltic activity,** which moves the contents of the lumen along

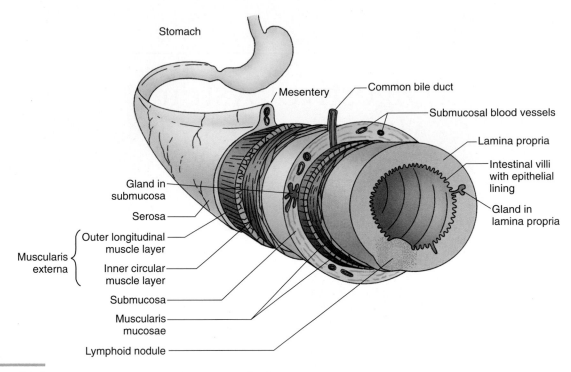

Figure 17–1 Alimentary tract. Layer contents are generalized.

the alimentary tract. The muscularis externa is composed of smooth muscle (except in the esophagus) and is usually organized in an inner circular layer and an outer longitudinal layer. Certain smooth muscle-like cells, the **interstitial cells of Cajal,** undergo rhythmic contractions and, therefore, are considered to be the pacemakers for the contraction of the muscularis externa. A second component of the enteric nervous system, known as **Auerbach's myenteric plexus,** is situated between these two muscle layers and regulates the activity of the muscularis externa (and, to a limited extent, the activity of the mucosa). Auerbach's plexus also houses postganglionic parasympathetic nerve cell bodies.

Three-dimensional reconstruction of the muscularis mucosae and of the muscularis externa shows that both the inner circular layer and the outer longitudinal layer are arranged helically. The pitch of the helices differs, however; the inner circular layer displays a tight helix, whereas the outer longitudinal layer presents a loose helix.

Serosa and Adventitia

The muscularis externa is enveloped by a thin connective tissue layer that may or may not be surrounded by the simple squamous epithelium of the visceral peritoneum. If the region of the alimentary canal is intraperitoneal, it is invested by peritoneum, and the covering is known as the *serosa.* If the organ is retroperitoneal, it adheres to the body wall by its dense irregular connective tissue component and is known as the *adventitia.*

Innervation of the Digestive Tract

The enteric nervous system, innervating the alimentary canal, is modulated by sympathetic and parasympathetic nervous systems.

The innervation of the alimentary canal is composed of two parts: the enteric nervous system and the sympathetic and parasympathetic components. The major controlling factor resides in the enteric nervous system, which is self-sufficient; however, its functions are normally modified by the sympathetic and parasympathetic components. In fact, if the sympathetic and parasympathetic connections to the entire gut are severed, the alimentary canal can perform all of its functions without any major problems.

Enteric Nervous System

The enteric nervous system is self-contained and comprises numerous repeating ganglia known as Meissner's submucosal plexus and Auerbach's myenteric plexus.

The digestive tract has its own self-contained nervous system (the enteric nervous system), which extends the entire length of the alimentary canal from the esophagus to the anus. The enteric nervous system is thus dedicated to controlling the secretory and motile functions of the alimentary canal. The 100 million or so neurons of the enteric nervous system are distributed in a large number of small clusters of nerve cell bodies and associated nerve fibers, in **Auerbach's myenteric plexus** and in **Meissner's submucosal plexus.** It is interesting that the number of neurons associated with the enteric nervous system approximates the total number of neurons contained within the spinal cord, suggesting that the enteric nervous system is an exceptionally important entity. Some investigators have proposed that it should be considered the third component of the autonomic nervous system (sympathetic, parasympathetic, and enteric nervous systems).

Although the two plexuses have numerous interconnections, they serve different functions. Generally speaking, the peristaltic motility of the digestive tract is under the direction of the myenteric plexus, whereas its secretory function and mucosal movement as well as the regulation of localized blood flow are governed by the submucosal plexus. Moreover, the myenteric plexus is concerned not only with local conditions but also with conditions along much of the digestive tract, whereas the submucosal plexus is attentive primarily to local conditions in the vicinity of the particular cluster of nerve cells in question. As with all generalizations, there are exceptions to the rules; therefore, it must be appreciated that there is a great deal of interaction between the two sets of plexuses, and the possibility of cross-controls has been suggested.

Sensory components have also been described in the wall of the alimentary canal. They convey information concerning the luminal contents, muscular status, and secretory status of the gut to the plexuses in the vicinity of the information as well as to plexuses at considerable distances from the location of the source of the information. In fact, some of the information is transmitted to sensory ganglia as well as to the central nervous system by nerve fibers that accompany fibers of the sympathetic and parasympathetic nerve supplies of the gut.

Parasympathetic and Sympathetic Supply to the Gut

Parasympathetic innervation stimulates peristalsis, inhibits sphincter muscles, and triggers secretory activity; sympathetic nerves inhibit peristalsis and activate sphincter muscles.

The digestive tract receives its parasympathetic nerve supply from the vagus nerve, except for the descending colon and rectum, which are innervated by the **sacral (spinal) outflow.** Most of the fibers of the vagus nerve are sensory and deliver information from receptors in the mucosa and muscularis of the alimentary canal to the central nervous system. Frequently, responses to the information are then conveyed by the vagal fibers to the alimentary canal. This process is known as the **vagovasal reflex.** The parasympathetic fibers synapse with postganglionic parasympathetic nerve cell bodies as well as with nerve cell bodies of the enteric nervous system in both plexuses. The parasympathetic innervation is responsible for inducing secretions from the glands of the digestive tract as well as for smooth muscle contraction.

The sympathetic innervation is derived from the splanchnic nerves. Sympathetic fibers are vasomotor, controlling blood flow to the alimentary canal.

As a generalization, it may be stated that parasympathetic innervation **stimulates peristalsis**, **inhibits sphincter muscles,** and **triggers secretory activity,** whereas sympathetic innervation **inhibits peristalsis** and **activates sphincter muscles.**

The remainder of this chapter discusses the various regions of the alimentary canal and examines how they differ from the general plan.

ESOPHAGUS

The esophagus is a muscular tube, approximately 25 cm in length, that conveys the bolus (masticated food) from the oral pharynx to the stomach. Along its entire length, its mucosa presents numerous longitudinal folds with intervening grooves that cause the lumen to appear to be obstructed; however, when the esophagus is distended the folds disappear and the lumen becomes patent.

Esophageal Histology
Mucosa

The esophageal mucosa is composed of a stratified squamous epithelium, fibroelastic lamina propria, and a smooth muscle layer that is the longitudinally disposed muscularis mucosae.

The mucosa of the esophagus is composed of three layers: epithelium, lamina propria, and muscularis mucosae (Fig. 17-2).

The lumen of the esophagus, lined by a 0.5-mm-thick, **stratified squamous nonkeratinized epithelium,** is usually collapsed and opens only during the process of swallowing. The epithelium presents a well-developed rete apparatus as it interdigitates with the underlying connective tissue. The epithelium is regenerated at a much slower rate than the remainder of the gastrointestinal tract; the newly formed cell in the basal

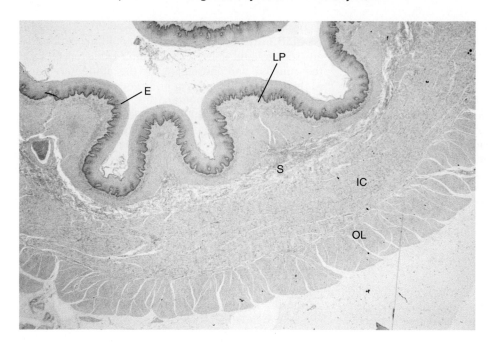

Figure 17-2 Light micrograph of the esophagus (×17). Note that the lumen is lined by a relatively thick stratified squamous epithelium (E) that forms a well-developed rete apparatus with the underlying lamina propria (LP). The submucosa (S) is surrounded by a thick muscularis externa, composed of inner circular (IC) and outer longitudinal (OL) muscle layers.

layer of the epithelium reaches the free surface in about 3 weeks after formation. Interspersed within the keratinocytes of the epithelium are antigen-presenting cells, known as **Langerhans cells,** which phagocytose and degrade antigens into small polypeptides known as epitopes. These cells also synthesize major histocompatibility complex (MHC) II molecules, attach the epitopes to these molecules, and place the MHC II–epitope complex on the external aspect of their plasmalemmae. Langerhans cells then migrate to lymph nodes, where they present the MHC II–epitope complex to lymphocytes (see Chapter 12).

The **lamina propria** is unremarkable. It houses **esophageal cardiac glands,** which are located in two regions of the esophagus, one cluster near the pharynx and the other near its juncture with the stomach. It also houses occasional lymphoid nodules, members of the MALT system. The **muscularis mucosae** is unusual in that it consists only of a single layer of longitudinally oriented smooth muscle fibers that become thicker in the vicinity of the stomach.

The esophageal cardiac glands produce mucus that coats the lining of the esophagus, lubricating it to protect the epithelium as the bolus is passed into the stomach. Because these glands resemble glands from the cardiac region of the stomach, some investigators suggest that they are ectopic patches of gastric tissue.

Submucosa

The submucosa of the esophagus houses mucous glands known as the esophageal glands proper.

The submucosa of the esophagus is composed of a dense, fibroelastic connective tissue, which houses the **esophageal glands proper.** The esophagus and the duodenum are the only two regions of the alimentary canal with glands in the submucosa. Electron micrographs of these tubuloacinar glands indicate that their secretory units are composed of two types of cells, mucous cells and serous cells.

Mucous cells have basally located, flattened nuclei and apical accumulations of mucus-filled secretory granules. The second cell type is **serous cells,** with round, centrally placed nuclei. The secretory granules of these cells contain the proenzyme **pepsinogen** and the antibacterial agent **lysozyme.** The ducts of these glands deliver their secretions into the lumen of the esophagus.

The submucosal plexus is in its customary location within the submucosa, in the vicinity of the inner circular layer of the muscularis externa.

Muscularis Externa and Adventitia

The muscularis externa of the esophagus is composed of both skeletal and smooth muscle cells.

The muscularis externa of the esophagus is arranged in two layers, inner circular and outer longitudinal. However, these muscle layers are unusual in that they are composed of both skeletal and smooth muscle fibers. The muscularis externa of the upper third of the esophagus has mostly skeletal muscle; the middle third has both skeletal and smooth muscle; and the lowest third has only smooth muscle fibers. Auerbach's plexus occupies its usual position between the inner circular and outer longitudinal smooth muscle layers of the muscularis externa.

The esophagus is covered by an **adventitia** until it pierces the diaphragm, after which it is covered by a **serosa.**

Esophageal Histophysiology

The esophagus does not have an anatomical sphincter but does have two physiological sphincters—the **pharyngoesophageal sphincter** and the **internal and external gastroesophageal sphincters**—which prevent reflux into the pharynx from the esophagus and into the esophagus from the stomach, respectively. The internal gastroesophageal sphincter, composed of smooth muscle fibers, is located at the region where the esophagus pierces the diaphragm and joins the stomach. The muscle fibers of this sphincter are always in tonus except at those times when a bolus is about to pass into the stomach or if a person is vomiting. Additionally, skeletal muscle fibers from the diaphragm encircle the esophagus and close it during inspiration and during elevation of the intra-abdominal pressure (as during defecation). A bolus entering the esophagus is conveyed, via peristaltic action of the muscularis externa, into the stomach at a rate of about 50 mm/sec.

CLINICAL CORRELATIONS

As the esophagus passes through the diaphragm, it is reinforced by fibers of that muscular structure. In some people, development is abnormal, causing a gap in the diaphragm around the wall of the esophagus that permits herniation of the stomach into the thoracic cage. This condition, known as **hiatal hernia,** weakens the gastroesophageal sphincter, allowing reflux of the stomach contents into the esophagus.

Barrett's syndrome is probably a premalignant condition due, initially, to gastroesophageal reflux. Part of the stratified squamous nonkeratinized epithelium of the esophagus, usually in the lowest region, is replaced by a simple columnar epithelium that resembles the lining of the stomach. Endoscopically, this metaplastic area is reddish in color, and at least 3 cm of the esophagus must be involved to be considered as Barrett's syndrome. If there are numerous red patches in the lower esophagus, esophageal resection may be necessary.

STOMACH

The stomach is responsible for the formation and processing of the ingested food into a thick acidic fluid known as chyme.

The stomach, the most dilated region of the alimentary canal, is a sac-like structure that, in the resting state, in the average adult has a volume of only 50 mL; however, it can accommodate approximately 1500 mL of food and gastric juices at maximal distention. As the stomach expands, its intraluminal pressure remains relatively constant due to the hormone **ghrelin,** which not only induces the sensation of hunger but also modulates receptive relaxation of the smooth muscle fibers of the muscularis externa. The bolus passes from the esophagus through the gastroesophageal junction into the stomach, where it is churned into a viscous fluid known as **chyme.** Intermittently, the stomach empties small aliquots of its contents through the **pyloric valve** into the duodenum. The stomach liquefies the food, continuing its digestion via the production of hydrochloric acid and the enzymes **pepsin, rennin,** and **gastric lipase** and via production of paracrine hormones.

Anatomically, the stomach has a concave lesser curvature and a convex greater curvature. Gross observations disclose that the stomach has four regions:

- **Cardia:** a narrow region at the gastroesophageal junction, 2 to 3 cm wide
- **Fundus:** a dome-shaped region to the left of the esophagus, frequently filled with gas
- **Body (corpus):** the largest portion, responsible for the formation of chyme
- **Pylorus (pyloric antrum):** a funnel-shaped, constricted portion equipped with a thick pyloric sphincter that controls the intermittent release of chyme into the duodenum

Histologically, the fundus and body are identical. All the gastric regions display **rugae,** longitudinal folds of the mucosa and submucosa (but transverse in the antrum), which disappear in the distended stomach. Rugae permit expansion of the stomach as it fills with food and gastric juices. Additionally, the epithelial lining of the stomach invaginates into the mucosa, forming **gastric pits (foveolae),** which are shallowest in the cardiac region and deepest in the pyloric region. Gastric pits increase the surface area of the gastric lining. Five to seven **gastric glands** of the lamina propria empty into the bottom of each gastric pit.

Gastric Histology

The ensuing discussion of the stomach details the fundic region (Fig. 17-3), because the microscopic

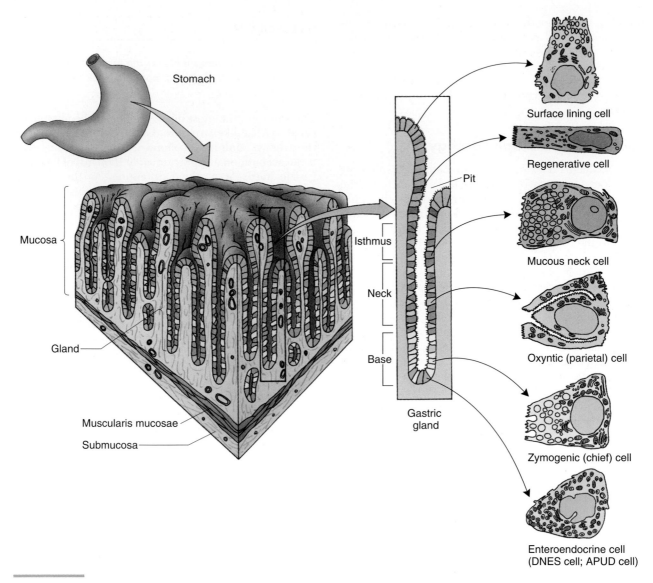

Figure 17–3 Cellular composition of the fundic stomach and fundic gland. The fundic glands open into the bottom of the gastric pits, and each gland is subdivided into an isthmus, a neck, and a base.

anatomy of each of the remaining regions is a variation of that of the fundic region.

Fundic Mucosa

The mucosa of the fundic stomach is composed of the usual three components: (1) an epithelium lining the lumen; (2) an underlying connective tissue, the lamina propria; and (3) the smooth muscle layers forming the muscularis mucosae.

Epithelium of the Stomach

The epithelial lining of the stomach secretes visible mucus that adheres to and protects the stomach lining.

The lumen of the fundic stomach is lined by a simple columnar epithelium composed of **surface-lining cells,** which manufacture a thick layer of mucus, known as **visible mucus** (Fig. 17-4A), a gel-like substance that adheres to the lining of the stomach and protects it from autodigestion. Moreover, bicarbonate ions trapped in this layer of mucus are able to maintain a relatively neutral pH at its interface with the surface-lining cell membrane, despite the low (acidic) pH of the luminal contents. Surface-lining cells continue into the gastric pits, forming their epithelial lining. **Regenerative cells** are also present in the base of these pits, but because they are more numerous in the neck of the gastric glands, they are discussed along with the glands.

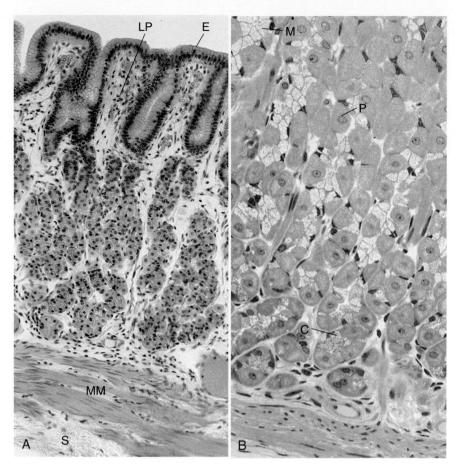

Figure 17–4 A, Light micrograph of the mucosa of the fundic stomach (×132). The mucosa is composed of the simple columnar epithelium (E), the connective tissue lamina propria (LP), and the muscularis mucosae (MM). A little section of the submucosa (S) is evident at the bottom left hand corner of the light micrograph. **B,** Light micrograph of fundic glands (×270). Note that the glands are very tightly packed, and much of the connective tissue is compressed into thin wafers occupied by capillaries. C, chief cell; M, mucous neck cell; P, parietal cell.

Electron micrographs of surface-lining cells display glycocalyx-covered, short, stubby microvilli on their apical surfaces. Their apical cytoplasm houses secretory granules containing a homogeneous substance, the precursor of visible mucus (Fig. 17-5). The lateral cell membranes of these surface lining cells form intricate zonulae occludentes and zonulae adherentes with those of neighboring cells. The cytoplasm between their basally placed nuclei and apical secretory granules is occupied chiefly by mitochondria and the protein synthesis and packaging apparatus of the cell.

Lamina Propria of the Stomach

The loose, highly vascularized connective tissue, the lamina propria, has a rich population of plasma cells, lymphocytes, mast cells, fibroblasts, and occasional smooth muscle cells. Much of the lamina propria is occupied by the 15 million closely packed gastric glands, known as fundic (oxyntic) glands in the fundic region (Fig. 17-4B).

FUNDIC GLANDS

Each fundic gland extends from the muscularis mucosae to the base of the gastric pit and is subdivided into three regions: the isthmus, the neck, and the base, of which the base is the longest (see Fig. 17-3). The simple columnar epithelium constituting the fundic gland is composed of six cell types: (1) surface-lining cells, (2) mucous neck cells, (3) regenerative (stem) cells, (4) parietal (oxyntic) cells, (5) chief (zymogenic) cells, and (6) diffuse neuroendocrine system (DNES) cells (also known as amine precursor uptake and decarboxylation [APUD] and enteroendocrine cells). The distribution of these cells within the three regions of the gland is presented in Table 17-1.

The surface-lining cells in the isthmus region are similar to those in the epithelium described earlier. The structure and function of the five other cell types are discussed next.

Mucous Neck Cells

Mucous neck cells produce soluble mucus that is mixed with and lubricates the chyme, reducing friction as it moves along the digestive tract.

Mucous neck cells are columnar and resemble surface-lining cells, but they are distorted by pressures from

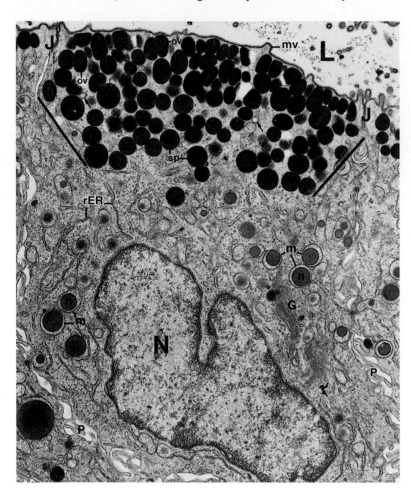

Figure 17–5 Electron micrograph of a surface lining cell from the body of a mouse stomach (×11,632). G, Golgi apparatus; J, junctional complex; L, lumen; m, mitochondria exhibiting large spherical densities known as nodules (n); mv, microvillus; N, nucleus; ov, oval secretory granules; P, intercellular projections; rER, rough endoplasmic reticulum; sp, spherical granules. (From Karam SF, Leblond CP: Identifying and counting epithelial cell types in the "corpus" of the mouse stomach. Anat Rec 232:231-246, 1992.)

TABLE 17–1 Distribution of Cell Types in Fundic Glands

Region	Cell Types
Isthmus	Surface lining cells and few DNES cells
Neck	Mucous neck cells, regenerative cells, parietal cells, and few DNES cells
Base	Chief cells, occasional parietal cells, and few DNES cells

DNES, diffuse neuroendocrine system.

neighboring cells. Thus, they have short microvilli, basally located nuclei, and a well-developed Golgi apparatus and rough endoplasmic reticulum (RER) (Fig. 17-6). Their mitochondria are located mainly in the basal region of the cell. The apical cytoplasm is filled with secretory granules containing a homogeneous secretory product, which differs from the mucus synthesized by surface-lining cells; this mucus is soluble and functions to lubricate the gastric contents. The lateral membranes of mucous neck cells form zonulae occludentes and zonulae adherentes with the surrounding cells.

Regenerative (Stem) Cells

A relatively few, thin regenerative cells are interspersed among the mucous neck cells of fundic glands (see Fig. 17-3). These columnar stem cells do not have many organelles but do have a rich supply of ribosomes. Their nuclei are basally located, have little heterochromatin, and display a large nucleolus. The lateral cell membranes of these cells also form zonulae occludentes and zonulae adherentes with those of neighboring cells.

Regenerative cells proliferate to replace all of the specialized cells lining the fundic glands, gastric pits, and luminal surface. Newly formed cells migrate to their new locations either deep into the gland or up into the gastric pit and gastric lining. Surface-lining cells, DNES cells, and mucous neck cells are replaced every 5 to 7 days; thus, regenerative cells have a high proliferative rate.

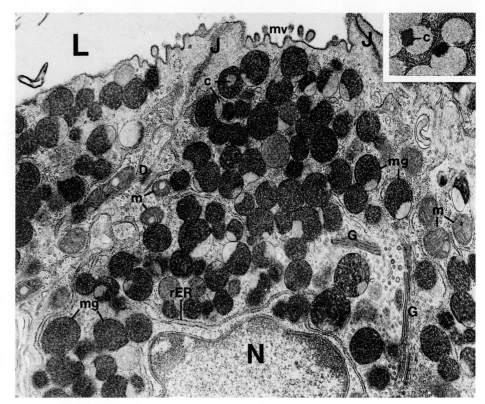

Figure 17–6 Electron micrograph of a mucous neck cell from the body of a mouse stomach. *Inset:* Secretory granule, (c). c, dense-cored granule; D, desmosome; G, Golgi apparatus; J, junctional complex; L, lumen; m, mitochondria; mg, mucous granules; mv, microvillus; N, nucleus; rER, rough endoplasmic reticulum. (From Karam SF, Leblond CP: Identifying and counting epithelial cell types in the "corpus" of the mouse stomach. Anat Rec 232:231-246, 1992.)

Parietal (Oxyntic) Cells

Parietal cells manufacture hydrochloric acid and gastric intrinsic factor; both products are released into the lumen of the stomach.

Large, round to pyramid–shaped parietal cells are located mainly in the upper half of the fundic glands and only occasionally in the base (see Figs. 17-3 and 17-4). They are about 20 to 25 μm in diameter and are situated at the periphery of the gland. These cells produce **hydrochloric acid (HCl)** and **gastric intrinsic factor.**

CLINICAL CORRELATIONS

Gastric intrinsic factor, a glycoprotein secreted into the lumen of the stomach, is necessary for vitamin B_{12} absorption from the ileum. Absence of this factor results in deficiency of vitamin B_{12} with the consequent development of **pernicious anemia.** Because the liver stores high quantities of vitamin B_{12}, a deficiency of this vitamin may take several months to develop after production of gastric intrinsic factor ceases.

Parietal cells have round, basally located nuclei, and their cytoplasm is eosinophilic. Their most remarkable characteristic is the invaginations of their apical plasmalemma to form deep **intracellular canaliculi** lined by microvilli (Figs. 17-7 and 17-8). The cytoplasm bordering these canaliculi is richly endowed by round and tubular vesicles, the **tubulovesicular system.** Additionally, parietal cells are rich in mitochondria, whose combined volume constitutes almost half that of the cytoplasm. The protein synthetic apparatus, the RER and the Golgi apparatus, are present but only to a limited extent.

The number of microvilli and the abundance of vesicles of the tubulovesicular system are indirectly related to each other and vary with the HCl secretory activity of parietal cells. During active HCl production, the number of microvilli increases and the tubulovesicular system decreases. Thus, the membrane, being stored as tubules and vesicles, is probably used for microvillar assembly, increasing the surface area of the cell by four to five times in preparation for HCl production.

The process of microvillus formation requires energy and involves polymerization of soluble forms of actin and myosin into filaments, which then interact to transport membranes from the tubulovesicular system to that of the intracellular canaliculus. The stored membranes have a high content of H^+,K^+-ATPase (a protein

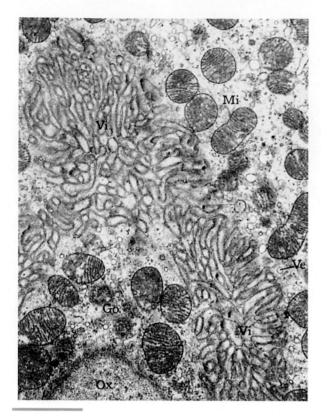

Figure 17–7 Electron micrograph of a parietal cell from the body of a mouse stomach (×14,000). Go, Golgi apparatus; Mi, mitochondria; Ox, nucleus of oxyphil cell; Ve, tubulovesicular apparatus; Vi, microvilli. (From Rhodin JAG.: An Atlas of Ultrastructure. Philadelphia, WB Saunders, 1963.)

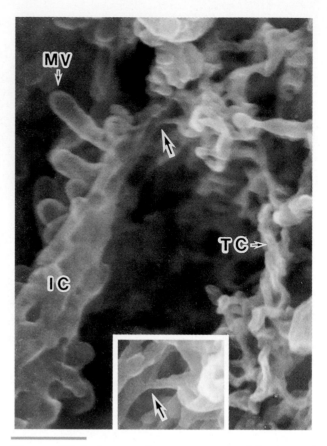

Figure 17–8 Scanning electron microscopy of the fractured surface of a resting parietal cell (×50,000). The cytoplasmic matrix is removed by the aldehyde-osmium-DMSO-osmium method (or A-ODO method), exposing the cytoplasmic membranes. The tubulocisternal network (TC) is connected to the intracellular canaliculus (IC) lined with microvilli (MV). *Inset:* A higher magnification of the area indicated by the *arrow* (×100,000). (From Ogata T, Yamasaki Y: Scanning EM of the resting gastric parietal cells reveals a network of cytoplasmic tubules and cisternae connected to the intracellular canaliculus. Anat Rec 258:15-24, 2000.)

that pumps protons from the cytoplasm into the intracellular canaliculus). The formation of hydrochloric acid is detailed later.

Chief (Zymogenic) Cells

Chief cells manufacture the enzymes pepsinogen, rennin, and gastric lipase and release them into the lumen of the stomach.

Most of the cells in the base of fundic glands are chief cells (see Figs. 17-3 and 17-4). These columnar cells display a basophilic cytoplasm, basally located nuclei, and apically situated secretory granules that house the proenzyme **pepsinogen** (as well as rennin and gastric lipase). Electron micrographs of chief cells exhibit a rich supply of RER, an extensive Golgi apparatus, and numerous apical secretory granules interspersed with a few lysosomes (Fig. 17-9). Short, blunt, glycocalyx-covered microvilli project from the apical aspect of the cell into the lumen of the gland.

Exocytosis of pepsinogen from chief cells is induced by both neural and hormonal stimulation. Neural stim-

ulation by the vagus nerve is the main contributor to pepsinogen release. Binding of **secretin** to receptors in the basal plasma membrane of chief cells triggers a second messenger system that also leads to exocytosis of pepsinogen.

DNES Cells (APUD or Enteroendocrine Cells)

DNES cells may be open or closed. They manufacture endocrine, paracrine, and neurocrine hormones.

A group of small cells that are individually dispersed among the other epithelial cells of the gastric mucosa are known collectively by several names:

■ Argentaffin and argyrophilic cells, because they stain with silver stains

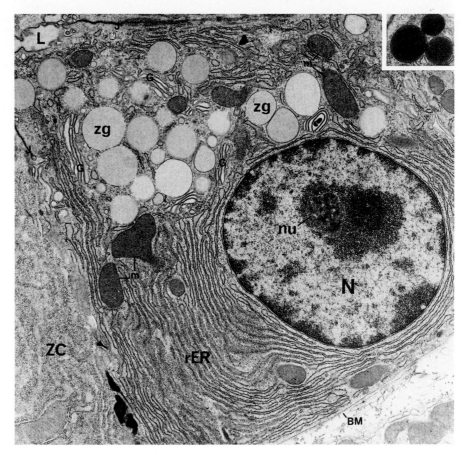

Figure 17–9 Electron micrograph of a chief cell from the fundus of a mouse stomach (×11,837). BM, basement membrane; G, Golgi apparatus; L, lumen; m, mitochondria; N, nucleus; nu, nucleolus; rER, rough endoplasmic reticulum; ZC, zymogenic (chief) cell; zg, zymogen granules;. (From Karam SF, Leblond CP: Identifying and counting epithelial cell types in the "corpus" of the mouse stomach. Anat Rec 232: 231-246, 1992.)

- APUD cells, because some of them can take up the precursors of amines and decarboxylate them
- DNES cells, because they are members of the diffuse neuroendocrine system of cells
- Enteroendocrine cells because they secrete hormone-like substances and are located in the epithelium of the enteric (alimentary) canal.

Some of these cells are individually designated according to the substance that they produce. Generally, a single type of DNES cell secretes only one agent, although occasional cell types may secrete two different agents. There are at least 13 different DNES cell types, only some of which are located in the mucosa of the stomach (Table 17-2). Cells of the DNES have been identified not only in the digestive tract but also in the respiratory system and in the endocrine pancreas. Additionally, some of the secretory products synthesized and released by these DNES cells are identical to neurosecretions localized in the central nervous system. The significance of their diverse location and the substances they produce is only incompletely understood.

Electron micrographs of DNES cells reveal that these small cells, which sit on the basal lamina, are of two types: those that reach the lumen of the gut (the

open type) and those that do not (the **closed type**). The open type reach the lumen via long, thin apical processes with microvilli, which may serve to monitor the contents of the gastric lumen. The cytoplasm of DNES cells has a well-developed RER and Golgi apparatus and numerous mitochondria. Additionally, small secretory granules are evident, disposed basally in most cells (Fig. 17-10).

All DNES cells release the contents of their granules basally into the lamina propria. The substances that cells release either travel short distances in the interstitial tissue to act on target cells in the immediate vicinity of the signaling cell (paracrine effect) or enter the circulation and travel a distance to reach their target cell (endocrine effect). Furthermore, the substance released may be identical to neurosecretions. Because of these three possibilities, some researchers have used the terms **endocrine, paracrine,** and **neurocrine** to differentiate among the three variations of the secreted substances.

Muscularis Mucosae of the Stomach

The smooth muscle cells that compose the muscularis mucosae are arranged in three layers. The inner

TABLE 17–2 Diffuse Neuroendocrine System (DNES) Cells and Hormones of the Gastrointestinal Tract

Cell*	Location	Hormone Produced	Granule Size (nm)	Hormonal Action
A	Stomach and small intestine	Glucagon (enteroglucagon)	250	Stimulates glycogenolysis by hepatocytes, thus elevating blood glucose levels
D	Stomach, small and large intestines	Somatostatin	350	Inhibits release of hormones by DNES cells in its vicinity
EC	Stomach, small and large intestines	Serotonin Substance P	300	Increases peristaltic movement
ECL	Stomach	Histamine	450	Stimulates HCl secretion
G	Stomach and small intestine	Gastrin	300	Stimulates HCl secretion, gastric motility (especially contraction of the pyloric region and relaxation of pyloric sphincter to regulate stomach emptying), and proliferation of regenerative cells in the body of the stomach
GL	Stomach, small and large intestines	Glicentin	400	Stimulates hepatocyte glycogenolysis, thus elevating blood glucose levels
I	Small intestine	Cholecystokinin	250	Stimulates the release of pancreatic enzymes and contraction of the gallbladder
K	Small intestine	Gastric inhibitory peptide	350	Inhibits HCl secretion
Mo	Small intestine	Motilin		Increases intestinal peristalsis
N	Small intestine	Neurotensin	300	Increases blood flow to ileum and decreases peristaltic action of small and large intestines
PP (F)	Stomach and large intestine	Pancreatic polypeptide	180	Stimulates release of enzymes by chief cells; depresses release of HCl by parietal cells; inhibits exocrine release of pancreas
S	Small intestine	Secretin	200	Stimulates release of bicarbonate-rich fluid from pancreas
VIP	Stomach, small and large intestines	Vasoactive intestinal peptide		Increases peristaltic action of small and large intestines and stimulates elimination of water and ions by GI tract

*This table lists most of the better-known DNES cells.

ECL, enterochromaffin-like cell; EC, enterochromaffin cell; G, gastrin-producing cell; GI, gastrointestinal; GL, glicentin-producing cell; HCl, hydrochloric acid; MO, motilin-producing cell; N, neurotensin-producing cell; PP (F), pancreatic polypeptide–producing cell (F cell); VIP, vasoactive intestinal peptide–producing cell.

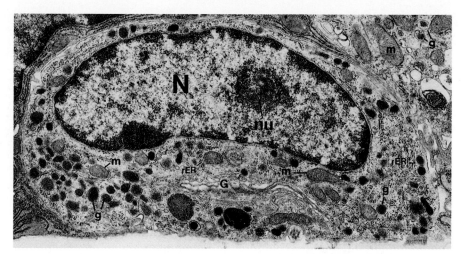

Figure 17–10 Electron micrograph of a DNES cell from the body of a mouse stomach. G, Golgi apparatus; g, secretory granules; N, nucleus; nu, nucleolus; m, mitochondria; rER, rough endoplasmic reticulum; (From Karam SF, Leblond CP: Identifying and counting epithelial cell types in the "corpus" of the mouse stomach. Anat Rec 232: 231-246, 1992)

circular and outer longitudinal layers are well defined; however, an occasional third layer, whose fibers are disposed circularly (outermost circular), is not always evident.

Differences in the Mucosa of the Cardiac and Pyloric Regions

The mucosa of the **cardiac region** of the stomach differs from that of the fundic region, in that the gastric pits are shallower and the base of its glands is highly coiled. The cell population of these cardiac glands is composed mostly of surface-lining cells, some mucous neck cells, a few DNES cells and parietal cells, and *no chief cells* (Table 17-3).

The glands of the **pyloric region** contain the same cell types as those in the cardiac region, but the predominant cell type in the pylorus is the mucous neck cell. In addition to producing mucus, these cells secrete **lysozyme,** a bactericidal enzyme. Pyloric glands are highly convoluted and tend to branch. Additionally, the gastric pits of the pyloric region are deeper than in both the cardiac and pyloric regions, extending approximately halfway down into the lamina propria (Fig. 17-11; also see Table 17-3).

Submucosa of the Stomach

The dense, irregular collagenous connective tissue of the gastric submucosa has a rich vascular and lymphatic network that supplies and drains the vessels of the lamina propria. The cell population of the submucosa resembles that of any connective tissue proper. The submucosal plexus is in its accustomed location, within the submucosa in the vicinity of the muscularis externa.

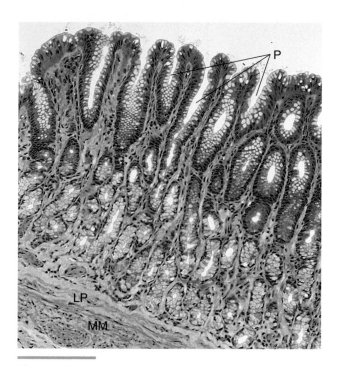

Figure 17–11 Light micrograph of the pyloric stomach (×132). The gastric pits are much deeper here than in the cardiac or fundic regions of the stomach. P, gastric pits; LP, lamina propria; MM, muscularis mucosae.

Muscularis Externa

The muscularis externa of the stomach is composed of three layers of smooth muscle: the innermost oblique layer, middle circular layer, and outer longitudinal layer.

The smooth muscle cells of the gastric muscularis externa are arranged in three layers. The **innermost oblique layer** is not well defined except in the cardiac

TABLE 17–3 Histology of the Alimentary Canal

Organ	Epithelium	Cell Type of Epithelium	Lamina Propria	Cells of Glands	Muscularis Mucosae	Submucosa	Muscularis Externa	Serosa or Adventitia
Esophagus	Stratified squamous nonkeratinized		Esophageal cardiac glands	Mucus-secreting	Longitudinal layer only	Esophageal glands proper	Inner circular and outer longitudinal	Adventitia (except serosa in abdominal cavity)
Cardiac stomach	Simple columnar	Surface lining cells (no goblet cells)	Cardiac glands; shallow gastric pits	Surface lining cells, mucous neck cells, regenerative cells, DNES cells, parietal cells	Inner circular, outer longitudinal and, in places, outermost circular	No glands	Inner oblique, middle circular, outermost longitudinal	Serosa
Fundic stomach	Simple columnar	Surface lining cells (no goblet cells)	Fundic glands	Surface lining cells, mucous neck cells, parietal cells, regenerative cells, chief cells DNES cells	Inner circular, outer longitudinal and, in places, outermost circular	No glands	Inner oblique, middle circular, outermost longitudinal	Serosa
Pyloric stomach	Simple columnar	Surface lining cells (no goblet cells)	Pyloric glands; deep gastric pits	Mucous neck cells, surface lining cells, parietal cells, regenerative cells, DNES cells	Inner circular, outer longitudinal and, in places, outermost circular	No glands	Inner oblique, middle circular (well developed to form pyloric sphincter), outermost longitudinal	Serosa
Duodenum	Simple columnar (goblet cells)	Surface absorptive cells, goblet cells, DNES cells	Crypts of Lieberkühn	Surface absorptive cells, goblet cells, regenerative cells, DNES cells, Paneth cells	Inner circular, outer longitudinal	Brunner's glands	Inner circular, outer longitudinal	Serosa and adventitia

Region	Epithelium	Surface cells	Glands	Cell types	Muscularis mucosae	Submucosa	Muscularis externa	Serosa/Adventitia
Jejunum	Simple columnar (goblet cells)	Surface absorptive cells, goblet cells, DNES cells	Crypts of Lieberkühn	Surface absorptive cells, goblet cells, regenerative cells, DNES cells, Paneth cells	Inner circular, outer longitudinal	No glands	Inner circular, outer longitudinal	Serosa
Ileum	Simple columnar (goblet cells)	Surface absorptive cells, goblet cells, DNES cells	Crypts of Lieberkühn; Peyer's patches	Surface absorptive cells, goblet cells, regenerative cells, DNES cells, Paneth cells	Inner circular, outer longitudinal	No glands (Peyer's patches may extend into this layer)	Inner circular, outer longitudinal	Serosa
Colon*	Simple columnar (goblet cells)	Surface absorptive cells, goblet cells, DNES cells	Crypts of Lieberkühn	Surface absorptive cells, goblet cells, regenerative cells, DNES cells	Inner circular, outer longitudinal	No glands	Inner circular, outer longitudinal modified to form taeniae coli	Serosa and adventitia
Rectum	Simple columnar (goblet cells)	Surface absorptive cells, goblet cells, DNES cells	Shallow crypts of Lieberkühn	Surface absorptive cells, goblet cells, regenerative cells, DNES cells, Paneth cells	Inner circular, outer longitudinal	No glands	Inner circular, outer longitudinal	Adventitia
Anal canal	Simple cuboidal; stratified squamous nonkeratinized; stratified squamous keratinized		Rectal columns; circumanal glands; *at anus*: hair follicles and sebaceous glands		Inner circular, outer longitudinal	No glands; internal and external hemorrhoidal plexuses	Inner circular (forms internal and sphincter), outer longitudinal (becomes fibroelastic sheet)	Adventitia
Appendix	Simple columnar (goblet cells)	Surface absorptive cells, goblet cells, DNES cells	Shallow crypts of Lieberkühn; lymphoid nodules	Surface absorptive cells, goblet cells, regenerative cells, DNES cells, Paneth cells	Inner circular, outer longitudinal	No glands; occasional lymphoid nodules; possible fatty infiltration	Inner circular, outer longitudinal	Serosa

*Includes cecum.
DNES, diffuse neuroendocrine system.

region. The **middle circular layer** is clearly evident along the entire stomach and is especially pronounced in the pyloric region, where it forms the **pyloric sphincter.** The **outer longitudinal muscle layer** is most evident in the cardiac region and the body of the stomach but is poorly developed in the pylorus. The myenteric plexus is located between the middle circular and outer longitudinal layers of smooth muscle.

The entire stomach is invested by a **serosa,** composed of a thin, loose, subserous connective tissue covered by a smooth, wet, simple squamous epithelium. This external covering provides an almost friction-free environment during the churning movements of the stomach.

Gastric Histophysiology

The lining and glands of the stomach produce and release secretions into the lumen of the stomach. These secretions are composed of water, hydrochloric acid, gastric intrinsic factor, pepsinogen, rennin, gastric lipase, visible mucus, and soluble mucus.

The gastric glands of the stomach produce approximately 2 to 3 L of gastric juices a day. These secretions are composed of (1) **water** (derived from the extracellular fluid in the interstitial connective tissue and delivered via parietal cells); (2) **hydrochloric acid (HCl)** and **gastric intrinsic factor** (manufactured by parietal cells); (3) the enzymes **pepsinogen, rennin,** and **gastric lipase** (manufactured by chief cells); (4) a glycoprotein, **visible mucus** (manufactured by surface-lining cells) which forms a coat of mucus that lines and protects the epithelium of the stomach and serves as a favorable, mostly neutral pH, environment for the bacterium *Helicobacter pylori*; and (5) **soluble mucus** that becomes part of the gastric content (produced by mucous neck cells). Little absorption of food products occurs in the stomach, although some substances, such as alcohol, can be absorbed by the gastric mucosa.

The three muscle layers of the muscularis externa interact such that during the contraction, the contents of the stomach are churned and the ingested food is liquefied to form **chyme,** a viscous fluid with the consistency of split pea soup. Independent contraction of the muscularis mucosae exposes the chyme to the entire surface area of the gastric mucosa.

Emptying of Gastric Contents

Interaction between neurons of the myenteric and submucosal plexuses, and mostly due to the effect of the hormone ghrelin, a constant intraluminal pressure is maintained, irrespective of the degree of distention of the stomach. In the empty stomach the pylorus is always open; however, during peristalsis the pyloric sphincter is closed. Coordinated contraction of the muscularis externa and momentary relaxation of the pyloric sphincter permit emptying of the stomach by intermittently delivering small aliquots of the chyme into the duodenum. The rate at which the stomach releases its chyme into the duodenum is a function of the acidity, the caloric and fat content, and the osmolality of the chyme. The production of the peristaltic waves occurs in a rhythmic fashion and is generated by the gastric pacemaker at a rate of about three per minute. Receptors in the duodenum, in response to the arrival of the chyme, cause a sudden closure of the pyloric sphincter and contraction of the muscularis externa of the pyloric antrum, driving the chyme back into the body of the stomach for a thorough mixing of the chyme with the digestive enzymes.

The factors that facilitate emptying of the stomach are the degree of its distention and the action of **gastrin,** a hormone that stimulates contraction of the muscularis externa of the pyloric region and relaxation of the pyloric sphincter. Factors that inhibit gastric emptying include distention of the duodenum; overabundance of fat, proteins, or carbohydrates; and increased osmolarity and excessive acidity of the chyme in the duodenum. These factors activate a neural feedback mechanism by stimulating release of cholecystokinin, which counteracts the action of gastrin, and stimulating the release of gastric inhibitory peptide, which also inhibits gastric contractions.

Gastric Hydrochloric Acid (HCl) Production

The three phases in the production of hydrochloric acid are cephalic, gastric, and intestinal.

Hydrochloric acid not only breaks down food material but also activates the proenzyme pepsinogen to become the active proteolytic enzyme **pepsin.** Because pepsin requires a low pH for its activity, the presence of HCl also provides the necessary acidic conditions (pH 1 to pH 2).

HCl secretion occurs in three phases as a result of different stimuli:

- **Cephalic:** Secretion caused by psychological factors (e.g., the thought, smell, or sight of food; stress) is elicited by parasympathetic impulses from the vagus nerve, which cause the release of **acetylcholine**
- **Gastric:** Secretion resulting from the presence of certain food substances in the stomach as well as from the stretching of the stomach wall is elicited by the paracrine hormones **gastrin** and **histamine** and by the neurocrine substance **acetylcholine;** gastrin and histamine are released by the DNES cells—G cells and enterochromaffin-like (ECL) cells—of the

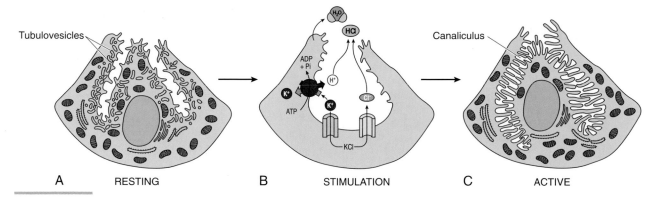

Figure 17–12 Parietal cell. **A,** Well-developed tubulovesicular apparatus in the resting cell. **B,** Mechanism of hydrochloric acid release. **C,** Numerous microvilli in the active cell.

stomach, respectively, and acetylcholine is released by the vagus nerve

- **Intestinal:** Secretion due to the presence of food in the small intestine is elicited by the endocrine hormone **gastrin,** released by G cells of the small intestine

Mechanism of Gastric Hydrochloric Acid Production

> *HCl production is initiated when gastrin, histamine, and acetylcholine bind to their respective receptors in the basal plasma membrane of parietal cells.*

Parietal cells have receptors for gastrin, histamine, and acetylcholine on their basal plasmalemma. Binding of these signaling molecules to the appropriate receptors causes the cells to manufacture and release HCl into the intracellular canaliculus. The process occurs as follows (Fig. 17-12):

1 The enzyme **carbonic anhydrase** facilitates the production of carbonic acid (H_2CO_3) (from water [H_2O] and carbon dioxide [CO_2]), which then dissociates into hydrogen ions (H^+) and bicarbonate (HCO_3^-) within the cytoplasm of the parietal cell.

2 An H^+,K^+-ATPase, using adenosine triphosphate (ATP) as an energy source, pumps intracellular H^+ out of the cell into the intracellular canaliculi and transfers extracellular potassium ion (K^+) into the cell.

3 Carrier proteins, utilizing ATP as an energy source, pump K^+ and chloride ion (Cl^-) out of the cell and into the intracellular canaliculus. Thus **Cl^-** and **H^+** enter the lumen of the intracellular canaliculus separately to combine as HCl.

4 K^+ is actively transported into the cell at the basal plasmalemma as well as at the microvilli jutting into the intracellular canaliculi, thus increasing the intracellular level of K^+. The high intracellular K^+ con-

centration forces K^+ to leave the cell via ion channels located in the basal plasmalemma and in the plasma membrane of the microvilli. Thus, K^+ is constantly recirculated in and out of the parietal cell.

5 Water, derived from the extracellular fluid, enters the parietal cell and then leaves the cytoplasm to enter the intracellular canaliculus as a consequence of the osmotic forces generated by the movement of ions just described. Because the intracellular canaliculus is an extension of the lumen of the stomach, HCl manufactured by the parietal cells enters the gastric lumen.

The lining of the stomach is protected from the high acidic content by the buffering activity of the HCO_3^- present in the layer of mucus manufactured by the surface-lining cells and, to a certain limited extent, by mucous neck cells. Additionally, the zonulae occludentes of the epithelial cells prevent the influx of HCl into the lamina propria, thus protecting the mucosa from damage. Moreover, evidence suggests that **prostaglandins** not only protect the cells lining the gastric lumen but also increase local circulation, especially when the integrity of the epithelial barrier is compromised. This increased blood flow removes the H^+ from the lamina propria.

Inhibition of Hydrochloric Acid Release

The hormones **somatostatin, prostaglandin,** and **gastric inhibitory peptide (GIP)** inhibit gastric HCl production. Somatostatin acts on G cells and ECL cells, inhibiting their release of gastrin and histamine, respectively. Prostaglandins and GIP act directly on parietal cells and inhibit their ability to produce HCl.

Additionally, **urogastrone,** produced by Brunner's glands of the duodenum, acts directly on parietal cells to inhibit HCl production.

CLINICAL CORRELATIONS

Possibly the most common cause of **ulcers** in the United States is the prevalent use of the non-steroidal anti-inflammatory drugs (NSAIDs) **ibuprofen** and **aspirin.** Both of these drugs inhibit the manufacture of prostaglandins, thus precluding their protective effects on the stomach lining.

The bacterium *Helicobacter pylori,* which is localized in the layer of mucus protecting the gastric epithelium, has also been implicated as a possible factor in ulcer formation.

Almost 12% of cancer-related fatalities are due to **gastric carcinoma,** one of the most common gastrointestinal malignancies. Although the cancer may be localized to any region of the stomach, the region of the lesser curvature and the pyloric antrum are the sites that are most generally involved.

SMALL INTESTINE

The small intestine has three regions: duodenum, jejunum, and ileum.

Digestion begins in the oral cavity and continues in the stomach and in the small intestine, which at 7 m is the longest region of the alimentary tract. The small intestine is divided into three regions: duodenum, jejunum, and ileum. Although these regions are similar histologically, their minor differences permit their identification.

The small intestine digests food material and absorbs end products of the digestive process. To perform its digestive functions, the first region of the small intestine, the duodenum, receives enzymes and an alkaline buffer from the pancreas and bile from the liver. Additionally, epithelial cells and glands of the mucosa contribute buffers and enzymes to facilitate digestion.

Common Histological Features

Because the three regions of the small intestine are similar histologically, their common features are described first. Following this discussion, variations from this plan are described for each segment (see Table 17-3), and then functional aspects are considered.

Modifications of the Luminal Surface

The surface area of the intestinal lumen is enlarged by the formation of plicae circulares, villi, microvilli, and crypts of Lieberkühn.

The luminal surface of the small intestine is modified to increase its surface area. Three types of modifications have been noted:

- **Plicae circulares (valves of Kerckring)** are transverse folds of the submucosa and mucosa that form semicircular to helical elevations, some as large as 8 mm tall and 5 cm long. Unlike rugae of the stomach, these are permanent fixtures of the duodenum and jejunum and end in the proximal half of the ileum. They not only increase the surface area of the small intestine by a factor of 2 to 3 but also decrease the velocity of the movement of chyme along the alimentary canal.
- **Villi** are epithelially covered, finger-like or oak leaf–like protrusions of the lamina propria. The core of each villus contains capillary loops, a blindly ending lymphatic channel **(lacteal),** and a few smooth muscle fibers, embedded in loose connective tissue and rich in lymphoid cells. Villi are permanent structures ranging from 10 to 40 per mm^2 (Figs. 17-13 to 17-15). Their numbers are greater in the duodenum than in the jejunum or the ileum, and their height decreases from 1.5 mm in the duodenum to about 0.5 mm in the ileum. These delicate structures confer a velvety appearance to the lining of the living organ. Villi increase the surface area of the small intestine by a factor of 10.
- **Microvilli,** modifications of the apical plasmalemma of the epithelial cells covering the intestinal villi, increase the surface area of the small intestine by a factor of 20.

Thus, the three types of intestinal surface modifications increase the total surface area available for absorption of nutrients by a factor of 400 to 600.

Invaginations of the epithelium into the lamina propria between the villi form intestinal glands, **crypts of Lieberkühn,** which also augment the surface area of the small intestine.

Intestinal Mucosa

The mucosa of the small intestine is composed of the usual three layers: a simple columnar epithelium, the lamina propria, and the muscularis mucosae.

Epithelium

The simple columnar epithelium covering the villi and the surface of the intervillar spaces is composed of surface absorptive cells, goblet cells, and DNES cells.

SURFACE ABSORPTIVE CELLS

Surface absorptive cells are tall columnar cells that function in terminal digestion and absorption of water and nutrients.

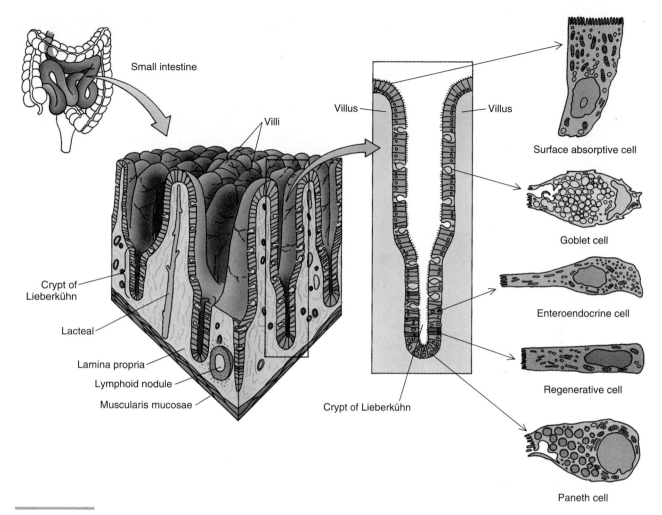

Figure 17–13 Mucosa, villi, crypts of Lieberkühn, and component cells of the small intestine. Note that the crypts of Lieberkühn open into the intervillar spaces. There is a solitary lymphoid nodule in the lamina propria.

The most numerous cells of the epithelium are surface absorptive cells (Fig. 17-16; also see Figs. 17-13 and 17-15). They are tall cells, about 25 μm in length, with basally located oval nuclei. Their apical surface presents a **brush border,** and in good tissue preparations, terminal bars are also evident. The principal functions of these cells are terminal digestion and absorption of water and nutrients. Additionally, these cells reesterify fatty acids into triglycerides, form chylomicrons, and transport the bulk of the absorbed nutrients into the lamina propria for distribution to the rest of the body. The process of absorption is discussed later in the chapter.

Electron micrographs of surface absorptive cells sport as many as 3000 **microvilli,** approximately 1 μm long, whose tips are covered with a thick **glycocalyx** layer. The glycocalyx coat not only protects the microvilli from autodigestion, but its enzymatic compo-

nents also function in terminal digestion of dipeptides and disaccharides into their monomers. The actin core of the microvilli is anchored into the actin and intermediate filaments of the cell web. The cytoplasm of surface absorptive cells is rich in organelles, especially endosomes, smooth endoplasmic reticulum (SER), RER, and Golgi apparatus.

The lateral cell membranes of these cells form zonulae occludentes, zonulae adherentes, desmosomes, and gap junctions with adjacent cells. The tight junctions prevent the passage of material via a paracellular route to or from the lumen of the gut.

GOBLET CELLS

Goblet cells are unicellular glands (see Figs. 17-13 and 17-15; also see Chapter 5). The duodenum has the smallest number of goblet cells, and their number

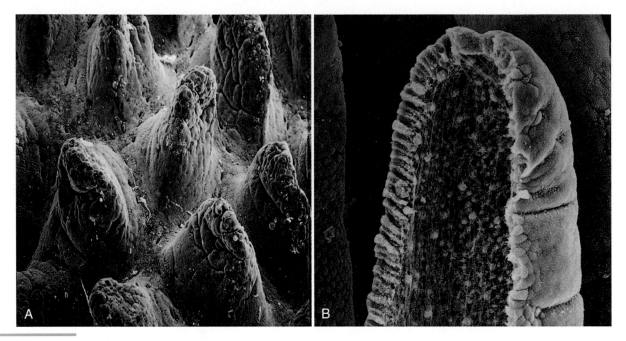

Figure 17–14 Scanning electron micrographs of villi from the mouse ileum. **A,** Observe the villi and the openings of the crypts of Lieberkühn in the intervillar spaces (×160). **B,** Note that the villus is fractured, revealing its core of connective tissue and migrating cells (×500). (From Magney JE, Erlandsen SL, Bjerknes ML, Cheng H: Scanning electron microscopy of isolated epithelium of the murine gastrointestinal tract: Morphology of the basal surface and evidence for paracrine-like cells. Am J Anat 177:43-53, 1986.)

increases toward the ileum. These cells manufacture **mucinogen,** whose hydrated form is **mucin,** a component of **mucus,** a protective layer lining the lumen.

DNES CELLS

The small intestine has various types of DNES cells that produce paracrine and endocrine hormones (see the earlier section on the stomach and Table 17-2). Approximately 1% of the cells covering the villi and intervillar surface of the small intestine are composed of DNES cells.

M CELLS (MICROFOLD CELLS)

Microfold cells phagocytose and transport antigens from the lumen to the lamina propria.

The simple columnar epithelial lining of the small intestine is replaced by squamous-like **M cells** in regions where lymphoid nodules abut the epithelium. These M cells, which are believed to belong to the mononuclear phagocyte system of cells, sample, phagocytose, and transport antigens present in the intestinal lumen.

Lamina Propria

The loose connective tissue of the lamina propria forms the core of the villi, which like trees of a forest rise above the surface of the small intestine (Fig. 17-17; also see Figs. 17-14 and 17-15). The remainder of the lamina propria, extending down to the muscularis mucosae, is compressed into thin sheets of highly vascularized connective tissue by the numerous tubular intestinal glands, the crypts of Lieberkühn. The lamina propria also is rich in lymphoid cells and contains occasional lymphoid nodules, which, as discussed later, help protect the intestinal lining from invasion by microorganisms.

CRYPTS OF LIEBERKÜHN

Crypts of Lieberkühn increase the surface area of the intestinal lining. They are composed of DNES cells, surface absorptive cells, goblet cells, regenerative cells, and Paneth cells.

Crypts of Lieberkühn are simple tubular (or branched tubular) glands (see Fig. 17-13) that open into the intervillar spaces as perforations of the epithelial lining. Scanning electron micrographs indicate that the base of each villus is surrounded by the openings of several crypts (see Fig. 17-14). These tubular glands are composed of surface absorptive cells, goblet cells, regenerative cells, DNES cells, and Paneth cells.

Surface absorptive and goblet cells occupy the upper half of the gland. Goblet cells have a short life span; it

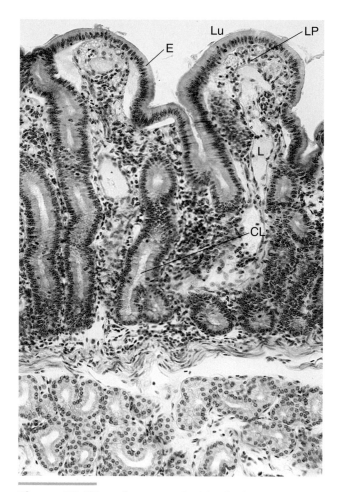

Figure 17–15 Light micrograph of the duodenal mucosa, displaying the simple columnar epithelium (E), the cellular lamina propria (LP) with its lacteals of villi, and the muscularis mucosae (×132). The submucosa houses Brunner's glands, a clear indication that this is a section of the duodenum. CL, crypts of Lieberkühn; Lu, lumen.

Electron micrographs of these undifferentiated cells display few organelles but many free ribosomes. Their single, basally located, oval nuclei are electron-lucent, indicating the presence of a large amount of euchromatin.

Paneth cells are clearly distinguishable because of the presence of large, eosinophilic, apical secretory granules (Fig. 17-18; also see Fig. 17-13). These pyramid-shaped cells occupy the bottom of the crypts of Lieberkühn and manufacture the antibacterial agent **lysozyme,** defensive proteins **(defensin),** and **tumor necrosis factor-α.** Unlike the other cells of the intestinal epithelium, Paneth cells have a comparatively long life span of 20 days and secrete lysozyme continuously. Electron micrographs of these cells display a well-developed Golgi apparatus, a large complement of RER, numerous mitochondria, and large apical secretory granules housing a homogeneous secretory product.

Muscularis Mucosae

The muscularis mucosae of the small intestine is composed of an inner circular layer and an outer longitudinal layer of smooth muscle cells (see Fig. 17-17). Muscle fibers from the inner circular layer enter the villus and extend through its core to the tip of the connective tissue, as far as the basement membrane. During digestion, these muscle fibers rhythmically contract, shortening the villus several times a minute.

Submucosa

The submucosa of the small intestine is composed of dense, irregular fibroelastic connective tissue with a rich lymphatic and vascular supply. The intrinsic innervation of the submucosa is from the parasympathetic **submucosal (Meissner's) plexus.** The submucosa of the **duodenum** is unusual because it houses glands known as Brunner's glands (duodenal glands).

BRUNNER'S GLANDS

Brunner's glands produce a mucous, bicarbonate-rich fluid as well as urogastrone (human epidermal growth factor).

Brunner's glands are branched, tubuloalveolar glands whose secretory portions resemble mucous acini (see Fig. 17-15). The ducts of these glands penetrate the muscularis mucosae and usually pierce the base of the crypts of Lieberkühn to deliver their secretory product into the lumen of the duodenum. Occasionally, their ducts open into the intervillar spaces. Electron micrographs of the acinar cells display a well-developed RER and Golgi apparatus, numerous mitochondria, and flattened to round nuclei.

is believed that after they disgorge their mucinogen they die and are desquamated. The basal half of the gland has no surface absorptive cells and only a few goblet cells; instead, most of the cells are regenerative cells (and their progeny), DNES cells, and Paneth cells. Only regenerative cells and Paneth cells are described here; the others have been discussed earlier.

Regenerative cells of the small intestine are stem cells that undergo extensive proliferation to repopulate the epithelium of the crypts, mucosal surface, and villi. These narrow cells appear to be wedged into limited spaces among the newly formed cells (see Fig. 17-13). Their rate of cell division is high, with a relatively short cell cycle of 24 hours. It has been suggested that 5 to 7 days after the appearance of a new cell, the cell has progressed to the tip of the villus and has been exfoliated.

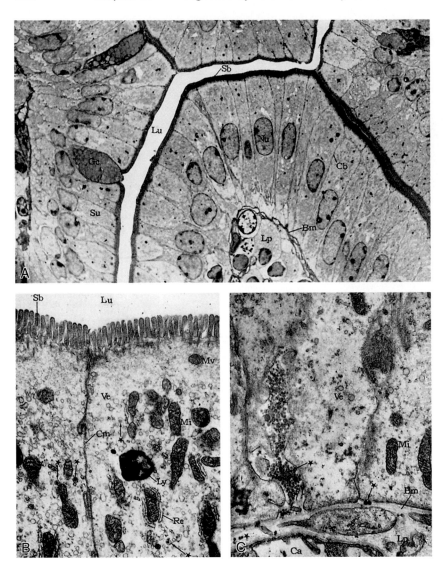

Figure 17–16 Surface absorptive cells from a villus of the mouse jejunum. **A,** Low-magnification electron micrograph displaying two goblet cells (Gc) and numerous surface absorptive cells (Su) (×1744). Note the striated border (Sb) facing the lumen (Lu). Nuclei (Nu) and cell boundaries (Cb) are clearly evident. Observe also that the epithelium is separated from the lamina propria by a well-defined basement membrane (Bm). **B,** A higher-magnification electron micrograph of two adjoining surface absorptive cells (×10,500). The striated border (Sb) is clearly composed of numerous microvilli that project into the lumen (Lu). The adjoining cell membranes (Cm) are close to each other. Mi, mitochondria; Ly, lysosomes; Re, rough endoplasmic reticulum; Ve, vesicles; *asterisk* indicates membrane-bound lipid droplets. **C,** Electron micrograph of the basal aspect of the surface absorptive cells (×11,200). Bm, basement membrane; Lp, lamina propria; Mi, mitochondria; Ve, vesicles; *asterisk* indicates chylomicrons. (From Rhodin JAG: An Atlas of Ultrastructure. Philadelphia, WB Saunders, 1963.)

Brunner's glands secrete a mucous, alkaline fluid in response to parasympathetic stimulation. This fluid helps neutralize the acidic chyme that enters the duodenum from the pyloric stomach. The glands also manufacture the polypeptide hormone **urogastrone** (also known as **human epidermal growth factor**), which is released into the duodenal lumen along with the alkaline buffer. Urogastrone inhibits production of HCl (by directly inhibiting parietal cells) and amplifies the rate of mitotic activity in epithelial cells.

Muscularis Externa and Serosa

The muscularis externa of the small intestine is composed of an inner circular layer and an outer longitudinal smooth muscle layer. **Auerbach's myenteric plexus,** located between the two muscle layers, is the intrinsic neural supply of the external muscle coat. The muscularis externa is responsible for the peristaltic activity of the small intestine.

Except for the second and third parts of the duodenum, which have **adventitia,** the entire small intestine is invested by a **serosa.**

Lymphatic and Vascular Supply of the Small Intestine

Lymph drainage in the small intestine begins as blindly ending lymphatic vessels known as lacteals.

The small intestine has a well-developed lymphatic and vascular supply. Blindly ending lymph capillaries called **lacteals,** which are located in the cores of villi, deliver

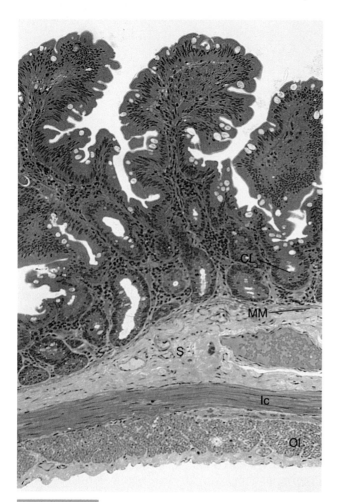

Figure 17–17 Light micrograph of the mucosa of a monkey jejunum (×132). Observe the well-developed villi, and note that there are no Peyer's patches in the lamina propria nor are there any Brunner's glands in the submucosa; therefore, this must be a section of the jejunum. CL, crypts of Lieberkühn; Ic, inner circular muscle layer; MM, muscularis mucosae; Ol, outer longitudinal muscle layer; S, submucosa.

their contents into the **submucosal lymphatic plexus.** From here, lymph passes through a series of lymph nodes to be delivered to the thoracic duct, the largest lymph vessel in the body. The thoracic duct empties its contents into the circulatory system at the junction of the left internal jugular and subclavian veins.

Capillary loops adjacent to the lacteals are drained by blood vessels that are tributaries of the **submucosal vascular plexus.** Blood from here is delivered to the hepatic portal vein to enter the liver for processing.

Regional Differences

The **duodenum** is the shortest segment of the small intestine, only 25 cm in length. It receives bile from the liver and digestive juices from the pancreas via the common bile duct and pancreatic duct, respectively. These ducts open into the lumen of the duodenum at the **duodenal papilla (of Vater).** The duodenum differs from the jejunum and ileum in that its villi are broader, taller, and more numerous per unit area. It has fewer goblet cells per unit area than the other segments, and there are **Brunner's glands** in its submucosa.

The villi of the **jejunum** are narrower, shorter, and sparser than those of the duodenum. The number of goblet cells per unit area is greater in the jejunum than in the duodenum.

The villi of the **ileum** are the sparsest, shortest, and narrowest of the three regions of the small intestine. The lamina propria of the ileum houses permanent clusters of lymphoid nodules, known as **Peyer's patches.** These structures are located in the wall of the ileum that is opposite the attachment of the mesentery. In the region of Peyer's patches the villi are reduced in height and may even be absent.

CLINICAL CORRELATIONS

Meckel's diverticulum is a very common congenital anomaly occurring in about 2% of the Caucasian population. The diverticulum, a remnant of the vitelline duct—an embryonic connection between the midgut and the yolk sac—is a short, wide-mouthed extension of the distal aspect of the ileum about 100 cm from the cecum. Most Meckel's diverticula are asymptomatic, but some can cause bleeding and intestinal obstruction. The obstruction is usually due to intussusception—that is, the prolapse of the ileum into the diverticulum.

Small Intestine Histophysiology

In addition to its roles in digestion and absorption, the small intestine exhibits immunological and secretory activities. These activities are considered first, after which the primary function of the small intestine is described.

Immunological Activity of the Lamina Propria

Immunoglobulin A produced by plasma cells in the lamina propria is recirculated through the liver and gallbladder.

The lamina propria is rich in plasma cells, lymphocytes, mast cells, extravasated leukocytes, and fibroblasts.

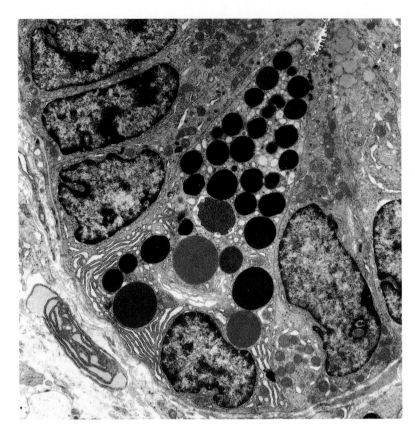

Figure 17–18 Electron micrograph of a Paneth cell from the rabbit ileum (×5900). Note the large, round granules in the cytoplasm of the Paneth cell. (From Satoh Y, Yamano M, Matsuda M, Ono K: Ultrastructure of Paneth cell in the intestine of various mammals. J Electron Microsc Tech 16:69-80, 1990.)

Additionally, solitary lymphoid nodules are frequently present in the lamina propria, adjacent to the epithelial lining of the mucosa. Moreover, as described previously, the ileum has permanent clusters of lymphoid nodules collectively known as Peyer's patches.

Where these lymphoid nodules come into contact with the epithelium, the columnar cells are replaced by M cells, which phagocytose luminal antigens (Figs. 17-19 and 17-20). Endocytosed antigens enter the endosomal system of these cells; however, instead of being processed, they are packaged in clathrin-coated vesicles, transferred to the basal aspect of the cell, and released into the lamina propria. Antigen-presenting cells and dendritic cells of the lymphoid nodule endocytose the transferred antigens, process them, and present the epitopes to lymphocytes for the initiation of an immune response.

Activated lymphocytes migrate to mesenteric lymph nodes, where they form germinal centers, regions where B cells proliferate. The newly formed B cells return to the lamina propria, where they differentiate into plasma cells that produce immunoglobulin A (IgA).

Some of the released antibodies bind to IgA receptors of epithelial cells and are complexed to **secretory component** (proteins manufactured by these cells) within the epithelial cells. The IgA-protein complex is transported into the lumen, a process known as **transcytosis,** and bound to the glycocalyx to defend the body against antigenic onslaught.

Most of the IgA produced in the lamina propria enters the circulatory system, is transported to the liver, where hepatocytes complex it with secretory component, and is released as a complex into bile. Thus, much of the luminal IgA enters the intestine through the common bile duct, as a constituent of bile.

Secretory Activity of the Small Intestine

Glands of the small intestine secrete mucus and a watery fluid in response to neural and hormonal stimulation. Neural stimulation, originating in the submucosal plexus, is the principal trigger, but the hormones secretin and cholecystokinin also play a part in regulating the secretory activities of Brunner's glands in the duodenum and of the crypts of Lieberkühn, which collectively produce almost 2 L of slightly alkaline fluid per day.

The DNES cells of the small intestine produce numerous hormones that affect movement of the small intestine and help regulate gastric HCl secretion and the release of pancreatic secretions (see Table 17-2).

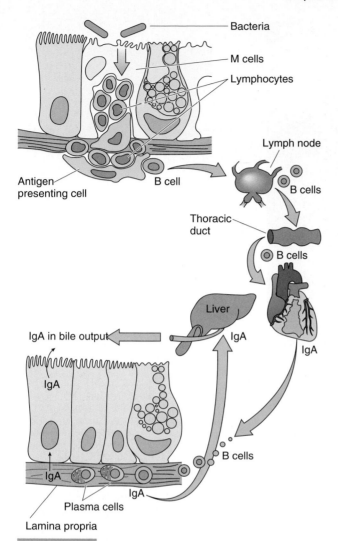

Figure 17–19 An M cell and its immunological relationship to the alimentary canal. Immunoglobulin A (IgA) is produced by plasma cells in the lamina propria. Some IgA then enters the lumen of the duodenum directly via the surface absorptive cells. Most of the IgA enters the hepatic portal system and hepatocytes of the liver complex it with secretory protein and deliver it into the gallbladder, where it is stored with bile. As bile is released into the duodenum, it will be rich in IgA. Therefore, most of the IgA enters the lumen of the duodenum via the bile.

CLINICAL CORRELATIONS

The rate of fluid secretion into the small intestine is greatly increased in response to **cholera toxin.** The amount of fluid lost as diarrhea may amount to as much as 10 L/day and, if not replaced, may lead to circulatory shock and death within a few hours. The fluid loss is accompanied by electrolyte imbalance, a contributory factor in the lethal effect of cholera.

Movement of the Small Intestine

The small intestine participates in two types of contraction: mixing and propulsive.

Movement of the small intestine may be subdivided into two interrelated phases:

- **Mixing contractions** are more localized and sequentially redistribute the chyme to expose it to the digestive juices.
- **Propulsive contractions** occur as **peristaltic waves** that facilitate the movement of the chyme along the small intestine. Because the chyme moves at an average of 1 to 2 cm/min, it spends several hours in the small intestine. The rate of peristalsis is controlled by neural impulses and hormonal factors. In response to gastric distention, a **gastroenteric reflex** mediated by the **myenteric plexus** provides the neural impetus for peristalsis in the small intestine. The hormones cholecystokinin, gastrin, motilin, substance P, and serotonin increase intestinal motility, whereas secretin and glucagon decrease it.

CLINICAL CORRELATIONS

If the intestinal mucosa is exposed to profound irritation by toxic substances, the muscularis externa can undergo intense, swift contractions of long duration known as **peristaltic rush.** These strong contractions propel the chyme into the colon within minutes for elimination as diarrhea.

Digestion

The chyme that enters the duodenum is in the process of being digested by enzymes produced by glands of the oral cavity and stomach. The process of digestion is intensified in the duodenum by enzymes derived from the exocrine pancreas. The final breakdown of proteins and carbohydrates occurs at the microvilli, where **dipeptidases** and **disaccharidases,** adherent to the glycocalyx, liberate individual amino acids and monosaccharides. These monomers are transported into the surface absorptive cells by specific carrier proteins; however, dipeptides and tripeptides are also endocytosed by the surface absorptive cells. Lipids are **emulsified** by bile salts into small fat globules that are split into monoglycerides and fatty acids. Bile salts segregate monoglycerides and free fatty acids into **micelles,** 2 nm in diameter, which diffuse into the surface absorptive cells through their plasmalemma.

Absorption

Approximately 6 to 7 L of fluid, 30 to 35 g of sodium, 0.5 kg of carbohydrates and proteins, and 1 kg of fat

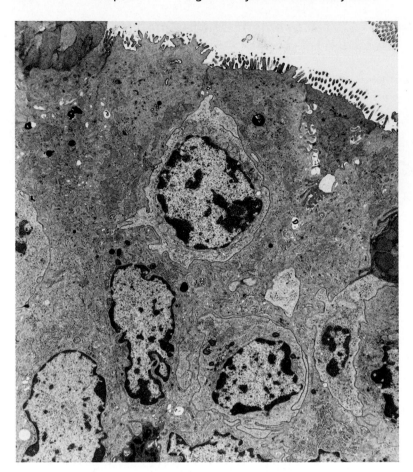

Figure 17–20 Electron micrograph of M cells of the mouse colon (×6665). Observe the electron-dense M cells surrounding the electron-lucent lymphocytes. (From Owen RL, Piazza AJ, Ermak TH: Ultrastructural and cytoarchitectural features of lymphoreticular organs in the colon and rectum of adult BALB/c mice. Am J Anat 190:10-18, 1991.)

are absorbed by the surface absorptive cells of the small intestine each day. Water, amino acids, dipeptides and tripeptides, ions, and monosaccharides enter the surface absorptive cells and are released into the intercellular space at the basolateral membrane. These nutrients then enter the capillary bed of the villi and are transported to the liver for processing.

Long-chain fatty acids and monoglycerides enter the SER of the surface absorptive cell, where they are reesterified to triglycerides (Fig. 17-21). The triglycerides are transferred to the Golgi apparatus, where they are combined with a β-lipoprotein coat, manufactured on the RER, to form **chylomicrons.** These large lipoprotein droplets, packaged by and released from the Golgi apparatus, are transported to the basolateral cell membrane to be released into the lamina propria. The chylomicrons enter the lacteals, filling these blindly ending lymphatic vessels with a lipid-rich substance known as **chyle.** Rhythmic contractions of the smooth muscle cells located in the cores of the villi cause shortening of each villus, which acts as a syringe, injecting the chyle from the lacteal into the submucosal plexus of lymph vessels.

Short-chain fatty acids (<12 carbons in length) do not enter the SER for reesterification. These free fatty acids, which are short enough to be somewhat water-soluble, progress to the basolateral membrane of the surface absorptive cell, diffuse into the lamina propria, and enter the capillary loops to be delivered to the liver for processing.

CLINICAL CORRELATIONS

Malabsorption in the small intestine may occur even though the pancreas delivers its normal complement of enzymes. The various diseases that result in malabsorption are called **sprue.** An interesting form of sprue, **gluten enteropathy (nontropical sprue),** is caused by **gluten,** a substance present in rye and wheat, that destroys the microvilli and even the villi of susceptible persons. These effects may result from an allergic response to gluten. In people with this disorder, the surface area available for absorption of nutrients is reduced. Treatment involves elimination of gluten-containing grains from the diet.

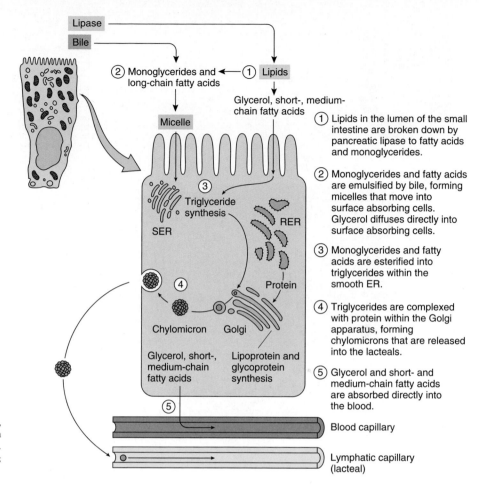

Figure 17–21 Fat absorption, fat processing, and chylomicron release by surface absorptive cells. SER, smooth endoplasmic reticulum; RER, rough endoplasmic reticulum.

The following labels appear in the figure:

Lipase

Bile

② Monoglycerides and long-chain fatty acids ◄── ① Lipids

Glycerol, short-, medium-chain fatty acids

Micelle

③ Triglyceride synthesis

SER

RER

④

Chylomicron   Golgi

Protein

Glycerol, short-, medium-chain fatty acids

Lipoprotein and glycoprotein synthesis

⑤

Blood capillary

Lymphatic capillary (lacteal)

① Lipids in the lumen of the small intestine are broken down by pancreatic lipase to fatty acids and monoglycerides.

② Monoglycerides and fatty acids are emulsified by bile, forming micelles that move into surface absorbing cells. Glycerol diffuses directly into surface absorbing cells.

③ Monoglycerides and fatty acids are esterified into triglycerides within the smooth ER.

④ Triglycerides are complexed with protein within the Golgi apparatus, forming chylomicrons that are released into the lacteals.

⑤ Glycerol and short- and medium-chain fatty acids are absorbed directly into the blood.

LARGE INTESTINE

The large intestine is subdivided into the cecum, colon, rectum, and anus; the appendix is a small, blind outpouching of the cecum.

The large intestine, composed of the cecum, colon (ascending, transverse, descending, and sigmoid), rectum, and anus, is approximately 1.5 m long (see Table 17-3). Its absorbs most of the water and ions from the chyme it receives from the small intestine and compacts the chyme into feces for elimination. The cecum and the colon are indistinguishable histologically and are discussed as a single entity called the **colon.** The **appendix,** a blind outpocketing of the cecum, is described separately.

Colon

The colon accounts for almost the entire length of the large intestine. It receives chyme from the ileum at the **ileocecal valve,** an anatomical as well as a physiologi-

cal sphincter that prevents reflux of the cecal contents into the ileum.

Colon Histology

The colon has no villi but is richly endowed with **crypts of Lieberkühn** that are similar in composition to those of the small intestine, except for the absence of Paneth cells (Figs. 17-22 to 17-25). The number of goblet cells increases from the cecum to the sigmoid colon, but, throughout most of the colon, the surface absorptive cells are the most numerous cell type. DNES cells are also present, although they are few in number. Rapid mitotic activity of the regenerative cells replaces the epithelial lining of the crypts and of the mucosal surface every 6 to 7 days.

The lamina propria, muscularis mucosae, and submucosa of the colon resemble those of the small intestine. The **muscularis externa** is unusual in that the outer longitudinal layer is not of continuous thickness along the surface; instead, most of it is gathered into three narrow ribbons of muscle fascicles

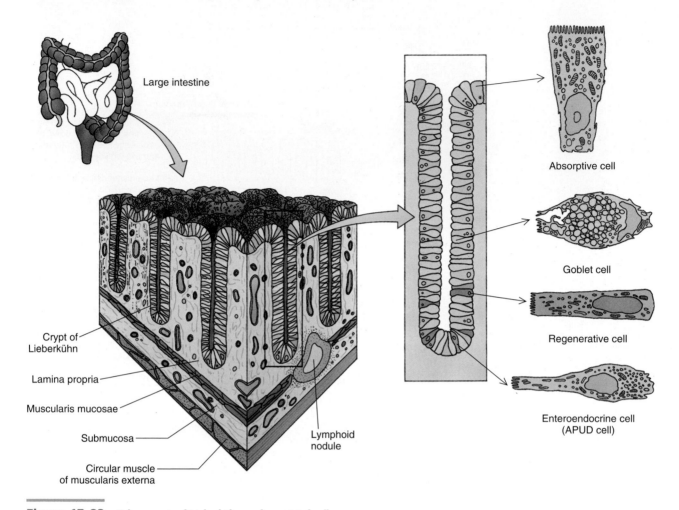

Large intestine

Absorptive cell

Goblet cell

Regenerative cell

Enteroendocrine cell
(APUD cell)

Crypt of
Lieberkühn

Lamina propria

Muscularis mucosae

Submucosa

Circular muscle
of muscularis externa

Lymphoid
nodule

Figure 17–22 Colon, crypts of Lieberkühn, and associated cells.

CLINICAL CORRELATIONS

Intense irritation of the colonic mucosa, as in **enteritis,** results in the secretion of large quantities of mucus, water, and electrolytes. Voiding of copious quantities of liquid stool, known as **diarrhea,** protects the body by diluting and eliminating the irritant. Long-term diarrhea and loss of a large amount of fluid and electrolytes, without a regimen of replacement therapy, may result in circulatory shock and even death.

Pseudomembranous colitis, an inflammatory disease of the bowel, may result from mercury poisoning, intestinal ischemia, and bronchopneumonia, but most frequently it is due to prolonged antibiotic therapy. Patients most at risk are those who are weak and/or elderly. As the intestinal flora is disrupted due to antibiotic therapy, *Clostridium difficile* plays a major role in the genesis of this disease. Clinical manifestations include fluid accumulation in the small intestine as well as epithelial shedding and the formation of a thick, viscous membrane composed of fibrin, mucus, neutrophils, and mononuclear cells. Symptoms include a low-grade fever (38°-40°C), copious watery diarrhea, severe abdominal cramps and abdominal tenderness. Mortality is relatively high (10%-15% of affected individuals) if the condition is not treated in a timely manner by fluid replacement therapy (as much as 10-15 L per 24 to 36 hours) to restore electrolyte balance and maintain adequate fluid volume.

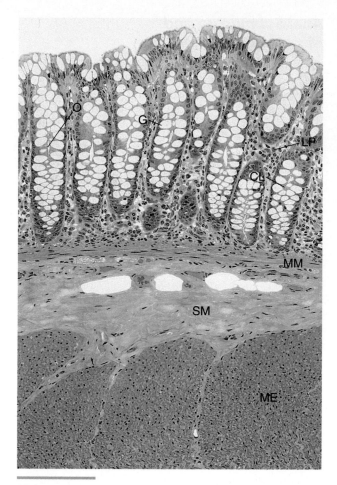

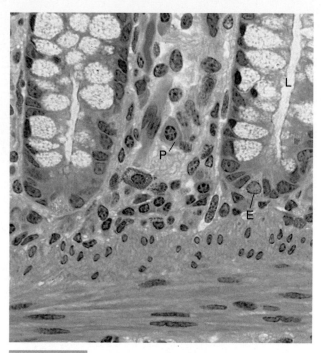

Figure 17–23 Light micrograph of the monkey colon (×132). It appears as if most of the cells of the epithelial lining are goblet cells (G), but in fact the surface absorptive cells constitute the largest population of this epithelium. CL, crypts of Lieberkühn; LP, lamina propria; ME, muscularis externa; MM, muscularis mucosae; O, open lumen of crypts of Lieberkühn; SM, submucosa.

Figure 17–24 Light micrograph of the crypts of Lieberkühn of the monkey colon (×270). Observe that the base of the crypt displays DNES cells whose granules are basally oriented. E, diffuse neuroendocrine system (DNES) cell; L, lumen of crypt; P, plasma cell.

known as **taeniae coli.** The constant tonus maintained by the taeniae coli puckers the large intestine into sacculations called **haustra coli.** The **serosa** displays numerous fat-filled pouches called **appendices epiploicae.**

Colon Histophysiology

The colon functions in absorption of water, electrolytes, and gases as well as in the compaction and elimination of feces.

The colon absorbs water and electrolytes (~1400 mL/day) and compacts and eliminates feces (~100 mL/day). Feces are composed of water (75%), dead bacteria (7%), roughage (7%), fat (5%), inorganic substances (5%), and undigested protein, dead cells, and bile

pigment (1%). The odor of feces varies with the individual and is a function of the diet and bacterial flora, which produce varied amounts of **indole, hydrogen sulfide,** and **mercaptans.** Bacterial by-products include riboflavin, thiamin, vitamin B_{12}, and vitamin K.

Bacterial action in the colon produces gases, released as **flatus,** composed of CO_2, methane, and H_2, which then is mixed with nitrogen and oxygen from swallowed air. The gas is combustible and, very infrequently, it may explode when electrical cauterization is used during sigmoidoscopy. The large intestine holds 7 to 10 L of gases each day, of which only 0.5 to 1 L is expelled as flatus; the remainder is absorbed through the lining of the colon.

The colon also secretes mucus and HCO_3^-. Mucus not only protects the mucosa of the colon but also facilitates the compaction of feces, because it is the mucus that permits adherence of the solid wastes into a compact mass. HCO_3^- adheres to the mucus and acts as a buffer, protecting the mucosa from the acid by-products of bacterial metabolism within the feces.

Rectum and Anal Canal

Histologically, the rectum resembles the colon, but the crypts of Lieberkühn are deeper and number fewer per unit area (see Table 17-3). The anal canal, the

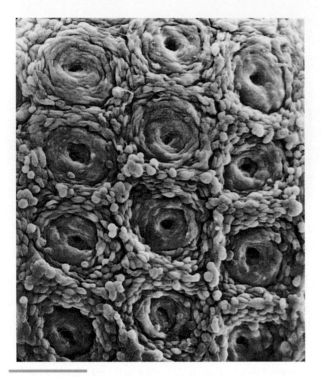

Figure 17–25 Scanning electron micrograph of a monkey colon (×516). Observe the opening of the crypts. (From Specian RD, Neutra MR: The surface topography of the colonic crypt in rabbit and monkey. Am J Anat 160:461-472, 1981.)

constricted continuation of the rectum, is about 3 to 4 cm long. Its crypts of Lieberkühn are short and few and are no longer present in the distal half of the canal. The mucosa displays longitudinal folds, the **anal columns (rectal columns of Morgagni).** These meet one another to form pouch-like outpocketings, the **anal valves,** with intervening **anal sinuses.** The anal valves assist the anus in supporting the column of feces.

Anal Mucosa

The **epithelium** of the anal mucosa is *simple cuboidal* from the rectum to the **pectinate line** (at the level of the anal valves), *stratified squamous nonkeratinized* from the pectinate line to the external anal orifice, and *stratified squamous keratinized* (epidermis) at the anus. The **lamina propria,** a fibroelastic connective tissue, houses **anal glands** at the rectoanal junction and **circumanal glands** at the distal end of the anal canal. Additionally, hair follicles and sebaceous glands are present at the anus. The **muscularis mucosae** is composed of an inner circular layer and an outer longitudinal layer of smooth muscle. These muscular layers do not extend beyond the pectinate line.

Anal Submucosa and Muscularis Externa

The **submucosa** of the anal canal is composed of fibroelastic connective tissue. It houses two venous plexuses, the **internal hemorrhoidal plexus,** situated above the pectinate line, and the **external hemorrhoidal plexus,** located at the junction of the anal canal with its external orifice, the **anus.**

The **muscularis externa** consists of an inner circular and an outer longitudinal smooth muscle layer. The inner circular layer becomes thickened as it encircles the region of the pectinate line to form the **internal anal sphincter muscle.** The smooth muscle cells of the outer longitudinal layer continue as a fibroelastic sheet surrounding the internal anal sphincter.

Skeletal muscles of the floor of the pelvis form an **external anal sphincter muscle** that surrounds the fibroelastic sheet and the internal anal sphincter. The external sphincter is under voluntary control and exhibits a constant tonus.

CLINICAL CORRELATIONS

An increase in the size of the vessels of the submucosal venous plexuses of the anal canal results in the formation of **hemorrhoids,** a condition common in pregnancy and in persons older than 50 years of age. This condition may manifest as painful defecation, the appearance of fresh blood with defecation, and anal itching.

As a **rectal examination** is performed by insertion of the index finger through the external anal orifice, the external anal sphincter tightens around the finger. Continued penetration results in activation of the internal anal sphincter, which also tightens around the finger. In males, structures that may be palpated through the anal canal include the bulb of the penis, the prostate, enlarged seminal vesicles, the inferior aspect of the distended bladder, and enlarged iliac lymph nodes; in females, palpable structures include the cervix of the uterus and, in pathological conditions, the ovaries and broad ligament.

Appendix

The histological appearance of the appendix resembles that of the colon, except that it is much smaller in diameter, has a richer supply of lymphoid elements and contains many more DNES cells in its crypts of Lieberkühn.

The **vermiform appendix** is a 5- to 6-cm-long diverticulum of the cecum with a stellate lumen that usually is occupied by debris. The mucosa of the appendix is composed of a simple columnar epithelium, consisting of surface absorptive cells, goblet cells, and M cells where lymphoid nodules adjoin the epithelium (see Table 17-3). The lamina propria is a loose connective tissue with numerous lymphoid nodules and shallow crypts of Lieberkühn. The cells composing these crypts are surface absorptive cells, goblet cells, regenerative cells, numerous DNES cells, and infrequent Paneth cells. The muscularis mucosae, submucosa, and muscularis externa do not deviate from the general plan of the alimentary canal, although lymphoid nodules and occasional fatty infiltration are present in the submucosa. The appendix is invested by a serosa.

CLINICAL CORRELATIONS

The incidence of inflammation of the appendix, **appendicitis,** is greater in teenagers and young adults than in older people; it also occurs more frequently in men than in women. Appendicitis usually is caused by obstruction of the lumen, which results in inflammation accompanied by swelling and an unremitting, severe pain in the lower right quadrant of the abdomen. Additional clinical signs are nausea and vomiting, fever (usually below 102° F), tense abdomen, and elevated leukocyte count. If the condition is not treated within 1 to 2 days, the appendix may rupture, leading to the onset of peritonitis, which may result in death if untreated.

Digestive System: Glands

18...

Extramural glands of the digestive system include the major salivary glands associated with the oral cavity (parotid, submandibular, and sublingual glands), the pancreas, and the liver and gallbladder. Each of these glands has numerous functions aiding the digestive process, and their secretory products are delivered to the lumen of the alimentary tract by a system of ducts.

Saliva produced by salivary glands facilitate the process of tasting food, initiate its digestion, and permit its deglutition (swallowing). These glands also protect the body by secreting the antibacterial agents lysozyme and lactoferrin as well as the secretory immunoglobulin IgA.

The pancreas manufactures a bicarbonate-rich fluid that buffers the acid chyme and produces enzymes necessary for the digestion of fats, proteins, and carbohydrates. The exocrine secretions of the pancreas are released into the lumen of the duodenum as necessary. In addition, the pancreas synthesizes and releases endocrine hormones, including insulin, glucagon, somatostatin, gastrin, and pancreatic polypeptide.

Bile, the exocrine secretion of the liver, is required for proper absorption of lipids, whereas many of the liver's endocrine functions are essential for life. These include metabolism of proteins, lipids, and carbohydrates; synthesis of blood proteins and coagulation factors; manufacture of vitamins; and detoxification of blood-borne toxins. The gallbladder concentrates bile and stores it until its release into the lumen of the duodenum.

MAJOR SALIVARY GLANDS

There are three pairs of major salivary glands: parotid, sublingual, and submandibular.

The major salivary glands are the paired parotid, sublingual, and submandibular glands. They are branched **tubuloalveolar glands** whose connective tissue capsule provides septa that subdivide the glands into lobes and lobules. Individual acini are also invested by thin connective tissue elements. The vascular and neural components of the glands reach the secretory units via the connective tissue framework.

Anatomy of Salivary Glands

Each of the major salivary glands has a secretory and a duct portion (Fig. 18-1). Note that according to some authors, the acinus, intercalated duct, and striated duct together constitute the **salivon,** the functional unit of a salivary gland.

Secretory Portions

The secretory portions of salivary glands are composed of serous and/or mucous secretory cells arranged in acini (alveoli) or tubules that are couched by myoepithelial cells.

The secretory portions, arranged in tubules and acini, are composed of three types of cells:

- **Serous cells** are seromucous cells because they secrete both proteins and a considerable amount of polysaccharides. These cells resemble truncated pyramids and have single, round, basally located nuclei, a well-developed rough endoplasmic reticulum (RER) and Golgi complex, numerous basal mitochondria, and abundant apically situated secretory granules rich in ptyalin (salivary amylase), which they secrete along with kallikrein, lactoferrin, and lysozyme. The basal aspects of the lateral cell membranes form tight junctions with each other. Apical to the tight junctions, intercellular canaliculi communicate with the lumen. The plasmalemma basal to the tight junctions forms many processes that interdigitate with those of neighboring cells.

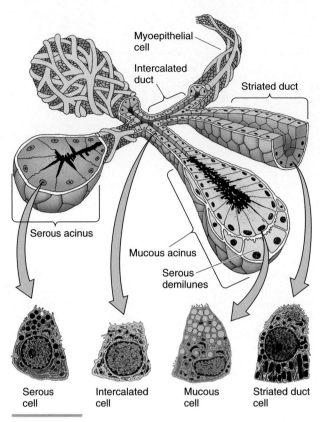

Figure 18–1 Salivary gland acini, ducts, and cell types.

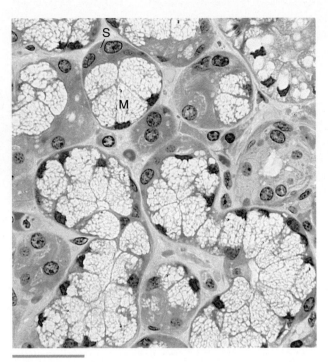

Figure 18–2 Light micrograph of the monkey sublingual gland displaying mucous acini (M) with serous demilunes (S). Note that serous demilunes may be fixation artifacts (×540).

- **Mucous cells** are similar in shape to the serous cells. Their nuclei are also basally located but are flattened instead of being round (Fig. 18-2). The organelle population of these cells differs from that of the serous cells in that mucous secretory cells have fewer mitochondria, a less extensive RER, and a considerably greater Golgi apparatus, indicative of the greater carbohydrate component of their secretory product (Fig. 18-3). The apical region of the cytoplasm is occupied by abundant secretory granules. The intercellular canaliculi and processes of the basal cell membranes are much less extensive than those of serous cells.
- **Myoepithelial cells (basket cells)** share the basal laminae of the acinar cells. They have a cell body that houses the nucleus and several long processes that envelop the secretory acinus and intercalated ducts (see Fig. 18-1). The cell body houses a small complement of organelles in addition to the nucleus and makes hemidesmosomal attachments with the basal lamina. The cytoplasmic processes, which form desmosomal contacts with the acinar and duct cells, are rich in actin and myosin; in electron micrographs these processes resemble smooth muscle cells. As the processes of myoepithelial cells contract, they press

on the acinus, facilitating release of the secretory product into the duct of the gland.

Duct Portions

The ducts of major salivary glands are highly branched and range from very small intercalated ducts to very large principal (terminal) ducts.

The duct portions of the major salivary glands are highly branched structures. The smallest branches of the system of ducts are the **intercalated ducts,** to which the secretory acini (and tubules) are attached. These small ducts are composed of a single layer of small cuboidal cells and possess some myoepithelial cells. Several intercalated ducts merge with each other to form **striated ducts,** composed of a single layer of cuboidal to low columnar cells (see Fig. 18-1). The basolateral membranes of these cells are highly folded, subdividing the cytoplasm into longitudinal compartments that are occupied by elongated mitochondria. The basolateral cell membranes of these cells have sodium adenosine triphosphatase (Na⁺-ATPase) that pumps sodium out of the cell into the connective tissue, thus conserving these ions and reducing the tonicity of saliva. Striated ducts join with each other, forming **intralobular ducts** of increasing caliber, which are surrounded by more abundant connective tissue elements.

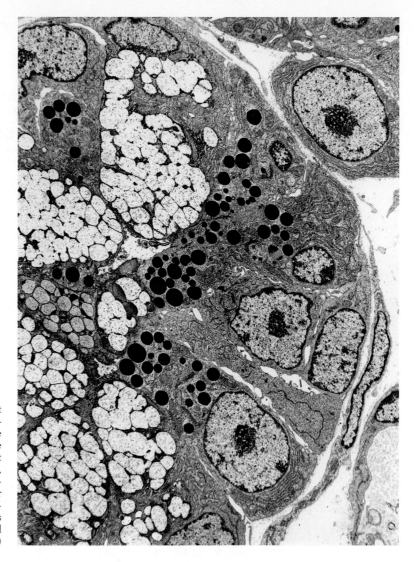

Figure 18–3 Electron micrograph of the rat sublingual gland displaying serous and mucous granules in the cytoplasm of the acinar cells (×5400). Note that the nuclei of serous cells are round, whereas the nuclei of mucous cells are flattened. Also observe that the serous secretory products are present as round, dense, dark structures. The mucous secretory products are mostly dissolved and appear light in color and spongy. (From Redman RS, Ball WD: Cytodifferentiation of secretory cells in the sublingual glands of the prenatal rat: A histological, histochemical, and ultrastructural study. Am J Anat 153:367-390, 1978.)

Ducts arising from lobules unite to form **interlobular ducts,** which in turn form **intralobar** and **interlobar ducts.** The **terminal (principal) duct** of the gland delivers saliva into the oral cavity.

Histophysiology of the Salivary Glands

Secretory cells of acini produce primary saliva that is modified by striated ducts to form secondary saliva.

The major salivary glands produce approximately 700 to 1100 mL of saliva per day. Minor salivary glands are located in the mucosa and submucosa of the oral cavity, but they contribute only 5% of the total daily salivary output. To perform at this level, salivary glands have an extraordinarily rich vascular supply. In fact, it has been

estimated that the basal rate of blood flow to salivary glands is 20 times greater than the flow of blood to skeletal muscle. During maximal secretion, the blood flow is correspondingly increased.

Saliva has numerous functions: lubricating and cleansing of the oral cavity, antibacterial activity, participating in the taste sensation by dissolving food material, initial digestion via the action of ptyalin (salivary amylase) and salivary lipase, aiding swallowing by moistening the food and permitting the formation of bolus, and participating in the clotting process and wound healing because of the clotting factors and epidermal growth factor present in saliva.

The saliva manufactured by the acinar cells, called **primary saliva,** is isotonic with plasma. The primary saliva, is modified by the cells of the striated ducts by removing sodium and chloride ions from it and secreting potassium and bicarbonate ions into it. Thereafter, the altered secretion, called **secondary saliva,** is hypotonic.

Acinar cells and duct cells also synthesize the secretory component required to transfer IgA from the connective tissue into the lumen of the secretory acinus (or duct). **Secretory IgA** complexes with antigens in the saliva, mitigating their deleterious effects. Saliva also contains lactoferrin, lysozyme, and thiocyanate ions. **Lactoferrin** binds iron, an element essential for bacterial metabolism; **lysozyme** breaks down bacterial capsules, permitting the entry of **thiocyanate ions,** a bactericidal agent, into the bacteria.

Salivary glands also secrete the enzyme **kallikrein** into the connective tissue. Kallikrein enters the bloodstream, where it converts kininogens, a family of plasma proteins, into **bradykinin,** a vasodilator that dilates blood vessels and enhances blood flow to the region.

Role of Autonomic Nerve Supply in Salivary Secretion

The major salivary glands do not secrete continuously. Secretory activity is stimulated via parasympathetic and sympathetic innervation. Innervation may be intraepithelial (i.e., formation of a synaptic contact between the end-foot and acinar cell) or subepithelial. In subepithelial innervation, the end-feet of axons do not make synaptic contact with the acinar cells; instead, they release their acetylcholine in the vicinity of the secretory cell, at a distance of approximately 100 to 200 nm from its basal plasmalemma. The cell thus activated stimulates neighboring cells via **gap junctions** to release their serous secretory product into the lumen of the acinus.

Parasympathetic innervation is the major initiator of salivation and is responsible for the formation of a serous saliva. Acetylcholine, released by the postganglionic parasympathetic nerve fibers, binds muscarinic cholinergic receptors, with consequent release of inositol trisphosphate. This effects the liberation of calcium ions, a second messenger, into the cytosol, which facilitates the secretion of serous saliva from the acinar cells.

Initially, **sympathetic innervation** reduces blood flow to the salivons, but that reduction is reversed in short order. Norepinephrine, released by the postganglionic sympathetic fibers, binds to β-adrenergic receptors, resulting in the formation of cyclic adenosine monophosphate (cAMP). This secondary messenger activates a cascade of kinases that result in the secretion of the mucous and enzymatic components of saliva by the acinar cells. The mucus is responsible for the adhesion of food particles in the bolus as well as for the creation of a slippery surface, facilitating swallowing.

Salivary output is enhanced by the taste and smell of food as well as by the process of chewing. A copious flow of saliva is also produced just before, during, and subsequent to vomiting. Inhibitors of salivation include fatigue, fear, and dehydration; moreover, salivary flow is greatly reduced while we are asleep.

Properties of Individual Salivary Glands
Parotid Gland

Although physically the largest of the salivary glands, the parotid gland produces only about 30% of the total salivary output; the saliva it produces is serous.

The parotid gland, the largest salivary gland, weighs about 20 to 30 g but produces only approximately 30% of the total output of saliva. Although this gland is said to produce a purely **serous secretion,** the secretory product has a mucous component. Electron micrographs of the apical regions of serous cells display numerous secretory granules filled with an electron-dense product that has an even more electron-dense core of unknown composition.

The saliva produced by the parotid gland has high levels of the enzyme **salivary amylase (ptyalin)** and secretory IgA. Salivary amylase is responsible for digestion of most of the starch in food, and this digestion continues in the stomach until the acidic chyme inactivates the enzyme. Secretory IgA inactivates antigens located in the oral cavity.

The connective tissue capsule of the parotid gland is well developed and forms numerous septa, which subdivide the gland into lobes and lobules. The duct system follows the distribution detailed earlier. By the 40th year of age, the gland becomes invaded by adipose tissue, which spreads from the connective tissue into the glandular parenchyma.

Sublingual Gland

The sublingual gland is very small, is composed mostly of mucous acini with serous demilunes, and produces a mixed saliva.

The sublingual gland, the smallest of the three major salivary glands, is almond-shaped, weighs only 2 to 3 g, and produces only about 5% of the total salivary output. The gland is composed of mucous tubular secretory units, many of which are capped by a small cluster of serous cells, known as serous demilunes (see Fig. 18-2). Although routine light microscopy demonstrates the presence of serous demilunes, if the tissue is quick-frozen, these are absent, indicating that they may be fixation artifacts and are merely small clusters of serous cells that deliver their secretion into a lumen in common with the mucous tubular secretory units. These serous cells have been shown to secrete lysozyme. The sublingual gland produces a mixed, but mostly mucous, saliva. The intercellular canaliculi are well developed between the mucous cells of the secretory units. Electron micrographs of the cells of the serous demilunes display apical accumulations of secretory vesicles; however, unlike the cells of the parotid and submandibular glands, these vesicles do not have an electron-dense core (see Fig. 18-3).

The sublingual gland has a scant connective tissue capsule, and its duct system does not form a terminal duct. Instead, several ducts open into the floor of the mouth and into the duct of the submandibular gland. Because of the organization of the ducts, some authors consider the sublingual gland to be composed of several smaller glandular subunits.

Submandibular Gland

The submandibular gland produces 60% of the total salivary output; although it manufactures a mixed saliva, the major portion is serous.

The submandibular gland (Fig. 18-4), although only 12 to 15 g in weight, produces approximately 60% of the total salivary output. About 90% of the acini produce serous saliva, whereas the remainder of the acini manufacture a mucous saliva. Electron micrographs of the apical aspects of the serous cells of this gland display electron-dense secretory products, with a denser core, within membrane-bound secretory granules. The number of serous demilunes is limited. The striated ducts of the submandibular gland are much longer than those of the parotid or sublingual glands; therefore, his-tological sections of this gland display many cross-sectional profiles of these ducts, a characteristic feature of the submandibular gland.

The connective tissue capsule of the submandibular gland is extensive and forms abundant septa, which subdivide the gland into lobes and lobules. Fatty infiltration of the connective tissue elements into the parenchyma is evident by midlife.

CLINICAL CORRELATIONS

Benign pleomorphic adenoma, a nonmalignant salivary gland tumor, usually affects the parotid and the submandibular glands. Surgical removal of the parotid gland must be performed with care because of the presence of the facial nerve plexus within the substance of the gland.

The parotid gland (and occasionally other major salivary glands) is also affected by viral infections, causing **mumps,** a painful disease that usually occurs in children and that may result in sterility when it affects adults.

PANCREAS

The pancreas is both an exocrine gland that produces digestive juices and an endocrine gland that manufactures hormones.

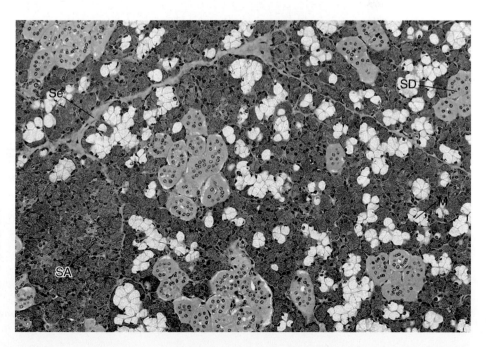

Figure 18–4 In this light micrograph, the submandibular gland is characterized by the numerous cross-sectional profiles of striated ducts (×132). Note that the ducts appear pale pink in color, and many display a very small but clear lumen. The mucous secretory product has a frothy appearance. Se, septum; SA, serous acinus; SD, serous demilune; M, mucous cells of an acinus.

The pancreas, situated on the posterior body wall, deep to the peritoneum, has four regions: uncinate process, head, body, and tail. It is about 25 cm long, 5 cm wide, and 1 to 2 cm thick, and it weighs approximately 150 g. Its flimsy connective tissue capsule forms septa, which subdivide the gland into lobules. The vascular and nerve supply of the pancreas, as well as its system of ducts, travels in these connective tissue compartments. The pancreas produces exocrine and endocrine secretions. The endocrine components of the pancreas, **islets of Langerhans,** are scattered among the exocrine secretory acini.

Exocrine Pancreas

The exocrine pancreas is a compound tubuloacinar gland that produces daily about 1200 mL of a bicarbonate-rich fluid containing digestive proenzymes. Forty to 50 acinar cells form a round to oval **acinus** whose lumen is occupied by three or four **centroacinar cells,** the beginning of the duct system of the pancreas (Fig. 18-5). The presence of centroacinar cells in the center of the acinus is a distinguishing characteristic of this gland.

Secretory and Duct Portions

The acinar cells of the pancreas have receptors for cholecystokinin and acetylcholine, whereas the centroacinar cells and intercalated ducts have receptors for secretin and perhaps for acetylcholine.

Each **acinar cell** is shaped like a truncated pyramid, with its base positioned on the basal lamina separating the acinar cells from the connective tissue compartment. The round nucleus of the cell is basally located and is surrounded by basophilic cytoplasm (Fig. 18-6). The apex of the cell, facing the lumen of the acinus, is

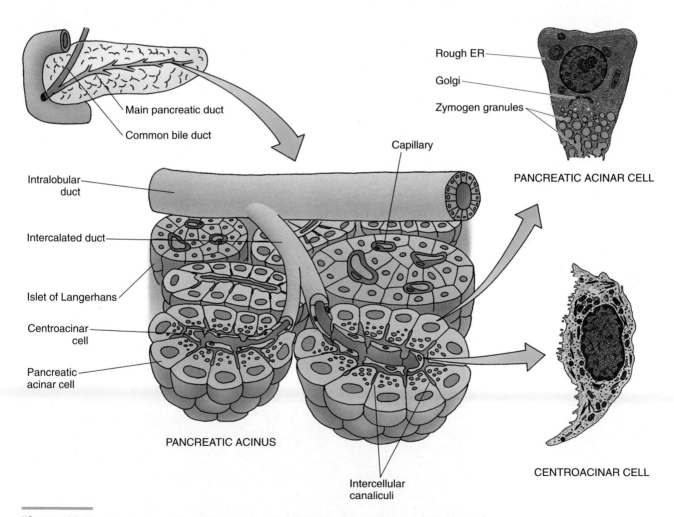

Figure 18–5 The pancreas with secretory acini, their cell types, and the endocrine islets of Langerhans.

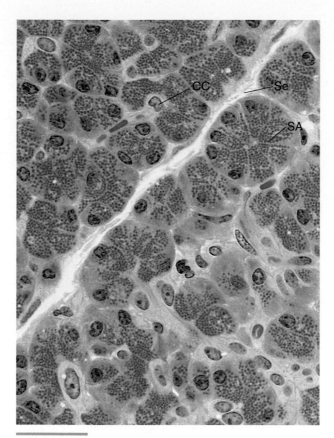

Figure 18–6 Light micrograph of the monkey exocrine pancreas (×540). Observe that the acini in section appear to be round structures and that much of the acinar cells have many secretory granules, known as zymogen granules. CC, centroacinar cells; Se, septum; SA, serous acinus.

The **duct system** of the pancreas begins within the center of the acinus with the terminus of the **intercalated ducts,** composed of pale, low cuboidal **centroacinar cells** (see Figs. 18-5 and 18-6). Centroacinar cells and intercalated ducts both have receptors on their basal plasmalemma for the hormone **secretin** and possibly for **acetylcholine,** released by postganglionic parasympathetic fibers. Intercalated ducts join each other to form larger **intralobular ducts,** several of which converge to form **interlobular ducts.** These ducts are surrounded by a considerable amount of connective tissue and deliver their contents into the **main pancreatic duct,** which joins the **common bile duct** before opening in the duodenum at the **papilla of Vater.**

Histophysiology of the Exocrine Pancreas

The acinar cells manufacture and release digestive enzymes, whereas the centroacinar cells and intercalated duct cells release a bicarbonate-rich buffer solution.

The acinar cells of the exocrine pancreas manufacture, store, and release a large number of enzymes: pancreatic amylase, pancreatic lipase, ribonuclease, deoxyribonuclease (DNase), and the proenzymes trypsinogen, chymotrypsinogen, procarboxypeptidase, and elastase. The cells also manufacture **trypsin inhibitor,** a protein that protects the cell from accidental intracellular activation of trypsin.

Release of the pancreatic enzymes is effected by the hormone **cholecystokinin** (pancreozymin) manufactured by DNES cells of the small intestine (especially of the duodenum) as well as by **acetylcholine** released by the postganglionic parasympathetic fibers.

The centroacinar cells and intercalated ducts manufacture a serous, bicarbonate-rich alkaline fluid, which neutralizes and buffers the acid chyme that enters the duodenum from the pyloric stomach. This fluid is enzyme-poor, and its release is effected by the hormone **secretin,** produced by enteroendocrine cells of the small intestine in conjunction with **acetylcholine,** released by the postganglionic parasympathetic fibers. Thus the enzyme-rich and enzyme-poor secretions are regulated separately, and the two secretions may be released at different times or concomitantly.

The assumed mechanism of bicarbonate ion secretion is facilitated by the enzyme **carbonic anhydrase,** which catalyzes the formation of carbonic acid (H_2CO_3) from water (H_2O) and carbon dioxide (CO_2). In the aquatic medium of the cytosol, H_2CO_3 dissociates to form H^+ and HCO_3^-; the HCO_3^- is actively transported into the lumen of the duct, whereas the hydrogen (H^+) ion is transported into the connective tissue elements.

filled with proenzyme-containing **secretory granules (zymogen granules),** whose number diminishes after a meal. The Golgi region, located between the nucleus and the zymogen granules, varies in size in inverse relation to the zymogen granule concentration.

The basal cell membranes of acinar cells have receptors for the hormone **cholecystokinin** and for the neurotransmitter **acetylcholine,** released by postganglionic parasympathetic nerve fibers. Electron micrographs of acinar cells display an abundance of basally located RER, a rich supply of polysomes, and numerous mitochondria exhibiting matrix granules. The Golgi apparatus is well developed but fluctuates in size, being smaller when the zymogen granules are numerous and larger after the granules release their contents.

The zymogen granules may release their contents individually, or several secretory vesicles may fuse with each other, forming a channel to the lumen of the acinus from the apical cytoplasm.

CLINICAL CORRELATIONS

Occasionally, the pancreatic digestive enzymes become active within the cytoplasm of the acinar cells, resulting in **acute pancreatitis,** which is often fatal. The histological changes involve an inflammatory reaction, necrosis of the blood vessels, proteolysis of the pancreatic parenchyma, and enzymatic destruction of adipose cells not only within the pancreas but also in the surrounding region of the abdominal cavity.

Pancreatic cancer is the fifth leading cause of mortality from all cancers, killing about 25,000 people in the United States per year. Fewer than 50% of patients survive more than 1 year, and fewer than 5% survive 5 years. Men are more susceptible to this disease than are women. Cigarette smokers have a 70% greater risk for development of pancreatic cancers than nonsmokers.

Endocrine Pancreas

The endocrine pancreas is composed of spherical aggregates of cells, known as islets of Langerhans, that are scattered among the acini.

Each **islet of Langerhans** is a richly vascularized spherical conglomeration of approximately 3000 cells. The approximately 1 million islets distributed throughout the human pancreas constitute the endocrine pancreas. A somewhat greater number of islets are present in the tail than in the remaining regions. Each islet is surrounded by reticular fibers, which also enter the substance of the islet to encircle the network of capillaries that pervade it (Fig. 18-7; also see Fig. 18-5).

Cells Composing the Islets of Langerhans

Five types of cells compose the parenchyma of each islet of Langerhans: beta (β) cells, alpha (α) cells, delta (δ) cells (D and D_1 cells), PP (pancreatic polypeptide–producing) cells, and G (gastrin-producing) cells. These cells cannot be differentiated from one another by routine histological examination, but immunocytochemical procedures allow them to be recognized. Electron micrographs also display the features that distinguish the various cells, especially the size and electron density of their granules (Fig. 18-8). Otherwise, the cells do not exhibit any unusual morphological features but resemble cells that specialize in protein synthesis. The characteristic features, locations, and hormones synthesized by these cells are presented in Table 18-1.

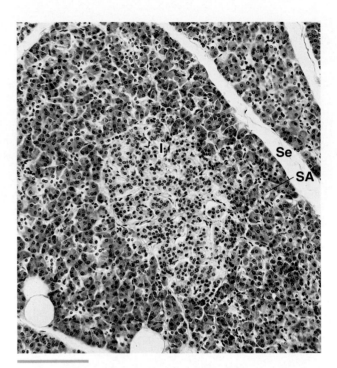

Figure 18–7 Light micrograph of the human pancreas displaying secretory acini and an islet of Langerhans (I) (×132). The histologic difference between the exocrine and endocrine pancreas is very evident in this photomicrograph because the islet is much larger than individual acini and is much lighter in color. Se, septum; SA, serous acinus.

Histophysiology of the Endocrine Pancreas

The cells of the islets of Langerhans produce insulin, glucagon, somatostatin, gastrin, and pancreatic polypeptide.

The two hormones produced in the greatest amounts by the endocrine pancreas—insulin and glucagon—act to decrease and increase blood glucose levels, respectively.

Insulin production begins with synthesis of a single polypeptide chain, **preproinsulin,** on the RER of β **cells.** Within the RER cisternae, this initial product is converted to **proinsulin** by enzymatic cleavage of a polypeptide fragment. Within the *trans* Golgi network, proinsulin is packaged into clathrin-coated vesicles, which lose their clathrin coat as they travel toward the plasmalemma. A segment of the proinsulin molecule near its center is removed by self-excision, thus forming insulin, which is composed of two short polypeptide chains linked by disulfide bonds. Insulin is released into the intercellular space in response to increased blood glucose levels, as occurs after consumption of a carbohydrate-rich meal.

TABLE 18–1 Cells and Hormones of the Islets of Langerhans

Cell	% of Total	Location	Fine Structure of Granules	Hormone and Molecular Weight (Da)	Function
β Cell	70%	Scattered throughout islet (but concentrated in center)	300 nm in diameter; dense core granule surrounded by wide electron-lucent halo	Insulin, 6000	Decreases blood glucose levels
α Cell	20%	Islet periphery	250 nm in diameter; dense core granule with narrow electron-lucent halo	Glucagon, 3500	Increases blood glucose levels
δ Cell (D and D₁)	5%	Scattered throughout islet	350 nm in diameter; electron-lucent homogeneous granule	*D cell:* Somatostatin, 1640	*Paracrine:* inhibits hormone release from endocrine pancreas and enzymes from exocrine pancreas *Endocrine:* reduces contractions of alimentary tract and gallbladder smooth muscles
				D₁ cell: Vasoactive intestinal peptide (VIP), 3800	Induces glycogenolysis; regulates smooth muscle tonus and motility of gut; controls ion and water secretion by intestinal epithelial cells
G cell	1%	Scattered throughout islet	300 nm in diameter	Gastrin, 2000	Stimulates production of hydrochloric acid by parietal cells of stomach
PP cell (F cell)	1%	Scattered throughout islet	180 nm in diameter	Pancreatic polypeptide, 4200	Inhibits exocrine secretions of pancreas

The released insulin binds to cell-surface insulin receptors on many cells, especially skeletal muscle, liver, and adipose cells. The plasma membranes of these cells also have glucose transport proteins, **glucose permease (glucose transport units),** which are activated to take up glucose, thus decreasing blood glucose levels. It is interesting that subplasmalemmal vesicles, rich in glucose permease, are added to the cell membrane during insulin stimulation and returned to their intracellular position when insulin levels are reduced.

Glucagon, a peptide hormone produced by **α cells,** is released in response to low blood glucose levels as well as by the consumption of a meal low in carbohydrate and high in protein. As in insulin production, a prohormone is produced first, and it undergoes proteolytic cleavage to yield the active hormone. Glucagon acts mainly on hepatocytes, causing these cells to activate glycogenolytic enzymes. These enzymes break

glycogen down to glucose, which is released into the bloodstream, increasing blood glucose levels. Glucagon also activates the hepatic enzymes responsible for **gluconeogenesis** (the synthesis of glucose from noncarbohydrate sources) if the intracellular glycogen depot of the hepatocytes is depleted.

Somatostatin, manufactured by one of the two types of **δ cells (D cells)** has both paracrine and endocrine effects. The hormone's paracrine effects are inhibition of the release of endocrine hormones by nearby **α** cells and **β** cells. Its endocrine effects are on smooth muscle cells of the alimentary tract and gallbladder, reducing the motility of these organs. Somatostatin is released in response to the increased levels of blood glucose, amino acids, or chylomicrons that occur after a meal. **Vasoactive intestinal peptide (VIP)** is produced by the second type of δ cells known as **D₁ cells.** This hormone induces glycogenolysis and

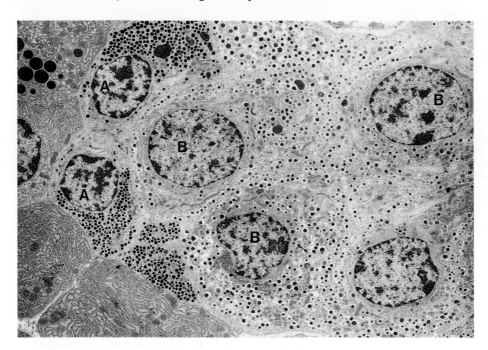

Figure 18–8 Electron micrograph of α cells (A) and β cells (B) in the rabbit islet of Langerhans (×5040). Note that the granules of α cells are much more numerous, more tightly packed, smaller, and denser than those of β cells. (From Jorns A, Grube D: The endocrine pancreas of glucagon-immunized and somatostatin-immunized rabbits. Cell Tissue Res 265:261-273, 1991.)

hyperglycemia and also regulates intestinal motility and the tone of smooth muscle cells of the wall of the gut. Additionally, VIP controls the secretion of ions and water by intestinal epithelial cells .

Gastrin, released by **G cells,** stimulates gastric release of HCl, gastric motility and emptying, and the rate of cell division in gastric regenerative cells.

Pancreatic polypeptide, a hormone produced by **PP cells,** inhibits the exocrine secretions of the pancreas and also stimulates the release of enzymes by the gastric chief cells while depressing the release of HCl by the parietal cells of the stomach.

LIVER

The liver, weighing approximately 1500 g, is the largest gland in the body. It is located in the upper right-hand quadrant of the abdominal cavity, just inferior to the diaphragm. The liver is subdivided into four lobes—right, left, quadrate, and caudate—the first two of which constitute its bulk (Fig. 18-9A).

Similar to the pancreas, the liver has both endocrine and exocrine functions; unlike the pancreas, however, the same cell (the **hepatocyte**) in the liver is responsible for the formation of **bile**—the liver's exocrine secre-

---

CLINICAL CORRELATIONS

Diabetes mellitus is a hyperglycemic metabolic disorder that results from (1) lack of insulin production by β cells of the islets of Langerhans or (2) defective insulin receptors on the target cells. There are two major forms of diabetes mellitus, type 1 and type 2 (Table 18-2). The incidence of type 2 is about five to six times that of type 1. If uncontrolled, both types of diabetes may have debilitating sequelae, including circulatory disorders, renal failure, blindness, gangrene, stroke, and myocardial infarcts. The most significant laboratory result indicative of diabetes is elevated blood glucose levels after an overnight fast.

Type 1 diabetes (insulin-dependent diabetes; juvenile-onset diabetes) usually affects persons younger than 20 years of age. It is characterized by the three cardinal signs of **polydipsia** (constant thirst), **polyphagia** (undiminished hunger), and **polyuria** (excessive urination).

Type 2 diabetes (non–insulin-dependent diabetes) is the *most common type* and usually affects persons older than 40 years of age.

Verner-Morrison syndrome (pancreatic cholera) is characterized by explosive, watery diarrhea that results in hypokalemia and hypochlorhydria. It is caused by the excessive manufacture and release of vasoactive intestinal peptide due to adenoma of the D_1 cells that produce this hormone. Frequently, tumors of D_1 cells are malignant.

TABLE 18–2 Comparison of Type 1 and Type 2 Diabetes Mellitus

Type	Common Synonyms	Clinical Characteristics	Patient Weight	Hereditary Component	Islets of Langerhans
Type 1 (insulin-dependent)	Juvenile-onset diabetes; juvenile diabetes; idiopathic diabetes	Abrupt onset of symptoms; age younger than 20 years; decreased blood insulin level; ketoacidosis is common; antibodies present against β cells; possible autoimmune disease; reacts to insulin; polyphagia, polydipsia, polyuria	Normal (or weight loss in spite of increase in food intake)	About 50% concordance in identical twins; environmental factors important in the development of the disease	Decrease in the size and number of β cells; islets are atrophied and fibrotic
Type 2 (non-insulin-dependent)	Adult-onset diabetes; ketosis-resistant diabetes	Onset after 40 years of age; mild decrease in blood insulin levels; ketoacidosis is rare; no antibodies against β cells; impaired insulin release; insulin-resistant; decrease in number of insulin receptors; impaired postreceptor signaling	80% of affected individuals are obese	About 90%-100% concordance in identical twins	Some decrease in number of β cells; amylin present in the tissue surrounding β cells

tion—and its numerous endocrine products. In addition, hepatocytes convert noxious substances into nontoxic materials that are excreted in bile.

General Hepatic Structure and Vascular Supply

The inferior, concave aspect of the liver houses the porta hepatis, through which the portal vein and hepatic artery bring blood into the liver and through which the bile ducts drain bile from the liver.

With the exception of the bare area, the liver is completely enveloped by peritoneum, which forms a simple squamous epithelium covering over the dense, irregular connective tissue **capsule (Glisson's capsule)** of the gland. Glisson's capsule is loosely attached over the entire circumference of the liver except at the porta hepatis, where it enters the liver, forming a conduit for the blood and lymph vessels and bile ducts. The liver is unusual in that its connective tissue elements are sparse; thus, the bulk of the liver is composed of uniform parenchymal cells, the **hepatocytes.**

The superior aspect of the liver is convex, whereas its inferior region presents a hilum-like indentation, the **porta hepatis.** The liver has a dual blood supply, receiving oxygenated blood from the **left hepatic artery** and the **right hepatic artery** (25%) and nutrient-rich blood via the **portal vein** (75%). Both vessels enter the liver at the porta hepatis. Blood leaves the liver at the posterior aspect of the organ through the **hepatic veins,** which deliver their contents into the inferior vena cava. Bile also leaves the liver at the porta hepatis, by way of the right and left hepatic ducts, to be delivered to the **gallbladder** for concentration and storage.

Because the liver occupies a central position in metabolism, all nutrients (except for chylomicrons and lipids less than 12 carbons in length) absorbed in the alimentary canal are transported directly to the liver via the portal vein. In addition, iron-rich blood from the spleen is routed, by way of the portal vein, directly to the liver for processing. Much of the nutritive material delivered to the liver is converted by the **hepatocytes** into storage products, such as glycogen, to be released as glucose when required by the body.

Hepatocytes are arranged in hexagon-shaped lobules **(classical lobules)** about 2 mm in length and 700 μm in diameter. These lobules are clearly demarcated by slender connective tissue elements (known as portal tracts) in animals such as the pig and the camel. However, because of the scarcity of connective tissue and the closely packed arrangement of the lobules in humans, the boundaries of the classical lobules can only be approximated.

Where three classical lobules are in contact with each other, the connective tissue elements are increased, and these regions are known as **portal areas**

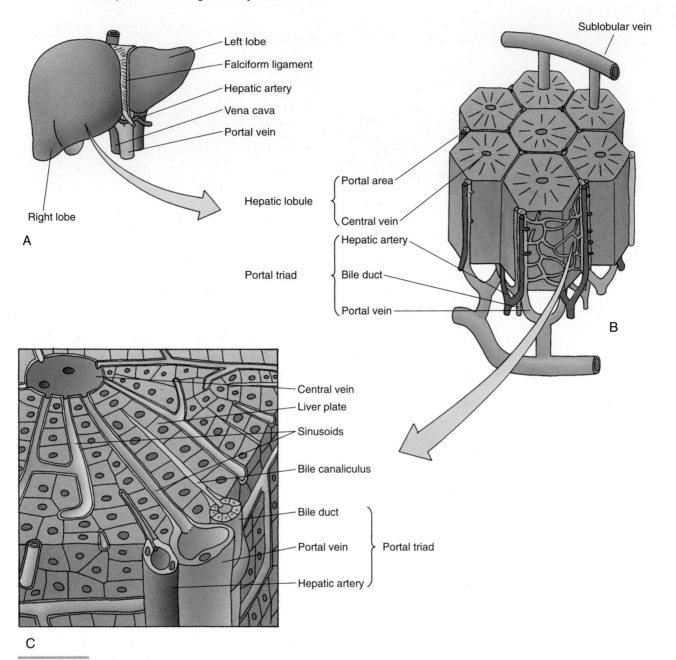

Figure 18–9 Liver. **A,** Gross anatomy of the liver. **B,** Liver lobules displaying the portal areas and the central vein. **C,** Portion of the liver lobule displaying the portal area, liver plates, sinusoids, and bile canaliculi.

(triads). In addition to lymph vessels, portal areas house the following three structures, each of which follows the longitudinal axis of each lobule (Fig. 18-9B):

- Slender branches of the hepatic artery
- Tributaries of the relatively large portal vein
- Interlobular bile ducts (recognized by their simple cuboidal epithelium).

The portal areas are isolated from the liver parenchyma by the **limiting plate,** a sleeve of modified hepatocytes. A narrow space, the **space of Möll,** separates the limiting plate from the connective tissue of the portal area.

Although one would expect to find six portal areas around each classical lobule, usually only *three* equally distributed portal areas are present in a random section (see Fig. 18-9B). Along the length of each slender branch of the hepatic artery within the portal area, fine branches, known as **distributing arterioles,** arise; like outstretched arms, they reach toward their counterparts in the neighboring portal areas. Smaller vessels, known as **inlet arterioles,** branch from the distributing arterioles (or from the parent vessel). In addition, the interlobular bile ducts are vascularized by a **peribiliary capillary plexus.** Venules are of two sizes: the larger **distributing veins** and the smaller **inlet venules.**

The longitudinal axis of each classical lobule is occupied by the **central vein,** the initial branch of the hepatic vein. Hepatocytes radiate, like spokes of a wheel, from the central vein, forming anastomosing, fenestrated plates of liver cells, separated from each other by large vascular spaces known as **hepatic sinusoids** (Fig. 18-10; also see Fig. 18-9C). **Inlet arterioles, inlet venules,** and branches from the **peribiliary capillary plexus** pierce the limiting plate (of modified hepatocytes) to join the hepatic sinusoids (see Fig. 18-10). As blood enters the sinusoids, its flow slows considerably and it slowly percolates into the central vein.

Because there is only one central vein in each lobule, it receives blood from every sinusoid of that lobule and its diameter increases as it progresses through the lobule. As the central vein leaves the lobule, it termi-

nates in the **sublobular vein.** Numerous central veins deliver their blood into a single sublobular vein; sublobular veins join each other to form **collecting veins,** which in turn form the right and left hepatic veins.

The Three Concepts of Liver Lobules

The three types of liver lobules are the classical lobules, portal lobules, and the hepatic acinus (acinus of Rappaport).

There are three basic conceptualizations of the liver lobule (Fig. 18-11). The **classical liver lobule** was the first to be defined histologically because the connective tissue arrangement in the pig liver afforded an obvious rationale. In this concept, blood flows from the periphery to the *center of the lobule* into the central vein. Bile, manufactured by liver cells, enters into small intercellular spaces, **bile canaliculi,** located between hepatocytes, and flows to the *periphery of the lobule* to the interlobular bile ducts of the portal areas.

The concept of an exocrine secretion flowing to the periphery of a lobule was not consistent with the situation in the acini of most glands, where the secretion enters a central lumen of the acinus. Therefore, histologists suggested that all hepatocytes that deliver their bile to a particular interlobular bile duct constitute a lobule, called the **portal lobule.** In histological sections, the portal lobule is defined as the triangular region whose center is the portal area and whose periphery is bounded by imaginary straight lines

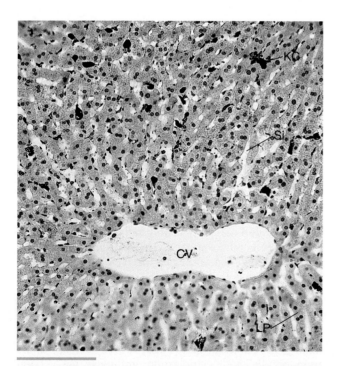

Figure 18–10 Light micrograph of a dog liver displaying the central vein (CV), liver plates (LP), and sinusoids (Si) (×270). This animal was injected with India ink that was phagocytosed by Kupffer cells (KC), which consequently appear as black spots.

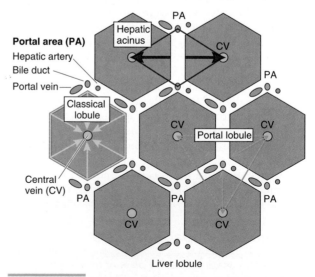

Figure 18–11 The three types of lobules in the liver: classical lobule, portal lobule, and hepatic acinus.

connecting the three surrounding central veins that form the three apices of the triangle.

A third conceptualization of hepatic lobules is based on blood flow from the distributing arteriole and, consequently, on the order in which hepatocytes degenerate subsequent to toxic or hypoxic insults. This ovoid to diamond-shaped lobule is known as the **hepatic acinus (acinus of Rappaport).** It is viewed as three poorly defined, concentric regions of hepatic parenchyma surrounding a distributing artery in the center. The outermost layer, zone 3, extends as far as the central vein and is the most oxygen-poor of the three zones. The remaining region is divided into two equal zones (1 and 2); zone 1 is the richest in oxygen.

Hepatic Sinusoids and Hepatocyte Plates

Plates of liver cells delineate vascular spaces between them that are lined by sinusoidal lining cells. The vascular spaces are known as hepatic sinusoids.

Anastomosing **plates of hepatocytes,** no more than two cells thick prior to the age of 7 years and one cell thick after that age, radiate from the central vein toward the periphery of the classical lobule (see Fig. 18-9*C*). The spaces between the plates of hepatocytes are occupied by hepatic sinusoids, and the blood flowing in these wide vessels is prevented from coming in contact with the hepatocytes by the presence of an endothelial lining composed of **sinusoidal lining cells.** Often, the cells of this endothelial lining do not make contact with each other, leaving gaps of up to 0.5 μm between them. The sinusoidal lining cells also have fenestrae that are present in clusters, known as **sieve plates.** Thus, particulate matter less than 0.5 μm in diameter may leave the lumen of the sinusoid with relative ease.

Resident macrophages, known as **Kupffer cells,** are associated with the sinusoidal lining cells in the sinusoids (Figs. 18-12 and 18-13). Frequently, phagosomes of Kupffer cells contain endocytosed particulate matter and cellular debris, especially defunct erythrocytes that are being destroyed by these cells. Electron micrographs of Kupffer cells display numerous filopodia-like projections, mitochondria, some RER, a small Golgi apparatus, and an abundance of lysosomes and late endosomes. Because these cells do not make intercellular junctions with the neighboring cells, it has been suggested that they may be migratory scavengers.

Perisinusoidal Space of Disse

The narrow space between a plate of hepatocytes and sinusoidal lining cells is known as the perisinusoidal space of Disse.

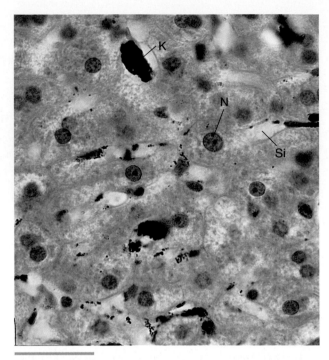

Figure 18–12 Light micrograph of a canine liver demonstrating plates of hepatocytes, sinusoids (Si), and India ink–containing Kupffer cells (K) (×540). N, nucleus.

The sinusoidal lining cells are separated from the hepatocytes by a narrow space of Disse (perisinusoidal space), and plasma escaping from the sinusoids has free access to this space (Fig. 18-14; also see Fig. 18-13). Microvilli of the hepatocytes occupy much of the space of Disse; the extensive surface area of the microvilli facilitates exchange of materials between the bloodstream and the hepatocytes. Hepatocytes do *not* come into contact with the bloodstream; instead, the space of Disse acts as an intermediate compartment between them.

Although the perisinusoidal space contains type III collagen fibers (reticular fibers) that support the sinusoids, as well as a limited amount of type I and type IV collagen fibers, a basal lamina is absent. Occasionally, nonmyelinated nerve fibers and stellate-shaped **hepatic stellate cells** (also known as **Ito cells** and **fat storing cells**) have been noted in this space (see Fig. 18-13). It is believed that hepatic stellate cells store vitamin A, manufacture and release type III collagen into the space of Disse, secrete growth factors required by the liver for generating new hepatocytes, and form fibrous connective tissue to replace hepatocytes damaged by toxins. In addition, **pit cells,** which display short pseudopodia and cytoplasmic granules, have been noted in the perisinusoidal space of mice and rats. These cells, believed to be natural killer cells, are also assumed to be in the human liver.

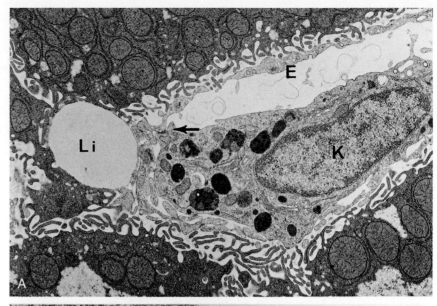

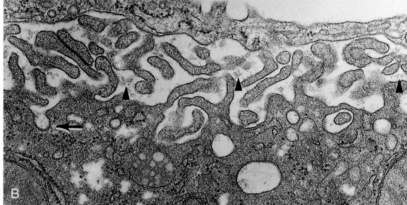

Figure 18–13 Electron micrograph of the shrew liver. **A,** Observe the sinusoid, with its sinusoidal lining cell (E), Kupffer cell (K), and a small region of a lipid droplet (Li)–containing Ito cell (×8885). **B,** A higher magnification of the hepatocyte displays its numerous microvilli (*arrowheads*) protruding into the space of Disse and the process of pinocytosis (*arrow*) (×29,670). (From Matsumoto E, Hirosawa K: Some observations on the structure of *Suncus* liver with special reference to the vitamin A–storing cell. Am J Anat 167:193-204, 1983.)

Hepatic Ducts

The system of hepatic ducts is composed of cholangioles, canals of Hering, and bile ducts leading to larger and larger bile ducts that finally culminate in the right and left hepatic ducts.

Bile canaliculi anastomose with one another, forming labyrinthine tunnels among the hepatocytes. As these bile canaliculi reach the periphery of the classic lobules, they merge with **cholangioles,** short tubules composed of a combination of hepatocytes and low cuboidal cells, and occasional oval cells. Bile from cholangioles enters the **canals of Hering,** slender branches of the **interlobular bile ducts,** that radiate parallel to the inlet arterioles and inlet venules. Interlobular bile ducts merge to form increasingly larger conduits, which eventually unite to form the **right hepatic duct** and the **left hepatic duct.** The extrahepatic system of bile ducts is described later. Most of the cells of the canals of Hering are composed of

low **cuboidal cells,** but interspersed among them are some **ovoid cells** that are capable of proliferation. The progeny of these oval cells may give rise to cuboidal cells of the bile duct system as well as to hepatocytes.

The cuboidal epithelial cells of the cholangioles, canals of Hering, and interlobular bile ducts secrete a bicarbonate-rich fluid similar to that produced by the duct system of the pancreas. The formation and release of this alkaline buffer are controlled by the hormone secretin, produced by diffuse neuroendocrine system (DNES) cells of the duodenum. This fluid acts, with fluid from the pancreas, to neutralize the acidic chyme that enters the duodenum.

Hepatocytes

Hepatocytes are 5- to 12-sided polygonal cells, approximately 20 to 30 μm in diameter, that are closely packed together to form anastomosing plates of liver cells, one cell in thickness. These cells exhibit variations in their

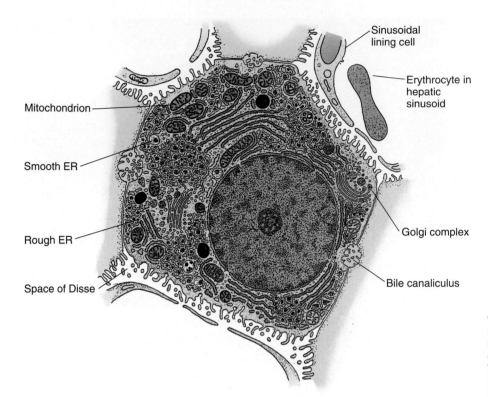

Figure 18–14 A hepatocyte and its sinusoidal and lateral domains. ER, endoplasmic reticulum. (From Lentz TL: Cell Fine Structure: An Atlas of Drawings of Whole-Cell Structure. Philadelphia, WB Saunders, 1971.)

structural, histochemical, and biochemical properties, depending on their location within liver lobules.

Domains of Hepatocyte Plasmalemma

The plasma membranes of hepatocytes are said to have two domains: lateral and sinusoidal.

Hepatocytes are arranged in such a manner that each cell not only comes in contact with other hepatocytes but also borders a space of Disse. Thus, the plasmalemma of hepatocytes is said to have lateral domains and sinusoidal domains.

LATERAL DOMAINS

The lateral domains are responsible for the formation of bile canaliculi.

The lateral domains of the hepatocyte cell membrane form elaborate, labyrinthine intercellular spaces, 1 to 2 μm in diameter, known as bile canaliculi, channels that conduct bile between hepatocytes to the periphery of the classical lobules (see Fig. 18-9C). Leakage of bile from bile canaliculi is prevented by the formation of tight junctions (fasciae occludentes) between adjoining liver cells, isolating these conduits from the remaining extracellular space.

Short, blunt microvilli project from the hepatocyte into the bile canaliculi, thus increasing the surface areas through which bile can be secreted (see Fig. 18-14). The actin cores of these microvilli mingle with the thickened network of actin and intermediate filaments that reinforce the region of the hepatocyte plasmalemma, which participates in the formation of bile canaliculi.

The cell membranes that form the walls of bile canaliculi display high levels of **Na⁺, K⁺-ATPase** activity and the enzyme **adenylate cyclase.** The lateral domains also have isolated gap junctions, whereby hepatocytes are able to communicate with each other.

SINUSOIDAL DOMAINS

The sinusoidal domains form microvilli that protrude into the perisinusoidal space of Disse.

The sinusoidal domains of hepatocyte plasma membranes also have microvilli that project into the space of Disse (see Figs. 18-13 and 18-14). It has been calculated that these microvilli increase the surface area of the sinusoidal domain by a factor of 6, facilitating the exchange of material between the hepatocyte and the plasma in the perisinusoidal space. This cell membrane is rich in mannose-6-phosphate receptors, Na⁺,K⁺-ATPase, and adenylate cyclase because it is here that the endocrine secretions of the hepatocyte are released and enter the sinusoidal blood and that material carried by the bloodstream is transported into the hepatocyte cytoplasm.

Hepatocyte Organelles and Inclusions

Hepatocytes are large, organelle-rich cells that manufacture the exocrine secretion bile as well as a large number of endocrine secretions; in addition, these cells can perform a large array of metabolic functions.

Although hepatocytes constitute only 60% of the total cell number, they compose about 75% of the weight of the liver. These cells manufacture **primary bile,** which is modified by the epithelial cells lining the bile ducts and gallbladder and becomes **bile.** Approximately 75% of the hepatocytes have a single nucleus, and the remainder have two nuclei. The nuclei vary in size, the smallest ones (50% of the nuclei) being diploid and the larger ones being polyploid, with the largest nuclei reaching 64 N.

Hepatocytes actively synthesize proteins for their own use as well as for export. Thus, they have an abundance of free ribosomes, RER, and Golgi apparatus (Figs. 18-15 and 18-16). Each cell houses several sets of Golgi apparatuses, located preferentially in the vicinity of bile canaliculi.

Because of the high energy requirements of hepatocytes, each cell contains as many as 2000 mitochondria. Cells near the central vein (zone 3 of the liver acinus) have nearly twice as many, but considerably smaller, mitochondria as hepatocytes in the periportal area (zone 1 of the liver acinus). Liver cells also have a rich complement of endosomes, lysosomes, and peroxisomes.

The complement of smooth endoplasmic reticulum (SER) of hepatocytes varies not only by region but also by function. Cells in zone 3 of the liver acinus have a much richer endowment of SER than those in the periportal area. Moreover, the presence of certain drugs and toxins in the blood induces an increase in the SER content of liver cells because detoxification occurs within the cisternae of this organelle.

CLINICAL CORRELATIONS

Persons who have consumed hepatotoxic substances, such as alcohol, display an increased number of lipid deposits in their zone 3 hepatocytes. In addition, persons who are taking barbiturates display an increase in the SER content of zone 3 liver cells. Since this zone has the lowest oxygen levels of the three zomes, this is the region of the liver acinus that is most susceptible to necrosis in case of severe liver injury.

Alcoholics and people who suffer from obstruction of the biliary tract or chronic poisoning are at risk for development of **cirrhosis,** a disease characterized by fibrosis, degeneration of hepatocytes, and disintegration of the normal organization of the liver.

Wilson's disease is a hereditary condition in which the liver does not eliminate copper by transferring it into bile. Instead copper accumulates in the eyes, where it appears as green to gold rings in the cornea; in the brain, where it interferes with normal brain function, causing tremors, aphasia, and, occasionally, psychosis; and in the liver, where it causes cirrhosis. If left untreated the disease is fatal, but the use of a chelating agent, usually penicillamine, binds with copper and facilitates its elimination from the body.

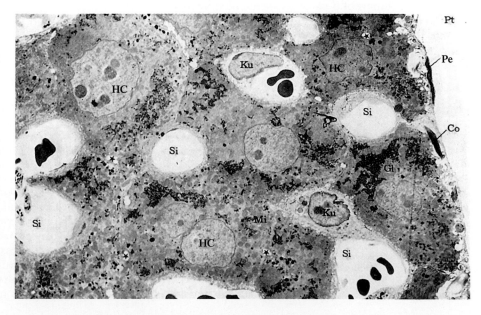

Figure 18–15 Low-magnification electron micrograph of a mouse liver (×2535). Most of the liver's surface is covered by peritoneum (Pe), which overlies the collagenous capsule (Co) of the liver. Observe the sinusoids (Si), Kupffer cells (Ku), and glycogen deposits (Gl) in the hepatocyte (HC) cytoplasm. Bile canaliculi are denoted by *asterisks* (°). Mi, mitochondria; Pt, peritoneal cavity. (From Rhodin JAG: An Atlas of Ultrastructure. Philadelphia, WB Saunders, 1963.)

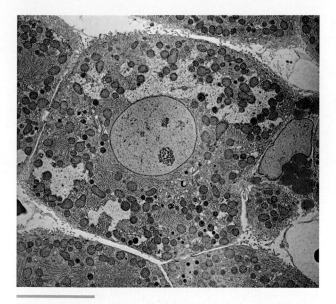

Figure 18–16 Electron micrograph of a rat hepatocyte (×2500). (From Tandler B, Krahenbuhl S, Brass EP: Unusual mitochondria in the hepatocytes of rats treated with a vitamin B$_{12}$ analogue. Anat Rec 231:1-6, 1991.)

Hepatocytes contain varying amounts of inclusions in the form of lipid droplets and glycogen (Fig. 18-17). The lipid droplets are mostly **very-low-density-lipoproteins (VLDLs)** and are especially prominent after the consumption of a fatty meal.

Glycogen deposits are present as accumulations of electron-dense granules 20 to 30 nm in size, known as **β particles,** in the vicinity of the SER. The distribution of glycogen varies with hepatocyte location. Liver cells in the vicinity of the portal area (zone 1 of liver acinus) display large clumps of β particles surrounded by SER, whereas pericentral hepatocytes (zone 3 of liver acinus) exhibit diffuse glycogen deposits (see Fig. 18-17). The number of these particles varies with the dietary state of the individual. They are abundant subsequent to eating and fewer after fasting.

Histophysiology of the Liver

The liver has both exocrine and endocrine roles as well as the protective function of detoxification of toxins and elimination of defunct erythrocytes.

The liver may have as many as 100 different functions, most of which are performed by the hepatocytes. Each of these liver cells produces not only the exocrine secretion bile but also various endocrine secretions. Hepatocytes metabolize the end products of absorption from the alimentary canal, store them as inclusion products, and release them in response to hormonal and nervous signals. Liver cells also detoxify drugs and toxins (pro-

tecting the body from their deleterious effects) and transfer secretory IgA from the space of Disse into bile. In addition, Kupffer cells phagocytose blood-borne foreign particulate matter and defunct erythrocytes.

Bile Manufacture

Bile, a fluid manufactured by the liver, is composed of water, bile salts, phospholipids, cholesterol, bile pigments, and IgA.

The liver produces approximately 600 to 1200 mL of bile/day. This fluid, which is mostly water, contains bile salts (bile acids), bilirubin glucuronide (bile pigment), phospholipids, lecithin, cholesterol, plasma electrolytes (especially sodium and bicarbonate), and IgA. It absorbs fat, eliminates approximately 80% of the cholesterol synthesized by the liver, and excretes blood-borne waste products such as bilirubin.

Bile salts constitute almost half of the organic components of bile. Most of the bile salts are resorbed from the lumen of the small intestine, enter the liver via the portal vein, are endocytosed by hepatocytes, and are transported into the bile canaliculi for subsequent re-release back into the duodenum **(enterohepatic recirculation of bile salts).** The remaining 10% of bile salts are manufactured de novo in the SER of hepatocytes by the conjugation of cholic acid, a metabolic by-product of cholesterol, to either taurine (tauricholic acid) or glycine (glycocholic acid).

CLINICAL CORRELATIONS

Because bile salts are amphipathic molecules, their *hydrophilic* regions are dissolved in aqueous media and their *hydrophobic* (*lipophilic*) regions surround lipid droplets. In the lumen of the duodenum, therefore, bile salts emulsify fats and facilitate their digestion. Absence of bile salts prevents fat digestion and absorption, resulting in **fatty stool.**

Bilirubin, a water-insoluble, yellowish green pigment, is the toxic degradation product of hemoglobin. As defunct erythrocytes are destroyed by macrophages in the spleen and by Kupffer cells in the liver, bilirubin is released into the bloodstream and is bound to plasma albumin. In this form, known as **free bilirubin,** it is endocytosed by hepatocytes. The enzyme **glucuronyltransferase,** located in the SER of the hepatocyte, catalyzes the conjugation of bilirubin with glucuronide to form the water-soluble **bilirubin glucuronide (conjugated bilirubin).** Some of the bilirubin glucuronide is released into the bloodstream,

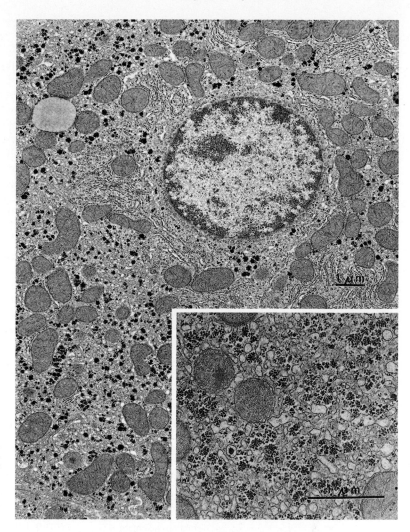

Figure 18–17 Electron micrograph of glycogen and lipid deposits in the pericentral hepatocyte of a rat. Bar = 1 μm. *Inset:* Glycogen particles at a higher magnification. Bar = 1 μm. (From Cardell RR, Cardell EL: Heterogeneity of glycogen distribution in hepatocytes. J Electron Microsc Techn 14:126-139, 1987.)

but most of it is excreted into the bile canaliculi for delivery into the alimentary canal for subsequent elimination with the feces (Fig. 18-18).

Lipid Metabolism

Hepatocytes remove chylomicrons from the space of Disse and degrade them into fatty acids and glycerol.

Chylomicrons released by surface-absorbing cells of the small intestine enter the lymphatic system and reach the liver through branches of the hepatic artery. Within hepatocytes they are degraded into fatty acids and glycerol. The fatty acids are subsequently desaturated and are used to synthesize phospholipids and cholesterol or are degraded into acetyl coenzyme A. Two molecules of acetyl coenzyme A are combined to form acetoacetic acid. Much of the acetoacetic acid is converted into β-hydroxybutyric acid and some into acetone. These three compounds—acidoacetic acid, β-hydroxybutyric acid, and acetone—are known as **ketone bodies.** Phospholipids, cholesterol, and ketone bodies are stored in hepatocytes until their release into the space of Disse. In addition, the liver manufactures **VLDLs,** which are also released into the space of Disse as droplets 30 to 100 nm in diameter.

Carbohydrate and Protein Metabolism

Additional responsibilities of the liver include the maintenance of normal blood glucose levels, deamination of amino acids, and the synthesis of many blood proteins.

The liver maintains normal levels of glucose in the blood by transporting glucose from the blood into the

A Protein synthesis and carbohydrate storage in the liver

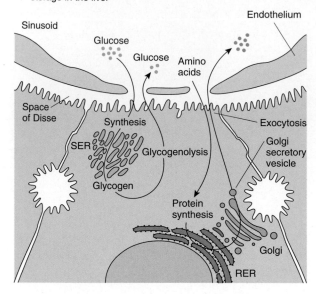

B Secretion of bile acids and bilirubin

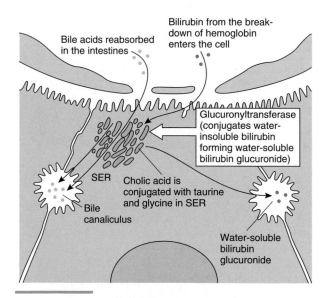

Figure 18–18 Hepatocyte function. SER, smooth endoplasmic epithelium. **A,** Protein synthesis and carbohydrate storage. **B,** Secretion of bile acids and bilirubin.

CLINICAL CORRELATIONS

The yellowish discoloration of the skin that is the hallmark of **jaundice** results from excessively high levels of free or conjugated bilirubin (which is yellowish green) in the bloodstream. The two primary types of jaundice have different causes. A decrease in bilirubin conjugation, because of either hepatocyte malfunction (as in hepatitis) or, more commonly, obstruction of the bile ducts, causes **obstructive jaundice.** Increased hemolysis of erythrocytes, producing so much free bilirubin that hepatocytes, even though unimpaired, cannot eliminate bilirubin rapidly enough, causes **hemolytic jaundice.**

Ketosis occurs when the concentration of ketone bodies in the blood becomes too high (as in persons suffering from diabetes or starvation). It is recognizable by the typical acetone breath of affected persons. If untreated, ketosis results in decreased blood pH **(acidosis),** possibly leading to death.

Excessive blood ammonia levels, indicative of impaired liver function or drastic reduction in blood flow to the liver, may lead to **hepatic coma,** a condition that is incompatible with life.

from noncarbohydrate sources (such as amino acids), a process known as **gluconeogenesis.**

One of the most essential roles of the liver is the elimination of blood-borne ammonia by converting it into **urea.** There are two major sources of ammonia in the body, the deamination of amino acids by hepatocytes and the synthesis of ammonia by bacterial action in the alimentary canal.

Approximately 90% of the blood proteins are manufactured by the liver (see Fig. 18-18). These proteins and related products include:

- Factors necessary for coagulation (such as fibrinogen, factor III, accelerator globulin, and prothrombin)
- Proteins required for the complement reactions
- Proteins that function in transport of metabolites
- Albumins
- All of the globulins except gamma (γ) globulins
- All of the nonessential amino acids that the body requires

Vitamin Storage

Vitamin A is stored in the greatest amount in the liver, but vitamins D and B_{12} are also present in substantial

hepatocytes and storing it in the form of glycogen. If blood glucose levels drop below normal, hepatocytes hydrolyze glycogen **(glycogenolysis)** into glucose and transport it out of the cells into the space of Disse (see Fig. 18-18). Hepatocytes can also synthesize glucose from other sugars (such as fructose and galactose) or

quantities. The liver contains enough vitamin stores to prevent deficiency of vitamin A for about 10 months, vitamin D for about 4 months, and vitamin B_{12} for more than 12 months.

Degradation of Hormones and Detoxification of Drugs and Toxins

The liver endocytoses and degrades hormones of the endocrine glands. The endocytosed hormones are transported into the bile canaliculi in their native form to be digested in the lumen of the alimentary canal or are delivered into late endosomes for degradation by lysosomal enzymes.

Drugs, such as barbiturates and antibiotics, and toxins are inactivated by **microsomal mixed-function oxidases** in hepatocytes. These drugs and toxins are usually inactivated in the cisterna of the SER by methylation, conjugation, or oxidation. Occasionally, detoxification occurs in peroxisomes rather than in the SER.

CLINICAL CORRELATIONS

Continued long-term use of certain drugs, such as barbiturates, decreases their effectiveness, requiring the prescription of increased doses. This **drug tolerance** is due to hypertrophy of the SER complement of hepatocytes and a concomitant increase in their mixed-function oxidases. The increase in the organelle size and the enzyme concentration is **induced** by the barbiturate, which is detoxified via oxidative demethylation. In addition, these hepatocytes concurrently become more efficient in detoxifying other drugs and toxins.

Immune Function

Hepatocytes complex IgA with secretory component and release the secretory IgA into the bile canaliculi.

Most of the IgA antibodies formed by plasma cells in the mucosa of the alimentary canal enter the circulatory system and are transported to the liver. Hepatocytes complex the IgA with secretory component and release the complex into bile, which then enters the lumen of the duodenum. Thus, much of the luminal IgA enters the intestine through the common bile duct, accompanying bile. The remainder of the luminal IgA is transported from the intestinal mucosa into the lumen by surface absorptive cells.

Kupffer cells, which are derived from monocyte precursors, are long-lived cells that are located within the hepatic sinusoids and adhere to the luminal surface of endothelial cells. Kupffer cells have Fc receptors as well as receptors for complement and thus can phagocytose foreign particulate matter. The importance of these cells is appreciable because blood from the portal vein contains a considerable number of microorganisms that enter the bloodstream from the lumen of the alimentary canal. These bacteria become opsonized in the lumen or mucosa of the gut or in the bloodstream. Kupffer cells recognize and endocytose at least 99% of these microorganisms. Kupffer cells also remove cellular debris and defunct erythrocytes from the blood.

Liver Regeneration

The liver has a great ability to regenerate after a hepatotoxic insult or even after a portion of the liver is excised.

Hepatocytes have a life span of approximately 150 days; thus, mitotic figures are present only infrequently. If hepatotoxic drugs are administered or a portion of the liver is excised, however, hepatocytes proliferate, and the liver regenerates its normal architecture and previous size.

The regenerative ability of the liver of rodents is so enormous that if 75% of the gland is excised, it regenerates to its normal size within 4 weeks. The human liver's regenerative capacity is much less than that of mice and rats. The mechanism of regeneration is controlled by transforming growth factor-α, transforming growth factor-β, epidermal growth factor, interleukin-6, and hepatocyte growth factor. Many of these factors are released by the hepatic stellate cells (Ito cells) located in the space of Disse, although hepatocyte growth factor is also present, bound to heparin, in the scant extracellular matrix of the liver. In most cases, the regeneration is due to the replicative capability of the remaining hepatocytes; however, if the hepatotoxic insult is too great, regeneration of the liver is due to the mitotic activity of the oval cells of cholangioles and canals of Hering.

GALLBLADDER

The gallbladder is a small, pear-shaped organ situated on the inferior aspect of the liver. It is about 10 cm in length and 4 cm in cross-section and can store about 70 mL of bile. This organ resembles a sack with a single opening. The bulk of the organ forms the **body,** and the opening, which is continuous with the **cystic duct,** is called the **neck.** The neck has an outpocketing known as Hartmann's pouch, a region where gallstones frequently lodge. The gallbladder stores and concentrates bile and releases it into the duodenum as required.

Structure of the Gallbladder

The wall of the gallbladder comprises four layers: epithelium, lamina propria, smooth muscle, and serosa/adventitia.

The mucosa of the empty gallbladder is highly folded into tall, parallel ridges (Fig. 18-19). As the gallbladder becomes distended with bile, the plication is reduced to a few short folds, and the mucosa becomes relatively smooth.

The lumen of the gallbladder is lined by a **simple columnar epithelium,** composed of two types of cells: the more common **clear cells** and the infrequent **brush cells** (Fig. 18-20). The oval nuclei of these cells are basally positioned and the supranuclear cytoplasm displays occasional secretory granules containing mucinogen. In electron micrographs, their luminal surface displays short microvilli coated by a thin layer of glycocalyx. The basal region of the cytoplasm is particularly rich in mitochondria, providing abundant energy for the Na⁺,K⁺-ATPase pump present in the basolateral cell membrane.

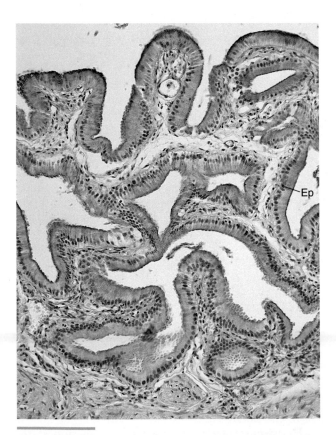

Figure 18–19 Light micrograph of an empty gallbladder (×132). Observe that the mucosa of the gallbladder is highly folded, indicating that it is empty. Note that the lumen of the gallbladder is lined by a simple columnar epithelium (Ep).

The lamina propria is composed of a vascularized loose connective tissue that is well endowed with elastic and collagen fibers. In the neck of the gallbladder, the lamina propria houses simple tubuloalveolar glands, which produce a small amount of mucus to lubricate the lumen of this constricted region. The thin, smooth muscle layer of the gallbladder is composed mostly of **obliquely oriented** fibers, whereas others are oriented longitudinally. Although the connective tissue adventitia is attached to Glisson's capsule of the liver, it may be separated from it with relative ease. The nonattached surface of the gallbladder is invested by peritoneum, providing it with a smooth, simple squamous epithelial serosa.

Extrahepatic Ducts

The right and left hepatic ducts unite to form the **common hepatic duct,** which is joined by the **cystic duct,** arising from the gallbladder. The merger of these two ducts forms the **common bile duct,** 7 to 8 cm long, which fuses with the pancreatic duct to form the **ampulla of Vater.** The ampulla opens at the duodenal papilla into the lumen of the duodenum.

The opening of the common bile duct and the pancreatic duct is controlled by a complex of four muscles—the sphincter choledochus, sphincter pancreaticus, sphincter ampullae, and fasciculus longitudinalis—collectively called the **sphincter of Oddi.** The locations and functions of these components are summarized in Table 18-3.

TABLE 18–3 The Sphincter of Oddi and Its Component Parts

Component	Location and Function
Sphincter choledochus	Surrounds and controls terminal region of common bile duct to stop bile flow into duodenum
Sphincter pancreaticus	Surrounds and controls terminal portion of pancreatic duct to stop pancreatic juices from entering duodenum and prevents entry of bile into pancreatic duct
Sphincter ampullae	Surrounds and controls ampulla of Vater and prevents entry of bile and pancreatic juices into duodenum
Fasciculus longitudinalis	Located in triangular interval delineated by ampulla of Vater, pancreatic duct, and common bile duct; facilitates entry of bile into lumen of duodenum

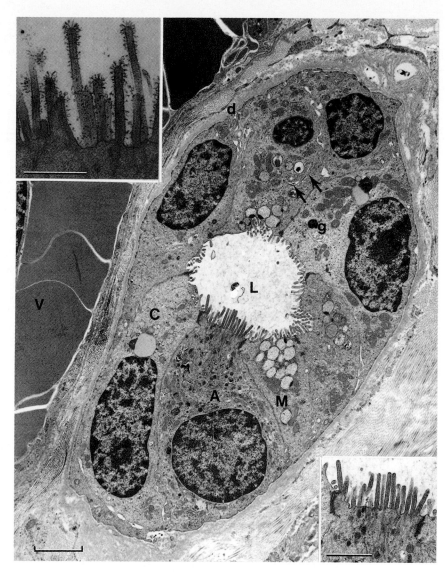

Figure 18–20 Electron micrograph of the human gallbladder diverticulum displaying brush cells (A) and clear cells (C) of the epithelium. d, interdigitations; g, granules; L, lumen; M, clear cells with mucoid granules; V, erythrocytes. *Arrows* indicate Golgi apparatus. Bar = 2 μm. *Upper inset:* Clear cell microvilli. Bar = 0.5 μm. *Lower inset:* Brush cell microvilli. Bar = 1.0 μm. (From Gilloteaux J, Pomerants B, Kelly T: Human gallbladder mucosa ultrastructure: Evidence of intraepithelial nerve structures. Am J Anat 184:321-333, 1989.)

Histophysiology of the Gallbladder

The gallbladder stores, concentrates, and releases bile. Bile release is triggered by cholecystokinin and vagal stimulation.

The primary functions of the gallbladder are to store, concentrate, and release bile. Bile is constantly manufactured by the liver and must make its way to the gallbladder. This activity requires that choledochus, pancreaticus, and ampullae sphincter muscles be maintained in a closed position so that the bile backs up the common bile duct and the cystic duct to enter the gallbladder.

Na$^+$ is actively transported from the basolateral region of the simple columnar epithelium of the gallbladder into the extracellular space and is passively followed by chloride (Cl$^-$) and water. To compensate for the loss of intracellular ions, apical ion channels permit Na$^+$ and Cl$^-$ to enter the simple columnar cells, reducing the salt (NaCl) concentration of bile. The requirement for osmotic equilibrium drives water from the bile into the simple columnar cell, thus concentrating bile.

The signaling molecule **cholecystokinin** is released by I cells (DNES cells) of the duodenum in response to a fatty meal. This molecule comes in contact with cholecystokinin receptors on the smooth muscle cells of the gallbladder and causes them to contract intermittently. Concurrently, contact of cholecystokinin receptors with the smooth muscle cells of the sphincter of Oddi causes the sphincter muscles to relax. As a result, the rhythmic contractile forces of the gallblad-der inject the bile into the lumen of the duodenum. In addition, **acetylcholine,** released by the vagal parasympathetic fibers, stimulates contraction of the gallbladder.

CLINICAL CORRELATIONS

Gallstones (cholelithiasis) are more common in women than in men and occur most frequently in the fourth decade in life. Approximately 20% of all women and 8% of all men have gallstones. Usually, people are unaware of their presence because gall-stones are either small enough to be eliminated with normal bile flow or too large to leave the gallblad-der. When they enter and become entrapped in the cystic or common hepatic ducts, gallstones obstruct bile flow and cause excruciating pain. Approximately 80% of gallstones are composed of cholesterol (**cho-lesterol stones);** most of the remainder are formed from the calcium salt of bile, calcium bilirubinate (**pigment stones),** or a combination of cholesterol and calcified bilirubinate. Cholesterol stones are large (1 to 3 cm) and pale yellow, have numerous facets, and are few in number. Pigment stones are smaller (1 cm), black, and ovoid, and they occur in large numbers. Usually, both types of stones are radiolucent.

Urinary System

19

The urinary system removes toxic by-products of metabolism from the bloodstream and removes urine from the body. These actions are performed by the two kidneys, which not only remove the toxins from the bloodstream but also conserve salts, glucose, proteins, and water as well as additional materials essential for proper health. Because of these eliminating and conserving functions, the kidneys also help to regulate blood pressure, hemodynamics, and the acid-base balance of the body. Urine is delivered from the kidneys into the two **ureters,** from which it passes to a storage organ, the **urinary bladder.** During voiding, the urinary bladder is emptied via the **urethra,** which delivers the urine to outside the body. In addition, the kidneys have an endocrine function in that they produce renin, erythropoietin, and prostaglandins, among others; they also convert a circulating precursor of vitamin D to the active vitamin.

KIDNEY

The kidneys have a concave region, known as the hilum, where the ureter, renal vein, renal artery, and lymph vessels pierce the kidney.

The kidneys are large, reddish, bean-shaped organs situated retroperitoneally on the posterior abdominal wall. Because of the position of the liver, the right kidney is approximately 1 to 2 cm lower than the left. Each kidney is about 11 cm long, 4 to 5 cm wide, and 2 to 3 cm thick. The kidney, embedded in perirenal fat, lies with its convex border situated laterally and its concave **hilum** facing medially. Branches of the renal artery and vein, lymph vessels, and ureter pierce the kidney at its hilum. The ureter is expanded at this region, forming the **renal pelvis.** A fat-filled extension of the hilum deeper into the kidney is called the **renal sinus.**

The kidney is invested by a thin, loosely adhering **capsule,** consisting mainly of dense, irregular collage-nous connective tissue with occasional elastic fibers and smooth muscle cells.

Overview of Kidney Structure

The kidney is subdivided into an outer cortex and an inner medulla.

A hemisected view of the kidney shows that it is separated into a cortex and a medulla (Fig. 19-1). The cortical region appears dark brown and granular, whereas the medulla contains 6 to 12 discrete, pyramid-shaped, pale striated regions, the **renal pyramids.** The base of each pyramid is oriented toward the cortex, constituting the corticomedullary border, whereas its apex, known as the **renal papilla,** points toward the hilum. The apex is perforated by 20 or so openings of the **ducts of Bellini;** this sieve-like region is known as the **area cribrosa.** The apex is surrounded by a cup-like **minor calyx,** which, joining two or three neighboring minor calyces, forms a **major calyx.** The three or four major calyces are larger subdivisions that empty into the **renal pelvis,** the expanded continuation of the proximal portion of the ureter. Neighboring pyramids are separated from each other by material resembling the cortex, the **cortical columns** (of Bertin).

The portion of the cortex overlying the base of each pyramid is known as a **cortical arch.** Macroscopically, three types of substances may be observed in the cortex: (1) red, dot-like granules, the **renal corpuscles;** (2) convoluted tubules, the **cortical labyrinth;** and (3) longitudinal striations, **medullary rays,** which are cortical continuations of material located in the renal pyramids.

A renal pyramid, with its associated cortical arch and cortical columns, represents a **lobe** of the kidney. Hence, the human kidney is a multilobar organ. Each medullary ray with part of the cortical labyrinth surrounding it is considered a kidney **lobule,** which continues into the medulla as a cone-shaped structure.

437

CLINICAL CORRELATIONS

During fetal development, the lobes of the kidney are accentuated by deep clefts, but this characteristic is normally obliterated in the adult. When the lobation is retained following infancy, the condition is known as **lobated kidney.**

Another anomalous kidney development is known as **polycystic kidney disease,** which presents varied morphological features according to the severity of the affliction; it involves the appearance of thin-walled cysts on and in the kidneys.

Uriniferous Tubules

The uriniferous tubule, the functional unit of the kidney, is composed of a nephron and a collecting tubule.

The functional unit of the kidney is the uriniferous tubule, a highly convoluted structure that modifies the fluid passing through it to form **urine** as its final output. This tubule consists of two parts, each with a different embryological origin, the **nephron** and the **collecting tubule** (see Fig. 19-1). There are approximately 1.3 million nephrons in each kidney. Several nephrons are drained by a single collecting tubule, and multiple collecting tubules join in the deeper aspect of the medulla to form larger and larger ducts. The largest of these

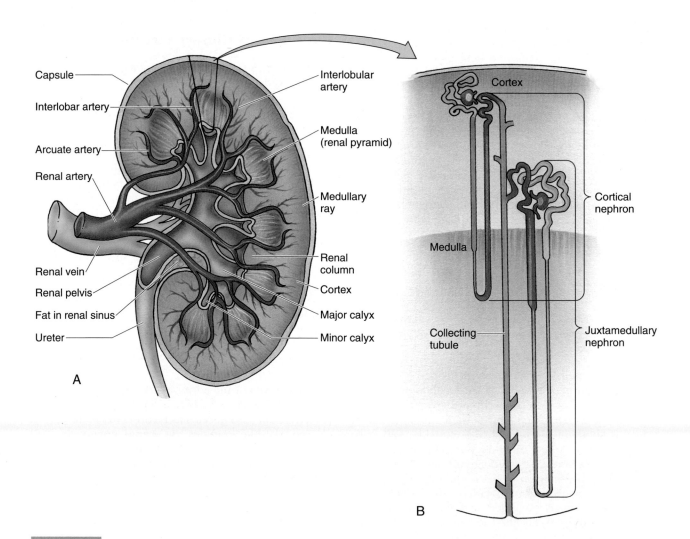

Figure 19–1 **A,** Hemisected kidney illustrating morphology and circulation. **B,** Arrangement of cortical and juxtamedullary nephrons.

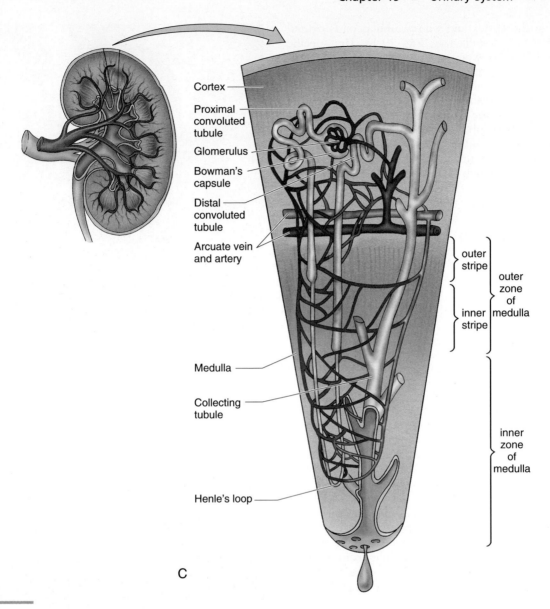

C

Figure 19–1, cont'd **C,** The uriniferous tubule and its vascular supply and drainage. The juxtamedullary nephron extends much deeper into the medulla than does the cortical nephron.

ducts, the **ducts of Bellini,** perforate the renal papilla at the area cribrosa.

Uriniferous tubules are densely packed so that the connective tissue **stroma** of the kidney is scant. The entire uriniferous tubule is epithelial in nature and is, therefore, separated from the connective tissue stroma by an intervening **basal lamina.** Much of the connective tissue is occupied by the rich vascular supply of the kidney. The functional relationship between the vascular supply and the uriniferous tubules is discussed later in this chapter.

Nephrons

There are two types of nephrons, depending on the location of their renal corpuscles and the length of their Henle's loop.

Two types of nephrons are found in the human kidney: shorter **cortical nephrons,** subdivided into two groups, superficial and midcortical nephrons, neither of which extend deep into the medulla, and the longer **juxtamedullary nephrons,** whose renal corpuscle is located in the cortex and whose tubular parts extend deep into the medulla (see Fig. 19-1). The specific locations of the two types of nephrons, the cellular composition of their various regions, and the specific alignments of these regions in register with one another permit the subdivision of the medulla into an **outer zone** and an **inner zone.** The outer zone of the medulla is further subdivided into an **outer stripe** and an **inner stripe.** Unless otherwise noted, all of the descriptions in this textbook refer to juxtamedullary nephrons, even though they constitute only 15% of all nephrons.

Each juxtamedullary nephron is about 40 mm long. The constituent parts of the nephron are modified to perform specific physiological functions. The renal corpuscle, with its attendant glomerulus, filters the fluid expressed from the bloodstream. The subsequent tubular portions of the nephron (i.e., the proximal tubule, the thin limbs of Henle's loop, and the distal tubule) modify the filtrate to form urine.

Renal Corpuscle

The renal corpuscle is composed of a tuft of capillaries, the glomerulus, surrounded by Bowman's capsule.

The renal corpuscle, an oval to round structure about 200 to 250 μm in diameter, is composed of a tuft of capillaries, the **glomerulus,** which is invaginated into **Bowman's capsule,** the dilated, pouch-like, proximal end of the nephron (Figs. 19-2 to 19-4; also see Fig. 19-1). During development, the capillaries become invested by the blind end of the tubular nephron, almost as if a hand were to push into the end of an expanded balloon. Hence, the space inside Bowman's capsule, known as **Bowman's space (urinary space),** is decreased in volume. The glomerulus is in intimate contact with the **visceral layer of Bowman's capsule,** composed of modified epithelial cells called **podocytes.** The outer wall surrounding Bowman's space, composed of simple squamous epithelial cells (sitting on a thin basal lamina), is the **parietal layer** (see Fig. 19-4).

The region where the vessels supplying and draining the glomerulus enter and exit Bowman's capsule is known as the **vascular pole,** whereas the region of continuation between the renal corpuscle and the proximal tubule, which drains Bowman's space, is called the **urinary pole.** The glomerulus is supplied by the short, straight **afferent glomerular arteriole** and drained by the **efferent glomerular arteriole;** thus the glomerulus is a completely arterial capillary bed. Although the outer diameter of the afferent arteriole is greater than that of the efferent arteriole, their luminal diameters are approximately equal.

The efferent glomerular arteriole presents greater resistance to blood flow, resulting in higher capillary

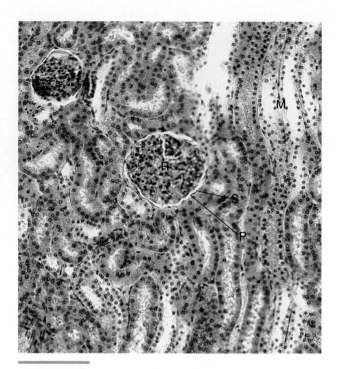

Figure 19–2 Light micrograph of the kidney cortex in a monkey, illustrating renal corpuscles (R), medullary ray (M), and cross-sectional profiles of the uriniferous tubules (×132). A portion of the urinary space (S) is clearly evident at the periphery of the renal corpuscle and is bound by the simple squamous epithelium composing the parietal layer (P) of Bowman's capsule.

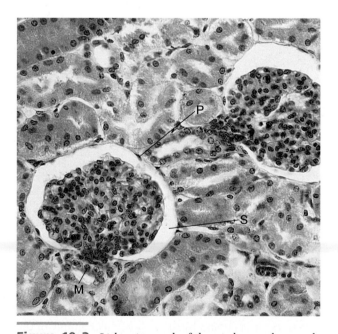

Figure 19–3 Light micrograph of the monkey renal corpuscle surrounded by cross-sectional profiles of proximal and distal tubules (×270). The macula densa (M) and the parietal layer (P) of Bowman's capsule are clearly evident as it encloses the clear space, a part of the urinary space (S).

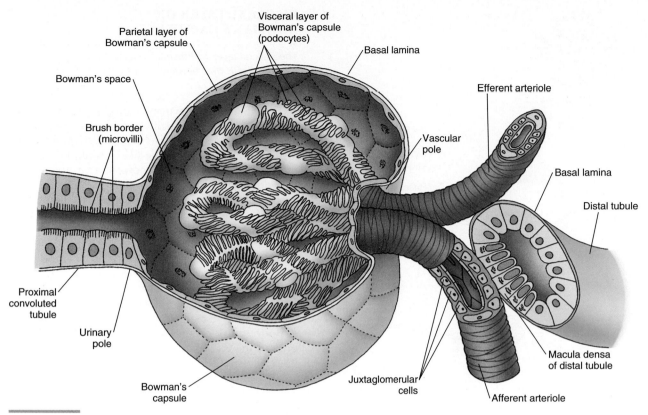

Figure 19–4 A renal corpuscle and its juxtaglomerular apparatus.

pressures in the glomerulus than in other capillary beds. Filtrate leaking out of the glomerulus enters Bowman's space through a complex **filtration barrier** composed of the endothelial wall of the capillary, the basal lamina, and the visceral layer of Bowman's capsule.

GLOMERULUS

The glomerulus is composed of tufts of fenestrated capillaries supplied by the afferent glomerular arteriole and drained by the efferent glomerular arteriole.

The glomerulus is formed as several tufts of anastomosing capillaries that arise from branches of the afferent glomerular arteriole. The connective tissue component of the afferent arteriole does not enter Bowman's capsule, and the normal connective tissue cells are replaced by a specialized cell type known as **mesangial cells.** There are two groups of mesangial cells: **extraglomerular mesangial cells** are located at the vascular pole, and pericyte-like **intraglomerular mesangial cells** are situated within the renal corpuscle (Figs. 19-5 and 19-6).

Intraglomerular mesangial cells are probably phagocytic and function in resorption of the basal lamina.

Mesangial cells may also be contractile because they have receptors for vasoconstrictors such as angiotensin II and thus reduce blood flow through the glomerulus. Moreover, they, along with podocytes and the glomerular basement membrane, provide physical support to the capillaries of the glomerulus. The glomerulus is composed of fenestrated capillaries (Fig. 19-7; also see Figs. 19-5 and 19-6) whose endothelial cells are highly attenuated, except for the region containing the nucleus; their fenestrae are usually not covered by a diaphragm. The pores are large, ranging between 70 and 90 nm in diameter; hence, these capillaries act as a barrier only to formed elements of the blood and to macromolecules whose effective diameter exceeds the size of the fenestrae.

Basal Lamina

Investing the glomerulus is a glomerular basal lamina (~300 nm thick), consisting of three layers (see Figs. 19-6 and 19-7). The middle dense layer, the **lamina densa,** is about 100 nm in thickness and consists of type IV collagen, composed of α_3, α_4, and α_5 chains (unlike the usual type, which is composed of α_1 and α_2 chains). Less electron-dense layers, the **laminae rarae**—which

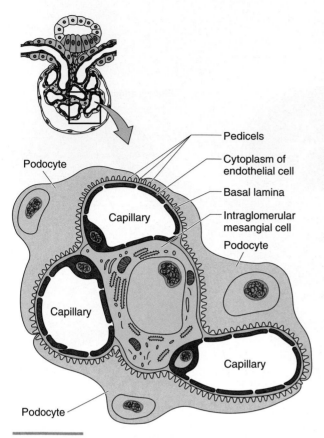

Figure 19–5 Relationship between the intraglomerular mesangial cell, podocytes, and glomerulus.

contain **laminin, fibronectin,** and the highly hydrated polyanionic proteoglycans perlacan and agrin—both rich in **heparan sulfate**—are located on either side of the lamina densa. Some refer to a **lamina rara interna,** between the endothelial cells of the capillary and the lamina densa, and the **lamina rara externa,** between the lamina densa and the visceral layer of Bowman's capsule. Fibronectin and laminin assist the pedicels and endothelial cells to maintain their attachment to the basal lamina.

CLINICAL CORRELATIONS

Mutations in the α_3 and α_4 chains of type IV collagen result in Alport's syndrome, an autosomal recessive disorder that is distinguished by loss of hearing, vision problems, and nephritis accompanied by microscopic hematuria. Persons with Alport's syndrome frequently suffer from kidney failure and may require a kidney transplant.

VISCERAL LAYER OF BOWMAN'S CAPSULE

The visceral layer of Bowman's capsule is composed of epithelial cells that become modified and are known as podocytes.

The visceral layer of Bowman's capsule is composed of epithelial cells that are highly modified to perform a filtering function. These large cells, called **podocytes,** have numerous long, tentacle-like cytoplasmic extensions, **primary (major) processes,** that follow but usually do not come in close contact with the longitudinal axes of the glomerular capillaries (see Fig. 19-7). Each primary process bears many **secondary processes,** known as **pedicels,** arranged in an orderly fashion. Pedicels completely envelop most of the glomerular capillaries by interdigitating with pedicels from neighboring major processes of different podocytes (Figs. 19-8 and 19-9).

Pedicels have a well-developed glycocalyx composed of the negatively charged sialoproteins **podocalyxin** and **podoendin.** Pedicels rest on the lamina rara externa of the basal lamina. Their cytoplasm is devoid of organelles but does house microtubules and microfilaments. Interdigitation occurs in such a fashion that narrow clefts, 20 to 40 nm in width, known as **filtration slits,** remain between adjacent pedicels. Filtration slits are not completely open; instead, they are covered by a thin **slit diaphragm** that extends between neighboring pedicels and acts as a part of the filtration barrier (Fig. 19-10; also see Fig. 19-7). The slit diaphragm has a central bar, on either side of which are rows of pores 14 nm² in area. The cell body of the podocyte is not at all unusual in organelle content. It houses the irregularly shaped nucleus as well as rough endoplasmic reticulum (RER), Golgi apparatus, and numerous free ribosomes.

Filtration Process

Fluid leaving the glomerular capillaries through the fenestrae is filtered by the basal lamina. The lamina densa traps larger molecules (>69,000 Da), whereas the polyanions of the laminae rarae impede the passage of negatively charged molecules and molecules that are incapable of deformation. The fluid, which contains small molecules, ions, and macromolecules, penetrates the lamina densa and must pass through the pores in the slit diaphragm of the filtration slits; if the macromolecules are uncharged and if they are 1.8 nm or less in diameter, they can pass without any hindrance through the slit diaphragm. However, if the uncharged macromolecules are greater than 4 nm in diameter they cannot pass through the slit diaphragm. The fluid entering Bowman's space is called the **glomerular ultrafiltrate.**

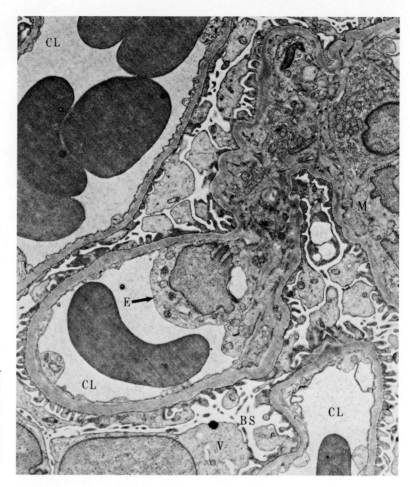

Figure 19–6 Electron micrograph of a region of the human kidney glomerulus containing red blood cells (×4594). Note the association between the intraglomerular mesangial cell and the podocytes around the glomerular capillaries. BS, Bowman's space; CL, capillary lumen; E, endothelial cell; M, mesangial cells; V, podocyte. (From Brenner BM, Rector FC: The Kidney, 4th ed. Vol 1. Philadelphia, WB Saunders, 1991.)

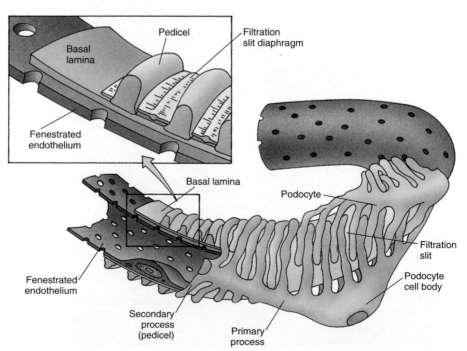

Figure 19–7 The interrelationship of the glomerulus, podocytes, pedicels, and basal laminae.

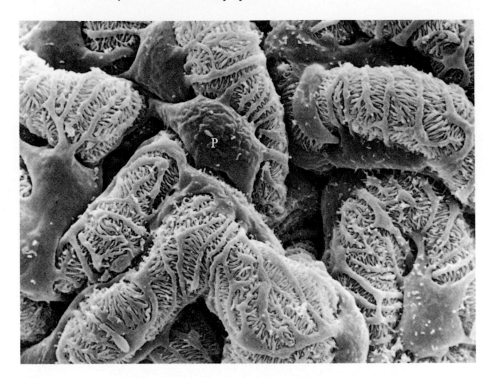

Figure 19–8 Scanning electron micrograph of podocytes (P) and their processes from the kidney of a rat (×4700). (From Brenner BM, Rector FC: The Kidney, 4th ed. Vol 1. Philadelphia, WB Saunders, 1991.)

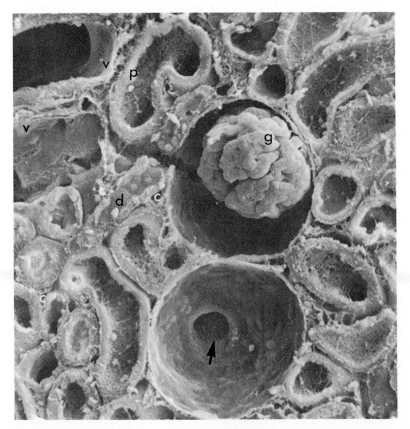

Figure 19–9 Scanning electron micrograph of the rat renal cortex displaying a renal corpuscle with its glomerulus (g) (×543). The renal corpuscle below it does not have its glomerulus, so the urinary pole (*arrow*) is evident. c, capillaries; d, distal convoluted tubule; p, proximal convoluted tubule; v, blood vessels. (From Leeson TS, Leeson CR, Paparo AA: Text/Atlas of Histology. Philadelphia, WB Saunders, 1988.)

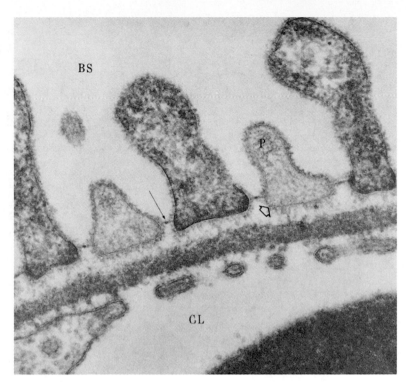

Figure 19–10 Electron micrograph of pedicels (P) and diaphragms bridging the filtration slits of a glomerulus in a rat (×86,700). BS, Bowman's space; CL, capillary lumen. Note the laminae rara externa (*short arrow*) and the filtration slit diaphragm (*long arrow*). (From Brenner BM, Rector FC: The Kidney, 4th ed, Vol 1. Philadelphia, WB Saunders, 1991.)

Because the basal lamina traps larger macromolecules, it would become clogged were it not continuously phagocytosed by **intraglomerular mesangial cells** and replenished by both the visceral layer of Bowman's capsule (podocytes) and glomerular endothelial cells.

CLINICAL CORRELATIONS

The presence of albumin in the urine (**albuminuria**) is the result of increased permeability of the glomerular endothelium. Among the causes of this condition are vascular injury, hypertension, mercury poisoning, and exposure to bacterial toxins.

The basal lamina may also become impaired because of the deposition of antigen-antibody complexes that are filtered from the glomeruli or from the reaction of antibasement membrane antibody with the basal lamina itself. Both of these instances produce types of **glomerulonephritis.**

In cases of **lipoid nephrosis,** the basal laminae are not congested with antibodies, but adjacent pedicels appear to fuse with one another. This disease is one of the most prevalent kidney disorders in children.

Proximal Tubule

The proximal tubule has two regions: the proximal convoluted tubule and the pars recta of the proximal tubule.

Bowman's space drains into the proximal tubule at the **urinary pole.** In this junctional region, sometimes called the neck of the proximal tubule (negligible in humans), the simple squamous epithelium of the parietal layer of Bowman's capsule joins the simple cuboidal epithelium of the proximal tubule (see Fig. 19-4). The proximal tubule, constituting much of the renal cortex, is approximately 60 μm in diameter and about 14 mm long. The tubule consists of a highly tortuous region, the **pars convoluta (proximal convoluted tubule),** located near renal corpuscles, and a straighter portion, the **pars recta (descending thick limb of Henle's loop),** which descends in medullary rays within the cortex and then in the medulla to become continuous with the loop of Henle at the junction of the outer and inner stripes.

Viewed with the light microscope, the convoluted portion of the proximal tubule is composed of a simple cuboidal type of epithelium with an eosinophilic, granular-appearing cytoplasm (Fig. 19-11; also see Fig. 19-3). The cells have an elaborate striated border and an intricate system of interlocking and interwoven lateral cell processes. Thus, the lateral cell membranes are usually

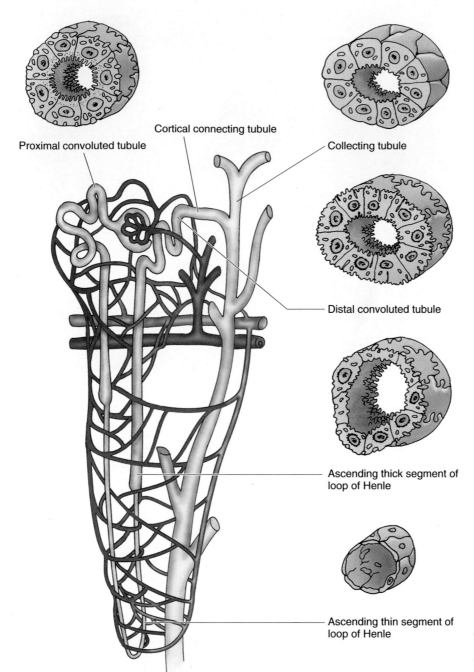

Proximal convoluted tubule

Cortical connecting tubule

Collecting tubule

Distal convoluted tubule

Ascending thick segment of loop of Henle

Ascending thin segment of loop of Henle

Figure 19–11 A drawing of the uriniferous tubule and its cross-sectional morphology.

indistinguishable with the light microscope. The height of the cells varies with their functional state—from a low cuboidal to an almost high cuboidal epithelium.

The method and rapidity of fixation modify the microscopic morphology of the proximal convoluted tubule because its lumen is kept open by fluid pressure. Ideal fixation demonstrates wide-open, empty lumina and no clumping of the striated border. However, paraffin sections usually display mostly occluded lumina;

fluted and ragged-appearing striated borders; few, basally placed nuclei per cross section of the tubule; and a lack of distinct lateral cell membranes. The cuboidal cells sit on a well-defined basement membrane, easily demonstrated by the periodic acid–Schiff (PAS) reaction. Each cross section is composed of approximately 10 to 20 cells, but because these cells are large, usually only six to eight nuclei are included in the plane of section (see Fig. 19-3).

On the basis of the ultrastructural features of its component cells, the proximal tubule can be subdivided into three regions:

- The first two thirds of the pars convoluta, designated S_1
- The remainder of the pars convoluta and much of the pars recta, designated S_2
- The remainder of the pars recta, designated S_3

Cells of the **S_1 region** have long (1.3 to 1.6 μm), closely packed microvilli and a system of intermicrovillar caveolae, known as **apical canaliculi,** that extend into the apical cytoplasm (Fig. 19-12). This system is more extensive during active diuresis, suggesting that it functions in resorption of proteins during tubular clearing of the **glomerular ultrafiltrate.** Mitochondria, Golgi apparatus, and other normal cellular components are present in these cells. Elaborate lateral and basal processes may extend almost the entire height of the cell. These processes are long and narrow and usually accommodate elongated, tubular mitochondria.

Cells composing the **S_2 region** are similar to those of the S_1 region, but they have fewer mitochondria and apical canaliculi, have less elaborate intercellular processes, and are lower in height.

Cells of the **S_3 region** are low cuboidal with few mitochondria. These cells have only infrequent intercellular processes and no apical canaliculi.

About 67% to perhaps as much as 80% of sodium, chloride (Cl^-), and water is resorbed from the glomerular ultrafiltrate and transported into the connective tissue stroma by cells of the proximal tubule. Sodium is actively pumped out of the cell at the basolateral cell membranes by a sodium pump associated with sodium-potassium adenosine triphosphatase (Na^+,K^+-ATPase). The sodium (Na^+) is followed by chloride to maintain electrical neutrality and by water to maintain osmotic equilibrium. The water passes through aquaporin-1 channels located in the basolateral cell membrane. In addition, all of the glucose, amino acids, and protein in the glomerular ultrafiltrate are resorbed by the vacuolar endocytic apparatus of the cells of the proximal tubule. Moreover, the proximal tubule also eliminates the organic solutes, drugs, and toxins that must be rapidly excreted from the body.

THIN LIMBS OF HENLE'S LOOP

The thin limbs of the loop of Henle have three regions: the descending thin limb, Henle's loop, and the ascending thin limb.

The pars recta of the proximal tubule continues as the thin limb of Henle's loop (see Fig. 19-11). This thin tubule, whose overall diameter is about 15 to 20 μm, is

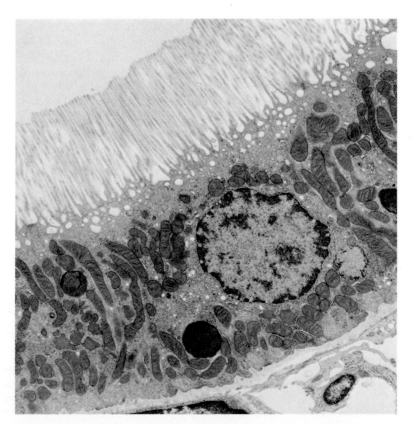

Figure 19–12 Electron micrograph of the S_1 segment of the rat proximal tubule (×7128). (From Brenner BM, Rector FC: The Kidney, 4th ed. Vol 1. Philadelphia, WB Saunders, 1991.)

composed of squamous epithelial cells with an average height of 1.5 to 2 μm. The length of the thin segments varies with the location of the nephron (see Fig. 19-1). In cortical nephrons, the thin segment is only 1 to 2 mm long or may be completely absent. Juxtamedullary nephrons have much longer thin segments, 9 to 10 mm in length, and they form a hairpin-like loop that extends deep into the medulla as far down as the renal papilla. The region of the loop continuous with the pars recta of the proximal tubule is called the **descending thin limb** (of Henle's loop), the hairpin-like bend is **Henle's loop,** and the region that connects Henle's loop to the pars recta of the **distal tubule** is known as the **ascending thin limb** of Henle's loop.

The nuclei of the cells composing the thin limbs bulge into the lumen of the tubule; hence, in paraffin section, these limbs resemble capillaries in cross section (see Fig. 19-11). They may be distinguished from capillaries in that their epithelial lining cells are slightly thicker, their nuclei stain less densely, and their lumina contain no blood cells.

The fine structure of the epithelial cells constituting the thin segments is not unusual. They present a few short, stubby microvilli on their luminal surfaces and a few mitochondria in the cytoplasm surrounding the nucleus. Numerous processes project from the basal portion of the cell to interdigitate with those of neighboring cells.

It is possible to differentiate among four types of epithelial cells composing different regions of Henle's loop according to their fine structural features. The locations and fine structural features of the four cell types are listed in Table 19-1.

The descending thin limb is highly permeable to water due to the presence of numerous aquaporin-1 water channels; it is reasonably permeable to urea,

sodium, chloride, and other ions. The major difference between the ascending and descending thin limbs is that the ascending thin limb is only moderately permeable to water. The significance of this difference in water permeability is discussed later.

Distal Tubule

The distal tubule has three regions: the pars recta (the ascending thick limb of Henle's loop), the macula densa, and the pars convoluta (the distal convoluted tubule).

The distal tubule is subdivided into the **pars recta,** which, as the continuation of the ascending thin limb of Henle's loop, is also known as the **ascending thick limb of Henle's loop,** and the **pars convoluta (distal convoluted tubule).** Interposed between the ascending thick limb and the distal convoluted tubule is a modified region of the distal tubule called the **macula densa.**

The ascending thick limb of Henle's loop is 9 to 10 mm in length and 30 to 40 μm in diameter. It joins the ascending thin limb of Henle's loop at the junction of the inner stripe with the inner zone of the medulla and ascends straight up through the medulla to reach the cortex. The low cuboidal epithelial cells composing the ascending thick segment have centrally placed, round to slightly oval nuclei and a few club-shaped, short microvilli. Although the lateral aspects of these cells interdigitate with each other, the interrelationships between neighboring cells are not nearly as elaborate as in the proximal convoluted tubules. Basal interdigitations are much more extensive, however, and the number of mitochondria is greater in these cells than in those of the proximal convoluted tubules. Moreover, these cells form highly efficient zonulae occludentes with their neighboring cells.

TABLE 19–1   Cell Types Composing the Thin Limbs of Henle's Loop

Cell Type	Location	Fine Structural Features
Type I	Cortical nephrons	Squamous cells with no lateral processes and no interdigitations
Type II	Juxtamedullary nephrons; descending thin limb of the outer zone of the medulla	Squamous cells with numerous long, radiating processes that interdigitate with those of neighboring cells; fascia occludentes between cells; infoldings of the basal plasmalemma
Type III	Juxtamedullary nephrons; descending thin limb of the inner zone of the medulla	Squamous cells with fewer processes and interdigitations than those of type II
Type IV	Juxtamedullary nephrons; ascending thin limb	Squamous cells with numerous long, radiating processes that interdigitate with those of neighboring cells as in type II cells; no infoldings of the basal plasmalemma

The thick ascending limb is not permeable to water or urea. In addition, its cells have chloride (and perhaps sodium) pumps that function in the active transport of chloride (and sodium) from the lumen of the tubule. Thus, as the filtrate reaches the cortex of the kidney within the lumen of the distal tubule, its salt concentration is low and its urea concentration remains high. These cells also manufacture Tamm-Horsfall protein, which they release into the lumen of the thick ascending limb to impede the formation of kidney stones.

As the ascending thick limb of the Henle loop passes near its own renal corpuscle, it lies between the afferent and efferent glomerular arterioles. This region of the distal tubule is called the **macula densa.** Because the cells of the macula densa are tall and narrow, the nuclei of these cells appear to be much closer together than those of the remainder of the distal tubule.

Distal convoluted tubules are short (4 to 5 mm) with an overall diameter of 25 to 45 μm. In paraffin sections, the lumina of these tubules are wide-open, the granular cytoplasm of the low cuboidal lining epithelium is paler than that of proximal convoluted tubules, and because the cells are narrower, more nuclei are apparent in tubular cross section. The ultrastructure of these cells demonstrates a clear, pale cytoplasm with a few, blunt apical microvilli (Fig. 19-13). Nuclei are more or less round and apically located, having one or two dense nucleoli. Mitochondria are not as numerous, and the basal interdigitations are not as extensive as those of the ascending thick limb of Henle's loop.

Because distal convoluted tubules are much shorter than proximal convoluted tubules, any section of the kidney cortex presents many more cross sections of proximal convoluted tubules than cross sections of distal convoluted tubules. Indeed, the ratio of cross sections of proximal to distal convoluted tubules surrounding any renal corpuscle is usually 7 : 1.

Distal convoluted tubules usually ascend slightly above their own renal corpuscles and drain into the arched portion of the collecting tubules.

Similar to the thick ascending limbs, the distal convoluted tubule is impermeable to water and urea. However, in the basolateral plasmalemma of its cells, high Na^+,K^+-ATPase activity powers sodium-potassium exchange pumps. Thus, in response to the hormone **aldosterone,** these cells can actively resorb almost all of the remaining sodium (and, passively, chloride) from the lumen of the tubule into the renal interstitium. In addition, potassium and hydrogen ions are actively secreted *into* the lumen, thus controlling the body's extracellular fluid potassium level and the acidity of urine, respectively.

Juxtaglomerular Apparatus

The juxtaglomerular apparatus has three components: the macula densa of the distal tubule, juxtaglomerular cells of the afferent glomerular arteriole, and extraglomerular mesangial cells.

The juxtaglomerular apparatus consists of the macula densa of the distal tubule, juxtaglomerular cells of the adjacent afferent (and, occasionally, efferent) glomerular arteriole, and the extraglomerular mesangial cells (also known as polkissen, lacis cells, and polar cushion) (Fig. 19-14).

The cells of the **macula densa** are tall, narrow, pale cells with centrally placed nuclei (Fig. 19-15; also see

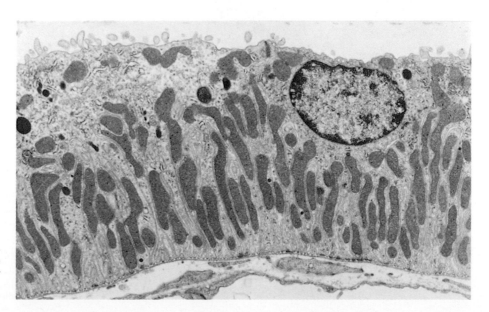

Figure 19–13 Electron micrograph of the distal convoluted tubule (×8100). (From Brenner BM, Rector FC: The Kidney, 4th ed. Vol 1. Philadelphia, WB Saunders, 1991.)

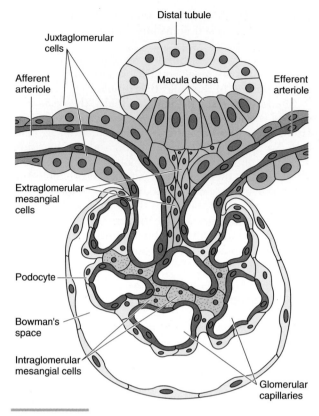

Figure 19–14 The juxtaglomerular apparatus.

Figs. 19-2 to 19-4 and Fig. 19-14). Because of the narrowness of these cells, the densely staining nuclei are near to each other; collectively, viewed with the light microscope, they appear as a dense spot. With the electron microscope, these cells demonstrate numerous microvilli, small mitochondria, and an infranuclearly located Golgi apparatus (see Fig. 19-15).

Juxtaglomerular cells, modified smooth muscle cells located in the tunica media of afferent (and, occasionally, efferent) glomerular arterioles, are richly innervated by sympathetic nerve fibers. The nuclei of these cells are round instead of elongated. Juxtaglomerular cells contain specific granules demonstrated to be the proteolytic enzyme **renin** (see Fig. 19-15). **Angiotensin-converting enzyme (ACE), angiotensin I,** and **angiotensin II** are also present in these cells (see later).

Juxtaglomerular cells and the cells of the macula densa have a special geographical relationship because the basal lamina, normally present in epithelium and other tissues, is absent at this point, permitting intimate contact between cells of the macula densa and the juxtaglomerular cells.

The extraglomerular mesangial cells, the third member of the juxtaglomerular apparatus, occupy the space bounded by the afferent arteriole, macula densa, efferent arteriole, and vascular pole of the renal corpuscle. These cells may contain occasional granules and are probably contiguous with the intraglomerular

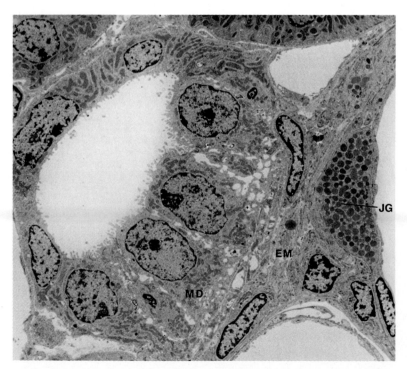

Figure 19–15 Electron micrograph of the juxtaglomerular apparatus from the kidney of a rabbit (×2552). The macula densa (MD), juxtaglomerular cells (JG) (containing electron-dense granules), and extraglomerular mesangial (EM) cells are displayed. (From Brenner BM, Rector FC: The Kidney, 4th ed. Vol 1. Philadelphia, WB Saunders, 1991.)

mesangial cells. The functional significance of the juxtaglomerular apparatus is discussed later.

Collecting Tubules

Collecting tubules, composed of a simple cuboidal epithelium, convey and modify the ultrafiltrate from the nephron to the minor calyces of the kidney.

Collecting tubules are not part of the nephron. They have different embryological origins, and it is only later in development that they meet the nephron and join it to form a continuous structure. The distal convoluted tubules of several nephrons join to form a short **connecting tubule** that leads into the collecting tubule (Fig. 19-16; also see Fig. 19-11). The glomerular ultrafiltrate that enters the collecting tubule is modified and delivered to the medullary papillae. Collecting tubules are about 20 mm long and have three recognized regions (see Fig. 19-1):

- Cortical
- Medullary
- Papillary

Cortical collecting tubules are located in the medullary rays and are composed of two types of cuboidal cells (see Figs. 19-2 and 19-11):

- Principal cells
- Intercalated cells

Principal cells have oval, centrally located nuclei, a few small mitochondria, and short, sparse microvilli.

The basal membranes of these cells display numerous infoldings. Because the lateral cell membranes are not plicated, they are clearly evident with the light microscope. These cells possess numerous aquaporin-2 channels that are very sensitive to antidiuretic hormone (ADH) and become completely permeable to water.

Intercalated cells display numerous apical vesicles 50 to 200 nm in diameter, microplicae on their apical plasmalemma, and an abundance of mitochondria. The nuclei of these cells are round and centrally located. There are two types of intercalated cells: **type A,** whose luminal membrane possesses H^+-ATPase that functions in transporting H^+ into the lumen of the tubule thus acidifying urine; and **type B,** whose basolateral membrane possesses H^+-ATPase and functions in resorbing H^+ and secreting HCO_3^-.

Medullary collecting tubules are of larger caliber because they are formed by the union of several cortical collecting tubules (see Fig. 19-11). Those in the outer zone of the medulla are similar to the cortical collecting tubules in that they display both principal and intercalated cells, whereas tubules of the inner zone of the medulla have principal cells only (Fig. 19-17).

Papillary collecting tubules (ducts of Bellini) are each formed by the confluence of several medullary collecting tubules. These are large ducts, 200 to 300 μm in diameter, and they open at the area cribrosa of the renal papilla to deliver the urine that they convey into the minor calyx of the kidney. These ducts are lined by tall columnar principal cells only.

Collecting tubules are impermeable to water. However, in the presence of ADH, they become

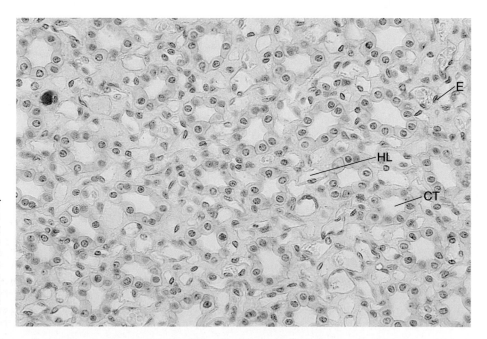

Figure 19–16 The medulla of the kidney displays the simple cuboidal epithelium of the collecting tubules (CT) as well as the simple squamous epithelium of the thin limbs of Henle's loop (HL) and the endothelial cells (E) of the vasa recta. Note that the connective tissue components are sparse and consist mostly of vascular elements (×270).

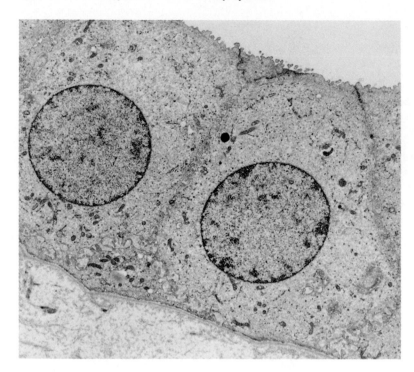

Figure 19–17 Electron micrograph of a collecting tubule from a rabbit kidney (×4790). (From Brenner BM, Rector FC: The Kidney, 4th ed. Vol 1. Philadelphia, WB Saunders, 1991.)

permeable to water (and, to a certain extent, urea). Thus, in the absence of ADH, urine is copious and hypotonic, and in the presence of ADH the volume of urine is low and concentrated.

Renal Interstitium

The renal interstitium is a very flimsy, scant amount of loose connective tissue housing three types of cells: fibroblasts, macrophages, and interstitial cells.

The kidney is invested by a dense, irregular collagenous type of connective tissue with some elastic fibers interspersed among the bundles of collagen. This capsule is not attached firmly to the underlying cortex. As blood vessels enter the hilum, they travel in a thin connective tissue cover, some of which is derived from the capsule. The cortical region has only delicate connective tissue elements that constitute less than 7% of the cortical volume and is associated mostly with the basement membranes investing the uriniferous tubules and their vascular supply. The two cellular components of the cortical connective tissue are **fibroblasts** and cells that are believed to be **interstitial dendritic cells,** members of the mononuclear phagocytic system.

The medullary interstitial connective tissue component is more extensive than that found in the cortex, in fact it occupies nearly 30% of the volume of the inner medulla. Embedded in this connective tissue are the various components of the uriniferous tubules as well as the extensive vascular network located in the medulla.

The cell population of this connective tissue consists of three cell types:

- Fibroblasts
- Macrophages
- Interstitial cells

Interstitial cells appear to be situated like the rungs of a ladder, one on top of the other, and are most numerous between straight collecting ducts and between the ducts of Bellini. Interstitial cells have elongated nuclei and numerous lipid droplets. It is believed that these cells synthesize **medullipin I,** a substance that is converted in the liver to **medullipin II,** a potent vasodilator that lowers blood pressure.

Renal Circulation
Arterial Supply

Each kidney receives 10% of the total blood volume per minute via a large branch of the abdominal aorta known as the renal artery.

The kidney receives an extremely extensive blood supply via the large **renal artery,** a direct branch of the abdominal aorta (see Fig. 19-1). Before entering the hilum of the kidney, the renal artery bifurcates into an anterior and a posterior division, which in turn subdivide to form a total of five **segmental arteries.** The branches of any one segmental artery do not form anastomoses with the branches of other segmental arteries. Hence, if blood flow through one of these arteries is blocked, circulation to the region of the kidney supplied by the affected vessel is interrupted. Therefore, the kidney is said to be subdivided into vascular segments, with each segment supplied by a specific artery.

The first subdivisions of the segmental arteries are called **lobar arteries,** one for each lobe of the kidney. These in turn branch to form two or three **interlobar arteries,** which travel between the renal pyramids to the corticomedullary junction. At the corticomedullary junction, these arteries form a series of vessels (perpendicular to the parent vessel) that, to a large extent, remain at that junction, occupying the same curved plane. Because these arteries describe a slight arc over the base of the renal pyramid, they are called **arcuate arteries.**

Although arcuate arteries once were believed to anastomose with each other, more recent studies suggest that terminal branches of these arteries do not join each other. Instead, terminal branches, as all other branches of the arcuate arteries, ascend into the cortex, forming interlobular arteries.

Interlobular arteries ascend within the cortical labyrinth approximately halfway between neighboring medullary rays. Hence, they travel in the interstices between any two lobules. Many branches arise from the interlobular arteries. These branches supply the glomeruli of renal corpuscles and are known as **afferent glomerular arterioles.** Some of the interlobular arteries ascend through the cortex to perforate the kidney capsule. Here they contribute to the formation of the capsular plexus. Most of the interlobular arteries, however, terminate as afferent glomerular arterioles.

Each glomerulus is drained by another arteriole, the **efferent glomerular arteriole.** There are two types of efferent glomerular arterioles, those draining glomeruli of cortical nephrons and those draining glomeruli of juxtamedullary nephrons.

Efferent glomerular arterioles from cortical nephrons are short and branch to form a system of capillaries, the **peritubular capillary network.** This capillary bed supplies the entire cortical labyrinth, with the obvious exception of the glomeruli. It is thought that the endothelial cells of the peritubular capillary network (and perhaps connective tissue cells of the cortex and outer medulla) manufacture and release the hormone **erythropoietin.**

The efferent glomerular arterioles, derived from glomeruli of juxtamedullary nephrons as well as from glomeruli located in the lower quadrant of the cortex, each give rise to 10 to 25 long, hairpin-like capillaries that dip deep into the medulla (Figs. 19-18 and 19-19). Their descending limbs have a narrow bore and are called **arteriolae rectae;** their ascending limbs are much greater in diameter and are called **venae rectae;**

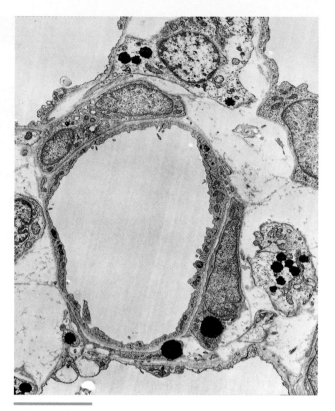

Figure 19–18 Electron micrograph of the arteria recta of a rat kidney. (From Takahashi-Iwanaga H: The three-dimensional cytoarchitecture of the interstitial tissue in the rat kidney. Cell Tissue Res 264:269-281, 1991.)

frequently, the arteriolae rectae and venae rectae together are referred to as the **vasa recta**—the term we shall use in this textbook. The hairpin-like shape of the vasa recta, which closely follows and wraps around the two limbs of Henle's loop and the collecting tubule, is essential in the physiology of urine concentration (see later.)

Venous Drainage

The arcuate veins receive blood from the cortex via the stellate veins and interlobular veins and from the medulla via the venae rectae; arcuate veins are drained by the interlobar veins that deliver their blood into the renal vein.

Venae rectae deliver their blood to **arcuate veins,** vessels that follow the paths of the same-named arteries. Blood is thus drained from the medulla. Cortical blood is collected into a star-shaped system of subcapsular veins called **stellate veins,** which are tributaries of the interlobular veins. Stellate veins also receive blood from the terminal portions of the efferent glomerular arterioles. The interlobular veins, paralleling the

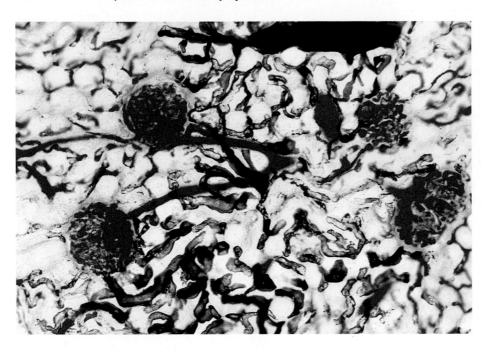

Figure 19–19 Light micrograph of injected kidney displaying the rich vascular supply of the kidney cortex (×132). The glomeruli (G) are clearly evident.

same-named arteries, deliver their blood to the arcuate veins. Hence, arcuate veins drain both the medulla and the cortex. Arcuate veins are tributaries of **interlobar veins** that unite, near the hilum, to form the **renal vein.** This large vein delivers the blood to the inferior vena cava. Note the absence of lobar and segmental veins in contrast to the presence of such named arteries in the arterial system of the kidney.

Lymphatic Supply of the Kidney

Lymph vessels of the kidney probably follow the larger arteries.

The lymphatic supply of the kidney is not completely understood. It is believed that most lymphatic vessels follow the larger arteries. According to most investigators, the lymphatic supply of the kidney may be subdivided into *superficial* and *deep* aspects located in the subcapsular region and in the medulla, respectively. The two systems may or may not join each other near the hilum, where they form several large lymphatic trunks. Lymph nodes in the vicinity of the vena cava and the abdominal aorta receive lymph from the kidneys. There are lymph vessels in the cortex that do not follow the larger arteries, but they do drain their lymph into a plexus of lymph vessels at the hilum.

Renal Innervation

Most nerve fibers that reach the kidney are unmyelinated, sympathetic fibers that form the renal plexus, traveling along the renal artery. The cell bodies of these fibers are probably located in the aortic and celiac plexuses. Sympathetic fibers are distributed by branches of the renal arterial tree, and these vessels are modulated by some of these fibers. Additional sympathetic fibers reach the epithelium of the renal tubules, the juxtaglomerular and interstitial cells, and the capsule of the kidney. Sensory fibers and parasympathetic fibers (probably from the vagus nerve) have also been described in the kidney.

General Functions of the Kidney

The kidneys play a role in excretion as well as in regulation of body fluid composition and volume. Specifically, they regulate solute components (e.g., sodium, potassium, chloride, glucose, amino acids) and acid-base balance. Thus, during the summer, when a great deal of fluid is lost through perspiration, the urinary output is reduced in volume and increased in osmolarity. During the winter months, when fluid loss through perspiration is minimal, the urinary output is increased in volume and the urine is dilute.

In addition, the kidneys excrete detoxified end products, regulate the osmolality of urine, and secrete substances such as erythropoietin, medullipin I, renin, and prostaglandins.

Finally, the kidneys regulate blood pressure and, in the presence of parathyroid hormone, aid in the conversion of a less active form of vitamin D to 1,25-dihydroxycholecalciferol, its most active form, which is responsible for the increased absorption of calcium and phosphate ions by the digestive system and their transport into the extracellular fluid compartment of the body. Although all of these functions are important aspects of kidney histophysiology, only the mechanism of urine formation is discussed in this chapter.

Mechanism of Urine Formation

The two kidneys receive about one fifth of the total blood volume (1220 mL) per minute, and they manufacture about 1 to 2 mL of urine per minute.

The two kidneys receive a large volume of circulating blood because the renal arteries are large and they are direct branches of the abdominal aorta. Inulin, a fructose polymer, can be used to measure the **glomerular filtration rate (GFR).** Such studies have shown that the entire blood supply circulates through the two kidneys every 5 minutes. Thus, approximately 1220 mL of blood enters the two kidneys each minute, from which 125 mL/min of glomerular filtrate is formed in the average male. Thus, 180 L of glomerular filtrate is formed each day, of which only 1.5 to 2.0 L is excreted as urine. Therefore, every day at least 178 L is resorbed by the kidneys, and only about 1% of the total glomerular filtrate is excreted.

Filtration in the Renal Corpuscle

Fluid component from the blood passes through the filtration barrier to become the ultrafiltrate.

As blood passes from the afferent glomerular arteriole into the glomerulus, it encounters a region of differential pressure, where the intracapillary blood pressure is greater than the opposing fluid pressure in Bowman's space, forcing fluid from the capillary into that space. An additional factor, colloid osmotic pressure of the blood proteins, opposes the entry of fluid into the Bowman space, but the net effect, the **filtration force,** is high (25 mm Hg). The fluid entering Bowman's space is called the **(glomerular) ultrafiltrate.**

Because of the tripartite **filtration barrier** (endothelial cell, basal lamina, filtration slit or diaphragm), cellular material and large macromolecules cannot leave the glomerulus; thus, the ultrafiltrate is similar to plasma (without its constituent macromolecules). Molecules greater than 69,000 Da (e.g., albumin) are trapped by the basal lamina. In addition to molecular weight, the molecular shape and charge of a molecule and the functional state of the filtration barrier all influence the ability of a molecule to traverse the filtration barrier. Because the filtration barrier has negatively charged components, macromolecules that are negatively charged are less able to cross it compared with positively charged or neutral macromolecules.

Resorption in the Proximal Tubule

The proximal tubule is the site of mass movement, where a tremendous amount of electrolytes, glucose, amino acids, protein, and water is conserved.

The **ultrafiltrate** leaves Bowman's space via the urinary pole to enter the proximal convoluted tubule, where modification of this fluid begins. Materials resorbed from the lumen of the proximal tubule enter the tubular epithelial cells, from which they are exocytosed into the interstitial connective tissue. Here, the resorbed substances gain entrance to the rich peritubular capillary network and thus are returned to the body via the bloodstream.

Most resorption of materials from the ultrafiltrate occurs in the proximal tubule. Normally, the following amounts are absorbed in the proximal tubule: 100% of proteins, glucose, amino acids, and creatine; almost 100% of bicarbonate ions; 67% to 80% of sodium and chloride ions; and 67% to 80% of the water.

The Na^+,K^+-ATPase-powered **sodium pumps** in the basolateral plasma membrane of the proximal tubule cell pump sodium into the renal interstitium. This movement of sodium ions out of the cell at the basolateral membrane causes sodium in the lumen of the tubule to leave the ultrafiltrate and enter the cell through its apical cell membrane. In this fashion, the net sodium movement is from the ultrafiltrate into the renal connective tissue. To maintain electrical neutrality, chloride ions passively follow sodium. Further, to maintain osmotic equilibrium, water passively follows sodium (by osmosis).

Additional energy-requiring pumps, located in the apical plasmalemma of proximal tubule cells, cotransport amino acids and glucose with sodium into the cell to be released into the renal interstitium. Proteins, brought into the cell by pinocytotic vesicles, are degraded by hydrolytic enzymes within late endosomes.

Each day, as much as 140 g of glucose, 430 g of sodium, 500 g of chloride, 300 g of bicarbonate, 18 g of potassium ions, 54 g of protein, and approximately 142 L of water are conserved by the proximal tubules of the kidney.

The proximal tubule also releases certain substances into the tubular lumen. These include hydrogen (H^+), ammonia, phenol red, hippuric acid, uric acid, organic bases, and ethylenediaminetetraacetate as well as certain drugs, such as penicillin.

Henle's Loop and the Countercurrent Multiplier System

The long Henle loop of the juxtamedullary nephron is responsible for the establishment of the countercurrent multiplier system.

The osmolarity of the glomerular ultrafiltrate is the same as that of circulating blood. This osmolarity is not altered by the proximal tubule because water has left its lumen in response to the movement of ions. However, the osmotic pressure of formed urine is different from that of blood. The osmotic pressure differential is established by the remaining regions of the uriniferous tubule. Interestingly, the osmolarity and volume of urine vary, indicating that the kidneys can modulate these factors.

A gradient of osmolarity, increasing from the corticomedullary junction to deep into the medulla, is maintained in the renal medullary interstitium. The long loops of Henle of **juxtamedullary nephrons** aid not only in the creation but also in the maintenance of this osmotic gradient via a **countercurrent multiplier system** (Fig. 19-20). The cells of the thin descending limb of Henle's loop are freely permeable to water and salts. Therefore, the movement of water reacts to the osmotic forces in its microenvironment. The thin ascending limb is relatively impermeable to water, but salts can enter or leave the tubule, depending on conditions in the interstitium. It is important to understand, at this point (to be explained later), that *urea enters* the lumina of the thin limbs of Henle's loop.

The thick ascending limb of Henle's loop is completely impermeable to water; however, a **chloride pump** actively removes chloride ions from the lumen of the tubules and these ions enter the renal interstitium. Sodium ions follow passively (although some suggest the presence of a sodium pump also) to preserve electrical neutrality. As the filtrate ascends, it contains fewer and fewer ions; hence, the amount of salts that may be transferred out into the interstitium decreases. Thus, a gradient of salt concentration is established in which the highest interstitial osmolarity is deep in the medulla, and the osmolarity of the interstitium decreases toward the cortex.

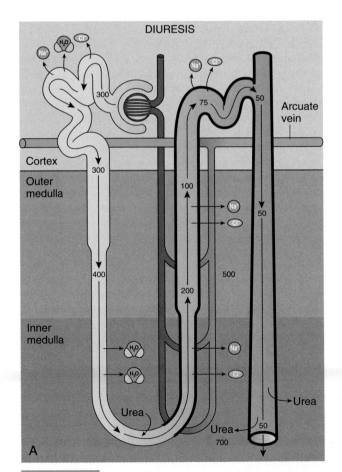

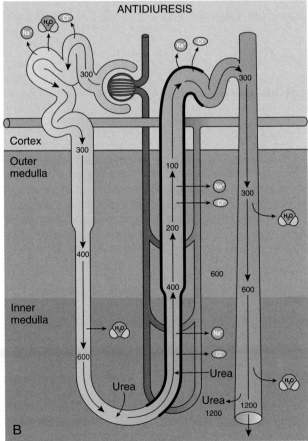

Figure 19–20 Histophysiology of the uriniferous tubule. **A,** Diuresis (in the absence of antidiuretic hormone [ADH]). **B,** Antidiuresis (in the presence of ADH). Numbers indicate milliosmoles per liter. Areas outlined by a *thick line* indicate that the tubule is impermeable to water. In the presence of ADH, the collecting tubule changes so that it becomes permeable to water and the concentration in the interstitium of the inner medulla increases. The vasa recta is simplified in this drawing because it encompasses the entire uriniferous tubule (see Fig. 19-1).

Because the medulla is tightly packed with thick and thin (ascending and descending) limbs of Henle's loop and collecting tubules, the gradient of osmolarity that is established is pervasive and affects all the tubules equally (see Fig. 19-20).

Therefore, keeping the foregoing in mind, we can recap the movement of ions and water, once again starting as the ultrafiltrate, which, as the student should recall, is isotonic with blood as it leaves the pars recta of the proximal tubule. As the ultrafiltrate descends in the thin descending limb of Henle's loop, it loses water (*reducing volume and increasing osmolarity*), reacting to the osmotic gradient of the interstitium, so that the intraluminal filtrate more or less becomes equilibrated with that of the surrounding connective tissue. This fluid of high osmolarity now ascends in the thin ascending limb of Henle's loop, which is mostly impermeable to water but not to salts. Thus, the volume of the ultrafiltrate does not change (i.e., the volume is the same when the ultrafiltrate leaves the ascending thin limb as when it entered it), but the osmolarity of the ultrafiltrate inside the tubule adjusts to the osmolarity of the interstitium.

The fluid entering the ascending thick limb of Henle's loop passes a region that is impermeable to water but has a chloride pump, which removes chloride ions from the lumen, followed passively (or perhaps also actively) by sodium ions. Because water cannot leave the lumen, the ultrafiltrate becomes *hypotonic but its volume remains constant* as it ascends to the cortex in the ascending thick limb. The chloride and sodium that were transferred from the lumen of the ascending thick limb into the connective tissue are responsible for the establishment of a concentration gradient in the renal interstitium of the outer medulla.

Monitoring the Filtrate in the Juxtaglomerular Apparatus

When cells of the macula densa detect a low sodium concentration in the ultrafiltrate, they cause juxtaglomerular cells to release the enzyme renin, which converts angiotensinogen to angiotensin I.

The cells of the macula densa probably monitor the filtrate volume and sodium concentration. If sodium concentration is below a specific threshold, macula densa cells do two things:

- They cause dilation of the afferent glomerular arterioles, thus increasing blood flow into the glomerulus.
- They instruct juxtaglomerular cells to release the enzyme renin into circulation.

The enzyme renin converts **angiotensinogen,** normally present in the bloodstream, into the decapeptide **angiotensin I,** a mild vasoconstrictor. In the capillaries

TABLE 19–2   Effects of Angiotensin II

Function	Result
Acts as a potent vasoconstrictor	Increased blood pressure
Facilitates synthesis and release of aldosterone	Resorption of sodium and chloride from lumen of distal convoluted tubule
Facilitates release of ADH	Resorption of water from lumen of collecting tubule
Increases thirst	Increased tissue fluid volume
Inhibits renin release	Feedback inhibition
Facilitates release of prostaglandins	Vasodilation of afferent glomerular arteriole, thus maintaining glomerular filtration rate

ADH, antidiuretic hormone.

of the lungs, and also to a lesser extent in those of the kidneys and other organs of the body, **angiotensin-converting enzyme (ACE)** converts angiotensin I to **angiotensin II,** an octapeptide hormone with numerous biological effects (Table 19-2). As a potent vasoconstrictor, angiotensin II reduces the luminal diameter of blood vessels, thus constricting the *efferent glomerular arterioles,* further increasing pressure within the glomerulus. The increased intraglomerular pressure along with the increased volume of blood flow results in the increased glomerular filtration rate of a larger volume of blood. Angiotensin II also influences the adrenal cortex to release **aldosterone,** a hormone that acts primarily on cells of the distal convoluted tubules, increasing their resorption of sodium and chloride ions.

CLINICAL CORRELATIONS

One of the causes contributing to **chronic essential hypertension** is the presence of elevated levels of angiotensin II. Elevated blood levels of angiotensin II were once believed to be due to the excessive release of renin from the juxtaglomerular cells of the juxtaglomerular apparatus. It is now realized that the increased activity of angiotensin-converting enzyme, rather than the renal release of renin, is directly responsible for elevating the concentration of angiotensin II.

Loss of Water and Urea from Filtrate in Collecting Tubules

Antidiuretic hormone (vasopressin) causes the conservation of water and the excretion of a concentrated urine.

The filtrate that leaves the distal convoluted tubule to enter the collecting tubule is hypotonic. As the collecting tubule passes through the medulla to reach the area cribrosa, it is also subject to the same osmotic gradients as the ascending and descending limbs of Henle's loop. In the absence of **antidiuretic hormone (ADH),** the cells of the collecting tubule and, to a lesser extent, of the distal convoluted tubule are completely impermeable to water (see Fig. 19-20). Therefore, the filtrate, or urine, is not modified in the collecting tubule and the urine remains dilute (hypotonic).

Under the influence of ADH, however, the cells of the collecting tubule (and, in animals other than humans and monkeys, the distal convoluted tubules) become freely permeable to water and urea. As the filtrate descends through the renal medulla in the collecting tubule, it is subject to the osmotic pressure gradients established by the hairpin-like loops of Henle and the vasa recta, and water leaves the lumina of the collecting tubules to enter the interstitium. Hence, the urine, in the presence of ADH, becomes concentrated and hypertonic.

In addition, the concentration of urea becomes extremely high in the lumen of the collecting tubule, and in the presence of ADH it passively enters the interstitium of the inner medulla. Thus, much of the concentration gradient of the renal interstitium in the inner medulla is due to the presence of urea rather than sodium and chloride.

The action of ADH is believed to be dependent on V_2 receptors located in the basolateral plasma membranes of principal cells of the collecting ducts. Once ADH binds to a V_2 receptor, the following occurs:

- Gs proteins are activated.
- Adenylate cyclase generates cyclic adenosine monophosphate (cAMP).
- Aquaporin-2 (AQP2) channels are inserted into the luminal plasma membrane (Table 19-3)
- Water, from the lumen of the collecting duct, enters the cell.
- Water leaves the cell via aquaporin 3 (AQP 3) and aquaporin 4 (AQP 4) channels (that are always present in the basolateral cell membranes) to enter the renal interstitium.

CLINICAL CORRELATIONS

Congenital nephrogenic diabetes insipidus is an X-linked disorder evidenced clinically only in male infants, although it may also have a certain degree of clinical penetrance in female infants. This condition, in affected males, manifests itself in the formation of copious quantities of dilute urine due to the malformation of the V_2 receptor. Additional symptoms include fever, vomiting, hypernatremia, and extreme dehydration. The blood level of ADH is normal or somewhat elevated, however, the aberrant ADH receptor cannot activate Gs proteins, and consequently aquaporins are not inserted into the luminal plasma membranes of collecting ducts, resulting in the inability to concentrate urine.

Vasa Recta and Countercurrent Exchange System

The lumen of the arterial limb of the vasa recta has a smaller diameter than that of the venous limb; both limbs are freely permeable to electrolytes and water.

The vasa recta helps maintain the osmotic gradient in the medulla because both arterial and venous limbs are freely permeable to water and salts (Fig. 19-21). Moreover, as indicated previously, the luminal diameter of the arterial limb is smaller than that of the venous limb. Therefore, as the blood courses down the arterial limb, it loses water and gains salts, and as it returns via the venous limb, it loses salts and gains water, thus acting as a countercurrent exchange system.

This mechanism ensures that the system of osmotic gradients remains undisturbed, because the osmolarity of the blood in the vessels is more or less equilibrated with that of the interstitium. However, the volume of salts and fluid being brought in by the arterial limb is less than that being taken away by the venous limb. This exchange system causes salt and water to be resorbed (returned back to the body) because of the concentration gradient in the renal medulla.

The structure and function of the various regions of the uriniferous tubule are presented in Table 19-4.

EXCRETORY PASSAGES

The excretory passages of the urinary system consist of the minor and major calyces, the pelvis of the kidney, the ureter, the single urinary bladder, and the single urethra.

TABLE 19–3 Structure and Function of the Uriniferous Tubule

Structure	Major Functions	Comments
Renal corpuscle: Simple squamous epithelium, fused basal laminae, podocytes	Filtration	Filtration barrier: endothelial cell, fused basal laminae, filtration slits
Proximal tubule: Simple cuboidal epithelium	Resorption of 67%–80% of water, sodium, and chloride (reducing volume of ultrafiltrate); resorption of 100% of protein, amino acids, glucose, and bicarbonate	Sodium pump in basolateral membrane; ultrafiltrate is isotonic with blood
Descending thin limb of Henle's loop: Simple squamous epithelium	Completely permeable to water and salts (reducing volume of ultrafiltrate)	Ultrafiltrate is hypertonic with respect to blood; urea enters lumen of tubule
Ascending thin limb of Henle's loop: Simple squamous epithelium	Impermeable to water, permeable to salts; sodium and chloride leave tubule to enter renal interstitium	Ultrafiltrate is hypertonic with respect to blood; urea leaves renal interstitium and enters the lumen of tubule
Ascending thick limb of Henle's loop: Simple cuboidal epithelium	Impermeable to water; chloride and sodium leave tubule to enter renal interstitium	Ultrafiltrate becomes hypotonic with respect to blood; chloride pump in basolateral cell membrane is responsible for establishment of osmotic gradient in interstitium of outer medulla
Macula densa: Simple columnar cells	Monitors sodium level and volume of ultrafiltrate in lumen of distal tubule	Contacts and communicates with juxtaglomerular cells
Juxtaglomerular cells: Modified smooth muscle cells	Synthesize and release renin into bloodstream	Renin initiates the reaction for the eventual formation of angiotensin II (see Table 19-2)
Distal convoluted tubule: Simple cuboidal epithelium	Responds to aldosterone by resorbing sodium and chloride from lumen	Ultrafiltrate becomes more hypotonic (in the presence of aldosterone); sodium pump in basolateral membrane; potassium is secreted into the lumen
Collecting tubule: Simple cuboidal epithelium	In the presence of ADH, water and urea leave the lumen to enter the urea interstitium	Urine becomes hypertonic in the presence of ADH; urea in interstitium is responsible for gradient of concentration in interstitium of the inner medulla

ADH, antidiuretic hormone.

Calyces

Each minor calyx accepts urine from the renal papilla of a renal pyramid; as many as four minor calyces may deliver their urine to a major calyx.

The renal papilla of each renal pyramid fits into a **minor calyx,** a funnel-shaped chamber that accepts urine leaving the ducts of Bellini at the area cribrosa (see Fig. 19-1). The portion of the apex of the pyramid that projects into the minor calyx is covered by **transitional epithelium,** which acts as a barrier, separating the urine from the underlying interstitial connective tissue. Deep to the lamina propria is a thin muscular coat composed entirely of smooth muscle. This muscular layer propels the urine into a **major calyx,** one of three or four larger, funnel-shaped chambers, each of which collects urine from two to four minor calyces. The major calyces are similar in structure to the minor calyces as well as to the expanded proximal region of the ureters,

TABLE 19–4 Types of Aquaporins and Their Locations In The Uriniferous Tubule

Aquaporin	Location	Function
Aquaporin-1 (AQP 1)	Proximal tubule and thin descending limb of Henle's loop	These segments are always permeable to water
Aquaporin-2 (AQP 2)	In the presence of ADH, is present in the luminal surface of principal cells of the collecting ducts In the absence of ADH, is stored in apically located vesicles of principal cells of collecting ducts	In the presence of ADH, AQP-2 channels are inserted into the luminal membranes of principal cells and water can traverse the cell to enter the renal interstitium
Aquaporin-3 and aquaporin-4 (AQP 3 and AQP 4)	Always present in the basolateral cell membranes of principal cells of collecting ducts	The basolateral cell membranes of principal cells of collecting ducts are always permeable to water

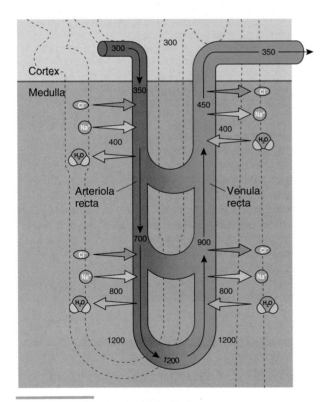

Figure 19–21 Histophysiology of the vasa recta. Numbers represent milliosmoles per liter. The arteriola recta is smaller in diameter than the venula recta.

the **renal pelvis.** The walls of the excretory passages thicken from the minor calyces to the urinary bladder.

Ureter

The ureters deliver urine from the kidneys to the urinary bladder.

Each ureter is about 3 to 4 mm in diameter, is approximately 25 to 30 cm long, and pierces the base of the urinary bladder. The ureters are hollow tubes consisting of:

- A mucosa, which lines the lumen
- A muscular coat (muscularis)
- A fibrous connective tissue covering

The **mucosa** of the ureter presents several folds, which project into the lumen when the ureter is empty but are absent when the ureter is distended. The **transitional epithelial lining,** three to five cell layers in thickness, overlies a layer of dense, irregular fibroelastic connective tissue, which constitutes the **lamina propria.** As always, the epithelium is separated from the underlying lamina propria by a basal lamina.

The **muscularis** of the ureter is composed of two predominantly inseparable layers of smooth muscle cells. The arrangement of the layers is opposite that found in the digestive tract, because the outer layer is arranged circularly and the inner layer is longitudinally disposed. This arrangement is true for the proximal two thirds of the ureter, but in the lower third, near the urinary bladder, a third muscle layer, whose fibers are oriented longitudinally, is added onto the existing surface of the existing muscle coat. Hence, the muscular fiber orientation in the lower one third of the ureter is **outer longitudinal, middle circular,** and **inner longitudinal.** However, it should be noted that, just as in the digestive tract, these muscle layers are arranged in a helical configuration, in which the pitch of the helices varies from short to long, thus giving the appearance of circular or longitudinal orientations.

The **fibrous outer coat** of the ureter is unremarkable. At its proximal and distal terminals, it blends with the capsule of the kidney and the connective tissue of the bladder wall, respectively. Contrary to expectation, urine does not pass down the ureter because of gravitational forces; instead, muscular contraction of the ureteric wall establishes peristalsis-like waves that convey urine to the urinary bladder. As the ureters pierce the posterior aspect of the base of the bladder, a valve-like flap of mucosa hangs over each ureteric orifice, preventing regurgitation of urine from the bladder back into the ureters.

Urinary Bladder

The urinary bladder stores urine until it is ready to be voided.

The urinary bladder is essentially an organ for storing urine until the pressure becomes sufficient to induce the urge for micturition, or voiding. Its mucosa also acts as an osmotic barrier between the urine and the lamina propria (Figs. 19-22 and 19-23). The mucosa of the bladder is arranged in numerous folds, which disappear when the bladder becomes distended with urine. During distention, the large, round, **dome-shaped cells** of the transitional epithelium become stretched and change their morphology to become flattened.

The accommodation of cell shape is performed by a unique feature of the **transitional epithelial cell** plasmalemma, which is composed of a mosaic of specialized, rigid, thickened regions, **plaques,** interspersed by normal cell membrane, **interplaque regions.** When the bladder is empty, the plaque regions are folded into irregular, angular contours, which disappear when the cell becomes stretched. These rigid plaque regions, anchored to intracytoplasmic filaments, resemble gap junctions, but this similarity is only superficial.

Plaques appear to be impermeable to water and salts; thus these cells act as osmotic barriers between the urine and the underlying lamina propria. The superficial cells of the transitional epithelium are held together by desmosomes and, possibly, by tight junctions, which also aid in the establishment of the osmotic barrier by preventing the passage of fluid between the cells.

The triangular region of the bladder, whose apices are the orifices of the two ureters and the urethra, is known as the **trigone.** The mucosa of the trigone is always smooth and is never thrown into folds. The embryonic origin of the trigone differs from that of the remainder of the bladder.

The lamina propria of the bladder may be subdivided into two layers: a more *superficial,* dense, irregular collagenous connective tissue and a *deeper,* looser layer of connective tissue composed of a mixture of collagen and elastic fibers. The lamina propria contains no glands except at the region surrounding the urethral orifice, where **mucous glands** may be found. Usually, these glands extend only into the superficial layer of the lamina propria. They secrete a clear viscous fluid that apparently lubricates the urethral orifice.

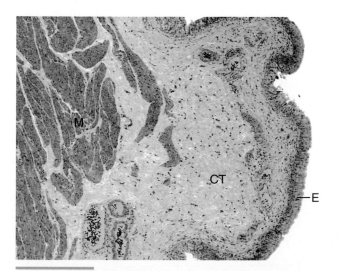

Figure 19–22 Low-power light micrograph of the monkey urinary bladder (×58). Observe the epithelium (E), the subepithelial connective tissue (CT), and the muscular coat (M) of the bladder.

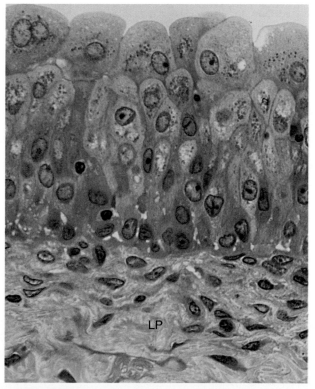

Figure 19–23 Light micrograph of transitional epithelium from the bladder of a monkey (×540). Observe the very large, dome-shaped cells abutting the lumen. LP, lamina propria.

The muscular coat of the urinary bladder is composed of three interlaced layers of smooth muscle, which can be separated only in the region of the neck of the bladder. Here, they are arranged as a thin inner longitudinal layer, a thick middle circular layer, and a thin outer longitudinal layer. The middle circular layer forms the **internal sphincter muscle** around the internal orifice of the urethra.

The adventitia of the bladder is composed of a dense, irregular collagenous type of connective tissue containing a generous amount of elastic fibers. Certain regions of the adventitia are covered by a serosa, a peritoneal reflection onto the wall of the bladder, whereas other regions may be surrounded by fat.

Urethra

The urethra conveys urine from the urinary bladder to outside the body.

The urinary bladder is drained by a single tubular structure, the urethra, which communicates with the outside, permitting elimination of urine from the body. As the urethra pierces the perineum, skeletal muscle fibers form the **external sphincter muscle** surrounding the urethra. This muscle permits voluntary control of micturition. The urethra of the male is longer than that of the female and has a dual function, acting as a route for semen as well as for urine.

CLINICAL CORRELATIONS

Loss of voluntary control over the **external sphincter muscle** of the urethra causes **urinary incontinence,** a condition affecting primarily older women.

Female Urethra

The female urethra is about 4 to 5 cm in length and 5 to 6 mm in diameter. It extends from the urinary bladder to the external urethral orifice just above and anterior to the opening of the vagina. Normally, the lumen is collapsed except during micturition. It is lined by a **transitional epithelium** near the bladder and by a **stratified squamous nonkeratinized epithelium** along the remainder of its length. Interspersed in the epithelium are patches of pseudostratified columnar epithelium. The mucosa is arranged in elongated folds because of the organization of the fibroelastic **lamina propria.** Along the entire length of the urethra are numerous clear, mucus-secreting **glands of Littre.**

A thin, vascular, erectile coat surrounds the mucosa, resembling the corpus spongiosum of the male. The muscular layer of the urethra is continuous with that of the bladder but is composed of two layers only, an inner longitudinal and an outer circular smooth muscle layer. As the urethra pierces the perineum (urogenital diaphragm), a sphincter of skeletal muscle surrounds it and permits voluntary control of micturition.

Male Urethra

The male urethra is 15 to 20 cm long, and its three regions are named according to the structures through which it passes:

- The **prostatic urethra,** 3 to 4 cm long, lies entirely in the prostate gland. It is lined by a transitional epithelium and receives the openings of many tiny ducts of the prostate, the prostatic utricle (a rudimentary homologue of the uterus), and the paired ejaculatory ducts.
- The **membranous urethra** is only 1 to 2 cm long. This segment is so-named because it passes through the perineal membrane (urogenital diaphragm). It is lined by stratified columnar epithelium interspersed with patches of pseudostratified columnar epithelium.
- The **spongy urethra (penile urethra),** the longest portion of the urethra (15 cm long), passes through the length of the penis, terminating at the tip of the glans penis as the external urethral orifice. This segment is so-named because it is located in the corpus spongiosum. It is lined by stratified columnar epithelium interspersed with patches of pseudostratified columnar and stratified squamous nonkeratinized epithelia. The enlarged terminal portion of the urethra in the glans penis (the **navicular fossa**) is lined by stratified squamous nonkeratinized epithelium.

The **lamina propria** of all three regions is composed of a loose fibroelastic connective tissue with a rich vascular supply. It houses numerous **glands of Littre,** whose mucous secretion lubricates the epithelial lining of the urethra.

20

Female Reproductive System

The female reproductive system consists of the internal reproductive organs (the paired ovaries and oviducts, the uterus, and the vagina; Fig. 20-1), and the the external genitalia (the clitoris, the labia majora, and the labia minora). Although the mammary glands are not considered part of the female reproductive system, their physiology and function are so closely associated with the reproductive system that they are discussed in this chapter.

The reproductive organs are incompletely developed and remain in a state of rest until **gonadotropic hormones** secreted by the pituitary gland signal the initiation of puberty. Thereafter, many changes take place in the entire reproductive system, including further differentiation of the reproductive organs, culminating in **menarche,** the first menstrual flow, occurring from about 9 to 15 years of age, with the average age 12.7 years. After the first menstrual flow, the menstrual cycle, which involves many hormonal, histological, and psychological changes, is repeated approximately each month (28 days) throughout the entire reproductive years, unless it is interrupted by pregnancy. As a woman nears the end of her reproductive years, her menstrual cycles become less regular as hormonal and neurological signals begin to change, initiating **menopause.** Eventually, menstrual cycles cease; after menopause, limited involution of the reproductive organs occurs. Thus, the female reproductive system is controlled by complex orchestrations of hormonal, neurological, and psychological factors.

OVARIES

The ovaries, covered by the germinal epithelium, are indistinctly divided into a cortex and a medulla.

The paired ovaries, located within the pelvis, are almond-shaped bodies 3 cm long, 1.5 to 2 cm wide, and 1 cm thick, each weighing approximately 14 g. The ovaries are suspended in the **broad ligament of the uterus** by an attachment called the **mesovarium,** a special fold of the peritoneum that conveys blood vessels to the ovaries (see Fig. 20-1).

The surface epithelium covering the ovaries, called the **germinal epithelium,** is a modified peritoneum. This low cuboidal epithelium, derived from the **mesothelial epithelium** covering the developing ovaries, was originally believed to give rise to the germ cells; although this is now known to be untrue, the name persists. Directly beneath this epithelium is the **tunica albuginea,** a poorly vascularized, dense, irregular collagenous connective tissue capsule whose collagen fibers are oriented more or less parallel to the ovary surface. Each ovary is subdivided into the highly cellular **cortex** and a **medulla,** which consists mostly of a richly vascularized loose connective tissue. The blood vessels of the medulla are derived from the ovarian arteries. Histologically, however, the division between the cortex and the medulla is indistinct.

Ovarian Cortex

The ovarian cortex is composed of the connective tissue stroma that houses ovarian follicles in various stages of development.

The ovarian cortex is composed of a connective tissue framework, the **stroma** (also known as the **interstitial compartment**), housing fibroblast-like **stromal cells** (also known as **interstitial cells**) as well as **ovarian follicles** in various stages of development (Fig. 20-2A).

Primordial germ cells, called **oogonia,** develop in the yolk sac endoderm shortly after the first month of

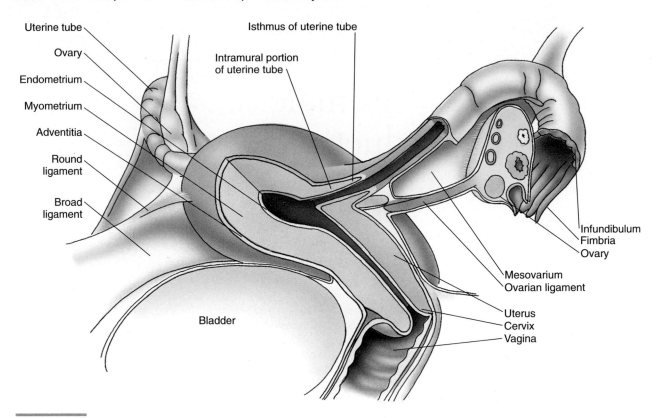

Figure 20–1 Female reproductive tract. The ovary is sectioned to show the developing follicles. The uterus and fallopian tube are both open to display their respective lumina.

gestation. They undergo several mitotic divisions and, during the 6th week after fertilization, migrate to the germinal ridges to populate the cortex of the developing ovaries. Here they continue to undergo mitotic divisions until near the end of the 5th fetal month. At this time, each ovary contains about 5 million to 7 million oogonia. About 1 million of the oogonia become surrounded by follicular cells and survive to the time of birth. The remaining oogonia do not become incorporated into follicles. Instead, they undergo **atresia;** that is, they degenerate and die.

The oogonia that survive enter the **prophase stage** of **meiosis I** and are known as **primary oocytes** (Fig. 20-3). Meiosis is then arrested in the diplotene stage by paracrine factors such as **meiosis-preventing substance,** produced by the follicular cells. Primary oocytes remain in that phase until just before ovulation, when they are triggered, in response to the surge of **luteinizing hormone (LH),** and by **meiosis-inducing substance** to complete their first meiotic division, forming the secondary oocyte and the first polar body.

Of the 1 million oogonia that survive to become incorporated into the primordial follicles, 600,000 become atretic over the next decade or so of life, and at menarche a young woman has only about 300,000 to 400,000

follicles. Generally, ovulation will occur every 28 days for the next 30 to 40 years, with one oocyte released each month, for a total of about 450 oocytes released over the reproductive period. The remaining follicles degenerate and die over the same period of time.

Phenotypic Sexual Development during Embryogenesis

The default phenotypic development is female.

During early embryogenesis, in the absence of both testosterone and antimüllerian hormone, the default phenotypic development is that of a female. The lack of testosterone does not permit the development of the wolffian ducts, the precursor of the male genital tract, and the lack of antimüllerian hormone permits the development of the müllerian ducts, the precursor of the female genital tract.

The Ovarian Cortex at Onset of Puberty

The pulsatile release of gonadotropin-releasing hormone has the major responsibility for the initiation of puberty.

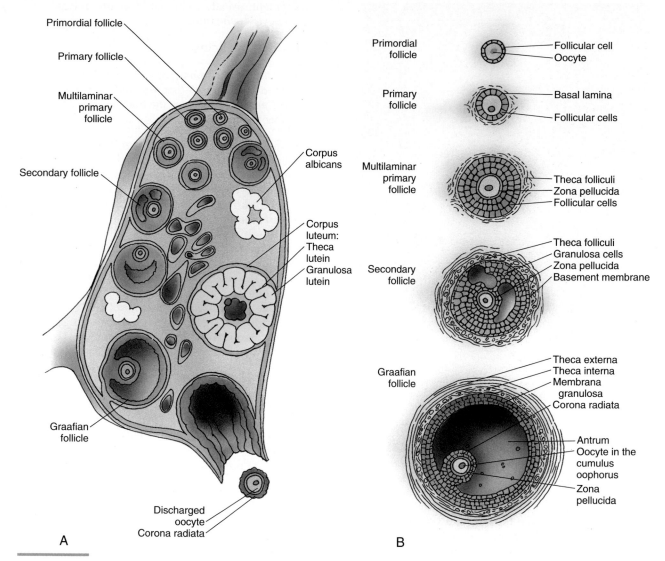

A

Primordial follicle

Primary follicle

Multilaminar primary follicle

Secondary follicle

Corpus albicans

Corpus luteum:
Theca lutein
Granulosa lutein

Graafian follicle

Discharged oocyte
Corona radiata

B

Primordial follicle — Follicular cell / Oocyte

Primary follicle — Basal lamina / Follicular cells

Multilaminar primary follicle — Theca folliculi / Zona pellucida / Follicular cells

Secondary follicle — Theca folliculi / Granulosa cells / Zona pellucida / Basement membrane

Graafian follicle — Theca externa / Theca interna / Membrana granulosa / Corona radiata / Antrum / Oocyte in the cumulus oophorus / Zona pellucida

Figure 20–2 Ovarian structure (**A**) and follicular development (**B**). Note the corpus luteum and corpus albicans. All the stages of follicular development, from the primordial follicle stage to the graafian follicle stage, are presented.

Before the onset of puberty, all of the follicles of the ovarian cortex are in the **primordial follicle** stage. The decapeptide **luteinizing hormone-releasing hormone (LHRH),** also known as **gonadotropin-releasing hormone (GnRH),** produced by the neurosecretory neurons of the arcuate nucleus and preoptic area of the hypothalamus, plays a major role in initiating puberty. It is interesting that release of LHRH is pulsatile, occurring approximately every 90 minutes, and that its half-life in the bloodstream is only about 2 to 4 minutes. The pulsatility of LHRH release is a prerequisite not only for the onset of menarche but also for the maintenance of the normal ovulatory and menstrual cycles throughout the reproductive life of the female.

The pulsatile release of LHRH results in a similar, pulsatile, release of gonadotropins (**follicle-stimulating hormone [FSH],** and **LH**) from the basophils of the anterior pituitary that culminates in the commencement of follicular development and the onset of the ovulatory cycle. The ovulatory cycle, follicular development, and the hormonal interrelationships are described next.

Ovarian Follicles

Ovarian follicles evolve through four developmental stages: primordial, primary, secondary, and graafian.

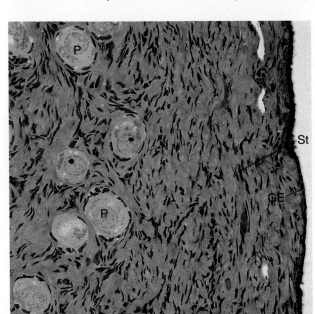

Figure 20–3 Light micrograph of the ovarian cortex demonstrating mostly primordial follicles (P), which are primary oocytes surrounded by follicular cells (×270). The germinal epithelium (GE) and the ovarian stroma (St) of the cortex also are evident in this micrograph.

Ovarian follicles are surrounded by stromal tissue and consist of a **primary oocyte** and its associated **follicular cells (granulosa cells)** arranged in a single spherical layer or several concentric layers around the primary oocyte. Follicular cells, similar to the germinal epithelium, are derived from the **mesothelial epithelium** and possibly also from a second source, the primitive sex cords of the **mesonephros,** a precursor of the metanephros, the structure that develops into the definitive kidney.

There are two stages of follicular development based on the growth of the follicle; the stages also are categorized by the development of the oocyte and of the follicular cells (Table 20-1; also see Fig. 20-2B):

■ Nongrowing, or *primordial*, follicles
■ Growing follicles
  ■ Unilaminar and multilaminar *primary* follicles
  ■ *Secondary* (antral) follicles
  ■ *Graafian* (mature) follicles

The development of the primary follicles is independent of FSH; instead, the differentiation and proliferation of the follicular cells are triggered by as yet uncharacterized local factors secreted probably by the follicular cells of the ovary. Secondary and later follicles, however, are under the influence of FSH. Follicular

development usually culminates in the release of a single oocyte (ovulation).

Primordial Follicles

Primordial follicles, composed of a single layer of flattened follicular cells that surround the primary oocyte, are separated from the ovarian stroma by a basement membrane.

Primordial follicles, the most primitive follicles, are abundant before birth, after which they become fewer in number. The primordial follicle is composed of a **primary oocyte** surrounded by a single layer of flattened **follicular cells** (Fig. 20-4; also see Fig. 20-3).

The **primary oocyte** (arrested in the **prophase stage** of **meiosis I**) is a spherical cell about 25 μm in diameter. It has a large, acentric nucleus containing a single nucleolus. The nucleoplasm appears vesicular because of the uncoiled chromosomes. The organelles include numerous mitochondria, abundant Golgi complexes, rough endoplasmic reticulum (RER) displaying only a few ribosomes, and occasional annulate lamellae.

The squamous **follicular cells** completely surround the primary oocyte and are attached to each other by desmosomes. They are separated from the connective tissue stroma by a basal lamina.

Primary Follicles

There are two types of primary follicles, unilaminar and multilaminar, depending on the number of layers of follicular cells that surround the primary oocyte.

Primordial follicles develop into primary follicles (see Fig. 20-3) distinguished as a result of changes in the primary oocyte, the follicular cells, and the surrounding stromal tissue.

The **primary oocyte** grows to about 100 to 150 μm in diameter with an enlarged nucleus (sometimes called the **germinal vesicle**). Several Golgi complexes are scattered throughout the cell, the RER becomes rich with ribosomes, free ribosomes are abundant, and mitochondria are numerous and dispersed throughout the cell.

Follicular cells become cuboidal in shape. As long as only a single layer of follicular cells encircles the oocyte, the follicle is called a **unilaminar primary follicle.** When the follicular cells proliferate and stratify, forming several layers of cells around the primary oocyte, the follicle is called a **multilaminar primary follicle,** and the follicular cells are more commonly referred to as **granulosa cells.** The proliferative activity of the granulosa cells is due to the signaling molecule **activin** produced by the primary oocyte.

During this stage, an amorphous substance (the **zona pellucida**) appears, separating the oocyte from

TABLE 20–1   Stages of Ovarian Follicular Development

Stage	FSH-Dependent	Oocyte	Zona Pellucida	Follicular Cells or Granulosa	Liquor Folliculi	Theca Interna	Theca Externa
Primordial follicle	No	Primary	None	Single layer of flat cells	None	None	None
Unilaminar primary follicle	No	Primary	Present	Single layer of cuboidal cells	None	None	None
Multilaminar primary follicle	No	Primary	Present; plasmalemma of primary oocyte forms gap junctions with filopodia of corona radiata cells	Several layers of follicular cells (now called granulosa cells)	None	Present	Present
Secondary follicle	Yes	Primary	Present with gap junctions	Spaces develop between granulosa cells	Accumulates in spaces between granulosa cells	Present	Present
Graafian follicle	Yes, until it becomes the dominant follicle	Primary, surrounded by corona radiata in cumulus oophorus	Present with gap junctions	Forms membrana granulosa and cumulus oophorus	Fills the antrum	Present	Present

FSH, follicle-stimulating hormone.

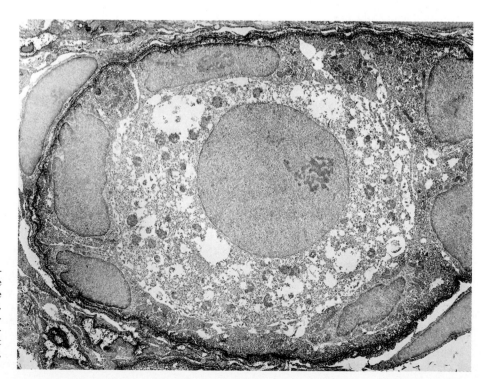

Figure 20–4 Electron micrograph of a primordial ovarian follicle of a rat ovary (×6200). Observe the oocyte surrounded by follicular cells. (From Leardkamolkarn V, Abrahamson DR: Immunoelectron microscopic localization of laminin in rat ovarian follicles. Anat Rec 233:4152, 1992.)

the surrounding follicular cells. The zonula pellucida is composed of three different glycoproteins, ZP_1, ZP_2, and ZP_3, secreted by the oocyte. Filopodia of the follicular cells invade the zonula pellucida, come in contact with the oocyte plasmalemma and form gap junctions through which they communicate with the oocyte throughout follicular development. The presence of gap junctions is necessary for the oocyte to be able to progress through meiosis.

Stromal cells begin to be organized around the multilaminar primary follicle, forming an inner **theca interna,** composed mostly of a richly vascularized cellular layer, and an outer **theca externa,** composed mostly of fibrous connective tissue. The cells composing the theca interna possess **LH receptors** on their plasmalemma, and these cells assume the ultrastructural characteristics of steroid-producing cells. Their cytoplasm accumulates numerous lipid droplets and has abundant smooth endoplasmic reticulum (SER), and the cristae of their mitochondria are tubular. These theca interna cells produce the male sex hormone **androstenedione,** which enters the granulosa cells where it is converted by the enzyme **aromatase** into the estrogen **estradiol.** The granulosa cells are separated from the theca interna by a thickened basal lamina.

Secondary (Antral) Follicles

Secondary follicles are similar to primary follicles except for the presence of accumulations of liquor folliculi among the granulosa cells.

The multilaminar primary follicle continues to develop and increase in size, reaching up to 200 µm in diameter. A large spherical follicle is formed with numerous layers of granulosa cells around the primary oocyte (whose size from this point on remains constant). Several intercellular spaces develop within the mass of granulosa cells and become filled with a fluid known as **liquor folliculi.** Once the multilaminar primary follicle displays the presence of liquor folliculi, it is known as a secondary follicle (Fig. 20-5; also see Fig. 20-2B).

Continued proliferation of the granulosa cells of the secondary follicle depends on **FSH** released by basophil cells of the anterior pituitary. Under the influence of FSH, the number of layers of the granulosa cells increases, as does the number of liquor folliculi– containing intercellular spaces. This fluid, an exudate of plasma, contains glycosaminoglycans, proteoglycans, and steroid-binding proteins produced by the granulosa cells. Moreover, it contains the hormones **progesterone, estradiol, inhibin, folliostatin (folliculostatin),** and **activin,** which regulate the release of LH and FSH. In addition, FSH (along with estrogen) induces

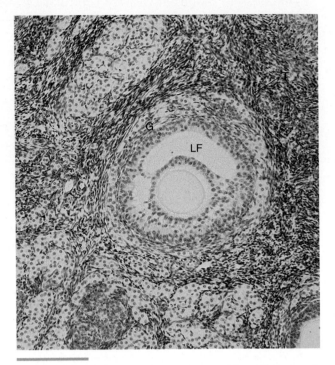

Figure 20–5 Light micrograph of a secondary follicle (×132). Observe the primary oocyte and the follicular fluid surrounded by membrana granulosa. Note also the presence of the basement membrane between the granulosa cells (G) and the theca interna (T). LF, liquor folliculi.

the granulosa cells to manufacture receptors for LH, which become incorporated into their plasmalemma.

As more fluid is produced, individual droplets of liquor folliculi coalesce to form a single, fluid-filled chamber, the **antrum.** The granulosa cells become rearranged so that the primary oocyte is now surrounded by a small group of granulosa cells that project out from the wall into the fluid-filled antrum. This structure is called the **cumulus oophorus.** The loosely arranged low cuboidal granulosa cells immediately adjacent to the zona pellucida move slightly away from the oocyte, but their filopodia remain within the zona pellucida, maintaining contact with the primary oocyte. This single layer of granulosa cells that immediately surrounds the primary oocyte is called the **corona radiata.** At this time two different types of granulosa cells may be distinguished: membrana granulosa and cumulus granulosa cells (Table 20-2).

Toward the end of this stage, stromal cells become enlarged and the theca interna is invaded by capillaries that nourish them as well as the avascular granulosa cells. Most of the follicles that reach this stage of development undergo atresia, but some of the granulosa cells associated with the atretic follicles do not degenerate; instead, they form **interstitial glands,** which secrete

TABLE 20–2	Types of Granulosa Cells
Cell Type	**Characteristics**
Membrana granulosa	
Granulosa mural cells	Abut the basement membrane
	Have LH and FSH receptors
	Function in steroidogenesis due to the presence of the enzyme aromatase (estradiol, progesterone)
	Produce the regulatory hormones activin, inhibin, folliculostatin, and insulin-like growth factor type I
	Form the bulk of the corpus luteum
Antral granulosa cells	Line the antrum
	Are not active in steroidogenesis
Cumulus oophorus granulosa cells	Surround the oocyte
	Contact the oocyte plasmalemma by their filopodia
	Do not possess many LH receptors
	Divide to form cells of the membrana granulosa
	Are ovulated along with the oocyte

FSH, follicle-stimulating hormone; LH, luteinizing hormone.

small amounts of androgens until menopause is concluded. A few secondary follicles continue to develop into mature follicles.

Graafian (Mature) Follicles

Graafian follicles, also known as mature follicles, may be as large as the entire ovary; it is these follicles that undergo ovulation.

Continued proliferation of the granulosa cells and continued formation of liquor folliculi result in the formation of a graafian (mature) follicle whose diameter may reach as much as 2.5 cm by the time of ovulation. The graafian follicle may be observed as a transparent bulge on the surface of the ovary, nearly as large as the ovary itself.

The follicular cells of the wall of the follicle compose the **membrana granulosa.** Continued formation of liquor folliculi causes the cumulus oophorus composed of the primary oocyte, the corona radiata, and associ-ated follicular cells to become detached from its base to float freely within the liquor folliculi (see Fig. 20-2B).

Ovulation

The process of releasing the secondary oocyte from the graafian follicle is known as ovulation.

By the 14th day of the menstrual cycle, estrogen produced mostly by the developing graafian follicle, but also by secondary follicles, causes elevation of blood estrogen to levels high enough to have the following effects:

■ Negative feedback inhibition shuts off FSH release by the anterior pituitary.
■ A sudden surge of LH is released by basophils of the anterior pituitary.

The surge in LH levels results in increased blood flow to the ovaries, and capillaries within the theca externa begin leaking plasma, resulting in edema. Concomitant with edema formation, histamine, prostaglandins, and collagenase are released in the vicinity of the graafian follicle. Additionally, plasminogen activator level, the enzyme that catalyzes the conversion of plasminogen to plasmin, increases in the follicle, and the newly formed plasmin facilitates the proteolysis of the membrana granulosa, permitting ovulation to occur.

In addition, the LH surge is responsible for the following events:

1 A local factor, **meiosis-inducing substance,** is released.
2 Under the influence of meiosis-inducing substance, the primary oocyte of the graafian follicle resumes and completes its first meiotic division, resulting in the formation of two daughter cells, the **secondary oocyte** and the **first polar body.** Because of the uneven distribution of the cytoplasm, the first polar body is composed of a nucleus surrounded by only a narrow rim of cytoplasm.
3 The newly formed secondary oocyte enters the **second meiotic division** and is arrested in **metaphase.**
4 The presence and continued formation of proteoglycans and hyaluronic acid by the granulosa cells attract water, thus causing an even greater increase not only in the size of the graafian follicle but also in the loosening of the membrana granulosa.
5 Just before ovulation, the surface of the ovary, where the graafian follicle is pressing against the tunica albuginea, loses its blood supply.
6 This thinned, avascular region becomes blanched and is known as the **stigma.** The connective tissue at the stigma degenerates, as does the wall of the graafian follicle in contact with the stigma, forming an opening between the peritoneal cavity and the antrum of the graafian follicle.

7 Through this opening, the secondary oocyte and its attendant follicular cells and some of the liquor folliculi are gently released from the ovary, resulting in **ovulation.** Although the average menstrual cycle is 28 days long, some cycles are longer and others are shorter; however, ovulation is always on the 14th day before the beginning of menstruation.

8 The remnants of the graafian follicle are converted into the corpus hemorrhagicum and then into the corpus luteum.

The distal, fimbriated end of the oviduct, which presses against the ovary, whisks the secondary oocyte and follicular cells into the **infundibulum** of the **oviduct** to begin the journey into the ampulla, where the oocyte may be fertilized (see Fig. 20-1). If it is not fertilized within approximately 24 hours, the secondary oocyte degenerates and is phagocytosed. The process of fertilization is discussed later in the chapter.

Corpus Luteum

The corpus luteum, formed from the remnants of the graafian follicle, is a temporary endocrine gland that manufactures and releases hormones that support the uterine endometrium.

After the secondary oocyte and its associated cells are ovulated, the remainder of the graafian follicle collapses and becomes folded; some of the ruptured blood vessels leak blood into the follicular cavity, forming a central clot. The resulting structure is known as the **corpus hemorrhagicum.** As the clot is removed by phagocytes, continued high levels of LH convert the corpus hemorrhagicum into a temporary structure known as the **corpus luteum,** which functions as an endocrine gland (Fig. 20-6). This highly vascularized structure is composed of granulosa-lutein cells (modified granulosa cells) and theca-lutein cells (modified theca interna cells).

Granulosa-Lutein Cells

Granulosa cells of the graafian follicle differentiate into hormone-producing granulosa-lutein cells.

The granulosa cells remaining in the central region of the follicle account for about 80% of the cell population of the corpus luteum. They become modified into large, pale-staining cells (30 to 50 μm in diameter) called **granulosa-lutein cells.** These cells have many long microvilli and develop all of the organelles necessary for steroid production, including abundant SER and RER, abundant mitochondria, several well-developed Golgi complexes, and some lipid droplets scattered throughout the cytoplasm (Fig. 20-7). The granulosa-lutein cells produce **progesterone** and convert androgens produced by the theca-lutein cells into **estrogens.**

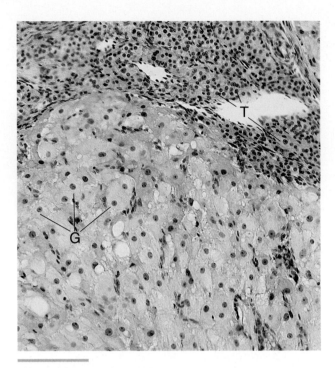

Figure 20–6 Light micrograph of the corpus luteum (×132). Note the difference between the large granulosa-lutein (G) and small theca-lutein (T) cells.

Theca-Lutein Cells

Theca-lutein cells, derived from the cells of the theca interna, secrete progesterone, androgens, and estrogens.

The **theca interna cells** at the periphery of the corpus luteum account for about 20% of the luteal cell population. These dark-staining cells remain small (15 μm in diameter) but become modified into hormone-secreting cells known as **theca-lutein cells.** They specialize in the production of **progesterone,** some estrogens, and **androgens.**

Degeneration of Corpus Luteum

The absence of LH leads to the degeneration of the corpus luteum.

Progesterone and estrogens secreted by granulosa-lutein and theca-lutein cells inhibit the secretion of LH and FSH, respectively. The absence of FSH prevents the development of new follicles, thus preventing a second ovulation. If pregnancy does not occur, the absence of LH leads to degeneration of the corpus luteum, forming the **corpus luteum of menstruation.** If pregnancy occurs, **human chorionic gonadotropin (hCG),** secreted by the placenta, maintains the corpus luteum for 3 months. Now called the **corpus luteum**

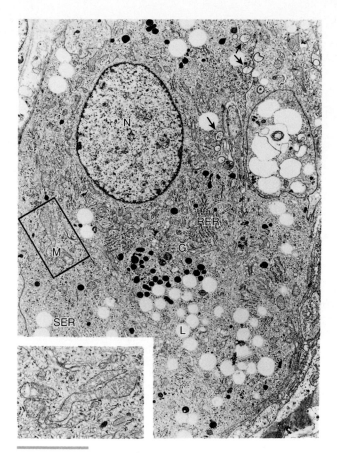

Figure 20–7 Electron micrograph of a rhesus monkey granulosa-lutein cell with its large acentric nucleus and numerous organelles (×6800). G, Golgi apparatus; L, lipid droplet; M, mitochondria (displayed at a higher magnification in *inset, lower left*); N, nucleus; RER, rough endoplasmic reticulum; SER, smooth endoplasmic reticulum. (From Booher C, Enders AC, Hendrick X, Hess DL: Structural characteristics of the corpus luteum during implantation in the rhesus monkey (*Macaca mulatta*). Am J Anat 160:1736, 1981.)

of pregnancy, it grows to a diameter of 5 cm and continues to secrete hormones necessary for the maintenance of pregnancy. Although the placenta becomes the main site of production of the various hormones involved in maintaining pregnancy 2 to 3 months after its formation, the corpus luteum continues to form these hormones for several months (see later).

Corpus Albicans

> As the corpus luteum degenerates and is being phagocytosed by macrophages, fibroblasts enter, manufacture type I collagen, and form a fibrous structure known as the corpus albicans.

The corpus luteum of menstruation (and also of pregnancy) is invaded by fibroblasts, becomes fibrotic, and ceases to function. Its remnants undergo autolysis, a process known as **luteolysis,** and are phagocytosed by macrophages. The fibrous connective tissue that forms in its place is known as the **corpus albicans** and persists for some time before being resorbed. The remnants of the corpus albicans persist as a scar on the surface of the ovary.

Atretic Follicles

> Follicles that undergo degeneration are known as atretic follicles.

The ovaries contain many follicles in various stages of development. Most follicles degenerate before reaching the mature stage, but multiple graafian follicles develop during each menstrual cycle. Nevertheless, once a single mature follicle ruptures and releases its secondary oocyte and associated cells, the remaining maturing follicles undergo atresia; the resulting **atretic follicles** are eventually phagocytosed by macrophages. Thus, normally, only a single follicle ovulates during each menstrual cycle. Occasionally, two separate follicles develop to maturity and ovulate, leading to fraternal twins if both oocytes are fertilized. Although about 2% of all follicles reach the mature stage and are primed to undergo ovulation, only 5% to 6% of these actually do. Of all the follicles present in the ovaries at menarche, just 0.1% to 0.2% develop to maturity and undergo ovulation.

Ovarian Medulla

> The ovarian medulla is a richly vascularized fibroelastic connective tissue housing connective tissue cells, interstitial cells, and hilar cells.

The central region of the ovary, the **medulla,** is composed of fibroblasts loosely embedded in a collagen-rich meshwork containing elastic fibers (see Fig. 20-2A). The medulla also contains large blood vessels, lymph vessels, and nerve fibers. The medulla of the premenstrual human ovary has a few clusters of epithelioid **interstitial cells** that secrete estrogens. In mammals having large litters, the ovaries contain many clusters of these interstitial cells, which collectively are called the **interstitial gland.** In humans, most of these interstitial cells involute during the first menstrual cycle and have little, if any, function.

Hilus cells constitute another group of epithelioid cells in the ovarian medulla. These cells have a similar configuration of organelles and contain the same substances in their cytoplasm as Leydig cells of the testes. These cells secrete androgens.

Summary of Hormonal Regulation of Ovarian Function

As mentioned previously, **FSH** and **LH** regulate maturation of ovarian follicles and ovulation. The pulsatile

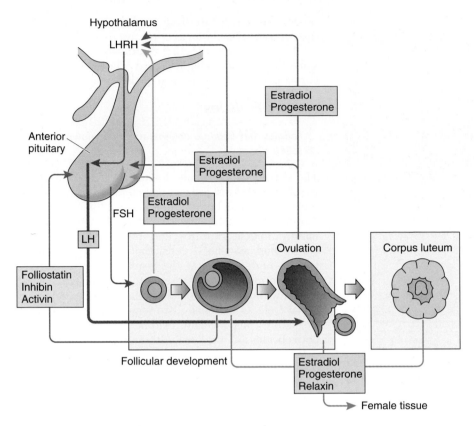

Figure 20–8 Hormonal interactions between the hypothalamo-pituitary axis and the female reproductive system. FSH, follicle-stimulating hormone; LH, luteinizing hormone; LHRH, luteinizing hormone–releasing hormone. Note that folliostatin and inhibin both suppress FSH release, whereas activin facilitates its release.

secretion of these gonadotropic hormones, which are produced in the pars distalis of the anterior pituitary, is in turn controlled by LHRH released in a pulsatile manner, every 90 minutes or so, by neurosecretory neurons located in the arcuate nucleus of the hypothalamus (Fig. 20-8 and Table 20-3). The pulsatility of LHRH release is essential for the normal functioning of the female ovulatory cycle because the up-regulation of LHRH receptors on basophils of the pars anterior of the pituitary gland can occur only if the pulsatility is maintained between 60 and 90 minutes (Table 20-4).

Although it is unclear what signal stimulates primordial and early (unilaminar) primary follicles to develop, it is known that the signaling molecule **activin,** produced by granulosa cells, stimulates release of FSH from the pituitary which, in turn, results not only in the proliferation of the granulosa cells of secondary and more developed follicles but also in enhancing the actions of FSH in those follicles. The development of the early follicles appears to be independent of FSH, whereas continued development of secondary follicles into graafian follicles depends on FSH.

Binding of LHRH to receptors on the basophils of the pars distalis induces the release of stored FSH and LH and stimulates continued FSH and LH synthesis. Subsequent binding of FSH to specific receptors on the granulosa cells of secondary follicles stimulates their development into graafian follicles. FSH also induces the theca interna cells of developing follicles to express LH receptors. LH binds to these receptors, thus inducing the theca interna cells to produce androgens from cholesterol. Androgens, released from the theca interna cells, cross the basement membrane and enter the granulosa cells. The enzyme **aromatase** of the granulosa cells converts androgens into **estrogens.** The granulosa cells of secondary follicles also produce several other hormones, (e.g., **inhibin, folliostatin, activin**) that help to regulate release of FSH (see Fig. 20-8).

As the blood levels of estrogen and other hormones produced by the granulosa cells rise, they continue to stimulate production of LH by the basophils of the anterior pituitary. When the blood concentration of estrogen reaches a threshold level, it restricts secretion of FSH in two ways: *indirectly*, by suppressing LHRH release from the hypothalamus, and *directly*, by inhibiting FSH release from the anterior pituitary.

Just before the midpoint of the menstrual cycle (the 14th day before onset of menstruation), the high estrogen level in the blood causes a surge of LH by gonadotrophs of the pituitary gland. The sudden high blood LH level stimulates the primary oocyte (by acti-

TABLE 20–3 Major Hormones Involved in the Female Reproductive System

Hormone	Source	Function
Luteinizing hormone–releasing hormone (LHRH)	Hypothalamus	Stimulates release of FSH and LH from anterior pituitary gland
Prolactin-inhibiting factor	Hypothalamus	Inhibits release of prolactin by acidophils of anterior pituitary gland
Follicle-stimulating hormone (FSH)	Basophils of anterior pituitary gland	Stimulates secretion of estrogen and development of ovarian follicles (from secondary follicle onward)
Luteinizing hormone (LH)	Basophils of anterior pituitary gland	Stimulates formation of estrogen and progesterone; promotes ovulation and formation of corpus luteum
Estrogens	Granulosa cells of ovary; granulosa-lutein cells of corpus luteum; and the placenta	Inhibits release of FSH and LHRH; triggers surge of LH; causes proliferation and hypertrophy of myometrium of uterus; causes development of female sexual characteristics, including breasts and body fat
Progesterone	Granulosa cells of ovary; theca-lutein and granulosa-lutein cells of corpus luteum; placenta	Inhibits release of LHRH from hypothalamus and of LH from basophils of the anterior pituitary; causes development of uterine endometrium and regulates viscosity of mucus produced by glands of uterine cervix; causes development of female sexual characteristics including breasts
Inhibin	Granulosa cells of ovary; granulosa-lutein cells of corpus luteum	Inhibits FSH secretion by basophils of the anterior pituitary
Activin	Oocyte	Promotes granulosa cell proliferation
Human chorionic gonadotropin (hCG)	Placenta	Assists in maintenance of corpus luteum; promotes release of progesterone
Human placental lactogen	Placenta	Promotes mammary gland development during pregnancy; promotes lactogenesis
Relaxin	Placenta	Facilitates parturition by softening the fibrocartilage of pubic symphysis; softens the cervix and facilitates its dilation in preparation for parturition
Oxytocin	Hypothalamus via the posterior pituitary	Stimulates smooth muscle contraction of uterus during orgasm and during parturition; stimulates contraction of myoepithelial cells of mammary gland, assisting in milk ejection

vating meiosis-inducing substance) to complete meiosis I, forming a secondary oocyte and the first polar body. The secondary oocyte then enters meiosis II and proceeds to metaphase. Meiosis II is interrupted in metaphase until fertilization triggers its completion.

This surge of **LH** also launches the process of ovulation, whereby the secondary oocyte is expelled from the mature follicle. The granulosa cells and theca interna cells of the remaining ovulated follicle, both of which have **LH receptors,** are activated by LH to form the **corpus luteum.** The granulosa cells and the theca interna cells are converted into granulosa-lutein cells and theca-lutein cells, respectively. Both of these luteal cell types now actively produce **progesterone,** although most of it is produced by the granulosa-lutein cell. In addition, inhibin, folliostatin, and activin-

TABLE 20–4   Pulsatility Rate of LHRH Release

Rate of Release	Direct Results	Effects of Direct Results
Less than 60 minutes	Down-regulates LHRH receptor formation	Anovulation due to lack of gonadotropin responsivity
Greater than 90 minutes	Inadequate stimulation of basophils	Anovulation and amenorrhea
Between 60 and 90 minutes	Adequate number of LHRH receptors on basophils	Normal ovulatory cycle

LHRH, luteinizing hormone–releasing hormone.

feedback regulators of FSH release continue to be produced by the corpus luteum.

If fertilization and implantation do not occur, the secretory activity of the corpus luteum continues for about 14 days and the organ is called the **corpus luteum of menstruation.** When fertilization and implantation occur, the corpus luteum increases in size and the organ is known as the **corpus luteum of pregnancy.** This organ continues its secretory function even though the placenta assumes the primary responsibility for hormonal regulation (see Fig. 20-8).

Progesterone stimulates development of the uterine endometrium during each menstrual cycle and inhibits the production of LH directly and indirectly (acting on both the hypothalamus and the pituitary gonadotrophs). In the absence of pregnancy, LH level soon falls below that required to maintain the corpus luteum, and the process of corpus luteum degeneration begins. If pregnancy occurs, **hCG** produced by the placenta provides positive feedback to the corpus luteum of pregnancy, thereby maintaining the production of progesterone early in pregnancy. By the 4th month of pregnancy, much of the hormonal control is assumed by the placenta. Another hormone, **relaxin,** produced by the placenta, facilitates parturition by softening of the fibrocartilage of the pubic symphysis to ease the widening of the pelvic outlet.

Although as many as 50 follicles begin to mature in each menstrual cycle and as many as five may reach the graafian follicle stage, usually only one of these follicles ovulates. The precise reason is not known; however, when a graafian follicle reaches a particular stage of development, when it is known as the **dominant follicle,** it is no longer FSH-dependent. The dominant follicle begins to produce large quantities of **inhibin,** the hormone that suppresses FSH release by the anterior pituitary. The lack of FSH, in turn, causes the remaining graafian follicles that are still FSH-dependent to atrophy, leaving only the dominant graafian follicle in the position of becoming ready for ovulation. In order for a multilaminar primary follicle to reach the dominant follicle stage, it has to pass through three ovulatory cycles; once the follicle becomes dominant, it still has to wait for about 15 days before it can become ovulated. Thus the period of time that has to pass between the multilaminar primary follicle stage and ovulation is approximately 100 days.

Oviducts (Fallopian Tubes)

The oviducts act as a conduit for spermatozoa to reach the primary oocyte and to convey the fertilized egg to the uterus.

The oviducts, or fallopian tubes, are paired, muscular-walled tubular structures approximately 12 cm long, each with an open end and an attached end (see Fig. 20-1). The oviducts become continuous with the wall of the uterus at their attached ends, where they traverse the uterine wall to open into its lumen. The free ends open into the peritoneal cavity close to the ovaries.

The oviducts are divided into four anatomical regions:

■ Beginning at the open end is the **infundibulum,** whose open end is fringed with projections called **fimbriae.** These fimbriae help to capture the secondary oocyte.
■ The expanded **ampulla** is where fertilization usually takes place.
■ The **isthmus** is the narrowed portion between the ampulla and the uterus.
■ The **intramural region** passes through the uterine wall to open into the lumen of the uterus.

The oviducts are covered by visceral peritoneum. Their walls are composed of three layers (Fig. 20-9):

■ Mucosa
■ Muscularis
■ Serosa

The **mucosa** is characterized by many longitudinal folds. These folds are present in all four regions of the

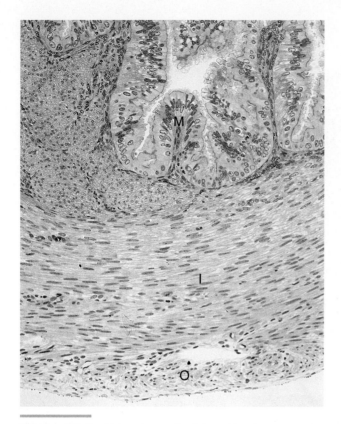

Figure 20–9 Light micrograph of the oviduct in cross section (×132). Observe the outer longitudinal (O) and inner circular (I) muscle layers and the mucosa (M). The mucosa is thrown into folds that reduce the size of the lumen.

oviduct but are most pronounced in the ampulla, where they branch; in the other regions, the mucosal folds are reduced to low elevations. The **simple columnar epithelium** that lines the lumen is tallest in the infundibulum and shortens as the oviduct approaches the uterus. Two different cell types constitute this epithelium:

- *Nonciliated* peg cells
- *Ciliated* cells

Peg cells have no cilia. They have a secretory function, providing a nutritive and protective environment for maintaining spermatozoa on their migration route to reach the secondary oocyte. Products within the secretions of the peg cells facilitate **capacitation** of spermatozoa, a process whereby spermatozoa become fully mature and capable of fertilizing the ovum. It is not known whether human spermatozoa require capacitation, because they are capable of in vitro fertilization of the ovum without being exposed to the female reproductive tract. If there is such a requirement, the sojourn in the female reproductive tract necessitates only a minimal amount of time. Secretory products also provide nutrition and protection to the ovum; if the

ovum is fertilized, the same secretions provide nutrients to the embryo during the initial phases of its development. The secretions of peg cells coupled with the movement of the fluid toward the uterus inhibit microorganisms in the uterus from moving to the oviduct and into the peritoneal cavity.

The **cilia** of the columnar **ciliated cells** beat in unison toward the uterus. As a result, the fertilized ovum, spermatozoa, and the viscous liquid produced by the peg cells are all propelled toward the uterus (Fig. 20-10).

The **lamina propria** of the oviduct mucosa is unremarkable; it is composed of loose connective tissue containing fibroblasts, mast cells, lymphoid cells, collagen, and reticular fibers. The **muscularis** consists of poorly defined inner circular and outer longitudinal layers of smooth muscle. Loose connective tissue also fills spaces between the bundles of muscle. A simple squamous epithelium provides the **serosal covering** of the oviduct. The loose connective tissue between the serosa and the muscularis contains many blood vessels and autonomic nerve fibers.

Because the oviducts are so richly vascularized with mostly large veins, contractions of the muscularis during ovulation constrict the engorged veins. This constriction causes distention of the entire oviduct and brings the fimbriae into contact with the ovary, thereby aiding the capture of the released secondary oocyte. Continued rhythmic contractions of the layers of the muscularis, coupled with the beating of the cilia within, help to propel the captured oocyte to the uterus.

Uterus

The uterus is a muscular organ consisting of a fundus, body, and cervix.

The uterus, a single, thick, pear-shaped structure located in the midline of the pelvis, receives at its broad, closed end the terminals of the paired oviducts. The uterus is a robust muscular organ about 7 cm long, 4 cm wide, and 2.5 cm thick. It is divided into three regions (see Fig. 20-1):

- The **body,** the broad portion into which the oviducts open
- The **fundus,** the rounded base located superior to the exit ports of the oviducts in the body
- The **cervix,** the narrow circular portion that protrudes and opens into the vagina

Body and Fundus

*The uterine wall of the body and the fundus is composed of an **endometrium, myometrium,** and either an **adventitia** or a **serosa.***

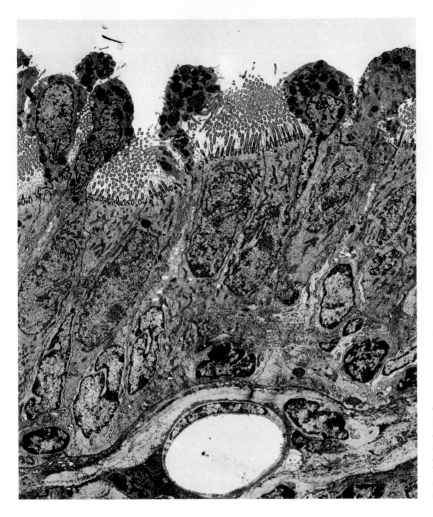

Figure 20–10 Electron micrograph of the oviduct epithelium (×40,000). Note the bulbous apices of the peg cells as well as the cilia of the ciliated cells. (From Hollis DE, Frith PA, Vaughan JD, et al: Ultrastructural changes in the oviductal epithelium of merino ewes during the estrous cycle. Am J Anat 171:441-456, 1984.)

Endometrium

The endometrium is the mucosal lining of the uterus, consisting of two layers, the superficial functionalis and the deeper located basalis.

The endometrium, or mucosal lining of the uterus, is composed of a simple columnar epithelium and a lamina propria. The epithelium is composed of **non-ciliated secretory columnar cells** and **ciliated cells,** whereas the lamina propria houses simple branched **tubular glands** that extend as far as the myometrium (Fig. 20-11). Although the glandular cells resemble those of the surface epithelium, there are no ciliated cells in the glands. The dense, irregular collagenous connective tissue of the **lamina propria** is highly cellular and contains star-shaped cells, macrophages, leukocytes, and an abundance of reticular fibers. The morphological and physiological alterations that occur in the endometrium during the phases of the menstrual cycle are controlled by various hormones (see later).

The endometrium consists of two layers (see Fig. 20-11):

- The **functionalis,** a thick, superficial layer that is sloughed at menstruation
- The **basalis,** a deep, narrow layer whose glands and connective tissue elements proliferate and thereby regenerate the functionalis during each menstrual cycle

The **functionalis** is vascularized by numerous coiled **helical arteries,** which originate from the **arcuate arteries** of the stratum vasculare, located in the middle layer of the myometrium. The coiled arteries give rise to a rich capillary network that supplies the glands and connective tissue of the functionalis. Another set of arteries, the **straight arteries,** also originate from the arcuate arteries but are much shorter and supply only the basalis.

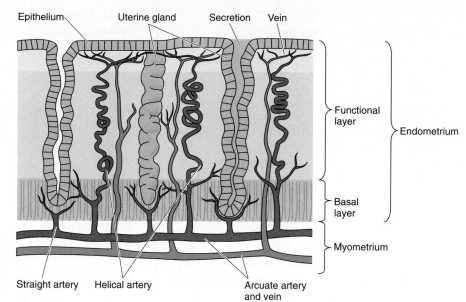

Epithelium Uterine gland Secretion Vein

Functional layer

Endometrium

Basal layer

Myometrium

Straight artery Helical artery Arcuate artery and vein

Figure 20–11 The uterine endometrium, showing the basal and functional layers. The basal layer is supplied by the straight arteries, whereas the functional layer is served by the coiled vessels known as helical arteries.

Myometrium

The myometrium is composed of inner longitudinal, middle circular, and outer longitudinal layers of smooth muscle.

The thick muscular wall of the uterus, the myometrium, is composed of *three layers* of smooth muscle. **Longitudinal muscle** makes up the *inner* and *outer layers,* whereas the richly *vascularized middle layer* contains mostly **circularly** arranged smooth muscle bundles. This richly vascularized region houses the **arcuate arteries** and is called the **stratum vasculare.** As the uterus narrows toward the cervix, the amount of muscle tissue diminishes and is replaced by fibrous connective tissue. At the cervix, the myometrium is composed of dense, irregular connective tissue containing elastic fibers and only a small number of scattered smooth muscle cells.

The size and number of the myometrial muscle cells are related to estrogen levels. The muscle cells are largest and most numerous during pregnancy, when estrogen levels are the highest; they are smallest after the conclusion of menstruation, when estrogen levels are low. When estrogen is absent, the myometrial muscle atrophies, with some cells succumbing to **apoptosis.** Although most of the increase in uterine size during pregnancy is related to **hypertrophy** of the smooth muscle cells, the smooth muscle cell population also increases, suggesting that **hyperplasia** also occurs. However, it is unclear whether the increase in cell number results only from division

of smooth muscle cells or also from differentiation of undifferentiated cells into smooth muscle fibers.

Sexual stimulation causes moderate uterine contractions. During menstruation, the contractions may be painful in some women. Powerful, rhythmic contractions of the pregnant uterus during delivery expel the fetus and later the placenta from the uterus. The process of uterine contractions during parturition is due to hormonal actions:

▪ Under the influence of **corticotropic hormone,** the myometrium and the fetal membranes produce **prostaglandins.**
▪ The posterior pituitary gland releases the hormone **oxytocin.**
▪ Prostaglandins and oxytocin stimulate uterine contractions.
▪ After delivery, oxytocin continues to stimulate uterine contractions, which inhibit excessive blood loss from the detachment site of the placenta.

Uterine Serosa and Adventitia

Because the uterus is tipped anteriorly and lies against the bladder, much of its anterior portion is covered by adventitia (connective tissue without an epithelial covering); thus, this area is **retroperitoneal.** The fundus and posterior portion of the body are covered by a serosa, composed of a layer of squamous mesothelial cells resting on areolar connective tissue; therefore this area is intraperitoneal.

Cervix

The cervix—the terminal end of the uterus—extends into the vagina.

The cervix is the terminal end of the uterus that protrudes into the vagina (see Fig. 20-1). The lumen of the cervix is lined by a **mucus-secreting simple columnar epithelium;** however, its external surface, where the cervix protrudes into the vagina, is covered by a **stratified squamous nonkeratinized epithelium** similar to that of the vagina. The wall of the cervix consists mostly of dense, collagenous connective tissue containing many elastic fibers and only a few smooth muscle fibers. Cervical mucosa contains branched **cervical glands.** Although the cervical mucosa changes during the menstrual cycle, it does not slough during menstruation.

At the midpoint in the menstrual cycle, around the time of ovulation, the cervical glands secrete a serous fluid that facilitates entry of the spermatozoa into the uterus. At other times, including during pregnancy, the secretions of the cervical glands become more viscous, forming a plug of thickened mucus in the orifice of the cervix, thus preventing the entry of sperm and microorganisms into the uterus. The hormone **progesterone** regulates the changes in the viscosity of the cervical gland secretions.

At the time of parturition, another luteal hormone, **relaxin,** induces lysis of collagen in the cervical walls. This results in a softening of the cervix, thus facilitating cervical dilation.

Menstrual Cycle

The menstrual cycle is divided into the menstrual, proliferative (follicular), and secretory (luteal) phases.

Normally, the average menstrual cycle is a 28-day cycle. Although the successive events constituting the cycle occur continuously, they can be described in three phases: **menstrual phase**, **proliferative (follicular) phase,** and **secretory (luteal) phase** (Fig. 20-12).

Menstrual Phase (Days 1 to 4)

The menstrual phase of the menstrual cycle is characterized by the desquamation of the functionalis layer of the endometrium.

Menstruation, which begins on the day that bleeding from the uterus starts, occurs when fertilization does not take place. In this case, the corpus luteum becomes nonfunctional about 14 days after ovulation, thus *reducing* the levels of **progesterone** and **estrogen.**

A couple of days before bleeding begins, the functionalis layer of the endometrium becomes deprived of

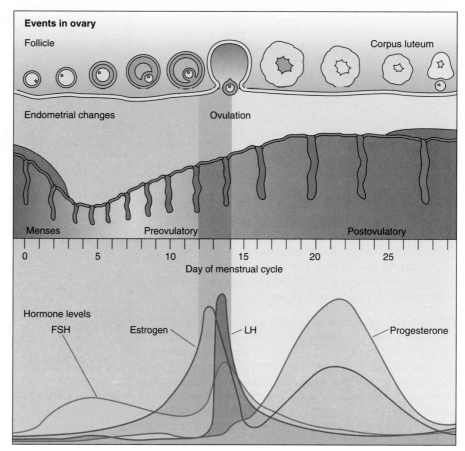

Events in ovary

Follicle

Corpus luteum

Endometrial changes

Ovulation

Menses

Preovulatory

Postovulatory

0   5   10   15   20   25

Day of menstrual cycle

Hormone levels

FSH   Estrogen   LH   Progesterone

Figure 20–12 Correlation of events in follicular development, ovulation, hormonal interrelationships, and the menstrual cycle. Note that the levels of estrogen and luteinizing hormone (LH) are highest at the time of ovulation. FSH, follicle-stimulating hormone.

blood as the coiled (helical) arteries are intermittently constricted. After 2 days or so, the coiled arteries become permanently constricted, reducing oxygen to the functionalis layer, leading to a shutdown of the glands, invasion by leukocytes, ischemia, and eventual **necrosis** of the **functionalis.** Shortly thereafter, the coiled arteries dilate once again; however, because these coiled arteries have been weakened by the previous events, they rupture. The disgorged blood removes patches of the functionalis to be discharged as a **hemorrhagic discharge (menses),** initiating menstruation on day 1.

Although the entire functionalis layer of the endometrium is sloughed, it is not completely released from the wall immediately; rather, this process continues for 3 to 4 days. During a normal menstrual period, the approximate blood loss is 35 mL, although in some women it may be greater.

Before and during the menstrual phase, the basalis layer of the endometrium continues to be vascularized by its own straight arteries and thus remains viable. The basal cells of the glands of the basalis begin to proliferate, and the newly formed cells migrate to the surface to begin reepithelialization of the connective tissue

wound of the uterine lumen. These events commence the proliferative phase of the menstrual cycle.

Proliferative (Follicular) Phase (Days 4 to 14)

The proliferative phase of the menstrual cycle is characterized by a reepithelialization of the lining of the endometrium and renewal of the functionalis.

The proliferative phase (also called the follicular phase because it occurs at the same time as the development of the ovarian follicles) begins when menstrual flow ceases, on about day 4, and continues through day 14. The proliferative phase is characterized by reepithelialization of the lining of the endometrium; reconstruction of the glands, connective tissue, and the coiled arteries of the lamina propria; and renewal of the functionalis.

During this phase, the functional layer becomes much thicker (up to 2 to 3 mm) because the proliferation of the cells in the base of the glands, whose blood supply remained intact, were unaffected during the menstrual phase. As stated before, it is these cells that are responsible for the formation of the epithelial lining of the uterus as well as for the establishment of new glands in the functionalis. These tubular glands are straight (not yet coiled), but their cells begin to accumulate glycogen, as do the cells of the stroma that proliferated to renew the stroma of the functionalis. The coiled arteries that were lost in the menstrual phase are replaced but are not tightly coiled and reach only two thirds of the way into the functionalis.

By the 14th day of the menstrual cycle (ovulation), the functionalis layer of the endometrium has been fully restored to its previous status with a full complement of epithelium, glands, stroma, and coiled arteries.

Secretory (Luteal) Phase (Days 15 to 28)

The secretory phase of the menstrual cycle is characterized by thickening of the endometrium as a result of edema and accumulated glycogen secretions of the highly coiled endometrial glands.

The secretory phase (or luteal phase) commences after ovulation. During this phase, the endometrium continues to thicken as a result of edema and accumulated glycogen secretions of the endometrial glands, which become highly convoluted and branched. The secretory products first accumulate in the basal region of the cytoplasm of the cells constituting the endometrial glands. As more secretory product is manufactured, the secretory granules move apically and are released into the lumen of the gland. This glycogen-rich material will nourish the conceptus before the formation of the placenta.

Most of the changes that result in the thickening of the endometrium are attributed to the functionalis, although the lumina of the glands located in the basalis are also filled with secretory product (Fig. 20-13). The coiled arteries of the functionalis attain full development, becoming more coiled and extending fully into the functional layer, by the 22nd day. Thus, at this point in the secretory phase, the endometrium is about 5 mm thick.

The secretory phase completes the cycle as the 28th day approaches, prestaging the menstrual phase of a new menstrual cycle.

Fertilization, Implantation, and Placental Development

Fertilization

Fertilization, the fusion of the sperm and the oocyte, occurs in the ampulla of the oviduct.

The oocyte and its attendant follicular cells are transported down the oviduct by the beating of the cilia of the ciliated cells of the epithelial lining and by rhythmic

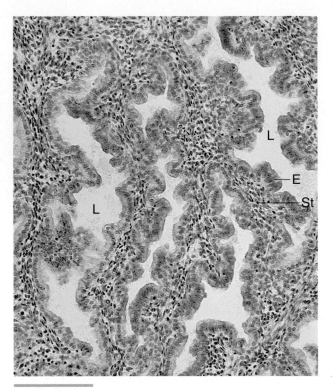

Figure 20–13 Light micrograph of the endometrium (E) of the uterus in the luteal phase (×132). Note the lumina (L) of the glands surrounded by stromal cells (St).

contractions of the smooth muscle of the oviduct (Fig. 20-14). The nutrient-rich fluid produced by peg cells of the mucosal epithelium nourishes the oocyte on its way to the uterus.

Spermatozoa, introduced into the vagina during sexual intercourse, pass through the cervix, the uterine lumen, and up the oviduct to the ampulla to encounter the secondary oocyte. Fertilization usually occurs in the ampulla (Fig. 20-15). At this time, the cells of the corona radiata still surround the **zona pellucida** and the secondary oocyte.

The ZP_3 molecules of the zona pellucida have two regions: (1) the sperm receptor that recognizes integral proteins of the sperm plasmalemma, and (2) the other region of the ZP_3 molecule that binds to receptor proteins located in the head of the sperm, triggering the **acrosome reaction.** This reaction results in the release of the acrosomal enzymes into the zona pellucida. The liberated enzymes, especially the inner acrosomal membrane–bound enzyme **acrosin,** digest the zona pellucida, permitting the flagellar movement of the spermatozoa to propel the sperm toward the oocyte. Once the spermatozoon penetrates the entire width of the zona pellucida, it enters the **perivitelline space,** located between the zona pellucida and the oocyte cell membrane, and can reach the oocyte.

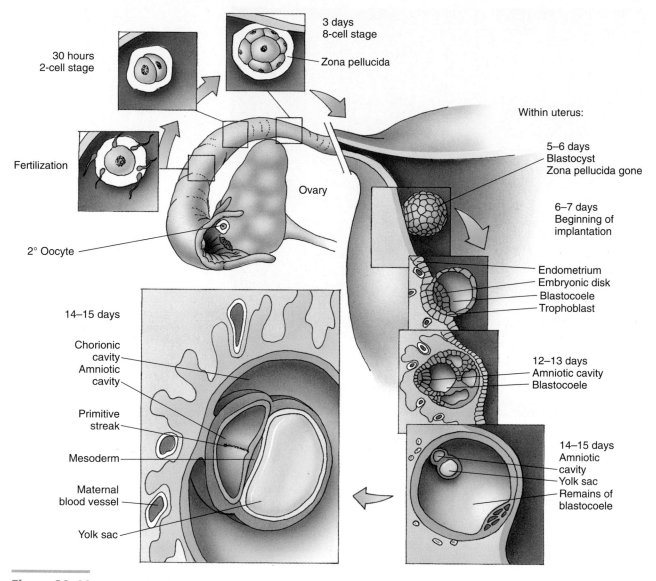

Figure 20–14 Process of fertilization, zygote formation, morula and blastocyst development, and implantation.

The contact between the sperm and the oocyte is responsible for the **cortical reaction,** which prevents **polyspermy,** the process by which more than a single sperm fuses with the egg. The cortical reaction has a fast and a slow component. The **fast component** involves a change in the resting membrane potential of the oocyte plasma membrane that prevents contact between the oocyte and another sperm. This alteration of the membrane potential lasts only a few minutes. The **slow component** involves the release of the contents of numerous cortical granules located in the oocyte's cytoplasm into the perivitelline space. Enzymes within the cortical granules act to hydrolyze ZP_3 molecules, the

sperm receptors, in the zona pellucida, thus preventing additional spermatozoa from reaching the oocyte.

At this time, entry of the sperm nucleus triggers the secondary oocyte to resume and complete its second meiotic division. This results in an unequal division of the cytoplasm, forming two haploid cells, the **ovum** and the **second polar body.** The nucleus of the ovum **(female pronucleus)** fuses with the nucleus of the spermatozoon **(male pronucleus),** forming a **zygote** with the diploid number of chromosomes and thus completing the event of fertilization.

The window of time between ovulation and fertilization is about 24 hours. If fertilization does not occur

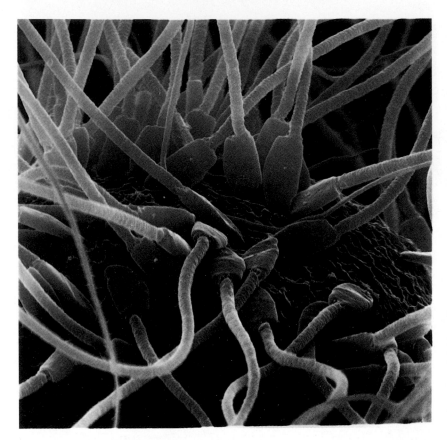

Figure 20–15 Scanning electron micrograph of fertilization (×5700). A large number of spermatozoa are trying to make their way through the cells of the corona radiata, but only a single spermatozoon will be able to fertilize the egg. (From Phillips DM, Shalgi R, Dekel N: Mammalian fertilization as seen with the scanning electron microscope. Am J Anat 174:357-372, 1985.)

during this period, the oocyte degenerates and is phagocytosed by macrophages.

Implantation

Implantation is the process that occurs as the blastocyst becomes embedded in the uterine endometrium.

As the zygote continues its journey through the oviduct on its way to the uterus, it undergoes numerous mitotic divisions, becoming the spherical cluster of cells known as the **morula** (see Fig. 20-14). With further divisions and modifications, the morula is transformed into the **blastocyst,** composed of a hollow ball of cells whose lumen contains a somewhat viscous fluid and a few cells at one pole. The peripheral cells are known as **trophoblasts,** and the cells trapped inside the blastocyst are the **embryoblasts.** The blastocyst enters the uterine cavity about 4 to 6 days after fertilization, and on the 6th or 7th day it begins to embed itself into the uterine wall, a process known as **implantation.** The trophoblasts of the blastocyst stimulate the transformation of the star-shaped **stromal cells** of the uterine endometrium into pale-staining **decidual cells,** whose stored glycogen probably provides nourishment for the developing embryo.

The embryoblasts develop into the embryo, whereas **trophoblast cells** give rise to the embryonic portion of the placenta. Trophoblast cells proliferate rapidly, forming an inner conglomeration of individual cells, which are mitotically active and are known as **cytotrophoblasts,** and a thicker outer syncytium of cells that do not undergo mitosis, called **syncytiotrophoblasts.**

The **cytotrophoblasts** proliferate, with the new cells joining the syncytiotrophoblasts. As the syncytiotrophoblasts increase in number, they form vacuoles that coalesce into large, labyrinthine spaces known as **lacunae.** Continued growth of the syncytium erodes the endometrium. This process permits deep penetration of the blastocyst into the wall of the endometrium, and by the 11th day of gestation the endometrial epithelium seals over the implantation site.

Placenta Development

The placenta is a vascular tissue derived from the uterine endometrium as well as from the developing embryo.

Continued erosion of the highly vascular endometrium by the **syncytiotrophoblasts** also erodes the maternal blood vessels. The blood from these vessels empties into

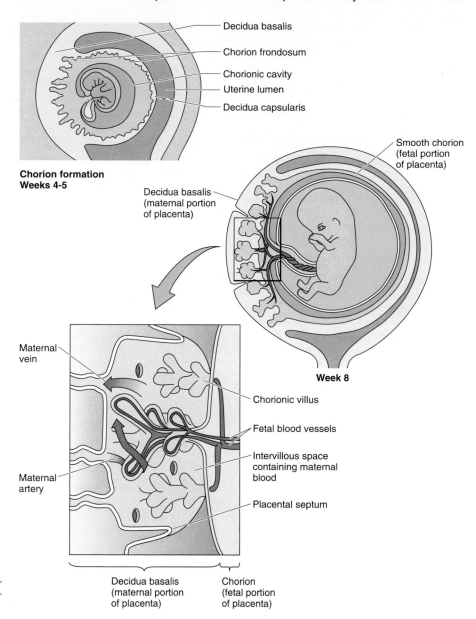

Figure 20–16 Chorion and decidua formation; *inset* shows circulation within the placenta.

the lacunae of the syncytiotrophoblasts that surround the embryo. Thus, the maternal blood provides nourishment for the developing embryo. With further growth and development, the **placenta** begins to be formed, with the resultant separation between the blood of the developing embryo and that of the mother (maternal blood). From the remainder of the trophoblast cells, the **chorion** develops and evolves into the **chorionic plate,** which gives rise to the **chorionic villi** (Fig. 20-16).

The developing trophoblasts induce changes in the endometrium in their vicinity, altering it to begin the formation of the maternal portion of the placenta. This

altered maternal tissue, called the **decidua,** is subdivided into three regions:

- The **decidua capsularis,** interposed between the uterine lumen and the developing embryo
- The **decidua basalis,** interposed between the developing embryo and the myometrium
- The **decidua parietalis,** which constitutes the balance of the decidua

Initially, the entire embryo is surrounded by decidua in order to nourish it. The region of the chorion in contact with the decidua capsularis forms short, insubstantial villi, thus remaining smooth-surfaced; this region of the chorion is known as the **chorion laeve.** The region of the decidua capsularis, however, becomes highly vascularized by maternal blood vessels; it is in this region that the placenta develops. The region of the chorionic plate in contact with the decidua basalis forms extensive chorionic villi, known as **primary villi;** thus, this region of the chorion is known as the **chorion frondosum.**

The primary villi are composed of both syncytiotrophoblasts and cytotrophoblasts. With further development, extraembryonic mesenchymal cells enter the core of the primary villi, converting them into **secondary villi** (Fig. 20-17). The connective tissue of the secondary villi becomes vascularized by extensive capillary beds, which are linked to the developing vascular supply of the embryo.

As development continues, the cytotrophoblast population decreases because these cells join the syncytium and contribute to its growth. The decidua basalis forms large vascular spaces, **lacunae,** that are compartmentalized into smaller regions by **placental septa,** extensions of the decidua. Secondary villi project into these vascular spaces and are surrounded by maternal blood

that is delivered to and drained from the lacunae by maternal blood vessels of the decidua basalis.

Most of the villi are not anchored to the decidua basalis but are suspended in maternal blood of the lacunae, similar to roots of vegetables grown in hydroponic environments; these are known as **free villi.** The villi anchored to the decidua basalis are called **anchoring villi.** Capillaries of free and anchoring villi are near the surface of the villi and are separated from the maternal blood by a slight amount of connective tissue and the syncytiotrophoblasts covering the secondary villus. Thus, maternal blood and fetal blood do not intermix; instead, nutrients and oxygen from maternal blood diffuse through the syncytiotrophoblasts, connective tissue, and endothelial cells of the capillaries of the villi to reach the fetal blood. These structures form the **placental barrier.** Certain substances, such as water, oxygen, carbon dioxide, small molecules, some proteins, lipids, hormones, drugs, and some antibodies (especially immunoglobulin G), can penetrate the placental barrier, whereas most macromolecules cannot.

In addition to being the site where nutritious substances, waste, and gases are exchanged between maternal and fetal blood, the placenta (specifically the syncytiotrophoblast) serves as an endocrine organ, secreting **hCG, chorionic thyrotropin, progesterone, estrogen,** and **chorionic somatomammotropin** (a growth-promoting and lactogenic hormone). Also, stromal connective tissue cells of the decidua form the **decidual cells,** which enlarge and synthesize **prolactin** and **prostaglandins.**

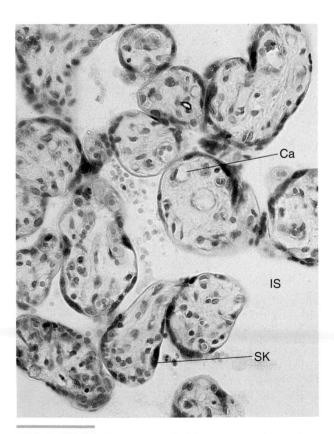

Figure 20–17 Light micrograph of cross sections of the chorionic villi of the placenta (×270). Observe the cytotrophoblasts and syncytiotrophoblasts covering the chorionic villi. Ca, capillary; IS, intervillous space; SK, syncytial knot.

CLINICAL CORRELATIONS

The blastocyst usually implants into the upper one third of the anterior or posterior wall of the uterus and it is in that location that the placenta will begin to develop. Occasionally, in 1 out of 200 pregnancies, implantation occurs lower down in the uterus, near the cervix, where the endometrium is much thinner and the connective tissue stroma is much denser. As the placenta begins to develop and enlarge, it covers partially or completely the opening of the cervix, making normal, vaginal delivery an untenable option. This condition is referred to as **placenta previa** and usually necessitates the delivery of the baby via a cesarean section.

Vagina

The vagina, a fibromuscular sheath, is composed of three layers: mucosa, muscularis, and adventitia.

The vagina is a fibromuscular tubular structure 8 to 9 cm in length connected to the uterus proximally and to the vestibule of the external genitalia distally. The vagina consists of three layers: **mucosa, muscularis,** and **adventitia.**

The lumen of the vagina is lined by a thick **stratified squamous nonkeratinized epithelium** (150 to 200 μm thick), although some of the superficial cells may contain keratohyalin. Langerhans cells in the epithelium function in antigen presentation to T lymphocytes housed in the inguinal lymph nodes. The epithelial cells are stimulated by estrogen to synthesize and store large deposits of **glycogen,** which is released into the lumen as the vaginal epithelial cells are sloughed. Naturally occurring vaginal bacterial flora metabolize the glycogen, forming **lactic acid,** which is responsible for the low pH in the lumen of the vagina, especially at the midpoint of the menstrual cycle. The lowered pH also helps to restrict pathogenic invasion.

The **lamina propria** of the vagina is composed of loose fibroelastic connective tissue containing a rich vascular supply in its deeper regions. It also contains numerous lymphocytes and neutrophils that reach the lumen by passing through intercellular spaces during certain periods in the menstrual cycle, where they participate in immune responses. Although the vagina does not contain glands, there is an increase in vaginal fluid during sexual stimulation, arousal, and intercourse that serves to lubricate its lining. This fluid is derived from the transudate present in the lamina propria combined with secretions from glands of the cervix.

The **muscularis** layer of the vagina is composed of smooth muscle cells arranged so that the mostly longitudinal bundles of the external surface intermingle with the more circularly arranged bundles near the lumen. A sphincter muscle, composed of skeletal muscle fibers, encircles the vagina at its external opening.

Dense, fibroelastic connective tissue constitutes the **adventitia** of the vagina, attaching it to surrounding structures. Contained within the adventitia is a rich vascular supply with a vast venous plexus and nerve bundles derived from the pelvic splanchnic nerves.

External Genitalia

The external genitalia (vulva) are composed of the labia majora, labia minora, vestibule, and clitoris.

The **labia majora** are two folds of skin heavily endowed with adipose tissue and a thin layer of smooth muscle. The homologue of these structures in the male is the scrotum, with the smooth muscle layer corresponding to the dartos muscle of the scrotum. The labia majora are covered with coarse hair on their external surface but are devoid of hair on their smooth inner surface.

Numerous sweat glands and sebaceous glands open on both surfaces.

The **labia minora,** located medial to and slightly deep to the labia majora, are the homologues of the urethral surface of the penis in the male. The labia minora are two smaller folds of skin devoid of hair follicles and adipose tissue. Their core is composed of a spongy connective tissue containing elastic fibers arranged in networks. They contain numerous sebaceous glands and are richly supplied with blood vessels and nerve endings.

The cleft situated between the right and left labia minora is the **vestibule,** a space that receives secretions of the **glands of Bartholin,** which are paired mucus-secreting glands, and many small **minor vestibular glands.** Also located in the vestibule are the orifices of the urethra and the vagina. In virgins, the orifice of the vagina is narrowed by a fold of epithelially enclosed fibrovascular tissue called the **hymen.**

The **clitoris** is located between the folds of the labia minora superiorly, where the two labia minora unite to form the prepuce over the top of the **glans clitoridis.** The **clitoris,** the female homologue of the penis, is covered by stratified squamous epithelium and is composed of two **erectile bodies** containing numerous blood vessels and sensory nerves, including Meissner's and pacinian corpuscles, which are sensitive during sexual arousal.

Mammary Glands

The mammary glands are compound tubuloalveolar glands that consist of 15 to 20 lobes radiating out from the nipple and are separated from each other by adipose and collagenous connective tissue.

Mammary glands secrete milk, a fluid containing proteins, lipids, and lactose as well as lymphocytes and monocytes, antibodies, minerals, and fat-soluble vitamins, to provide the proper nourishment for the newborn.

The mammary glands develop in the same manner and are of the same structure in both sexes until puberty, when changes in the hormonal secretions in females cause further development and structural changes within the glands. Secretions of **estrogen** and **progesterone** from the ovaries (and later from the placenta) and **prolactin** from the acidophils of the anterior pituitary gland initiate development of **lobules** and **terminal ductules.** Full development of the ductal portion of the breast requires **glucocorticoids** and further activation by **somatotropin.**

Concomitant with these events is an increase in connective tissue and adipose tissue within the stroma, causing the gland to enlarge. Full development occurs at about 20 years of age, with minor cyclic changes during each menstrual period, whereas major changes occur during pregnancy and in lactation. After age 40 or so, the secretory portions as well as some of the ducts and connective tissue elements of the breasts begin to atrophy, and they continue this process throughout menopause.

The glands within the breasts are classified as **compound tubuloalveolar glands,** consisting of 15 to 20 lobes radiating out from the nipple and separated from each other by adipose and collagenous connective tissue. Each lobe is drained by its own **lactiferous duct** leading directly to the **nipple,** where it opens onto its surface. Before reaching the nipple, each of the ducts is dilated to form a **lactiferous sinus** for milk storage and then narrows before passing through the nipple.

Resting (Nonsecreting) Mammary Glands

Alveoli are not developed in the resting mammary gland.

Resting, or nonsecreting, mammary glands of nonpregnant women have the same basic architecture as the lactating (active) mammary gland, except that they are smaller and without developed alveoli, which occur only during pregnancy. Near the opening at the nipple, lactiferous ducts are lined by a stratified squamous (keratinized) epithelium. The lactiferous sinus and the lactiferous duct leading to it are lined by stratified cuboidal epithelium, whereas the smaller ducts leading to the lactiferous duct are lined by a simple columnar epithelium. Stellate myoepithelial cells located between the epithelium and the basal lamina also wrap around the developing alveoli and become functional during pregnancy.

Lactating (Active) Mammary Glands

During pregnancy, the terminal portions of the ducts branch and grow and develop secretory units known as alveoli.

Mammary glands are activated by elevated surges of **estrogen** and **progesterone** during pregnancy to become lactating glands to provide milk for the newborn. At this time, the terminal portions of the ducts branch and grow and the alveoli develop and mature (Fig. 20-18). As pregnancy progresses, the breasts enlarge as a result of hypertrophy of the glan-

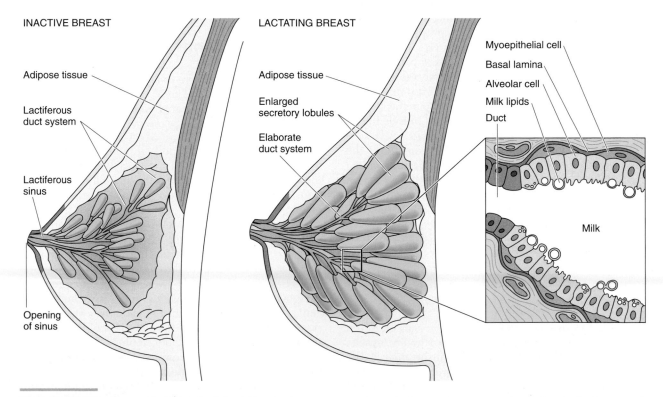

Figure 20–18 Comparison of the glandular differences between an inactive and a lactating breast. *Inset* shows a longitudinal section of a gland and duct of the active mammary gland.

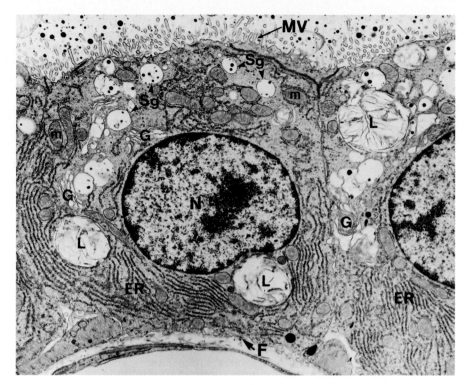

Figure 20–19 Electron micrograph of an acinar cell from the lactating mammary gland of the rat (×9000). Note the large lipid droplets (L), abundant rough endoplasmic reticulum (ER), and Golgi apparatus (G). F, folds of the basal plasmalemma; m, mitochondria; MV, microvilli; Sg, secretory granules; (From Clermont Y, Xia I, Rambourg A, et al: Structure of the Golgi apparatus in stimulated and nonstimulated acinar cells of mammary glands of the rat. Anat Rec 237:308-317, 1993.)

dular parenchyma and engorgement with **colostrum,** a protein-rich fluid, in preparation for the newborn. Within a few days after birth, when estrogen and progesterone secretions have subsided, **prolactin,** secreted by acidophils of the anterior pituitary gland, activates the secretion of milk, which replaces the colostrum.

The **alveoli** of the lactating (active) mammary glands are composed of cuboidal cells partially surrounded by a meshwork of myoepithelial cells. These secretory cells possess abundant RER and mitochondria, several Golgi complexes, many lipid droplets, and numerous vesicles (Fig. 20-19) containing caseins (milk proteins) and lactose. However, not all regions of the alveolus are in the same stage of production, because different acini display varying degrees of preparation for synthesis of milk substances (Fig. 20-20).

The secretions of the alveolar cells are of two kinds: lipids and proteins.

Lipids are stored as droplets within the cytoplasm. They are released from the secretory cells, possibly by the **apocrine** mode of exocytosis, whereby small droplets coalesce to form larger and larger droplets that move to the periphery of the cell. Once there, they project as cytoplasmic blebs into the lumen; eventually, the lipid droplets containing blebs are pinched off and become part of the secretory product. Each bleb then consists of a central lipid droplet surrounded by a narrow rim of cytoplasm and enclosed by a plasmalemma.

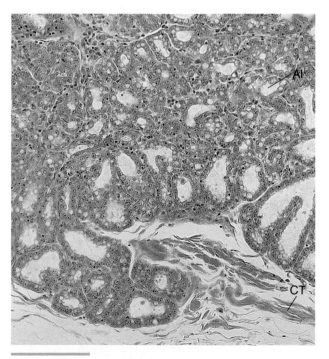

Figure 20–20 Light micrograph of the human mammary gland (×132). Observe the crowded alveoli (Al), and note that various regions of the gland are in different stages of the secretory process. CT, connective tissue.

Proteins synthesized within these secretory cells are liberated from the cells by the **merocrine** mode of exocytosis in much the same manner as would be expected of other cells that synthesize and release proteins into the extracellular space.

Areola and Nipple

The circular, heavily pigmented skin in the center of the breast is the areola. It contains sweat glands and sebaceous glands at its margin as well as **areolar glands (of Montgomery)** that resemble both sweat and mammary glands. In the center of the areola is the nipple, a protuberance covered by stratified squamous epithelium containing the terminal openings of the lactiferous ducts. In fair-skinned individuals, a pinkish color is imparted to the nipple as a result of the color of blood in the rich vascular supply within the long dermal papillae that extend near its surface. During pregnancy, the color becomes darker because of increased pigmentation of the areola and the nipple.

The core of the nipple is composed of dense collagenous connective tissue with abundant elastic fibers connected to the surrounding skin or interlaced within the connective tissue and a rich component of smooth muscle cells. The wrinkling of the skin on the nipple results from the attachments of the elastic fibers. The abundant smooth muscle fibers are arranged in two ways: circularly around the nipple and radiating longitudinally along the long axis of the nipple. The contraction of these muscle fibers is responsible for erection of the nipple.

Most of the sebaceous glands located around the lactiferous ducts open onto the surface or sides of the nipple, although some open into the lactiferous ducts just before those ducts open onto the surface.

Mammary Gland Secretions

Prolactin is responsible for the production of milk by the mammary glands; oxytocin is responsible for the milk ejection reflex.

Although the mammary gland is prepared to secrete milk even before birth, certain hormones prohibit this. However, when the placenta is detached in the adult female, **prolactin** from the anterior pituitary stimulates the production of milk, which reaches full capacity in a few days. Before that, for the first 2 or 3 days after birth, a protein-rich thick fluid called **colostrum** is secreted. This high-protein secretion, rich in vitamin A, sodium, and chloride, also contains lymphocytes and monocytes, minerals, lactalbumin, and antibodies (immunoglobulin A) to provide nutrition and passive immunity to the newborn.

Milk, usually produced by the 4th day after parturition, is a fluid that contains minerals, electrolytes, carbohydrates (including lactose), immunoglobulins (mostly immunoglobulin A), proteins (including caseins), and lipids. Production of milk results from the stimuli of sight, touch, handling of the newborn, and anticipation of nursing, events that create a surge in **prolactin** release. Once initiated, milk production is continuous, with the milk being stored within the duct system.

Concomitant with the production of prolactin, **oxytocin** is released from the posterior lobe of the pituitary. Oxytocin initiates the **milk ejection reflex** by inducing contractions of the myoepithelial cells around the alveoli and the ducts, thus expelling the milk.

CLINICAL CORRELATIONS

Mothers who cannot **breast-feed** their infants on a regular feeding schedule are inclined to suffer from poor lactation. This may motivate a decision to discontinue nursing altogether, with the result that the infant is deprived of the passive immunity conferred by ingesting antibodies from the mother.

Breast cancer, second only to lung cancer as one of the major causes of cancer-related death in women, may be of two different types: **ductal carcinoma** of the ductal cells and **lobular carcinoma** of the terminal ductules. Detection must be early, or the prognosis is poor because the carcinoma may **metastasize** to the axillary lymph nodes and from there to the lungs, bone, and brain. At the recommendation of the medical profession, early detection through self-examination and mammography has helped to reduce breast cancer mortality rates. In the year 2005, approximately 270,000 women and 1700 men were diagnosed with breast cancer in the United States and approximately 40,000 women and 500 men died of breast cancer. There is an inverse relationship between the age of the woman and her risk of contracting the disease, in that in 2005 1 out of 2200 women less than 30 years of age contracted breast cancer, whereas 1 out 54 and 1 out of 23 women less than 50 and 60 years of age, respectively, contracted breast cancer. Although breast cancer is more likely to occur at an older age, younger women tend to have more aggressive breast cancers.

21

Male Reproductive System

The male reproductive system consists of two **testes** suspended in the scrotum, a system of intratesticular and extratesticular **genital ducts,** associated **glands,** and the male copulatory organ, the **penis** (Fig. 21-1). The testes are responsible for the formation of the male gametes, known as **spermatozoa,** as well as for the synthesis, storage, and release of the male sex hormone, **testosterone.**

The glands associated with the male reproductive tract are the paired **seminal vesicles,** the single **prostate gland,** and the two **bulbourethral glands (of Cowper).** These glands form the noncellular portion of **semen** (spermatozoa suspended in the secretions of the accessory glands), which not only nourishes the spermatozoa but also provides a fluid vehicle for their delivery into the female reproductive tract. The **penis** has a dual function: It delivers semen to the female reproductive tract during copulation and serves as the conduit of urine from the urinary bladder to outside the body.

TESTES

The testes, located in the scrotum, are paired organs that produce spermatozoa and testosterone.

Each testis of a mature male is an oval organ approximately 4 cm long, 2 to 3 cm wide, and 3 cm thick. During embryogenesis, the testes develop retroperitoneally on the posterior wall of the abdominal cavity. As they descend into the scrotum, they carry with them a portion of the peritoneum. This peritoneal outpouching, the **tunica vaginalis,** forms a serous cavity that partially surrounds the anterolateral aspect of each testis, permitting it some degree of mobility within its compartment in the scrotum.

General Structure and Vascular Supply

Connective tissue septa divide the testis into lobuli testis, each of which houses one to four seminiferous tubules.

Each testis is surrounded by a capsule of dense, irregular collagenous connective tissue known as the **tunica albuginea.** Immediately deep to this layer is a highly vascularized loose connective tissue, the **tunica vasculosa,** which forms the vascular capsule of the testis. The posterior aspect of the tunica albuginea is somewhat thickened, forming the **mediastinum testis,** from which connective tissue septa radiate to subdivide each testis into approximately 250 pyramid-shaped intercommunicating compartments known as the **lobuli testis** (Fig. 21-2).

Each lobule has one to four blindly ending **seminiferous tubules,** which are surrounded by a richly innervated and highly vascularized loose connective tissue derived from the tunica vasculosa. Dispersed throughout this connective tissue are small conglomerations of endocrine cells, the **interstitial cells (of Leydig)** (see later), which are responsible for the synthesis of testosterone.

Spermatozoa are produced by the **seminiferous epithelium** of the seminiferous tubules. Spermatozoa enter short straight ducts, **tubuli recti,** that connect the open end of each seminiferous tubule to the **rete testis,** a system of labyrinthine spaces housed within the mediastinum testis. The spermatozoa leave the rete testis through 10 to 20 short tubules, the **ductuli efferentes,** which eventually fuse with the **epididymis.**

The vascular supply of each testis arises from the abdominal aorta as the **testicular artery,** which descends with the testis into the scrotum, accompanying the **ductus deferens (vas deferens).** The testicular artery forms several branches before it pierces the

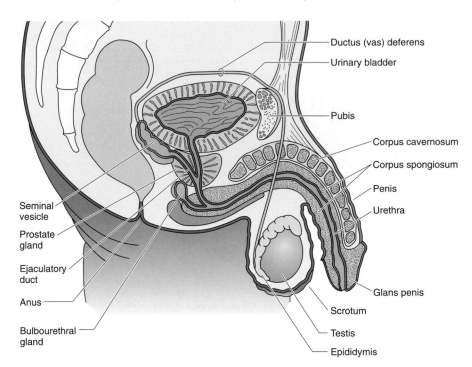

Figure 21–1 The male reproductive system.

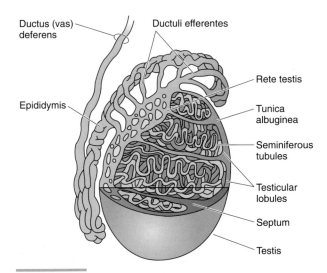

Figure 21–2 The testis and epididymis. Lobules and their contents are not drawn to scale.

capsule of the testis to form the intratesticular vascular elements. The capillary beds of the testes are collected into several veins, the **pampiniform plexus of veins,** which are wrapped around the testicular artery. The artery, veins, and ductus deferens together form the **spermatic cord,** which passes through the inguinal canal, the passageway from the abdominal cavity to the scrotum.

Blood in the pampiniform plexus of veins, which is cooler than that in the testicular artery, acts to reduce the temperature of the arterial blood, thus forming a **countercurrent heat exchange system.** In this fashion, it helps keep the temperature of the testes a few degrees lower than that of the remainder of the body. At this cooler temperature (95° F [35° C]), spermatozoa develop normally, whereas at body temperature, spermatozoa that may develop are sterile. The testes are maintained at a cooler temperature in the scrotum , thus aiding the cooling effect of the pampiniform plexus of veins.

Seminiferous Tubules

Seminiferous tubules are composed of a thick seminiferous epithelium surrounded by a thin connective tissue, the tunica propria.

Seminiferous tubules are highly convoluted hollow tubules, 30 to 70 cm long and 150 to 250 μm in diameter, that are surrounded by extensive capillary beds. About 1000 seminiferous tubules are present in the two testes, for a total length of nearly 0.5 km (0.3 mile), dedicated to the production of spermatozoa.

The wall of the seminiferous tubule is composed of a slender connective tissue layer, the **tunica propria,** and a thick seminiferous epithelium. The tunica propria and the seminiferous epithelium are separated from each other by a well-developed **basal lamina.** The connective tissue comprises mostly interlaced, slender, type I collagen fiber bundles housing several layers of fibroblasts. In some animals, but not in humans, **myoid cells,** similar to smooth muscle, are also present; the cells impart contractility to the seminiferous tubules of animals.

The seminiferous epithelium (or **germinal epithelium**) is several cell layers thick (Figs. 21-3 and 21-4) and is composed of two types of cells: Sertoli cells and spermatogenic cells (Fig. 21-5; also see Fig. 21-4). The latter cells are in various stages of maturation.

Sertoli Cells

Sertoli cells support, protect, and nourish spermatogenic cells; phagocytose cytoplasmic remnants of spermatids; secrete androgen-binding protein, hormones, and a nutritive medium; and establish the blood-testis barrier.

Sertoli cells are tall, columnar cells whose lateral cell membranes possess complex infoldings, which make it

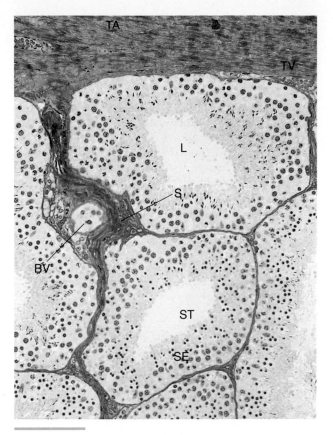

Figure 21–3 Light micrograph of the capsule of a monkey testis, with cross-sectional profiles of blood vessels (BV), lumen (L), septa (S), seminiferous epithelium (SE), seminiferous tubules (ST), tunica albuginea (TA), and tunica vasculosa (TV) (×132).

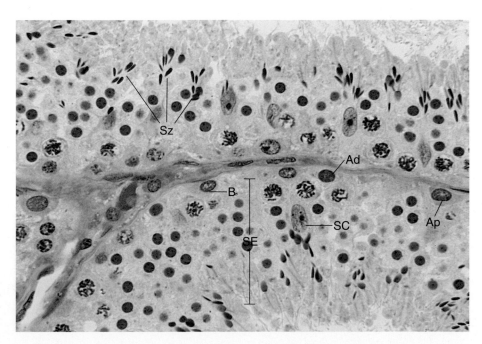

Figure 21–4 Seminiferous tubule (×540). Note the seminiferous epithelium (SE), pale spermatogonia A (Ap), dark spermatogonia A (Ad), spermatogonia B (B), Sertoli cell (SC), and spermatozoa (Sz).

impossible to distinguish their lateral cell boundaries using light microscopy. Their apical cell membranes are also highly folded and project into the lumina of the seminiferous tubules. These cells have a basally located, clear, oval nucleus with a large, centrally positioned nucleolus (see Fig. 21-5). The cytoplasm has been shown to house inclusion products known as **crystalloids of Charcot-Böttcher,** the composition and function of which are not known.

Electron micrographs reveal that the cytoplasm of Sertoli cells is replete with profiles of smooth endoplasmic reticulum (SER), but the amount of rough endoplasmic reticulum (RER) is limited. The cell also has numerous mitochondria, a well-developed Golgi apparatus, and numerous vesicles that belong to the endolysosomal complex. The cytoskeletal elements of Sertoli cells are also abundant, indicating that one of the functions of these cells is to provide structural support for the developing gametes.

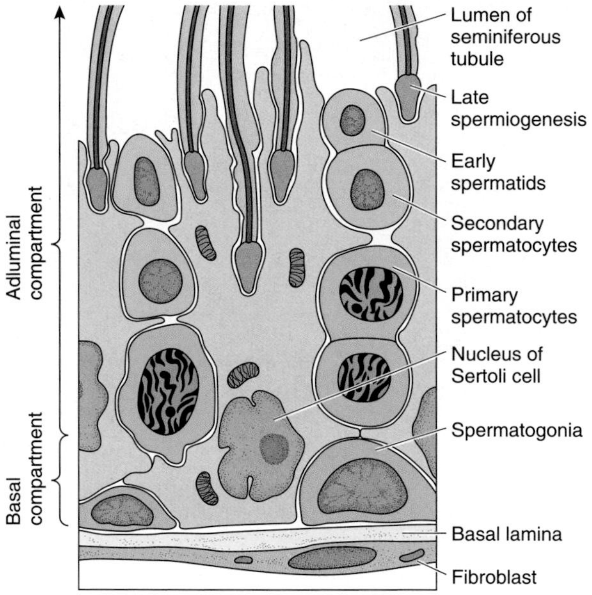
Lumen of seminiferous tubule
Late spermiogenesis
Early spermatids
Secondary spermatocytes
Primary spermatocytes
Nucleus of Sertoli cell
Spermatogonia
Basal lamina
Fibroblast
Adluminal compartment
Basal compartment

Figure 21–5 Seminiferous epithelium.

The lateral cell membranes of adjacent Sertoli cells form occluding junctions with each other, thus subdividing the lumen of the seminiferous tubule into two isolated, concentric compartments (Fig. 21-6; also see Fig. 21-5). The **basal compartment** is narrower, is located basal to the zonulae occludentes, and surrounds the wider **adluminal compartment.** Thus, the zonulae occludentes of these cells establish a blood-testis barrier that isolates the adluminal compartment from connective tissue influences, thereby protecting the developing gametes from the immune system. Because spermatogenesis begins after puberty, the newly differentiating germ cells, which have a different chromosome number as well as expressing different surface membrane receptors and molecules, would be considered "foreign cells" by the immune system. Were it not for the isolation of germ cells from the connective tissue compartments by the zonulae occludentes of the Sertoli cells, an immune response would be mounted against them.

Sertoli cells perform the following functions:

- Physical and nutritional support of the developing germ cells
- Phagocytosis of cytoplasm eliminated during spermiogenesis
- Establishment of a blood-testis barrier by the formation of zonulae occludentes between adjacent Sertoli cells

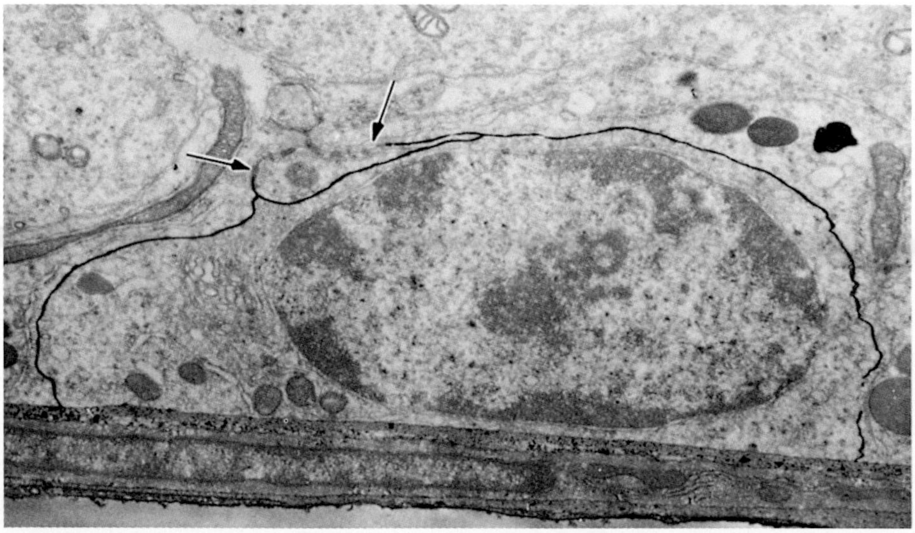

Figure 21–6 Electron micrograph of the basal compartmentof the seminiferous epithelium (×15,000). The testis has been perfused with an electron-dense tracer (lanthanum nitrate) to demonstrate that the occluding junctions *(arrows)* between adjacent Sertoli cells prevent the tracer from entering the adluminal compartment. (From Leeson TS, Leeson CR, Papparo AA: Text/Atlas of Histology. Philadelphia, WB Saunders, 1988.)

■ Synthesis and release of **androgen-binding protein (ABP),** a macromolecule that facilitates an increase in the concentration of testosterone in the seminiferous tubule by binding to it and preventing it from leaving the tubule

■ Synthesis and release (during embryogenesis) of **antimüllerian hormone,** which suppresses the formation of the müllerian duct (precursor of the female reproductive system) and thus establishes the "maleness" of the developing embryo

■ Synthesis and secretion of **inhibin,** a hormone that inhibits the release of follicle-stimulating hormone (FSH) by the anterior pituitary

■ Secretion of a fructose-rich medium that nourishes and facilitates the transport of spermatozoa to the genital ducts

■ Synthesis and secretion of **testicular transferrin,** an apoprotein that accepts iron from serum transferrin and conveys it to maturing gametes

Spermatogenic Cells

The process of spermatogenesis, whereby spermatogonia give rise to spermatozoa, is divided into three phases: spermatocytogenesis, meiosis, and spermiogenesis.

Most of the cells composing the thick seminiferous epithelium are **spermatogenic cells** in various stages of maturation (see Fig. 21-5). Some of these cells, **spermatogonia,** are located in the basal compartment, whereas most of the developing cells—**primary spermatocytes, secondary spermatocytes, spermatids,** and **spermatozoa**—occupy the adluminal compartment. Spermatogonia are diploid cells that undergo mitotic division to form more spermatogonia as well as primary spermatocytes, which migrate from the basal into the adluminal compartment. Primary spermatocytes enter the **first meiotic division** to form secondary spermatocytes, which undergo the **second meiotic division** to form **haploid** cells known as **spermatids.** These haploid cells are transformed into spermatozoa (mature sperm) through shedding of much of their cytoplasm, rearrangement of their organelles, and formation of flagella.

Various cell types that result from this process of cell maturation, called **spermatogenesis,** are diagrammed in Figure 21-7. The maturation process is divided into three phases:

■ **Spermatocytogenesis:** Differentiation of spermatogonia into primary spermatocytes

■ **Meiosis:** Reduction division whereby diploid primary spermatocytes reduce their chromosome complement, forming haploid spermatids

■ **Spermiogenesis:** Transformation of spermatids into spermatozoa (sperm)

Differentiation of Spermatogonia

Spermatogonia (2n) are influenced by testosterone at puberty to enter the cell cycle.

Spermatogonia are small, diploid germ cells located in the basal compartment of the seminiferous tubules (see Figs. 21-5 and 21-7). These cells lie on the basal lamina and, subsequent to puberty, become influenced by testosterone to enter the cell cycle. There are three categories of spermatogonia:

■ **Dark type A spermatogonia** are small (12 μm in diameter) dome-shaped cells. They have flattened, oval nuclei with abundant heterochromatin, imparting a dense appearance to the nucleus. Dark type A spermatogonia are **reserve cells** that have *not* entered the cell cycle but may do so. Once they undergo mitosis, they form additional dark type A spermatogonia as well as pale type A spermatogonia.

■ **Pale type A spermatogonia** are identical to the dark type A cells, except that their nuclei have abundant euchromatin, giving them a pale appearance. These cells have only a few organelles, including mitochondria, a limited Golgi complex, some RER, and numerous free ribosomes. These cells are induced by testosterone to *proliferate* and give rise, by mitosis, to additional pale type A spermatogonia and to type B spermatogonia.

■ **Type B spermatogonia** resemble pale type A spermatogonia, but usually their nuclei are round rather than flattened. These cells also divide mitotically to give rise to primary spermatocytes.

Meiotic Division of Spermatocytes

The first meiotic division of the primary spermatocyte, followed by the second meiotic division of the secondary spermatocyte, reduces the chromosome number and deoxyribonucleic acid (DNA) content to the haploid (n) state in the spermatids.

As soon as primary spermatocytes are formed, they migrate from the basal compartment into the adluminal compartment. As these cells migrate between adjacent Sertoli cells, they form zonulae occludentes with the Sertoli cells and thus help maintain the integrity of the blood-testis barrier. Primary spermatocytes are the largest cells of the seminiferous epithelium (see Fig. 21-5). They have large, vesicular-appearing nuclei whose chromosomes are in various stages of condensation. Shortly after their formation, primary spermatocytes duplicate their DNA to obtain a 4n DNA content; however, the chromosome number remains diploid (2n).

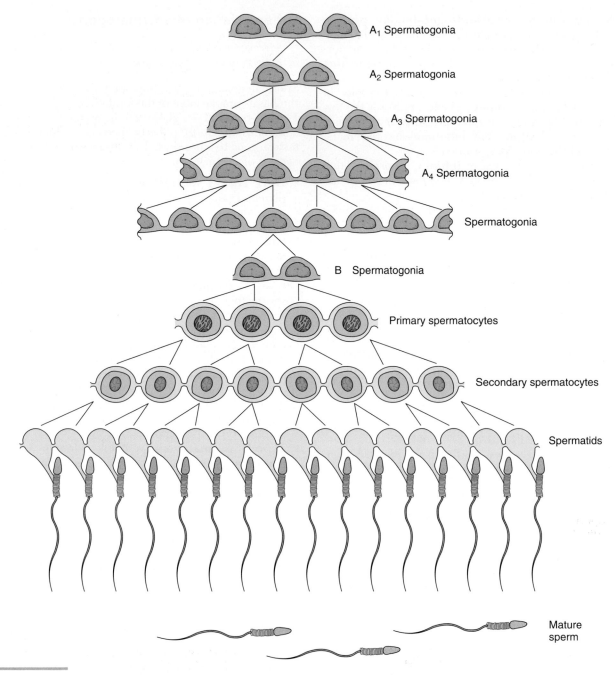

A₁ Spermatogonia

A₂ Spermatogonia

A₃ Spermatogonia

A₄ Spermatogonia

Spermatogonia

B Spermatogonia

Primary spermatocytes

Secondary spermatocytes

Spermatids

Mature sperm

Figure 21–7 Spermatogenesis, displaying the intercellular bridges that maintain the syncytium during differentiation and maturation. (Modified from Ren X-D, Russell L: Clonal development of interconnected germ cells in the rat and its relationship to the segmental and subsegmental organization of spermatogenesis. Am J Anat 192:127, 1991.)

During the **first meiotic division,** the DNA content is halved (to 2n DNA) in each daughter cell and the chromosome number is reduced to haploid (n). During the **second meiotic division,** the DNA content of each new daughter cell is reduced to haploid (1n DNA), whereas the chromosome number remains unaltered (haploid).

Prophase I of the first meiotic division lasts for 22 days and involves four stages:

■ Leptotene
■ Zygotene
■ Pachytene
■ Diakinesis

The chromosomes of a primary spermatocyte begin to condense, forming long threads during **leptotene** and pairing with their homologues during **zygotene**. Further condensation yields short, thick chromosomes, recognizable as **tetrads,** during **pachytene**. The exchange of segments (**crossing over**) of homologous chromosomes occurs during **diakinesis;** this random genetic recombination results in the unique genome of each gamete and contributes to the variation of the gene pool.

During **metaphase I,** the paired homologous chromosomes line up at the equatorial plate. The members of each pair pull apart and then migrate to opposite poles of the cell in **anaphase I,** and the daughter cells separate (although a cytoplasmic bridge remains), forming two secondary spermatocytes during **telophase I.**

Because the homologous chromosomes are segregated during anaphase, the X and Y chromosomes are sorted into separate secondary spermatocytes, eventually forming spermatozoa that carry either X or Y chromosomes. Thus, it is the spermatozoon that determines the chromosomal (genetic) sex of the future embryo.

Secondary spermatocytes are relatively small cells, and because they are short-lived, they are not readily seen in the seminiferous epithelium. These cells, which contain 2n DNA, do not replicate their chromosomes; they quickly enter the second meiotic division, forming two haploid (1n DNA) spermatids.

During mitosis of spermatogonia and meiosis of spermatocytes, nuclear division (**karyokinesis**) is accompanied by a **modified cytokinesis.** As each cell divides to form two cells, a **cytoplasmic bridge** remains between them, holding the newly formed cells tethered to each other (see Fig. 21-7). Because this incomplete division occurs over a number of mitotic and meiotic events, it results in the formation of a **syncytium** of cells, a large number of spermatids that are connected to one another. This connection enables the spermatogenic cells to communicate with each other and thus to synchronize their activities.

CLINICAL CORRELATIONS

The most common abnormality due to nondisjunction of the XX homologues is known as **Klinefelter syndrome.** Individuals afflicted with this syndrome usually have XXY chromosomes (an extra X chromosome). They are typically infertile, are tall and thin, exhibit various degrees of masculine characteristics (including small testes), and are somewhat retarded mentally.

Transformation of Spermatids (Spermiogenesis)

Spermatids discard much of their cytoplasm, rearrange their organelles, and form a flagellum to become transformed into spermatozoa; this process of transformation is known as spermiogenesis.

Spermatids are small, round haploid cells (8 μm in diameter). All the spermatids that are the progeny of a single pale type A spermatogonium are connected to one another by cytoplasmic bridges. They form small clusters and occupy a position near the lumen of the seminiferous tubule. These cells have abundant RER, numerous mitochondria, and a well-developed Golgi complex. During their transformation into spermatozoa, they accumulate hydrolytic enzymes, rearrange and reduce the number of their organelles, form flagella and associated skeletal apparatus, and shed some of their cytoplasm. This process of **spermiogenesis** is subdivided into four phases (Figs. 21-8 and 21-9):

■ Golgi phase
■ Cap phase
■ Acrosomal phase
■ Maturation phase

GOLGI PHASE

During the Golgi phase of spermiogenesis, hydrolytic enzymes are formed on the RER, modified in the Golgi apparatus, and packaged by the *trans* **Golgi network** as small, membrane-bound **preacrosomal granules.** These small vesicles fuse with one another, forming an **acrosomal vesicle.** The hydrolytic enzymes in this vesicle are visualized with the electron microscope as an electron-dense material known as the **acrosomal granule.** The acrosomal vesicle comes into contact with and becomes bound to the nuclear envelope, thus establishing the anterior pole of the developing spermatozoon.

As the acrosomal vesicle is being formed, the centrioles leave the vicinity of the nucleus, and one of them participates in the formation of the **flagellar axoneme.** After the generation of the microtubules is initiated, the centrioles return to the vicinity of the nucleus to assist in the formation of the **connecting piece,** a structure that will surround the centrioles (see later in the description of the spermatozoon).

CAP PHASE

During the cap phase, the acrosomal vesicle increases in size, and its membrane partially surrounds the nucleus (see Fig. 21-8). As this vesicle enlarges to its final size, it becomes known as the **acrosome (acrosomal cap).**

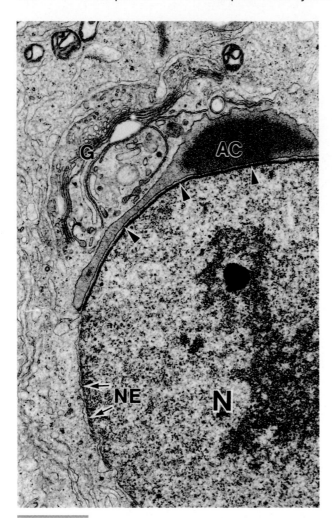

Figure 21–8 Electron micrograph of the cap stage of a rodent spermatid (×18,000). AC, acrosome; G, Golgi apparatus; N, nucleus; NE, nuclear envelope. (From Oshako S, Bunick D, Hess RA, et al: Characterization of a testis specific protein localized in the endoplasmic reticulum of spermatogenic cells. Anat Rec 238:335-348, 1994.)

ACROSOMAL PHASE

The acrosomal phase is characterized by several alterations in the morphology of the spermatid. The nucleus becomes condensed, the cell elongates, and the mitochondria shift location.

The chromosomes become tightly condensed and tightly packaged. As the chromosomal volume decreases, the volume of the entire nucleus is also reduced. Additionally, the nucleus becomes flattened and assumes its specific morphology.

Microtubules assemble to form a cylindrical structure, the **manchette,** which aids in the elongation of the spermatid. As the elongating cytoplasm reaches the microtubules of the flagellar axoneme, the manchette

microtubules disassemble. Their place is assumed by the **annulus,** an electron-dense, ring-like structure that delineates the junction of the spermatozoon's **middle piece** with its **principal piece** (see Fig. 21-9). A mitochondrial sheath forms around the axoneme of the middle piece of the tail of the spermatozoon.

During formation of the mitochondrial sheath and elongation of the spermatid, nine columns of **outer dense fibers** form around the axoneme. These dense fibers are attached to the connecting piece formed during the Golgi phase. After their establishment, the dense fibers become surrounded by ribs, a series of ring-like, dense structures known as the **fibrous sheath.**

MATURATION PHASE

The maturation phase is characterized by the shedding of spermatid cytoplasm. As the excess cytoplasm is released, the syncytium is disrupted and individual spermatozoa are liberated from the large cellular mass. The cytoplasmic remnants are phagocytosed by Sertoli cells, and the disengaged spermatozoa are released into the lumen of the seminiferous tubule (**spermiation**).

Note that the newly formed spermatozoa are **immotile** and cannot fertilize an oocyte. Spermatozoa gain motility while passing through the epididymis. Only after they enter the female reproductive system do spermatozoa become **capacitated** (i.e., capable of fertilization).

Structure of Spermatozoa

Spermatozoa are composed of a head, housing the nucleus, and a tail that is divided into four regions: neck, middle piece, principal piece, and end piece.

The spermatozoa (sperm), produced by spermatogenesis, are long cells (~65 μm). Each spermatozoon is composed of a head, housing the nucleus, and a tail, which accounts for most of its length (Fig. 21-10; also see Fig. 21-9).

HEAD OF THE SPERMATOZOON

The flattened head of the spermatozoon is about 5 μm long and is surrounded by plasmalemma (see Fig. 21-9). It is occupied by the condensed electron-dense nucleus, containing only 1 member of the 23 pairs of chromosomes (22 autosomes + the Y chromosome—or 22 autosomes + the X chromosome), and the **acrosome,** which partially surrounds the anterior aspect of the nucleus. The acrosome comes into contact with the cell membrane of the spermatozoon anteriorly. It houses various enzymes, including neuraminidase, hyaluronidase, acid phosphatase, aryl sulfatase, and a trypsin-like protease known as **acrosin.**

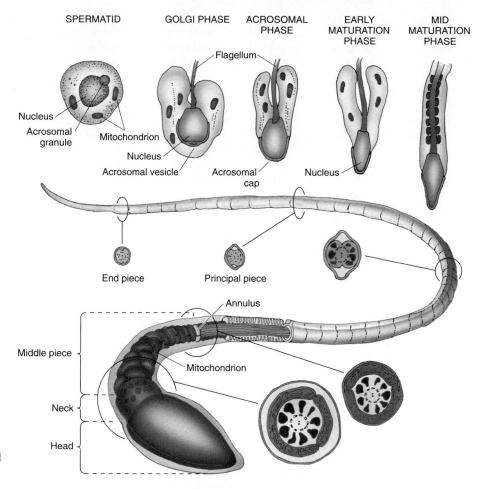

SPERMATID   GOLGI PHASE   ACROSOMAL PHASE   EARLY MATURATION PHASE   MID MATURATION PHASE

Figure 21–9 Spermiogenesis and a mature spermatozoon.

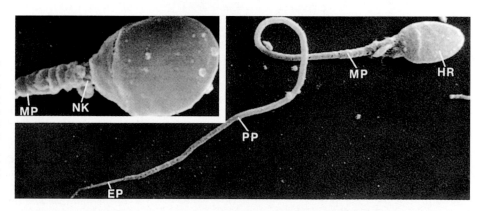

Figure 21–10 Scanning electron micrograph of human spermatozoa (×15,130). The entire spermatozoon is shown, including head region (HR), middle piece (MP), principal piece (PP), and end piece (EP) (×650). *Inset,* Head, neck (NK), and middle piece (MP). (From Kessel RG: Tissue and Organs: A Text Atlas of Scanning Electron Microscopy. San Francisco, WH Freeman, 1979.)

Binding of a spermatozoon to the ZP3 molecule of the zona pellucida triggers the **acrosomal reaction,** the release of the acrosomal enzymes that digest a path for the sperm to reach the oocyte, thereby facilitating the process of fertilization (see Chapter 20, Fig. 20-15). The acrosomal reaction as well as the process of fertilization is described in Chapter 20.

TAIL OF THE SPERMATOZOON

The tail of the spermatozoon is subdivided into four regions: neck, middle piece, principal piece, and end piece (see Fig. 21-9). The plasmalemma of the head is continuous with the tail's plasma membrane.

The **neck** (~5 μm long) connects the head to the remainder of the tail. It is composed of the cylindrical arrangement of the nine columns of the **connecting piece** that encircles the two centrioles, one of which is usually fragmented. The posterior aspects of the columnar densities are continuous with the nine **outer dense fibers.**

The **middle piece** (~5 μm long) is located between the neck and the principal piece. It is characterized by the presence of the mitochondrial sheath, which encircles the **outer dense fibers** and the centralmost **axoneme.** The middle piece stops at the **annulus,** a ring-like, dense structure to which the plasmalemma adheres, thus preventing the mitochondrial sheath from moving caudally into the tail. Also, two of the nine outer dense fibers terminate at the annulus; the remaining seven continue into the principal piece.

The **principal piece** (~45 μm long) is the longest segment of the tail and extends from the annulus to the end piece. The axoneme of the principal piece is continuous with that of the middle piece. Surrounding the axoneme are the seven outer dense fibers that are continuous with those of the middle piece and are surrounded, in turn, by the **fibrous sheath.** The principal piece tapers near its caudal extent, where both the outer dense fibers and the fibrous sheath terminate, and is continuous with the end piece.

The **end piece** (~5 μm long) is composed of the central axoneme surrounded by plasmalemma. The axoneme is disorganized in the last 0.5 to 1.0 μm, so that instead of the nine doublets and two singlets, 20 haphazardly arranged, individual microtubules are evident.

CYCLE OF THE SEMINIFEROUS EPITHELIUM

The seminiferous epithelium displays 16-day cycles; four cycles are required to complete spermatogenesis.

Because germ cells that arise from a single pale type A spermatogonium are connected by cytoplasmic bridges and constitute a syncytium, they can communicate with each other and synchronize their development. Careful examination of the human seminiferous epithelium reveals six possible characteristic associations of developing cell types, known as the six **stages of spermatogenesis** because they are undergoing transformations to form spermatozoa (Fig. 21-11). Each cross-sectional profile of a seminiferous tubule may be subdivided into three or more wedgeshaped areas, each displaying a different stage of spermatogenesis.

Studies following the fate of tritium-labeled thymidine (³H-thymidine) injected into the testes of human volunteers have demonstrated that radioactivity appears at 16-day intervals in the same stage of spermatogenesis. Each 16-day interval is known as a **cycle of the seminiferous epithelium,** and the process of spermatogenesis requires the passage of four cycles, or 64 days. Examination of serial cross sections of a single seminiferous tubule reveals that the same stage of the seminiferous epithelium continues to reappear at specific distances along the length of the tubule. The distance between two identical stages of the seminiferous epithelium is called the **wave of the seminiferous epithelium.** Thus, in humans there are six repeating waves of the seminiferous epithelium, corresponding to the six stages.

Interstitial Cells of Leydig

The interstitial cells of Leydig, scattered among connective tissue elements of the tunica vasculosa, secrete testosterone.

The seminiferous tubules are embedded in the **tunica vasculosa,** a richly vascularized, loose connective tissue housing scattered fibroblasts, mast cells, and other cellular constituents normally present in loose connective tissue. Also dispersed throughout the tunica vasculosa are small collections of endocrine cells, the interstitial cells of Leydig, which produce the hormone **testosterone.**

The interstitial cells of Leydig are polyhedral and are approximately 15 μm in diameter. They have a single nucleus, although occasionally they may be binucleate. They are typical steroid-producing cells that have mitochondria with tubular cristae, a large accumulation of SER, and a well-developed Golgi apparatus (Fig. 21-12). These cells also house some RER and numerous lipid droplets, but they contain no secretory vesicles, because testosterone is probably released as soon as its synthesis is complete. Lysosomes and peroxisomes are also evident, as are lipochrome pigments (especially in older men). The cytoplasm also contains crystallized proteins, the **crystals of Reinke,** a characteristic of human interstitial cells.

Histophysiology of the Testes

The principal functions of the testes are the production of spermatozoa and the synthesis and release of testosterone.

The two testes form about 200 million spermatozoa per day by a process that may be considered a holocrine type of secretion. Sertoli cells of the seminiferous epithelium also produce a fructose-rich fluid that acts to nourish and transport the newly formed spermatozoa from the lumen of the seminiferous tubule to the extratesticular genital ducts.

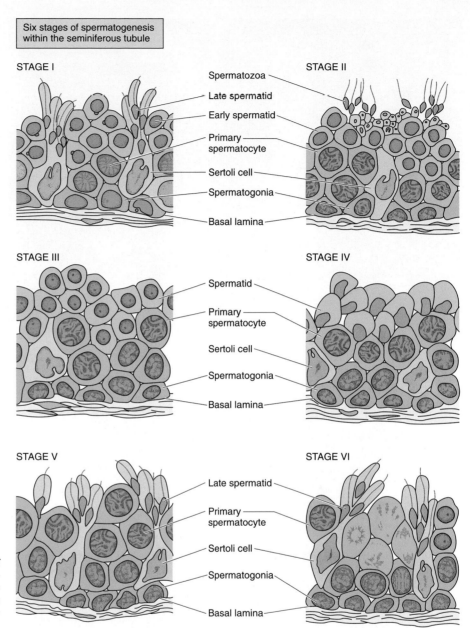

Figure 21–11 The six stages of spermatogenesis in the human seminiferous tubule. (Redrawn from Clermont Y: The cycle of the seminiferous epithelium in man. Am J Anat 112:35-52, 1963.)

Luteinizing hormone (LH), a gonadotropin released from the anterior pituitary gland, binds to LH receptors on the Leydig cells, activating adenylate cyclase to form cyclic adenosine monophosphate (cAMP). Activation of protein kinases of the Leydig cells by cAMP induces inactive **cholesterol esterases** to become active and cleave free cholesterol from intracellular lipid droplets. The first step in the pathway of testosterone synthesis is also LH-sensitive, because LH activates **cholesterol desmolase,** the enzyme that converts free cholesterol into pregnenolone. The various products of the synthetic pathway are shuttled between the smooth endo-plasmic reticulum and mitochondria until **testosterone,** the male hormone, is formed and is ultimately released by these cells (Fig. 21-13).

Because blood testosterone levels are not sufficient to initiate and maintain spermatogenesis, FSH, another anterior pituitary gonadotropin, induces Sertoli cells to synthesize and release **androgen-binding protein (ABP)** (Fig. 21-14). As its name implies, ABP binds testosterone, thereby preventing the hormone from leaving the region of the seminiferous tubule and elevating the testosterone levels in the local environment sufficiently to sustain spermatogenesis.

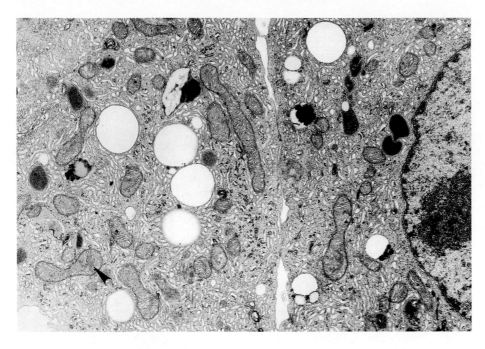

Figure 21–12 Low-magnification electron micrograph exhibits areas of two human Leydig cells (×18,150). Mitochondria are relatively uniform in diameter, and even at low magnification, stacked lamellae are an evident form of the cristae *(arrowhead)*. (From Prince FP: Mitochondrial cristae diversity in human Leydig cells: A revised look at cristae morphology in these steroid-producing cells. Anat Rec 254:534-541, 1999.)

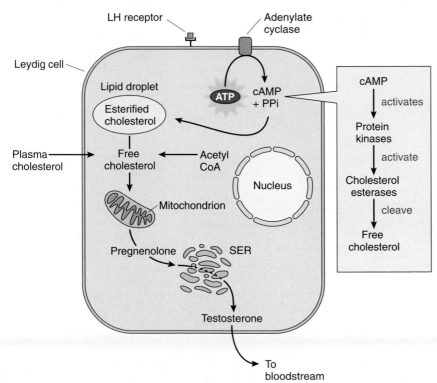

Figure 21–13 Testosterone synthesis by the interstitial cells of Leydig. ATP, adenosine triphosphate; cAMP, cyclic adenosine monophosphate; CoA, coenzyme A; LH, luteinizing hormone; SER, smooth endoplasmic reticulum.

Release of LH is inhibited by increased levels of testosterone and dihydrotestosterone, whereas release of FSH is inhibited by the hormone **inhibin,** produced by Sertoli cells (see Fig. 21-14). It is interesting to note that estrogens, female sex hormones, are also bound by ABP and thus can reduce the levels of spermatogenesis.

Testosterone is also required for the normal functioning of the seminal vesicles, prostate, and bulbourethral glands as well as for the appearance and

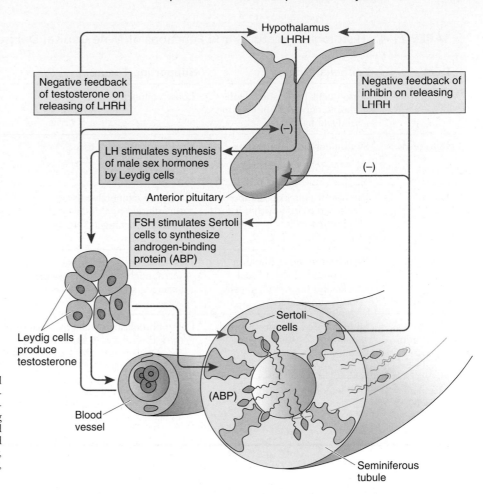

Figure 21–14 Hormonal control of spermatogenesis. FSH, follicle-stimulating hormone; LH, luteinizing hormone; LHRH, luteinizing hormone–releasing hormone. (Adapted from Fawcett, DW: Bloom and Fawcett's A Textbook of Histology, 10th ed. Philadelphia, WB Saunders, 1975.)

maintenance of the male secondary sexual characteristics. The cells that require testosterone possess **5α-reductase,** the enzyme that converts testosterone to its more active form, **dihydrotestosterone.**

GENITAL DUCTS

The genital ducts may be subdivided into two categories: those located within the testes (**intratesticular**) and those located external to the testes (**extratesticular**) (Table 21-1).

Intratesticular Genital Ducts

Intratesticular ducts include the tubuli recti and the rete testis.

The genital ducts located within the testis connect the seminiferous tubules to the epididymis. These intratesticular ducts are the tubuli recti and the rete testis (see Fig. 21-2).

Tubuli Recti

The tubuli recti deliver spermatozoa from the seminiferous tubules into the rete testis.

The tubuli recti are short, straight tubules that are continuous with the seminiferous tubules and deliver the spermatozoa, formed by the seminiferous epithelium, to the rete testis. These short tubules are lined by Sertoli cells in their first half, near the seminiferous tubule, and by a simple cuboidal epithelium in their second half, near the rete testis. The cuboidal cells have short, stubby microvilli, and most possess a single flagellum.

Rete Testis

Immature spermatozoa pass from the tubuli recti into the rete testis, labyrinthine spaces lined by cuboidal epithelium.

The rete testis consists of labyrinthine spaces, lined by a simple cuboidal epithelium, within the mediastinum

TABLE 21–1 Histological Features and Functions of Male Genital Ducts

Duct	Epithelial Lining	Supporting Tissues	Function
Tubuli recti	Sertoli cells in proximal half; simple cuboidal epithelium in distal half	Loose connective tissue	Convey spermatoza from seminiferous tubules to rete testis
Rete testis	Simple cuboidal epithelium	Vascular connective tissue	Conveys spermatozoa from tubuli recti to ductuli efferentes
Ductuli efferentes	Patches of nonciliated cuboidal cells alternating with ciliated columnar cells	Thin loose connective tissue surrounded by thin layer of circularly arranged smooth muscle cells	Convey spermatozoa from rete testis to epididymis
Epididymis	Pseudostratified epithelium composed of short basal cells and tall principal cells (with stereocilia)	Thin loose connective tissue surrounded by layer of circularly arranged smooth muscle cells	Conveys spermatoza from ductuli efferentes to ductus deferens
Ductus (vas) deferens	Stereociliated pseudostratified columnar epithelium	Loose fibroelastic connective tissue; thick three-layered smooth muscle coats; *inner* and *outer* longitudinal, *middle* circular	Delivers spermatozoa from tail of epididymis to ejaculatory duct
Ejaculatory duct	Simple columnar epithelium	Subepithelial connective tissue folded, giving lumen irregular appearance; no smooth muscle	Delivers spermatozoa and seminal fluid to prostatic urethra at colliculus seminalis

testis. These cuboidal cells, which resemble those of the tubuli recti, have numerous short microvilli with a single flagellum (Fig. 21-15).

Ductuli Efferentes

The ductuli efferentes are interposed between the rete testis and the epididymis.

The 10 to 20 ductuli efferentes are short tubules that drain spermatozoa from the rete testis and pierce the tunica albuginea of the testis to conduct the sperm to the epididymis (see Fig. 21-2). Thus, the ductuli efferentes become confluent with the epididymis at this point.

The simple epithelial lining of the lumen of each ductule consists of patches of **nonciliated cuboidal cells** alternating with regions of **ciliated columnar cells.** The successive clusters of short and tall epithelial cells impart the characteristic festooned appearance to the lumina of the ductuli efferentes. The cuboidal cells are richly endowed with lysosomes, and their apical plasmalemmae display numerous invaginations indicative of endocytosis. These cells are believed to resorb most of the luminal fluid elaborated by the Sertoli cells of the seminiferous tubule. The cilia of the columnar cells probably move the spermatozoa toward the epididymis.

The simple epithelium sits on a basal lamina that separates it from the thin, loose connective tissue wall of each ductule. The connective tissue is surrounded by a thin layer of smooth muscle whose cells are circularly arrayed.

Extratesticular Genital Ducts

The extratesticular genital ducts are the epididymis, ductus deferens, and ejaculatory duct.

The extratesticular genital ducts associated with each testis are the epididymis, the ductus deferens (vas deferens), and the ejaculatory duct (see Fig. 21-1). The epididymis secretes numerous factors that, in an unknown manner, facilitate maturation of spermatozoa. As noted previously, however, spermatozoa cannot fertilize a secondary oocyte until they undergo **capacitation,** a process triggered by secretions produced in the female genital tract.

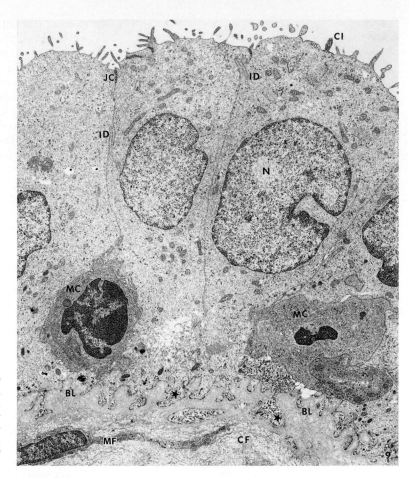

Figure 21–15 Electron micrograph of the epithelium of the bovine rete testis (×19,900). BL, basal lamina; CF, collagen fibers; CI, cilium; ID, interdigitation of the lateral plasmalemmae; JC, junctional complexes; MC, monocellular cell; MF, myofibroblast; N, nucleus. (From Hees H, Wrobel KH, Elmagd AA, Hees I: The mediastinum of the bovine testis. Cell Tissue Res 255:29-39, 1989.)

Epididymis

The epididymis, a highly convoluted tubule divided into a head, body, and tail, is continuous with the ductus deferens.

Each epididymis is a thin, long (4 to 6 m), highly convoluted tubule that is folded into a space only 7 cm long on the posterior aspect of the testis (see Fig. 21-2). The epididymis may be subdivided into three regions: head, body, and tail. The head, formed by the union of the 10 to 20 ductuli efferentes, becomes highly coiled and continues as the equally highly coiled body. The distal portion of the tail, which stores spermatozoa for a short time, loses its convolutions as it becomes continuous with the ductus deferens.

The lumen of the epididymis is lined by a **pseudostratified epithelium** composed of two cell types (Fig. 21-16):

■ Basal cells
■ Principal cells

The short **basal cells** of this epithelium are pyramidal to polyhedral. They have round nuclei in which

large accumulations of heterochromatin impart a dense appearance to this structure. The sparse cytoplasm of these cells is relatively clear, with a scarcity of organelles. It is believed that the basal cells function as stem cells, regenerating themselves as well as the principal cells as the need arises.

The tall **principal cells** of the epithelium of the epididymis have irregular, oval nuclei with one or two large nucleoli. These nuclei are much paler than those of the basal cells and are located basally within the cell.

The cytoplasm of the principal cell houses abundant RER located between the nucleus and the basal plasmalemma. The cytoplasm also has a large, supranuclearly positioned Golgi complex, numerous profiles of apically located SER, endolysosomes, and multivesicular bodies. The apical cell membranes of the principal cells display a profusion of pinocytotic and coated vesicles at the bases of the many **stereocilia** that project into the lumen of the epididymis. These long, branched, cellular extensions are clusters of nonmotile microvilli that appear to form clumps as they adhere to one another.

The principal cells resorb the luminal fluid, which is endocytosed by pinocytotic vesicles and delivered to the

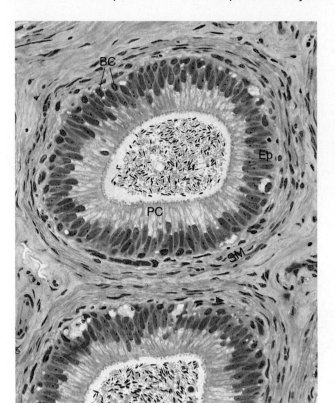

Figure 21–16 Light micrograph of the epididymis in a monkey (×270). Basal cells (BC), epithelium (Ep), principal cells (PC), smooth muscle (SM).

endolysosomes for disposal. Additionally, these cells phagocytose remnants of cytoplasm that were not removed by Sertoli cells. Principal cells also manufacture **glycerophosphocholine,** a glycoprotein that inhibits spermatozoon capacitation, thus preventing the spermatozoon from fertilizing a secondary oocyte until the sperm enters the female genital tract.

The epithelium of the epididymis is separated by a basal lamina from the underlying loose connective tissue. A layer of circularly arranged smooth muscle cells surrounds the connective tissue layer. **Peristaltic contractions** of this layer help conduct the spermatozoa to the ductus deferens.

Ductus Deferens (Vas Deferens)

The ductus deferens is a muscular tube that conveys spermatozoa from the tail of the epididymis to the ejaculatory duct.

Each ductus deferens is a thick-walled muscular tube with a small, irregular lumen that conveys spermatozoa

from the tail of the epididymis to the ejaculatory duct (see Figs. 21-1 and 21-2).

The stereociliated **pseudostratified columnar epithelium** of the ductus deferens is similar to that of the epididymis, although the principal cells are shorter. A basal lamina separates the epithelium from the underlying loose fibroelastic connective tissue, which has numerous folds, thus making the lumen appear irregular. The thick smooth muscle coat surrounding the connective tissue is composed of three layers: inner and outer longitudinal layers with an intervening middle circular layer. The smooth muscle coat is invested by a thin layer of loose fibroelastic connective tissue.

CLINICAL CORRELATIONS

Because the ductus deferens has a muscular wall 1 mm thick, it is easily perceptible through the skin of the scrotum as a dense, rolling tubule. **Vasectomy** (surgical removal of part of the ductus deferens) is performed via a small slit through the scrotal sac, thus sterilizing the person.

The dilated terminus of each ductus deferens, known as the **ampulla,** has a highly folded, thickened epithelium. As the ampulla approaches the prostate gland, it is joined by the seminal vesicle. The continuation of the junction of the ampulla with the seminal vesicle is called the **ejaculatory duct.**

Ejaculatory Duct

The ampulla of the ductus deferens joins the seminal vesicle to form the ejaculatory duct, which then enters the prostate gland and opens in the prostatic urethra.

Each ejaculatory duct is a short, straight tubule that enters the substance of and is surrounded by the prostate gland (see Fig. 21-1). The ejaculatory duct ends as it pierces the posterior aspect of the prostatic urethra at the **colliculus seminalis.** The lumen of the ejaculatory duct is lined by a simple columnar epithelium. The subepithelial connective tissue is folded, a feature responsible for the irregular appearance of its lumen. The ejaculatory duct has no smooth muscle in its wall.

ACCESSORY GENITAL GLANDS

The male reproductive system has five **accessory glands:** the paired seminal vesicles, the single prostate gland, and the paired bulbourethral glands (see Fig. 21-1).

Seminal Vesicles

The paired seminal vesicles, located adjacent to the posterior wall of the prostate gland, secrete a viscous fluid that constitutes about 70% of the ejaculate.

The paired seminal vesicles are highly coiled tubular structures about 15 cm long. They are located between the posterior aspect of the neck of the bladder and the prostate gland and join the ampulla of the ductus deferens just above the prostate gland.

The mucosa of the seminal vesicles is highly convoluted, forming labyrinth-like cul-de-sacs that, in three dimensions, are observed to open into a central lumen. The lumen is lined by a **pseudostratified columnar epithelium** composed of short basal cells and low columnar cells (Fig. 21-17).

Each **columnar cell** has numerous short microvilli and a single flagellum projecting into the lumen of the gland. The cytoplasm of these cells displays RER, Golgi apparatus, numerous mitochondria, some lipid and lipochrome pigment droplets, and abundant secretory granules. The height of the cells varies directly with blood testosterone levels. The subepithelial connective tissue is **fibroelastic** and is surrounded by smooth muscle cells, arranged as an inner circular layer and an outer longitudinal layer. The **smooth muscle coat** is, in turn, surrounded by a flimsy layer of fibroelastic connective tissue.

The seminal vesicles once were believed to store spermatozoa, some of which are always present in the lumen of this gland. It is now known that these glands produce a viscous, yellow **fructose-rich seminal fluid** that constitutes 70% of the volume of semen. Although seminal fluid also contains amino acids, citrates, prostaglandins, and proteins, fructose is its principal constituent, because it is the source of energy for spermatozoa. The characteristic pale yellow color of semen is due to the lipochrome pigment released by the seminal vesicles.

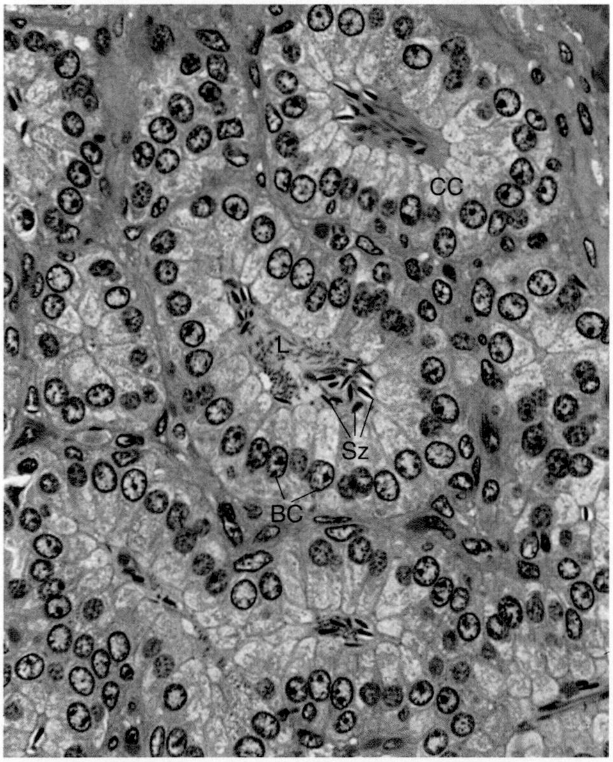

Prostate Gland

The prostate gland, surrounding a portion of the urethra, secretes acid phosphatase, fibrinolysin, and citric acid directly into the lumen of the urethra.

The prostate gland, the largest of the accessory glands, is pierced by the urethra and the ejaculatory ducts (Fig. 21-18). The slender **capsule** of the gland is composed of a richly vascularized, dense, irregular collagenous

Figure 21–17 Light micrograph of the monkey seminal vesicle (×270). Basal cells (BC), columnar cells (CC), lumen (L), spermatozoa (Sz).

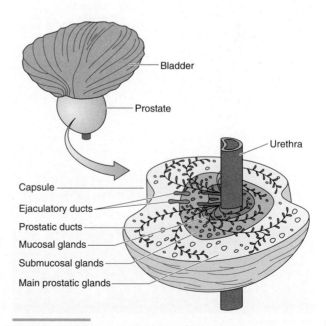

Figure 21–18 Human prostate gland.

connective tissue interspersed with **smooth muscle cells.** The connective tissue **stroma** of the gland is derived from the capsule and is, therefore, also enriched by smooth muscle fibers in addition to their normal connective tissue cells.

The prostate gland, a conglomeration of 30 to 50 individual **compound tubuloalveolar glands,** is arranged in three discrete, concentric layers:

■ Mucosal
■ Submucosal
■ Main

Each tubuloalveolar gland has its own duct that delivers the secretory product into the prostatic urethra.

The **mucosal glands** are closest to the urethra and thus are the shortest of the glands. The **submucosal glands** are peripheral to the mucosal glands and are consequently larger than the mucosal glands. The largest and most numerous of the glands are the peripheral-most **main glands,** which compose the bulk of the prostate.

The components of the prostate gland are lined by a **simple** to **pseudostratified columnar epithelium** (Fig. 21-19), the cells of which are well endowed with organelles responsible for the synthesis and packaging of proteins. Hence, these cells have an abundant RER, a large Golgi apparatus, numerous secretory granules (Fig. 21-20), and many lysosomes.

The lumina of the tubuloalveolar glands frequently house round to oval **prostatic concretions (corpora amylacea),** composed of calcified glycoproteins, whose numbers increase with a person's age (see Fig. 21-19). The significance of these concretions is not understood.

The **prostatic secretion** constitutes a part of semen. It is a serous, white fluid rich in lipids, proteolytic enzymes, acid phosphatase, fibrinolysin, and citric acid. The formation, synthesis, and release of the prostatic secretions are regulated by **dihydrotestosterone,** the active form of testosterone.

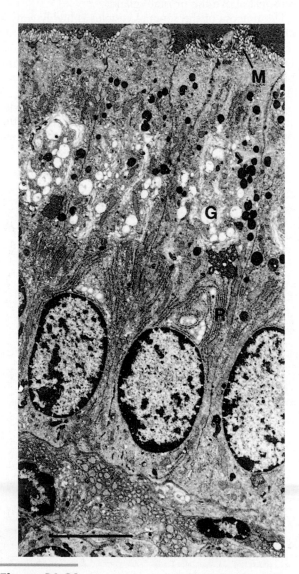

Figure 21–20 Electron micrograph of the prostate gland in a hamster. G, Golgi apparatus; M, microvilli; R, rough endoplasmic reticulum. Bar = 5 μm. (From Toma JG, Buzzell GR: Fine structure of the ventral and dorsal lobes of the prostate in a young adult Syrian hamster, *Mesocricetus auratus.* Am J Anat 181:132-140, 1988.)

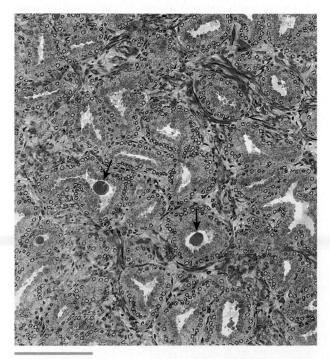

Figure 21–19 Light micrograph of the prostate gland of a monkey (×132). Note areas of prostatic concretion *(arrows).*

Bulbourethral Glands

The paired bulbourethral glands, located at the root of the penis, secrete a slippery lubricating solution directly into the urethra.

The bulbourethral glands (**Cowper's glands**) are small (3 to 5 mm in diameter) and are located at the root of the penis, just at the beginning of the membranous urethra (see Fig. 21-1). Their fibroelastic capsule contains not only fibroblasts and smooth muscle cells but also skeletal muscle fibers derived from the muscles of the urogenital diaphragm. Septa derived from the capsule divide each gland into several lobules. The epithelium of these compound tubuloalveolar glands varies from **simple cuboidal** to **simple columnar.**

The secretion produced by the bulbourethral glands is a thick, slippery fluid containing galactose and sialic acid that probably plays a role in lubricating the lumen of the urethra. During the process of ejaculation, this viscous fluid precedes the remainder of the semen.

Histophysiology of the Accessory Genital Glands

The bulbourethral glands secrete a viscous slippery fluid that lubricates the lining of the urethra. It is the first of the glandular secretions to be released subsequent to

erection of the penis. Just before ejaculation, secretions from the prostate are discharged into the urethra, as are the spermatozoa from the ampulla of the ductus deferens. The prostatic secretions apparently help the spermatozoa achieve motility. The final secretions arise from the seminal vesicles, which are responsible for a significant increase in the volume of the semen. Their fructose-rich fluid is used by the spermatozoa for energy.

The ejaculate, known as **semen,** is about 3 mL in volume in humans and consists of secretions from the accessory glands and 200 to 300 million spermatozoa.

PENIS

The penis functions as an excretory organ for urine and as the male copulatory organ for the deposition of spermatozoa into the female reproductive tract.

The penis is composed of three columns of **erectile tissue,** each enclosed by its own dense, fibrous connective tissue capsule, the **tunica albuginea** (Fig. 21-21).

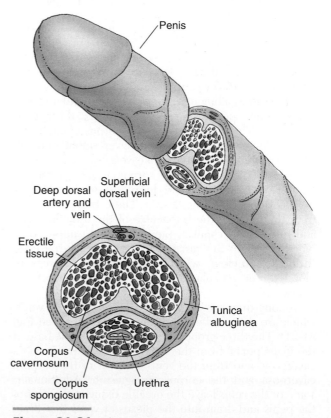

Figure 21–21 The penis in cross section.

Two of the columns of erectile tissue, the **corpora cavernosa,** are positioned dorsally; their tunicae albugineae are discontinuous in places, permitting communication between their erectile tissue. The third column of erectile tissue, the **corpus spongiosum,** is positioned ventrally. Because the corpus spongiosum houses the penile portion of the urethra, it is also called the **corpus cavernosum urethrae.** The corpus spongiosum ends distally in an enlarged, bulbous portion, the **glans penis** (head of the penis). The tip of the glans penis is pierced by the end of the urethra as a vertical slit.

The three corpora are surrounded by a common loose connective tissue sheath, but no hypodermis, and are covered by thin skin. The skin of the proximal portion of the penis has coarse pubic hairs and numerous sweat and sebaceous glands. The distal portion of the penis is hairless and has only a few sweat glands. Skin continues distal to the glans penis to form a retractable sheath, the **prepuce,** which is lined by a mucous membrane, a moist, stratified squamous nonkeratinized epithelium. When an individual is circumcised, it is the prepuce that is removed.

Structure of Erectile Tissue

Vascular spaces within the erectile tissues become engorged with blood, causing erection of the penis.

Erectile tissue of the penis contains numerous variably shaped, endothelially lined spaces that are separated from one another by trabeculae of connective tissue and smooth muscle cells. The vascular spaces of the corpora cavernosa are larger centrally and smaller peripherally, near the tunica albuginea. However, the vascular spaces of the corpus spongiosum are similar in size throughout its extent. The trabeculae of the corpus spongiosum contain more elastic fibers and fewer smooth muscle cells than those of the corpora cavernosa.

The erectile tissues of the corpora cavernosa receive blood from branches of the **deep and dorsal arteries of the penis** (see Fig. 21-21). These branches penetrate the walls of the trabeculae of the erectile tissue and form either capillary plexuses, which supply some blood flow into the vascular spaces, or coiled arteries **(helical arteries),** which are important sources of blood to the vascular spaces during erection of the penis.

Venous drainage occurs via three groups of veins, which are drained by the **deep dorsal vein** (see Fig. 21-21). The three groups of veins arise from the base of the glans penis, from the dorsal aspect of the corpora cavernosa, and from the ventral aspect of the corpora cavernosa and the corpus spongiosum. Additionally, some of the veins leave the erectile tissue at the root of the penis and drain into the plexus of veins that drain the prostate gland.

Mechanisms of Erection, Ejaculation, and Detumescence

Erection is controlled by the parasympathetic nervous system; it is a result of sexual, tactile, olfactory, visual, auditory, and/or psychological stimulation. Ejaculation is controlled by the sympathetic nervous system.

When the penis is flaccid, the vascular spaces of the erectile tissue contain little blood. In this condition, much of the arterial blood flow is diverted into arteriovenous anastomoses that connect the branches of the deep and dorsal arteries of the penis to veins that deliver their blood into the deep dorsal vein (Fig. 21-22A). Thus, the blood flow bypasses the vascular spaces of the erectile tissue.

Erection occurs when blood flow is shifted to the vascular spaces of the erectile tissues (the corpora cavernosa and, to a limited extent, the corpus spongiosum), causing the penis to enlarge and become turgid (Fig. 21-22B). During erection, the tunica albuginea surrounding the erectile tissues is stretched and decreases in thickness from 2 to 0.5 mm.

The shift in blood flow that leads to erection is controlled by the **parasympathetic nervous system** following sexual stimulation (e.g., pleasurable tactile, olfactory, visual, auditory, and psychological stimuli). The parasympathetic impulses trigger local release of **nitric oxide,** which causes relaxation of smooth muscles of the branches of the deep and dorsal arteries of the penis, increasing the flow of blood into the organ. Simultaneously, the arteriovenous anastomoses undergo constriction, diverting the flow of blood into the helical arteries of the erectile tissue. As these spaces become engorged with blood, the penis enlarges and becomes turgid, and erection ensues. The veins of the penis become compressed, and the blood is trapped in the vascular spaces of the erectile tissue, thus maintaining the penis in an erect condition (see Fig. 21-22).

Continued stimulation of the glans penis results in **ejaculation,** the forceful expulsion of **semen** from the male genital ducts. Each ejaculate, which has a volume of about 3 mL in humans, consists of secretions from the accessory genital glands and 200 to 300 million spermatozoa. Subsequent to erection, the bulbourethral glands release a viscous fluid that lubricates the lining of the urethra. Just before ejaculation, the prostate gland discharges its secretion into the urethra, and spermatozoa from the ampullae of the two ductus deferentes are released into the ejaculatory ducts. The prostatic secretion apparently helps the spermatozoa achieve motility. The final secretion added to semen is a fructose-rich fluid, released from the seminal vesicles, that provides energy to the spermatozoa. This secretion forms much of the volume of the ejaculate.

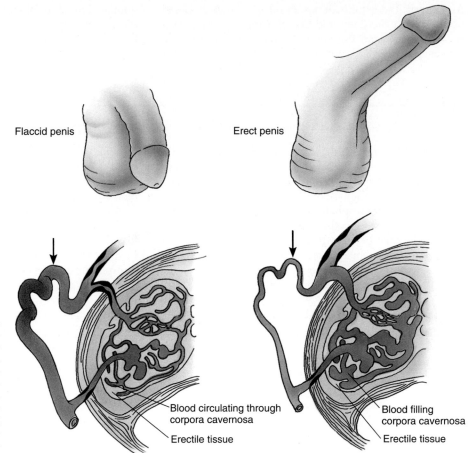

Flaccid penis

Erect penis

Blood circulating through
corpora cavernosa

Erectile tissue

Blood filling
corpora cavernosa

Erectile tissue

Figure 21–22 Circulation in the flaccid and erect penis. The arteriovenous anastomosis *(arrow)* in the flaccid penis is wide, diverting blood flow into the venous drainage. In the erect penis, the arteriovenous anastomosis is constricted and blood flow into the vascular spaces of the erectile tissue is increased, causing the penis to become turgid with blood. (Adapted from Conti G: Acta Anat 5:217, 1952.)

CLINICAL CORRELATIONS

A single ejaculate normally contains approximately 50 to 100 million spermatozoa per milliliter. A male whose sperm count is less than 20 million spermatozoa per milliliter of ejaculate is considered **sterile.**

The inability to achieve erection is known as **impotence.** Temporary erectile dysfunction can result from psychological factors or drugs (e.g., alcohol); whereas permanent impotence can be caused by many factors, including lesions in certain regions of the brain and hypothalamus, as well as spinal cord injuries, autonomic innervation malfunction, stroke, Parkinson's disease, diabetes, multiple sclerosis, and even psychological disorders.

Ejaculation, unlike erection, is regulated by the **sympathetic nervous system.** These impulses trigger the following sequence of events:

1 Contraction of the smooth muscles of the genital ducts and accessory genital glands forces the semen into the urethra.
2 The sphincter muscle of the urinary bladder contracts, preventing the release of urine (or the entry of semen into the bladder).
3 The bulbospongiosus muscle, which surrounds the proximal end of the corpus spongiosum (bulb of the penis), undergoes powerful, rhythmic contractions, resulting in forceful expulsion of semen from the urethra.

Ejaculation is followed by the cessation of parasympathetic impulses to the vascular supply of the penis.

As a result, the arteriovenous shunt is reopened, blood flow through the deep and dorsal arteries of the penis is diminished, and the vascular spaces of the erectile tissues are slowly emptied of blood by the venous drainage. As the blood leaves these vascular spaces, the penis undergoes **detumescence** and becomes flaccid.

CLINICAL CORRELATIONS

The neurotransmitter **nitric oxide (NO)** released by the endothelial cells of the sinusoids activate guanlyate cyclase of smooth muscle cells to produce cyclic guanosine monophosphate (cGMP) from guanosine triphosphate (GTP), thus relaxing the the smooth muscle cells. Relaxation of the smooth muscle cells permits the accumulation of blood in the sinusoids, and these enlarged vessels compress the small return venous channels that drain the sinusoids, resulting in erection of the penis.

After ejaculation or when the parasympathetic impulses cease and cGMP levels dwindle, another enzyme, **phosphodiesterase (PDE),** destroys the cGMP, permitting smooth muscle contraction to occur again; the sinusoids begin to be drained of blood and the erection is terminated.

Although **sildenafil (Viagra)** was originally developed as a treatment for heart failure, it was found to produce erections in many patients. Further study showed that the medication blocked phosphodiesterase from inhibiting cGMP degradation, thus leading to erection.

22

Special Senses

Peripheral nerve terminals are of two structural types: (1) terminals of axons, which transmit impulses from the central nervous system (CNS) to skeletal and smooth muscles **(motor endings)** or to glands **(secretory endings),** and (2) terminals of dendrites, called **sensory endings** or **receptors,** which perceive various stimuli and transmit this sensory input to the CNS. These sensory receptors are classified into three types, depending on the source of the stimulus, and are components of the general or special somatic and visceral afferent pathways:

- Exteroceptors
- Proprioceptors
- Interoceptors

Exteroceptors, located near the body surface, are specialized to perceive stimuli from the external environment. These receptors, sensitive to temperature, touch, pressure, and pain, are components of the **general somatic afferent** pathways and are described in the first part of this chapter. Other exteroceptors, specialized for perceiving light (sense of vision) and sound (sense of hearing), are components of the **special somatic afferent** pathways (discussed later). Smell and taste stimuli are perceived by unique nerve endings in the viscera of the respiratory and digestive systems, respectively; these exteroceptors are classified as the **special visceral afferent modality.** Receptors for olfaction (sense of smell) are discussed in Chapter 15, and receptors for taste are discussed in Chapter 16.

Proprioceptors are specialized receptors located in joint capsules, tendons, and intrafusal fibers within muscles (see Chapter 8). These **general somatic afferent** receptors transmit sensory input to the CNS, which is translated into information that relates to an awareness of the body in space and in movement. Certain receptors of the **vestibular (balance) mechanism** (see later), located within the inner ear, are specialized for receiving stimuli related to motion vectors within the head; this input is transmitted to the brain for processing into awareness of motion for corrective balancing.

Interoceptors are specialized receptors that perceive sensory information from within organs of the body; therefore, the modality serving this function is the **general visceral afferent** modality.

SPECIALIZED PERIPHERAL RECEPTORS

Certain peripheral receptors, specialized to receive particular stimuli, include mechanoreceptors, thermoreceptors, and nociceptors.

The dendritic endings of certain sensory receptors, located in various regions of the body, including muscles, tendons, skin, fascia, and joint capsules, are specialized to receive particular stimuli. These adaptations help the dendrite respond to a particular stimulus. Thus, these receptors are classified into three types:

- **Mechanoreceptors,** which respond to touch (Figs. 22-1 to 22-3)
- **Thermoreceptors,** which respond to cold and warmth
- **Nociceptors,** which respond to pain due to mechanical stress, extremes of temperature differences, and chemical substances

Although these specialized receptors generally are triggered only by a particular stimulus, any stimulus that is intense enough can trigger any receptor.

Mechanoreceptors

Mechanoreceptors respond to mechanical stimuli that may deform the receptor or the tissues surrounding the receptor. Stimuli that trigger the mechanoreceptors are touch, stretch, vibrations, and pressure.

Nonencapsulated Mechanoreceptors

Nonencapsulated mechanoreceptors are simple unmyelinated receptors present in the skin, connective tissues, and surrounding hair follicles.

Peritricial nerve endings, the simplest form of mechanoreceptors, are unmyelinated, lack Schwann cells, and are not covered by a connective tissue capsule. Such nerve endings are located in the epidermis of the skin, especially in regions of great sensitivity, such as the face and the cornea of the eye, where they respond to stimuli related to touch and pressure (see Fig. 22-1D). Additionally, peritricial nerve endings are wrapped around the base and shaft of hair follicles and function in touch perception related to the deformation of the hairs. Moreover, some naked nerve endings function as nociceptors or as thermoreceptors.

Merkel's disks are slightly more complex mechanoreceptors (see Fig. 22-1A). Specialized for perceiving discriminatory touch, these receptors are composed of an expanded unmyelinated nerve terminal associated with **Merkel cells,** specialized epithelial cells interspersed with keratinocytes in the stratum basale of the skin (see Fig. 14-1). These receptors are located mostly in nonhairy skin and regions of the body more sensitive to touch.

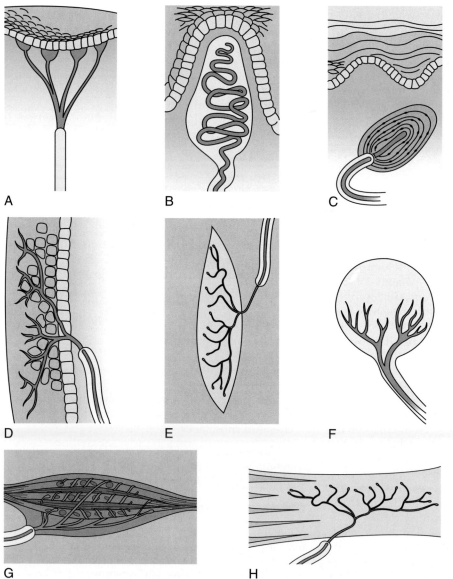

A

B

C

D

E

F

G

H

Figure 22–1 Various mechanoreceptors. **A,** Merkel's disk. **B,** Meissner's corpuscle. **C,** Pacinian corpuscle. **D,** Peritricial (naked) nerve endings. **E,** Ruffini's corpuscle. **F,** Krause's end bulb. **G,** Muscle spindle. **H,** Golgi tendon organ.

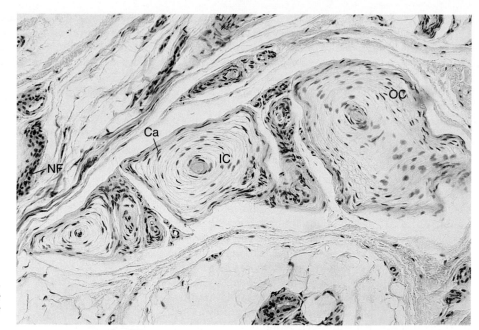

Figure 22–2 Pacinian corpuscles (×132). Ca, capsule; IC, inner core; NF, nerve fiber; OC, outer core.

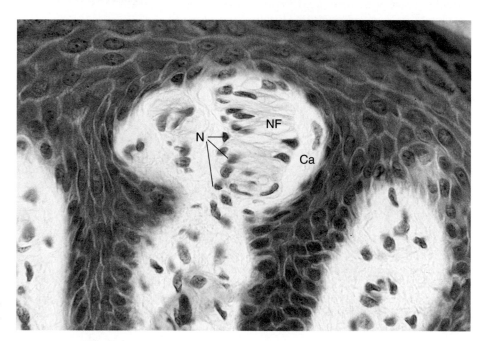

Figure 22–3 Meissner's corpuscle (×540). Ca, capsule; N, nuclei; NF, nerve fiber.

Encapsulated Mechanoreceptors

Encapsulated mechanoreceptors exhibit characteristic structures and are present in specific locations.

Meissner's corpuscles (see Fig. 22-3) are encapsulated mechanoreceptors specialized for **tactile discrimination.** These receptors are located in the dermal

papillae of the glabrous (nonhairy) portion of the fingers and palms of the hands, where they account for about half of the tactile receptors. They also are located in the eyelids, lips, tongue, nipples, and skin of the foot and forearm. Meissner's corpuscles, which measure 80 by 30 μm, are located in the dermal papillae, with their long axes oriented perpendicular to the skin surface (see Fig. 22-1B). Each Meissner's corpuscle is formed by three or four nerve terminals and their associated Schwann cells, all of which are encapsulated by connective tissue. Contained within the capsule are stacks of epithelioid cells, possibly modified Schwann cells or fibroblasts, that serve to separate the branching nerve terminals. Meissner's corpuscles are especially sensitive to edges and points and to movements of these objects.

Pacinian corpuscles, another example of the encapsulated mechanoreceptors, are located in the dermis and hypodermis in the digits of the hands and in the breasts, as well as in connective tissue of the joints, periosteum, and the mesentery. These mechanoreceptors are specialized to perceive pressure, touch, and vibration. Pacinian corpuscles are large, ovoid receptors 1 to 2 mm long by 0.1 to 0.7 mm in diameter (see Figs. 22-1C and 22-2). Each receptor is composed of a single unmyelinated fiber that courses the entire length of the corpuscle. The **core** of the corpuscle contains the nonmyelinated nerve terminal and its Schwann cells, surrounded by approximately 60 layers of modified fibroblasts, each layer separated from the next by a small fluid-filled space. An additional group of 30 less dense, modified fibroblasts surround the core and are, in turn, enveloped by connective tissue, forming the **capsule** around the core. The arrangement of the cells in the lamellae makes the histological section of a pacinian corpuscle resemble a sliced onion.

Ruffini's endings (corpuscles) are encapsulated endings located in the dermis of the skin, nail beds, periodontal ligaments, and joint capsules. These large receptors, 1 mm long by 0.2 mm in diameter (see Fig. 22-1E), are composed of branched, nonmyelinated terminals interspersed with collagen fibers and surrounded by four to five layers of modified fibroblasts. The connective tissue capsule surrounding each of these receptors is anchored at each end, increasing their sensibility to stretching and pressure in the skin and in the joint capsules.

Krause's end bulbs are spherical, encapsulated nerve endings located in the papillary region of the dermis, joints, conjunctiva, peritoneum, genital regions, and the subendothelial connective tissues of the oral and nasal cavities (see Fig. 22-1F). Originally, they were thought to be receptors sensitive to cold, but present evidence does not support this concept. Their function is unknown.

Both muscle spindles and Golgi tendon organs are encapsulated mechanoreceptors involved in proprioception. **Muscle spindles** (see Fig. 22-1G) provide feedback concerning the changes in muscle length as well as the rate of alteration in the length of the muscle, and **Golgi tendon organs** (see Fig. 22-1H) monitor the tension as well as the rate at which the tension is being produced during movement. Information from these two sensory structures is processed mostly at the unconscious levels within the spinal cord; however, the

information also reaches the cerebellum and even the cerebral cortex, so that the individual may sense muscle position. Golgi tendon organs and muscle spindles are discussed in Chapter 8.

Thermoreceptors

Thermoreceptors, which respond to temperature differences of about 2° C [35.6° F], are of three types: warmth receptors, cold receptors, and temperature-sensitive nociceptors.

Although specific receptors have not been identified for warmth, it is assumed that these receptors are naked endings of small nonmyelinated nerve fibers that respond to temperature increases. Cold receptors are derived from naked nerve endings of myelinated fibers that branch and penetrate the epidermis. Because thermoreceptors are not activated by physical stimulation, they are believed to respond to differing rates of temperature-dependent biochemical reactions.

Nociceptors

Nociceptors are receptors sensitive to pain caused by mechanical stress, extremes of temperature, and cytokines such as bradykinin, serotonin, and histamine.

Nociceptors are responsible for pain perception. These receptors are naked endings of myelinated nerve fibers that branch freely in the dermis before entering the epidermis. Nociceptors are divided into three groups: (1) those that respond to mechanical stress or damage; (2) those that respond to extremes in heat or cold; and (3) those that respond to chemical compounds such as bradykinin, serotonin, and histamine.

EYE

The bulb of the eye is composed of three tunics: fibrous, vascular, and neural.

The eyes (orbs), approximately 24 mm in diameter, are located within the hollow bony orbits of the skull . They are the **photosensory organs** of the body. Light passes through the cornea, lens, and several refractory structures of the orb; light is then focused by the lens on the light-sensitive portion of the neural tunic of the eye, the **retina,** which contains the photosensitive **rods and cones.** Through a series of several layers of nerve cells and supporting cells, the visual information is transmitted by the optic nerve to the brain for processing.

The eyes begin to develop from three different sources at about the 4th week of embryonic development. Outgrowths of the forebrain, the future retina and optic nerve, are the first to be observed. As a result of continued growth of this structure, the surface ecto-derm is induced to develop into the lens and some of the accessory structures of the anterior portion of the eye. Later in development, adjacent mesenchyme condenses to form the tunics and associated structures of the orb.

The bulb of the eye is composed of three tunics, or coats (Fig. 22-4):

- A **fibrous tunic,** forming the tough outer coat of the eye
- A **vascular tunic,** the pigmented and vascular middle coat
- A **neural tunic,** the retina, composing the innermost coat

The fibrous tunic of the eye also receives insertions of the **extrinsic muscles** of the eye, which are responsible for coordinated movements of the eyes to gain access to various visual fields. Smooth muscles located within the orb accommodate focusing of the lens and control the aperture of the pupil. Located outside the orb, but still within the orbit, is the **lacrimal gland** (tear gland), which secretes **lacrimal fluid** (tears) that moistens the anterior surface of the eye. The lacrimal fluid moistens the eye and the inner surface of the eyelids by passing through the **conjunctiva,** a transparent membrane that covers and protects the anterior surface of the eye.

Tunica Fibrosa

The tunica fibrosa is composed of the sclera and the cornea.

The external fibrous tunic of the eye, the tunica fibrosa, is divided into the sclera and the cornea (see Fig. 22-4). The white, opaque **sclera** covers the posterior five sixths of the orb, whereas the colorless, transparent **cornea** covers the anterior one-sixth of the orb.

Sclera

The white opaque sclera is composed of type I collagen fibers interlaced with elastic fibers.

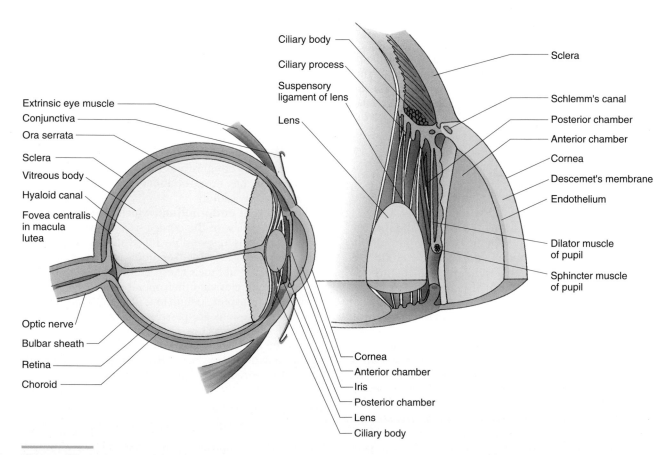

Figure 22–4 Anatomy of the eye (orb).

The sclera, the white of the eye, is nearly devoid of blood vessels. It is a tough, fibrous connective tissue layer, about 1 mm thick posteriorly, thinning at the equator and then thickening again near its junction with the cornea. It consists of interlacing type I collagen bundles alternating with networks of elastic fibers; this arrangement gives form to the orb, which is maintained by intraocular pressure from the aqueous humor (located anterior to the lens) and the vitreous body (located posterior to the lens).

Fibroblasts located in the connective tissue of the sclera are elongated, flat cells. Melanocytes are located in deeper regions of the sclera. Tendons of the extraocular muscles insert into the dense connective tissue surface layer of the sclera, which is enveloped by the **capsule of Tenon,** a fascial sheath that covers the optic nerve and the orb as far anteriorly as the ciliary region. This sheath, which separates the orb from the periorbital fat, is connected to the sclera by a thin layer of loose connective tissue called the **episclera.** The orb, along with its various parts and attached extraocular muscles, moves in unison within the periorbital fat–filled bony orbit.

Cornea

The cornea is the transparent bulging anterior sixth of the orb.

The cornea is the transparent, avascular, and highly innervated anterior portion of the fibrous tunic that bulges out anteriorly from the orb. It is slightly thicker than the sclera and is composed of five histologically distinct layers:

- Corneal epithelium
- Bowman's membrane
- Stroma
- Descemet's membrane
- Corneal endothelium

The **corneal epithelium,** the continuation of the conjunctiva (a mucous membrane covering the anterior sclera and lining the internal surface of the eyelids), is a stratified, squamous, nonkeratinized epithelium, composed of five to seven layers of cells, that covers the anterior surface of the cornea. The larger superficial cells have microvilli and exhibit zonulae occludentes. The remaining cells constituting the corneal epithelium interdigitate with and form desmosomal contacts with one another. Their cytoplasm contains the usual array of organelles along with intermediate filaments. The corneal epithelium is highly innervated by numerous free nerve endings. Mitotic figures are observed mostly near the periphery of the cornea, with a turnover rate of approximately 7 days. Damage to the cornea is repaired rapidly as cells migrate to the defect to cover the injured region. Subsequently, mitotic activity replaces the cells that migrated to the wound. The corneal epithelium also functions in transferring water and ions from the stroma into the conjunctival sac.

Bowman's membrane lies immediately deep to the corneal epithelium. Electron micrographs reveal it to be a fibrillar lamina, 6 to 30 μm thick, composed of type I collagen fibers arranged in an apparently random fashion. It is believed that Bowman's membrane is synthesized by both the corneal epithelium and cells of the underlying stroma. Sensory nerve fibers pass through this structure to enter and terminate in the epithelium.

The transparent **stroma** is the thickest layer of the cornea, constituting about 90% of its thickness. It is composed of collagenous connective tissue, consisting mostly of type I collagen fibers that are arranged in 200 to 250 lamellae, each about 2 μm in thickness. The collagen fibers within each lamella are arranged parallel to one another, but fiber orientation shifts in adjacent lamellae. The collagen fibers are interspersed with thin elastic fibers, embedded in ground substance containing mostly chondroitin sulfate and keratan sulfate. Long, slender fibroblasts are also present among the collagen fiber bundles. During inflammation, lymphocytes and neutrophils are also present in the stroma. At the **limbus** (sclerocorneal junction) is a scleral sulcus whose inner aspect at the stroma is depressed and houses endothelium-lined spaces, known as the **trabecular meshwork,** that lead to the canal of Schlemm. The **canal of Schlemm** is the site of outflow of the aqueous humor from the anterior chamber of the eye into the venous system.

Descemet's membrane is a thick basement membrane interposed between the stroma and the underlying endothelium. Although this membrane is thin (5 μm at birth) and homogeneous in younger persons, electron microscopy has demonstrated that it becomes thicker (17 μm) and has cross-striations and hexagonal fiber patterns in older adults.

The **corneal endothelium,** which lines the internal (posterior) surface of the cornea, is a simple squamous epithelium. It is responsible for synthesis of proteins that are necessary for secreting and maintaining Descemet's membrane. These cells exhibit numerous pinocytotic vesicles, and their membranes have sodium pumps that transport sodium ions (Na^+) into the anterior chamber; these ions are passively followed by chloride ions (Cl^-) and water. Thus, excess fluid within the stroma is resorbed by the endothelium, keeping the stroma relatively dehydrated, a factor that contributes to maintaining the refractive quality of the cornea.

Tunica Vasculosa

The vascular middle tunic of the eye, the tunica vasculosa (uvea), is composed of three parts: (1) the **choroid,** (2) the **ciliary body,** and (3) the **iris** (see Fig. 22-4).

Choroid

The choroid, the pigmented posterior portion of the middle vascular tunic, is loosely attached to the sclera and separated from the retina by Bruch's membrane.

The choroid is the well-vascularized, pigmented layer of the posterior wall of the orb that is loosely attached to the tunica fibrosa. It is composed of loose connective tissue containing numerous fibroblasts and other connective tissue cells, and it is richly supplied with blood vessels. The black color of the choroid is due to the myriad of melanocytes present in it. Because of the abundance of small blood vessels in the inner surface of the choroid, that region is known as the **choriocapillary layer** and is responsible for providing nutrients to the retina. The choroid is separated from the retina by **Bruch's membrane,** a membrane 1 to 4 μm thick composed of a network of elastic fibers located in the central region and sandwiched on both sides by collagen fiber layers. The outer aspect of each collagen fiber layer is covered by a basal lamina that belongs to capillaries on one side and the pigment epithelium of the retina on the other side.

Ciliary Body

The ciliary body is a wedge-shaped portion of the choroid located in the lumen of the orb between the iris and the vitreous body and projecting toward the lens.

The ciliary body, the wedge-shaped extension of the choroid that rings the inner wall of the eye at the level of the lens, occupies the space between the ora serrata of the retina (the junction between and anterior and posterior portions of the retina) and the iris. One surface of the ciliary body abuts the sclera at the sclerocorneal junction, another surface abuts the vitreous body, whereas the medial surface projects toward the lens, forming short, finger-like projections known as **ciliary processes.**

The ciliary body is composed of loose connective tissue containing numerous elastic fibers, blood vessels, and melanocytes. Its inner surface is lined by the **pars ciliaris of the retina,** a pigmented layer of the retina that is composed of two cell layers. The outer cell layer, which faces the lumen of the orb, is a nonpigmented columnar epithelium (**nonpigmented ciliary epithelium**), whereas the inner cell layer is composed of a pigmented simple columnar epithelium (**pigmented ciliary epithelium**), which is rich in melanin.

The anterior one third of the ciliary body has about 70 **ciliary processes,** which radiate out from a central core of connective tissue containing abundant fenestrated capillaries. Fibers, composed of fibrillin (**zonule fibers**), radiate from the ciliary processes to insert into the lens capsule, forming the **suspensory ligaments of the lens,** which anchor the lens in place.

The ciliary processes are covered by the same two layers of epithelium that cover the ciliary body. The inner nonpigmented layer has many interdigitations and infoldings; its cells transport a protein-poor plasma filtrate, the **aqueous humor,** into the posterior chamber of the eye. The aqueous humor flows from the posterior chamber into the anterior chamber by passing through the **pupillary aperture** between the iris and the lens. The aqueous humor exits the anterior chamber by passing into the trabecular meshwork near the limbus and, finally, as stated previously, into the canal of Schlemm, which leads directly into the venous system. Aqueous humor provides nutrients and oxygen for the lens and the cornea.

The bulk of the ciliary body is composed of three bundles of smooth muscle cells called the **ciliary muscle.** One bundle, because of its orientation, stretches the choroid, thus altering the opening of the canal of Schlemm for drainage of the aqueous humor. The remaining two muscle bundles, attached at the scleral spur, function in reducing tension on the zonulae. Contractions of this muscle, mediated by parasympathetic fibers of the oculomotor nerve (cranial nerve [CN] III), stretch the choroid body, thereby releasing tension on the suspensory ligaments of the lens. As a result, the lens becomes thicker and more convex. This action permits focusing on nearby objects, a process called **accommodation.** Relaxation of all three muscle bundles increases tension on the zonule, thereby flattening the lens enabling focusing on distant objects. Constant adjustments between various degrees of contraction and relaxation are required to permit focusing on objects distant, intermediate, and close.

CLINICAL CORRELATIONS

Glaucoma is a condition resulting from prolonged increased intraocular pressure caused by the failure of drainage of the aqueous humor from the anterior chamber of the eye. It is one of the world's leading causes of blindness. In **chronic glaucoma,** the most common condition, the continued increasing pressure causes progressive damage to the eye, particularly in the retina; if left untreated, blindness results.

Iris

The iris, the colored anterior extension of the choroid, is a contractile diaphragm that controls the pupillary aperture.

The iris, the anteriormost extension of the choroid, lies between the posterior and anterior chambers of the eye, completely covering the lens except at the **pupillary aperture (pupil).** The iris is thickest in the middle, thinning toward its junction with the ciliary body and at the rim of the pupil. The anterior surface consists of two concentric rings: the **pupillary zone,** lying nearest the pupil, and the wider **ciliary zone.** The anterior surface of the iris is irregular, with trenches extending into it; it also contains contraction furrows, which are easily distinguished when the pupil is dilated. An incomplete layer of pigmented cells and fibroblasts covers the anterior surface of the iris. Deep to this layer is a stroma of poorly vascularized connective tissue containing numerous fibroblasts and melanocytes, which gives way to a well-vascularized, loose connective tissue zone.

The posterior surface of the iris is smooth and is covered by the continuation of the two layers of retinal epithelium that cover the ciliary body. The surface facing the lens is composed of heavily pigmented cells, which block the light from passing through the iris except at the pupil. The epithelial cells facing the stroma of the iris have extensions that form the **dilator pupillae muscle.** Hence, this muscle is myoepithelial in nature. Another muscle, the **sphincter pupillae muscle,** is located in a concentric ring around the pupil. Contractions of these smooth muscles alter the diameter of the pupil. The diameter of the pupil changes inversely to the amount of light entering it. Thus, bright light causes constriction of pupillary diameter, whereas dim light dilates it. Pupil diameter is the result of the the functions of the two intrinsic muscles contained within the iris. The dilator pupillae muscle, innervated by the sympathetic nervous system, dilates the pupil; the sphincter pupillae muscle, innervated by parasympathetic fibers of the oculomotor nerve (CN III), constricts the pupil.

The abundant population of melanocytes in the epithelium and stroma of the iris not only blocks the passage of light into the eye (except at the pupil) but also imparts color to the eyes. The eyes are dark when the number of melanocytes is high, and they are blue when the number of melanocytes is low.

Lens

The lens, the transparent biconvex disk located directly behind the pupil, focuses light rays on the retina.

The lens of the eye is a flexible, biconvex, transparent disk composed of epithelial cells and their secretory products. The lens consists of three parts: lens capsule, subcapsular epithelium, and lens fibers (see Fig. 22-4).

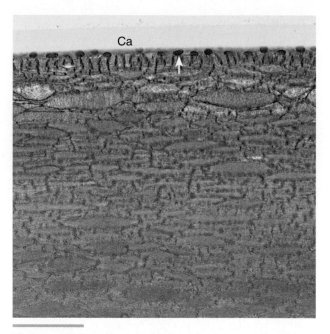

Figure 22–5 Light micrograph of the lens (×132). Note the simple cuboidal epithelium (*arrow*) on the anterior surface and the capsule (Ca) covering the epithelium.

The **lens capsule** is a basal lamina, 10 to 20 μm thick, containing mostly type IV collagen and glycoprotein that covers the epithelial cells and envelops the entire lens. This elastic, transparent, homogeneous structure, which refracts light, is thickest anteriorly.

The **subcapsular epithelium** is located only on the anterior and lateral surfaces of the lens, immediately deep to the lens capsule (Fig. 22-5). It is composed of a single layer of cuboidal cells, which communicate with each other via gap junctions. The apices of these cells are directed toward the lens fibers and interdigitate with them, especially in the vicinity of the equator, where they are elongated and are columnar in shape.

The bulk of the lens is composed of approximately 2000 long cells known as **lens fibers.** These cells lie immediately deep to the subcapsular epithelium and lens capsule (Fig. 22-6). The cells of the subcapsular epithelium give rise to these highly differentiated, hexagonal cells, the lens fibers, which lose their nuclei and organelles and continue elongating until they reach a length of 7 to 10 μm. This process of elongation, known as **maturation,** continues throughout the life of the individual. Eventually these long, hexagonal cells become filled with **crystallins,** which are lens proteins whose presence increases the refractory index of the lens fibers.

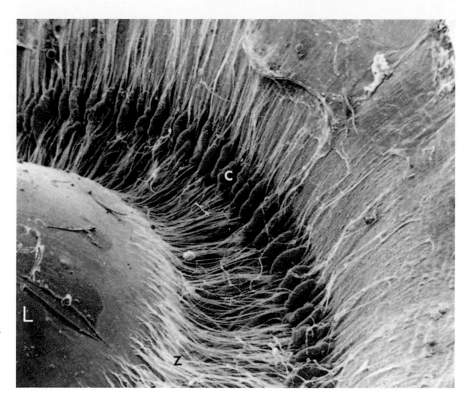

Figure 22–6 Scanning electron micrograph of the posterior surface of the lens (×28). C, ciliary body; L, lens; Z, zonula fibers. (From Leeson TS, Lee CR, Paparo AA: Text/Atlas of Histology. Philadelphia, WB Saunders, 1988.)

CLINICAL CORRELATIONS

Presbyopia is the inability of the eye to focus on near objects (accommodation) and is caused by an age-related decrease in the elasticity of the lens. As a result, the lens cannot become spherical for exact focusing. This condition can be corrected with eyeglasses.

Cataract is usually also an age-related condition in which the lens becomes opaque, thus impairing vision. This condition may be due to an accumulation of pigment or other substances as well as to excessive exposure to ultraviolet radiation. Although cataracts do not usually respond to medication and eventually lead to blindness, the opaque lens may be excised and replaced with a corrective lens.

Vitreous Body

The vitreous body is a transparent, refractile gel that fills the cavity of the eye **(vitreous cavity)** behind the lens. It is composed mostly (99%) of water containing a minute amount of electrolytes, collagen fibers, and hyaluronic acid. It adheres to the retina over its entire surface, especially at the ora serrata. Occasional macrophages and small cells called **hyalocytes** are observed at the periphery of the vitreous body; these are believed to synthesize collagen and hyaluronic acid. The fluid-filled **hyaloid canal,** a narrow channel that was occupied by the hyaloid artery in the fetus, extends through the entire vitreous body from the posterior aspect of the lens to the optic disk.

CLINICAL CORRELATIONS

Eye floaters (vitreous opacities)—specks, clouds, cobwebs, and so forth—that persons appear to see in front of their eyes represent small debris that is floating in the vitreous body, caused by its dehydration. These objects cast shadows on the retina that are translated by the brain as images in front of the eyes. Although most of the time these floaters naturally resolve, some persons find their presence disruptive, especially when they are reading or driving. Specialized laser treatments can obliterate the floaters.

Retina (Neural Tunic)

The retina, composed of 10 layers, possesses specialized receptors, called rods and cones, that are responsible for photoreception.

The retina, the third and innermost tunic of the eye, is its neural portion, which contains the photoreceptor cells, known as rods and cones (Figs. 22-7, 22-8, and 22-9; also see Fig. 22-4). The retina develops from the optic cup, an evagination of the diencephalon, which gives rise to the primary optic vesicle. Later in development, this structure invaginates to form a bilaminar, secondary optic vesicle from which the retina develops, whereas the stalk of the optic cup becomes the optic nerve.

The retina is formed of an outer **pigmented layer** that develops from the outer wall of the optic cup. The neural portion of the retina develops from the inner layer of the optic cup and is called the **retina proper.** The pigmented layer of the retina covers the entire internal surface of the orb, reflecting over the ciliary body and the posterior wall of the iris, whereas the retina proper stops at the ora serrata. The cells composing the retina proper constitute a highly differentiated extension of the brain.

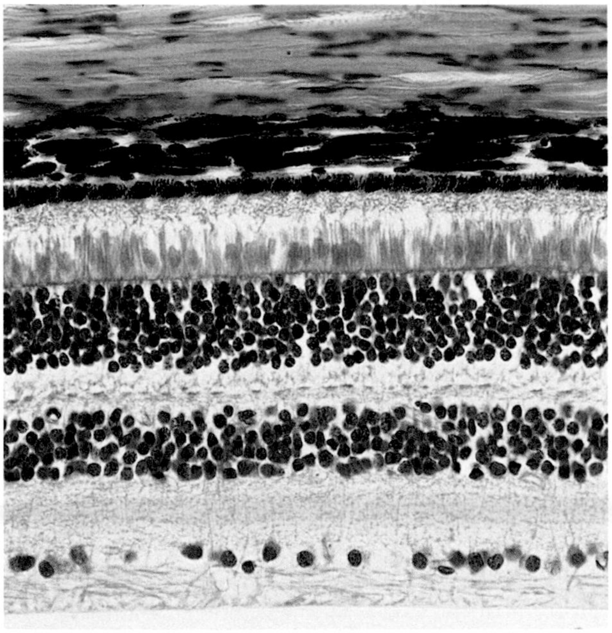

The **optic disk,** located on the posterior wall of the orb, is the exit site of the optic nerve. Because it contains no photoreceptor cells, it is insensitive to light and is therefore called the **"blind spot"** of the retina. Approximately 2.5 mm lateral to the **optic disk** is a yellow-pigmented zone in the retinal wall called the **macula lutea** (yellow spot). Located in the center of this spot is an oval depression, the **fovea centralis,** where visual acuity is greatest (see Fig 22-4). The fovea is a specialized area of the retina containing only cones, which are packed tightly as the other layers of the retina are pushed aside. As distance from the fovea increases, the number of cones decreases and the number of rods increases.

The portion of the retina that functions in photoreception lines (faces) the inner surface of the choroid

Figure 22–7 Light micrograph of the retina with its described ten layers (×270). (1) Pigment epithelium, (2) lamina of rods and cones, (3) external (outer) limiting membrane, (4) outer nuclear layer, (5) outer plexiform layer, (6) inner nuclear layer, (7) inner plexiform layer, (8) ganglion cell layer, (9) optic nerve fiber layer, (10) inner limiting membrane.

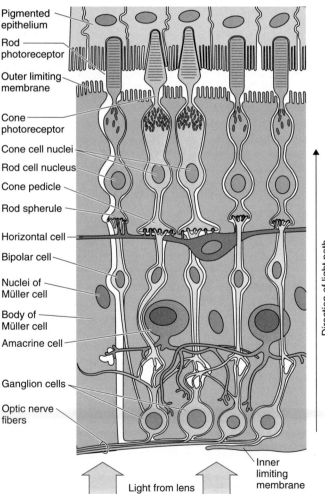

Pigmented epithelium
Rod photoreceptor
Outer limiting membrane
Cone photoreceptor
Cone cell nuclei
Rod cell nucleus
Cone pedicle
Rod spherule
Horizontal cell
Bipolar cell
Nuclei of Müller cell
Body of Müller cell
Amacrine cell
Ganglion cells
Optic nerve fibers
Inner limiting membrane
Direction of light path
Light from lens

Figure 22–8 Cellular layers of the retina. The space observed between the pigmented layer and the remainder of the retina is an artifact of development and does not exist in the adult except during detachment of the retina.

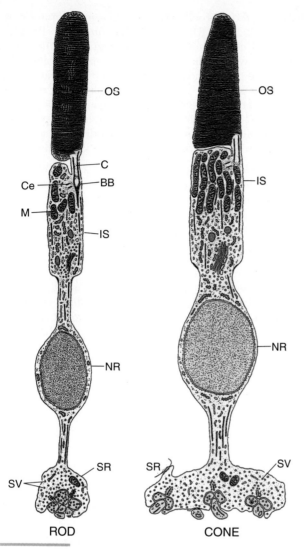

Figure 22–9 Morphology of a rod and a cone. BB, basal body; C, connecting stalk; Ce, centriole; IS, inner segment; M, mitochondria; NR, nuclear region; OS, outer segment; SR, synaptic region; SV, synaptic vesicles. (Modified from Lentz TL: Cell Fine Structure: An Atlas of Drawings of Whole-Cell Structure. Philadelphia, WB Saunders, 1971.)

layer from the optic disk to the ora serrata and is composed of 10 distinct layers (see Figs. 22-7 and 22-8). From outside, adjacent to the choroid, to inside, where they are continuous with the optic nerve, these layers are as follows:

1 Pigment epithelium
2 Layer of rods and cones
3 External (outer) limiting membrane
4 Outer nuclear layer
5 Outer plexiform layer
6 Inner nuclear layer
7 Inner plexiform layer
8 Ganglion cell layer
9 Optic nerve fiber layer
10 Inner limiting membrane.

Pigment Epithelium

The pigment epithelium, derived from the outer layer of the optic cup, is composed of cuboidal to columnar cells (14 μm wide and 10 to 14 μm tall) whose nuclei are located basally. The cells are attached to Bruch's membrane, which is located between the choroid and the pigment cells. Mitochondria are especially abundant in the cytoplasm near the numerous cell invaginations with Bruch's membrane, suggesting transport in this region. Desmosomes, zonulae occludentes, and zonulae adherentes are present on the lateral cell membranes, forming the blood-retina barrier. Moreover, gap junctions on the lateral cell membranes permit intercellular communication. The cell apices exhibit microvilli and sleeve-like structures that surround and isolate the tips of the individual photoreceptor cells.

The most distinctive feature of the pigment cells is their abundance of melanin granules, which these cells synthesize and store in their apical portions. The apical cytoplasm also contains residual bodies housing phagocytosed tips shed by the rods. Additionally, smooth endoplasmic reticulum (SER), rough endoplasmic reticulum (RER), and Golgi apparatus are abundant in the cytoplasm.

The pigmented epithelium has several functions. Pigmented epithelial cells absorb light after it has passed through and stimulated the photoreceptors, thus preventing reflections from the tunics, which would impair focus. These pigmented cells continually phagocytose spent membranous disks from the tips of the photoreceptor rods. Pigment epithelial cells also play an active role in vision by esterifying vitamin A derivatives in their SER.

CLINICAL CORRELATIONS

Because the sleeve-like extensions of the pigment epithelial cells merely surround the photoreceptor rod and cone tips, sudden hard jolts may disengage them, resulting in **detachment of the retina,** a common cause of partial blindness. The condition can be corrected surgically by "spot welding" the two structures back together. However, if this condition is left unattended, the rods and cones die because they will have lost the metabolic support normally provided by the pigment epithelium. Their death leaves a blind spot in the visual field corresponding to the area where the photoreceptors were lost.

Layer of Rods and Cones

The optical portion of the retina houses two distinct types of photoreceptor cells called rods and cones. Both rods and cells are polaarized cells whose apical portions, known as the **outer segments,** are specialized dendrites. The outer segments of the rods and cones are surrounded by pigmented epithelial cells (see Fig. 22-8). The bases of the rod and cone cells form synapses with the underlying cells of the bipolar layer. There are approximately 100 to 120 million rods and 6 million cones. Rods are specialized receptors for perceiving objects in dim light, whereas cones are specialized receptors for perceiving objects in bright light reception. Cones are further adapted for color vision, whereas rods perceive only light. Rods and cones are unevenly distributed in the retina, in that cones are highly concentrated in the fovea; thus, this is the area of the retina where high-acuity vision occurs.

Rods

Rods are the photoreceptors of the retina specialized for perceiving dim light.

Rods, which are activated in dim light only, are so sensitive that they can produce a signal from a single photon of light. However, they cannot mediate signals in bright light, and they cannot sense color. Rods are elongated cells (50 μm long by 3 μm in diameter) oriented parallel to one another but perpendicular to the retina. These are composed of an outer segment, an inner segment, a nuclear region, and a synaptic region (see Fig. 22-9).

The **outer segment of the rod,** its dendritic end, presents several hundred flattened membranous lamellae oriented perpendicular to its long axis (Fig. 22-10; also see Fig. 22-9). Each lamella represents an invagination of the plasmalemma, which is detached from the cell surface, thus forming a disk. Each disk is composed of two membranes separated from each other by an 8-nm space. The membranes contain **rhodopsin (visual purple),** a light-sensitive pigment. Because the outer segment is longer in rods than in cones, rods contain more rhodopsin, respond more slowly than cones, and have the capacity to collectively summate the reception.

The **inner segment of the rod** is separated from the outer segment by a constriction called the **connecting stalk.** Passing through the connecting stalk and into the outer segment of the rod is a modified cilium (lacking the central singlet microtubules) that arises from a basal body located at the apical end of the inner segment. Congregated near the interface with the connecting stalk are abundant mitochondria and cytoplasmic glycogen granules, both necessary for the production of energy for the visual process. The cytoplasm basal to the mitochondria is rich in microtubules, polysomes, SER, RER, and Golgi complexes. Proteins produced in the inner segment migrate to the outer segment, where they become incorporated into the disks. The disks gradually migrate to the apical end of the outer segment and are eventually shed into the sheaths of the pigment cells, where they will be phagocytosed. The length of time from protein incorporation, through migration, and finally to shedding is less than 2 weeks. The process of photoreception is as follows:

1 Photoreception by rods begins with absorption of light by the light-sensitive photopigment **rhodopsin,** composed of the transmembrane protein **opsin** bound to *cis* retinal, the aldehyde form of vitamin A.

2 Absorption of light causes isomerization of the retinal moiety into **all-*trans* retinal,** which then dissociates from opsin.

3 This **bleaching** yields activated opsin, which facilitates binding of guanosine triphosphate (GTP) to the α-subunit of **transducin,** a trimeric G protein.

4 The resulting **GTP-G$_\alpha$** activates cyclic guanosine monophosphate (cGMP) phosphodiesterase, an enzyme that catalyzes the breakdown of 3',5'-cGMP.

5 The decreasing cytosolic cGMP concentration results in closure of Na$^+$ channels in the plasma membrane of the rod so that Na$^+$ cannot leave the cell, and the **rod becomes hyperpolarized.**

6 Hyperpolarization of the rod results in the **inhibition of neurotransmitter release** into the synapse with the bipolar cells.

7 During the next dark phase, the level of cGMP is regenerated, the Na$^+$ channels are reopened, and the **Na$^+$ flow** resumes as before.

8 The **all-*trans* retinal** remaining from the breakdown **diffuses** and is carried to the retinal pigment epithelium via retinal binding proteins.

9 The **all-*trans* retinal is recycled** to its 11-*cis* retinal form.

10 Finally, *cis* retinal is returned to the rod, where it is once again bound to opsin to form **rhodopsin.**

When the rod is not activated by light, cGMP maintains open Na$^+$ channels in the plasmalemmae of rod cells. During the dark phase, sodium ions are pumped out of the inner segment and enter the outer segment of the rods through sodium-gated ion channels. The presence of sodium ions in the outer segment results in the release of neurotransmitter substance into the synapse with the bipolar cells.

The signal is not induced by depolarization, as it is in most cells; rather, light-induced hyperpolarization causes the signal to be transmitted through the various cell layers to the ganglion cells, where the signal generates an action potential along the axons to the brain.

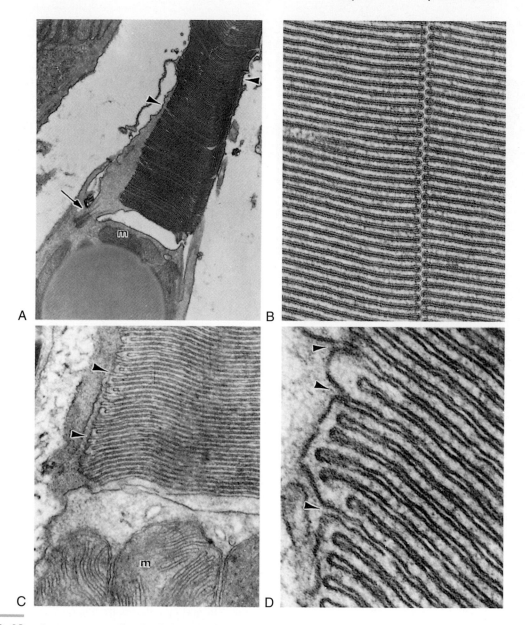

Figure 22–10 Electron micrographs of rods from the eye of a frog and cones from the eye of a squirrel. **A,** Disks in the outer segment (*arrowheads*) and mitochondria (m) in the inner segment of the rod of a frog (×16,200). Note the cilium (*arrow*) connecting the inner and outer segments. **B,** Higher magnification of the disks in the outer segment of the rod of a frog (×76,500). **C,** Junction of the outer and inner segments of the cone of a squirrel (*arrowheads,* disks in the outer segment). m, mitochondria. (×28,800). **D,** Higher magnification of the disks in the outer segment of a squirrel eye showing continuity of the lamellae with the plasmalemma (*arrowheads*). (×82,800). (From Leeson TS, Leeson CR, Paparo AA: Text-Atlas of Histology. Philadelphia, WB Saunders, 1988.)

Cones

Cones are specialized photoreceptors of the retina for perceiving bright light and color.

Although the mode of function of the cones is similar to that of rods, cones are activated in bright light and produce greater visual acuity compared with rods.

There are three types of cones, each containing a different variety of the photopigment **iodopsin.** Each variety of iodopsin has a maximum sensitivity to one of three colors of the spectrum—red, green, and blue—and the difference resides in the opsins rather than in the 11-*cis* retinal.

Cones are elongated cells (60 μm long by 1.5 μm in diameter), being longer and narrower at the fovea

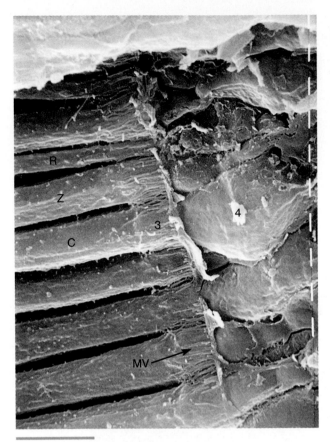

Figure 22–11 Scanning electron micrograph of the retina in a monkey in a displaying cones (C) and a few rods (R) (×5800). MV, microvilli belonging to the Müller cells; Z, inner segments; 3, external (outer) limiting membrane; 4, outer nuclear layer. (From Borwein B, Borwein D, Medeiros J, McGowan J: The ultrastructure of monkey foveal photoreceptors, with special reference to the structure, shape, size, and spacing of the foveal cones. Am J Anat 159:125-146, 1980.)

centralis. Their structure is similar to that of rods with the following few exceptions (Fig. 22-11; also see Figs. 22-9B and 22-10):

■ Their apical terminal (outer segment) is shaped more like a cone than a rod.
■ The disks of cones, although composed of lamellae of the plasmalemma, are attached to the plasma membrane, unlike the lamellae of the rods, which are separated from the plasma membrane.
■ Protein produced in the inner segment of cones is inserted into the disks throughout the entire outer segment; in the rods, it is concentrated in the most distal region of the outer segment.
■ Unlike rods, cones are sensitive to color and provide greater visual acuity.
■ Recycling of the cone photopigment does not require the retina pigment cells for the processing.

External (Outer) Limiting Membrane

Although the term *external limiting membrane* is still used in descriptions of the layers of the retina, this structure is not a membrane. Instead, electron micrographs have revealed that this "layer" is a region of zonulae adherentes between Müller cells (modified neuroglial cells) and the photoreceptors. Distal to this, microvilli of the Müller cells project into the interstices between the inner segments of the rods and cones.

Outer Nuclear Layer

The outer nuclear layer consists of a zone occupied mainly by the nuclei of the rods and cones. In histological sections, the nuclei of rods are smaller, more rounded, and more darkly stained than the nuclei of cones.

Outer Plexiform Layer

Axodendritic synapses between the photoreceptor cells and dendrites of bipolar and horizontal cells are located in the outer plexiform layer. There are two types of synapses in this layer: *flat synapses*, which display the usual synaptic histology, and *invaginated synapses.* Invaginated synapses are unique, in that they consist of a dendrite of a single bipolar cell and a dendrite from each of two horizontal cells, thus making a **triad.** Located within this invaginated synaptic region is a ribbon-like lamella **(synaptic ribbon)** containing neurotransmitter. It is believed that this structure captures and assists in distributing the neurotransmitter.

Inner Nuclear Layer

The nuclei of bipolar, horizontal, amacrine, and Müller cells compose the inner nuclear layer.

Bipolar neurons are interposed between photoreceptor cells and ganglion cells. These neurons may be contacted by many rods (10 near the macula to as many as 100 near the ora serrata), thus permitting summation of the signals, which is especially useful in low light intensity. Cones, however, do not converge, at least near the fovea; instead each cone synapses with several bipolar cells, thus further enhancing visual acuity. Axons of the bipolar cells synapse with dendrites of the ganglion cells.

Horizontal cells located in this layer synapse with the synaptic junctions between the photoreceptor cells and the bipolar cells. These cells function to modulate the synaptic activity.

Amacrine cells are located at the inner limits of this layer. Their dendrites all exit from one area of the cell and terminate on synaptic complexes between bipolar cells and ganglion cells. They also synapse on **interplexiform cells** that are interspersed with bipolar cell bodies. Amacrine cells function as a feedback mechanism by transferring neuronal information derived from the bipolar cell-ganglion synaptic complex to interplexiform cells, whose axons communicate with bipolar and horizontal cells.

Müller cells are neuroglial cells that extend between the vitreous body and the inner segments of the rods and cones, where Müller cells end by forming zonulae adherentes with the photoreceptor cells represented by the external limiting membrane. Microvilli extend from the apical surface. Thus, Müller cells function as supporting cells for the neural retina.

Inner Plexiform Layer

The processes of amacrine, bipolar, and ganglion cells are intermingled in the inner plexiform layer. **Axodendritic synapses** between the axons of bipolar cells and the dendrites of ganglion cells and amacrine cells also are located here. As in the outer plexiform layer, there are two types of synapses in this layer: *flat* and *invaginated*. Invaginated synapses consist of an axon of a single bipolar cell and two dendrites of either amacrine cells or ganglion cells or one dendrite from each of the two different cells, thus making a **dyad**. Also located within this synapse is a shortened version of the **synaptic ribbon**, which contains neurotransmitter.

Ganglion Cell Layer

Cell bodies of large multipolar neurons of the ganglion cells, up to 30 μm in diameter, are located in the ganglion cell layer. The axons of these neurons pass to the brain. Hyperpolarization of the rods and cones activates these ganglion cells, which then generate an action potential that is passed by their axons to the brain via the visual relay system.

Optic Nerve Fiber Layer

Nerve fibers are formed of unmyelinated axons of the ganglion cells in the optic nerve fiber layer. These axons become myelinated as the nerve pierces the sclera.

Inner Limiting Membrane

Basal laminae of the Müller cells compose the inner limiting membrane.

Accessory Structures of the Eye

Conjunctiva

The conjunctiva is the mucous membrane lining the eyelids and reflecting onto the sclera of the anterior surface of the eye.

A transparent mucous membrane, known as the conjunctiva, lines the inner surface of the eyelids (**palpebral conjunctiva**) and covers the sclera of the anterior portion of the eye (**bulbar conjunctiva**). The conjunctiva is composed of a stratified columnar epithelium that contains goblet cells overlying a basal lamina and a lamina propria composed of loose connective tissue. Secretions of the goblet cells become a part of the **tear film,** which aids in lubricating and protecting the epithelium of the anterior aspect of the eye. At the corneoscleral junction, where the cornea begins, the conjunctiva continues as the stratified squamous **corneal epithelium** and is devoid of goblet cells.

CLINICAL CORRELATIONS

Conjunctivitis is an inflammation of the conjunctiva usually associated with hyperemia and a discharge. It may be caused by a number of bacterial agents, viruses, allergens, and parasitic organisms. Some forms of conjunctivitis are extremely contagious, are damaging to the eye, and may cause blindness if untreated.

Eyelids

Eyelids, covered externally by skin and internally by the conjunctiva, provide a protective barrier for the anterior surface of the eye.

The eyelids are formed as folds of skin that cover the anterior surface of the developing eye. Accordingly, stratified squamous epithelium of skin covers their external surface; at the **palpebral fissure,** palpebral conjunctiva covers their inner surface. The eyelids are supported by a framework of **tarsal plates.** Sweat glands are located in the skin of the eyelids, as are fine hairs and sebaceous glands. The dermis of the eyelids is generally thinner than in most skin, contains numerous elastic fibers, and is without fat. The margins of the eyelids contain **eyelashes** arranged in rows of three or four, but they are without arrector pili muscles.

Modified sweat glands, called **glands of Moll,** form a simple spiral before opening into the eyelash follicles. **Meibomian glands,** modified sebaceous glands located in the tarsus of each lid, open on the free edge of the lids. The oily substance secreted by these glands becomes incorporated into the tear film and impedes evaporation of the tears. Other smaller, modified sebaceous glands, the **glands of Zeis,** are associated with the eyelashes and secrete their product into the eyelash follicles.

Lacrimal Apparatus

The lacrimal apparatus keeps the anterior surface of the eye lubricated with tears, thus preventing dehydration of the cornea.

The lacrimal apparatus consists of:

- The lacrimal gland, which secretes the lacrimal fluid (tears)
- The lacrimal canaliculi, which carry the lacrimal fluid away from the surface of the eye
- The lacrimal sac, a dilated portion of the duct system
- The nasolacrimal duct, which delivers the lacrimal fluid to the nasal cavity

The **lacrimal gland** lies in the lacrimal fossa located in the superolateral aspect of the orbit. It lies outside the conjunctival sac, although it communicates with the sac via 6 to 12 secretory ducts, which open into the sac at the lateral portion of the superior conjunctival fornix. The gland is a serous, compound tubuloalveolar gland that resembles the parotid gland. Myoepithelial cells completely surround its secretory acini.

Lacrimal fluid (tears) is composed mostly of water. This sterile fluid, containing the antibacterial agent **lysozyme,** passes through the secretory ducts to enter the conjunctival sac. The upper eyelids, by blinking, wash the tears over the anterior portion of the sclera and cornea, thus keeping them moist and protected from dehydration. The lacrimal fluid is wiped in a medial direction and enters the **lacrimal punctum,** an aperture located in each of the medial margins of the upper and lower eyelids. The punctum of each eyelid leads directly to **lacrimal canaliculi,** which join into a common conduit that leads to the lacrimal sac. The walls of the lacrimal canaliculi are lined by stratified squamous epithelium.

The **lacrimal sac** is the dilated superior portion of the nasolacrimal duct. It is lined by pseudostratified ciliated columnar epithelium.

The inferior continuation of the lacrimal sac is the **nasolacrimal duct,** also lined by pseudostratified ciliated columnar epithelium. This duct carries the lacrimal fluid into the inferior meatus located in the floor of the nasal cavity.

EAR (VESTIBULOCOCHLEAR APPARATUS)

The ear, the organ of hearing and balance, is composed of three regions: the outer ear, the middle ear, and the inner ear.

The ear, the organ of hearing as well as the organ of equilibrium, or balance, is divisible into three parts: (1) the external ear, (2) the middle ear (tympanic cavity), and (3) the inner ear (Fig. 22-12).

Sound waves received by the **external ear** are translated into mechanical vibrations by the tympanic membrane (eardrum). These vibrations then are amplified by the bony ossicles in the **middle ear (tympanic cavity)** and transferred to the fluid medium of the **inner ear** at the oval window. The inner ear, a perilymph-filled bony labyrinth in which is suspended a membranous labyrinth, regulates hearing (the cochlear portion) and maintains balance (the vestibular portion). Sensory input into the entire vestibulocochlear apparatus is transmitted to the brain by the two divisions of the vestibulocochlear nerve (CN VIII).

External Ear

The external ear comprises the auricle, the external auditory meatus, and the tympanic membrane.

The external ear is composed of the auricle (pinna), the external auditory meatus, and the tympanic membrane (see Fig. 22-12). The **auricle** develops from parts of the first and second branchial arches. Its general shape, size, and specific contours are usually distinctive in each person, with familial similarities. The pinna is composed of an irregularly shaped plate of elastic cartilage covered by thin skin that adheres tightly to the cartilage. The cartilage of the pinna is continuous with the cartilage lining the cartilaginous portion of the external auditory meatus.

The **external auditory meatus** is the canal that extends from the pinna into the temporal bone to the external surface of the tympanic membrane. Its superficial portion is composed of elastic cartilage, which is continuous with the cartilage of the pinna. Temporal bone replaces the cartilage as support within the inner two thirds of the canal. The external auditory meatus is covered with skin containing hair follicles, sebaceous glands, and modified sweat glands known as **ceruminous glands,** which produce a waxy material called **cerumen** (earwax). Hair and the sticky wax help prevent objects from penetrating deep into the meatus.

The **tympanic membrane** covers the deepest end of the external auditory meatus. It represents the closing plate between the first pharyngeal groove and the first pharyngeal pouch, where ectoderm, mesoderm, and endoderm are in close proximity. The external surface of the tympanic membrane is covered by a thin epidermis derived from ectoderm, whereas its internal surface is composed of a simple squamous to cuboidal epithelium derived from endoderm. A thin layer of mesodermal elements, including collagen fibers, elastic fibers, and fibroblasts, is interposed between the two epithelial layers of the tympanic membrane. This membrane receives sound waves transmit-

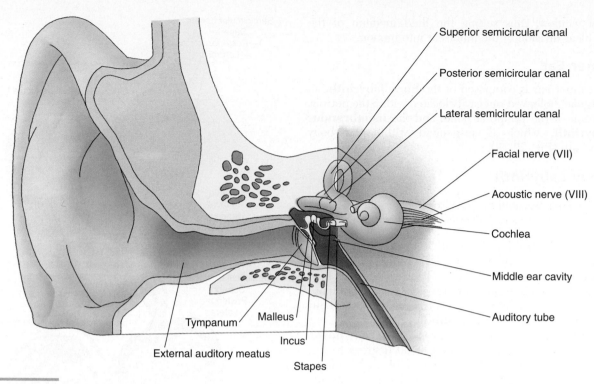

Figure 22–12 Anatomy of the ear.

ted to it by air through the external auditory meatus, which cause it to vibrate. In this fashion, the sound waves are converted into mechanical energy that is transmitted to the bony ossicles in the middle ear.

Middle Ear

The middle ear (tympanic cavity) houses the three bony ossicles: the malleus, the incus, and the stapes.

The middle ear, or **tympanic cavity,** is an air-filled space located in the petrous portion of the temporal bone. This space communicates posteriorly with the mastoid air cells and anteriorly, via the **auditory tube (eustachian tube),** with the pharynx (see Fig. 22-12). The three bony ossicles are housed in this space, spanning the distance between the tympanic membrane and the membrane at the oval window.

The tympanic cavity is lined by simple squamous epithelium, which is continuous with the internal lining of the tympanic membrane. In its deepest two thirds, however, the bone of the tympanic cavity gives way to cartilage as it approaches the auditory tube. Similarly, its epithelial covering becomes a pseudostratified ciliated columnar epithelium as it approaches the auditory tube. The lamina propria over the bony wall adheres to it tightly and does not contain glands, but the lamina propria overlying the cartilaginous portion contains

many mucous glands whose ducts open into the lumen of the tympanic cavity. Additionally, goblet cells and lymphoid tissue are found in the vicinity of the pharyngeal opening.

During swallowing, blowing the nose, and yawning, the orifice of the auditory tube at the pharynx opens, permitting an equalization of air pressure in the tympanic cavity with that in the external auditory meatus, which is located on the opposite side of the tympanic membrane. This is why swallowing, blowing one's nose, or yawning relieves the "ear pressure" that occurs during rapid descent when one is flying in an airplane.

Located within the medial wall of the tympanic cavity are the **oval window** and the **round window,** which connect the middle ear cavity to the inner ear. These two windows are formed by membrane-covered voids in the bony wall. The bony ossicles, the **malleus, incus,** and **stapes** are articulated in series by synovial joints lined with simple squamous epithelium. The malleus is attached to the tympanic membrane, with the incus interposed between it and the stapes, which in turn is attached to the oval window. Two small skeletal muscles, the **tensor tympani** and the **stapedius,** modulate movements of the tympanic membrane and the bony ossicles to prevent damage from loud sounds. Vibrations of the tympanic membrane set the ossicles into motion, and because of their lever action, the oscillations are magnified to vibrate the membrane of the oval window, thus setting the fluid medium of the cochlear division of the inner ear into motion.

Inner Ear

The inner ear is composed of the **bony labyrinth,** an irregular, hollowed-out cavity located within the petrous portion of the temporal bone, and the **membranous labyrinth,** which is suspended within the bony labyrinth (Fig. 22-13).

Bony Labyrinth

> *The bony labyrinth has three components: the semicircular canals, the vestibule, and the cochlea.*

The bony labyrinth is lined with endosteum and is separated from the membranous labyrinth by the **perilymphatic space.** This space is filled with a clear fluid called the **perilymph,** within which the membranous labyrinth is suspended. The central region of the bony labyrinth is known as the **vestibule.**

The three **semicircular canals (superior, posterior,** and **lateral)** are oriented at 90 degrees to one another (see Fig. 22-13). One end of each canal is enlarged; this expanded region is called the **ampulla.** All three semicircular canals arise and return to the vestibule, but one end of each of two of the canals shares an opening to the vestibule; consequently, there are only five orifices to the vestibule. Suspended within the canals are the **semicircular ducts,** which are regionally named continuations of the membranous labyrinth.

The **vestibule** is the central portion of the bony labyrinth located between the anteriorly placed cochlea and the posteriorly placed semicircular canals. Its lateral wall contains the **oval window (fenestra vestibuli),** covered by a membrane to which the footplate of the stapes is attached, and the **round window (fenestra cochleae),** covered only by a membrane. The vestibule also houses specialized regions of the membranous labyrinth (the **utricle** and the **saccule**).

The **cochlea** arises as a hollow bony spiral that turns upon itself, like a snail shell, two and one-half times around a central bony column, the **modiolus.** The modiolus projects into the spiraled cochlea with a shelf of bone called the **osseous spiral lamina,** through which traverse blood vessels and the **spiral ganglion,** the cochlear division of the vestibulocochlear nerve.

Membranous Labyrinth

> *The membranous labyrinth is filled with endolymph and possesses the following specialized areas: the saccule and utricle, the semicircular ducts, and the cochlear duct.*

The membranous labyrinth is composed of an epithelium derived from the embryonic ectoderm, which

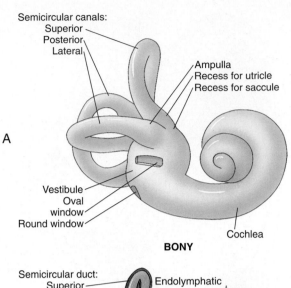

A

Semicircular canals:
Superior
Posterior
Lateral
Ampulla
Recess for utricle
Recess for saccule
Vestibule
Oval window
Round window
Cochlea

BONY

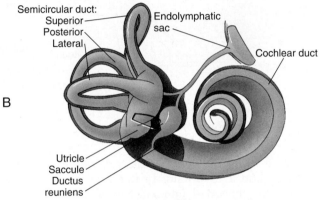

B

Semicircular duct:
Superior
Posterior
Lateral
Endolymphatic sac
Cochlear duct
Utricle
Saccule
Ductus reuniens

MEMBRANOUS

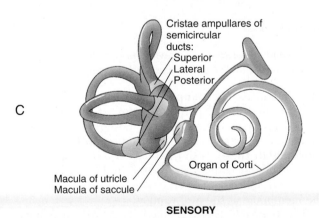

C

Cristae ampullares of semicircular ducts:
Superior
Lateral
Posterior
Organ of Corti
Macula of utricle
Macula of saccule

SENSORY

Figure 22–13 Cochlea of the inner ear. **A,** Anatomy of bony labyrinth. **B,** Anatomy of the membranous labyrinth. **C,** Sensory labyrinth.

invades the developing temporal bone and gives rise to two small sacs, the **saccule** and **utricle,** as well as to the **semicircular ducts** and the **cochlear duct** (see Fig. 22-13). Circulating through the entire membranous labyrinth is **endolymph,** a viscous fluid that resembles extracellular fluid in its ionic composition (i.e., it is sodium-poor but potassium-rich).

Thin strands of connective tissue attached to the endosteum of the bony labyrinth pass through the perilymph to be inserted into the membranous labyrinth. In addition to anchoring the membranous labyrinth to the bony labyrinth, these connective tissue strands carry blood vessels that nourish the epithelia of the membranous labyrinth.

Saccule and Utricle

The saccule and utricle, sac-like structures lying in the vestibule, contain neuroepithelial cells that are specialized to sense position of the head and linear movement.

The saccule and utricle are connected to each other by a small duct, the **ductus utriculosaccularis.** Additionally, small ducts from each join to form the **endolymphatic duct,** whose dilated blind end is known as the **endolymphatic sac.** Another small duct, the **ductus reuniens,** joins the saccule with the duct of the cochlea (see Fig. 22-13).

The walls of the saccule and utricle are composed of a thin outer vascular layer of connective tissue and an inner layer of simple squamous to low cuboidal epithelium. Specialized regions of the saccule and utricle act as receptors for sensing orientation of the head relative to gravity and acceleration, respectively. These receptors are called the **macula of the saccule** and the **macula of the utricle.**

The maculae of the saccule and utricle are located so that they are perpendicular to each other (i.e., the macula of the saccule is located predominantly in the wall, thus detecting linear vertical acceleration, whereas the macula of the utricle is located mostly in the floor, thus detecting linear horizontal acceleration). The epithelium of the nonreceptor regions of the saccule and utricle is composed of light and dark cells. **Light cells** have a few microvilli, and their cytoplasm contains a few pinocytotic vesicles, ribosomes, and only a small number of mitochondria. The cytoplasm of the **dark cells,** however, contains an abundance of coated vesicles, smooth vesicles, and lipid droplets as well as numerous elongated mitochondria located in compartments formed by infoldings of the basal plasma membrane. Nuclei of the dark cells are irregular in shape and are often located apically. Although the function of these two cell types is not known, it is thought that light cells play a role in absorption and that dark cells control endolymph composition.

The maculae are thickened areas of the epithelium, 2 to 3 mm in diameter. They are composed of two types of **neuroepithelial cells** called **type I and type II hair cells,** as well as of supporting cells that sit on a basal lamina (Figs 22-14 and 22-15). Nerve fibers from the vestibular division of the vestibulocochlear nerve supply the neuroepithelial cells.

Each type I or type II hair cell has a single kinocilium and 50 to 100 stereocilia arranged in rows according to length, with the longest (10 μm) being nearest the kinocilium.

Type I hair cells are plump cells with a rounded base that narrows toward the neck (see Fig. 22-15). Their cytoplasm contains occasional RER, a supranuclear Golgi complex, and numerous small vesicles. Each stereocilium, which is anchored in a dense terminal web, is a long microvillus with a core of many actin filaments cross-linked by **fimbrin.** The filamentous core imparts rigidity to the stereocilia, so that bending can occur only in the neck region, near their site of origin from the apical plasma membrane.

Type II hair cells are similar to type I hair cells with regard to the stereocilia and kinocilium, but their shape is more columnar and their cytoplasm contains a larger Golgi complex and more vesicles (see Fig. 22-15).

Supporting cells of the maculae, which are interposed between both types of hair cells, have a few microvilli. Thick junctional complexes bind these cells to each other and to the hair cells. They exhibit a well-developed Golgi complex and secretory granules, suggesting that they may help maintain the hair cells or may contribute to the production of endolymph.

Innervation of the hair cells is derived from the vestibular division of the vestibulocochlear nerve. The rounded bases of the type I hair cells are almost entirely surrounded by a cup-shaped afferent nerve fiber. Type II hair cells exhibit many afferent fibers synapsing on the basal area of the cell. Structures resembling **synaptic ribbons** are present near the bases of type I and type II hair cells. The synaptic ribbons of the type II hair cells probably function in synapses with efferent nerves, which are thought to be responsible for increasing the efficiency of synaptic release.

The stereocilia of the neuroepithelial hair cells are covered by and embedded in a thick, gelatinous glycoprotein mass, the **otolithic membrane.** The surface region of this membrane contains small calcium carbonate crystals known as **otoliths** or **otoconia** (see Figs. 22-14 and 22-15).

Semicircular Ducts

Each of the three semicircular ducts contains an expanded region, the ampulla, where specialized receptors (neuroepithelial hair cells) sense linear and angular movement.

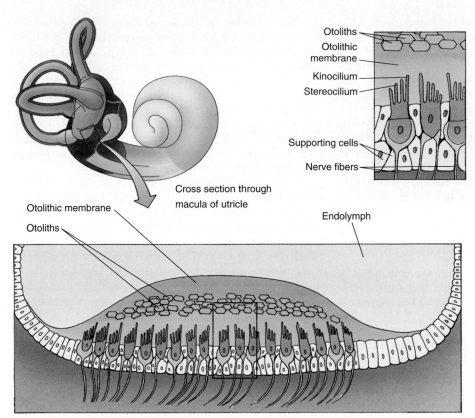

Otoliths
Otolithic membrane
Kinocilium
Stereocilium
Supporting cells
Nerve fibers

Cross section through macula of utricle

Otolithic membrane

Otoliths

Endolymph

Figure 22–14 Hair cells and supporting cells in the macula of the utricle.

Each semicircular duct, a continuation of the membranous labyrinth arising from the utricle, is housed within its semicircular canal and thus conforms to its shape. Each of the three ducts is dilated at its lateral end (near the utricle). These expanded regions, called the **ampullae,** contain the **cristae ampullares,** which are specialized receptor areas. Each crista ampullaris is composed of a ridge whose free surface is covered by sensory epithelium consisting of **neuroepithelial hair cells** and **supporting cells** (Fig. 22-16). The supporting cells sit on the basal lamina, whereas the hair cells do not; rather, the hair cells are cradled between the supporting cells. The neuroepithelial cells, also known as **type I** and **type II hair cells,** exhibit the same morphology as the hair cells of the maculae (discussed earlier). The **cupula,** a gelatinous glycoprotein mass overlying the cristae ampulares, is similar to the otolithic membrane in structure and function, but it is cone-shaped and does not contain otoliths.

Cochlear Duct and Organ of Corti

The cochlear duct and its organ of Corti are responsible for the mechanism of hearing.

The cochlear duct, a diverticulum of the saccule, is another regionally named portion of the membranous labyrinth. The cochlear duct is a wedge-shaped receptor organ housed in the bony cochlea and surrounded on two sides by perilymph but separated from it by two membranes (Figs. 22-17 and 22-18). The roof of the **scala media (cochlear duct)** is the **vestibular (Reissner's) membrane,** whereas the floor of the scala media is the **basilar membrane.** The perilymph-filled compartment lying above the vestibular membrane is called the **scala vestibuli,** whereas the perilymph-filled compartment lying below the basilar membrane is the **scala tympani.** These two compartments communicate at the **helicotrema,** near the apex of the cochlea.

The **vestibular membrane** is composed of two layers of squamous epithelia separated from each other by a basal lamina. The inner layer is the lining cells of the scala media, and the outer layer is the lining cells of the scala vestibuli. Numerous tight junctions seal both layers of cells, thus ensuring a high ionic gradient across the membrane. The **basilar membrane,** extending from the spiral lamina at the modiolus to the lateral wall, supports the organ of Corti and is composed of two zones: the zona arcuata and the zona pectinata. The **zona arcuata** is thinner, lies more medial, and supports the organ of Corti. The **zona pectinata** is similar to a fibrous meshwork containing a few fibroblasts.

The lateral wall of the cochlear duct, extending between the vestibular membrane and the spiral

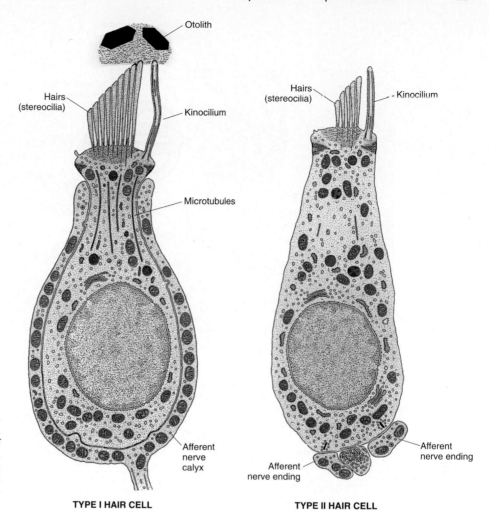

Otolith

Hairs (stereocilia)

Kinocilium

Microtubules

Afferent nerve calyx

TYPE I HAIR CELL

Hairs (stereocilia)

Kinocilium

Afferent nerve ending

Afferent nerve ending

TYPE II HAIR CELL

Figure 22–15 The morphology of type I and type II neuroepithelial (hair) cells of the maculae of the saccule and utricle. (From Lentz TL: Cell Fine Structure: An Atlas of Drawings of Whole-Cell Structure. Philadelphia, WB Saunders, 1971.)

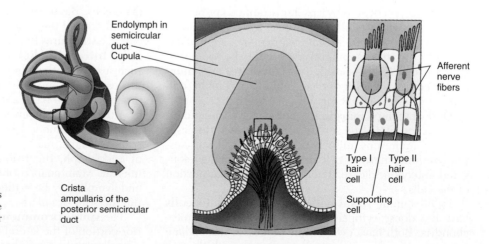

Endolymph in semicircular duct

Cupula

Afferent nerve fibers

Type I hair cell

Type II hair cell

Supporting cell

Crista ampullaris of the posterior semicircular duct

Figure 22–16 The hair cells and supporting cells in one of the cristae ampullares of the semicircular canals.

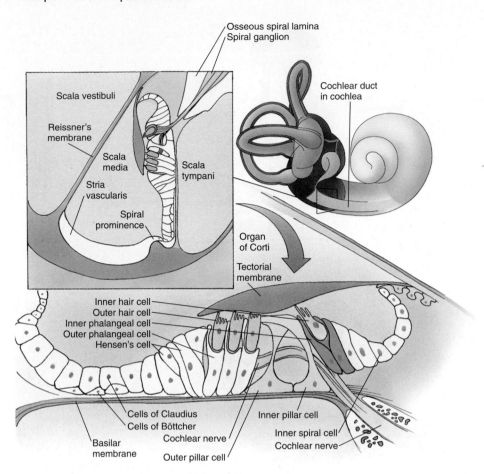

Figure 22–17 Organ of Corti.

prominence, is covered by a pseudostratified epithelium called the **stria vascularis.** Unlike most epithelia, it contains an *intraepithelial plexus of capillaries.* Although the stria vascularis is reported to be composed of three cell types—**basal, intermediate,** and **marginal cells**—the three types closely resemble one another in electron micrographs.

Dark-staining **marginal cells** have abundant microvilli on their free surfaces. Their dense cytoplasm contains numerous mitochondria and small vesicles. Labyrinthine, narrow cell processes containing elongated mitochondria are abundant on the basilar portion of the cells.

Light-staining **basal cells** and **intermediate cells** have less dense cytoplasm containing only a few mitochondria. Both have cytoplasmic processes that radiate out from the cell surfaces to interdigitate with the cell processes of the marginal cells and with other interme-

diate cells. Basal cells also have cellular processes that ascend around the bases of the marginal cells, forming cup-like structures that isolate and support the marginal cells. **Intraepithelial capillaries** are positioned in such a fashion that they are surrounded by the basal processes of the marginal cells and the ascending processes of the basal and intermediate cells.

Although it has been suggested that a number of cells in the membranous labyrinth, including those of the stria vascularis, may be responsible for the production of endolymph, the true nature of its origin remains unclear. Maintenance of the ionic composition of the endolymph may be a function of the marginal cells of the the stria vascularis.

The **spiral prominence** is also located on the inferior portion of the lateral wall of the cochlear duct. It is a small protuberance that juts out from the periosteum of the cochlea into the cochlear duct throughout its

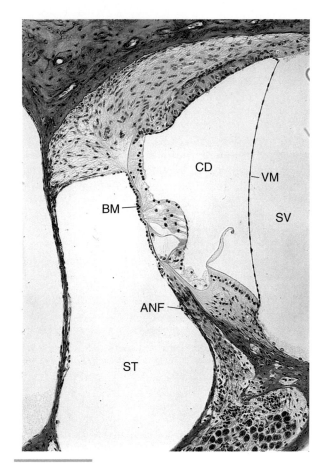

Figure 22–18 Light micrograph of the organ of Corti sitting on the basilar membrane (BM) within the cochlea (×180). The cochlear duct (CD), containing endolymph, is limited by the vestibular membrane (VM) and the BM. The scala vestibuli (SV) and the scala tympani (ST) contain perilymph. Observe the spiral ganglion and the vestibulocochlear (acoustic) nerve fibers (ANF) coming from the hair cells of the organ of Corti.

entire length. The basal cells of the stria vascularis are continuous with the vascular layer of cells covering the prominence. Inferiorly, these cells are reflected into the spiral sulcus, where they become cuboidal. Other cells of this layer continue onto the basilar lamina as the **cells of Claudius,** which overlie the smaller **cells of Böttcher** (see Fig. 22-17). The latter cells are located only in the basilar turns of the cochlea. The function of the cells of Claudius and Böttcher is unknown.

At the narrowest portion of the cochlear duct, where the vestibular and basilar membranes meet, periosteum covering the spiral lamina bulges out into the scala media, forming the **limbus of the spiral lamina.** Part of the limbus projects over the **internal spiral sulcus (tunnel).** The upper portion of the limbus is the **vestibular lip,** and the lower portion is called the **tym-**

panic lip of the limbus, a continuation of the basilar membrane. Numerous perforations in the tympanic lip accommodate branches of the cochlear division of the vestibulocochlear nerve (acoustic nerve). **Interdental cells** located within the body of the spiral limbus secrete the **tectorial membrane,** a proteoglycan-rich gelatinous mass containing numerous fine keratin-like filaments, that overlies the organ of Corti. Stereocilia of specialized receptor hair cells of the organ of Corti are embedded in the tectorial membrane (see Fig. 22-17).

The **organ of Corti,** the specialized receptor organ for hearing, lies on the basilar membrane and is composed of neuroepithelial hair cells and several types of supporting cells. Although the supporting cells of the organ of Corti have different characteristics, they all originate on the basilar membrane and contain bundles of microtubules and microfilaments, and their apical surfaces are all interconnected at the free surface of the organ of Corti. Supporting cells include **pillar cells, phalangeal cells, border cells,** and **cells of Hensen** (see Figs. 22-17 and 22-18).

SUPPORTING CELLS OF THE ORGAN OF CORTI

The supporting cells of the organ of Corti are the inner and outer pillar cells, the inner and outer phalangeal cells, the border cells, the cells of Hensen, and the cells of Böttcher.

Inner and **outer pillar cells** are tall cells with wide bases and apical ends; thus, they are shaped like an elongated "I." They are attached to the basilar membrane, and each one arises from a broad base. The central portions of both inner and outer pillar cells are deflected to form the walls of the **inner tunnel,** where the inner pillar cells form the medial wall of the tunnel and the outer pillar cells form the lateral wall of the tunnel. At their apices, both inner and outer pillar cells are again in contact with each other. Their cytoplasm contains bundles of microfilaments and microtubules. Inner pillar cells outnumber outer pillar cells, with three inner pillar cells usually abutting two outer pillar cells. The pillar cells support the hair cells of the organ of Corti.

Outer phalangeal cells are tall columnar cells that are attached to the basilar membrane. Their apical portions are cup-shaped to support the basilar portions of the outer hair cells along with bundles of efferent and afferent nerve fibers, which pass between them on their way to the hair cells. Because their cup-shaped apices cradle the hair cells, the outer phalangeal cells do not reach the free surface of the organ of Corti. However, originating from the lateral aspect of each of these cells is a small **phalangeal process** that extends to the reticular lamina. Microtubules and microfilaments within the phalangeal process add to its rigidity. The distal, flattened end of the phalangeal process is in contact with its cradled hair cell and an adjacent hair cell. There is a fluid-filled gap around unsupported regions of the outer hair cells. This space is called the **space of Nuel,** and it communicates with the inner tunnel.

Inner phalangeal cells are located deep to the inner pillar cells; unlike the outer phalangeal cells, they completely surround the inner hair cells they support.

Border cells delineate the inner border of the organ of Corti. They are slender cells that support the inner aspects of the organ of Corti.

Cells of Hensen define the outer border of the organ of Corti. These tall cells are located between the outer phalangeal cells and the shorter cells of Claudius, which rest on the underlying **cells of Böttcher.**

All of these cells support the outer aspects of the organ of Corti (see Fig. 22-17).

NEUROEPITHELIAL CELLS (HAIR CELLS) OF THE ORGAN OF CORTI

There are two types of neuroepithelial cells in the organ of Corti: inner hair cells and outer hair cells.

Neuroepithelial hair cells are specialized for transducing impulses for the organ of hearing. Depending on their locations, these cells are called inner hair cells and outer hair cells.

Inner hair cells, a single row of cells supported by inner phalangeal cells, extend the inner limit of the entire length of the organ of Corti. Inner hair cells are short and exhibit a centrally located nucleus, numerous mitochondria (especially beneath the terminal web), RER and SER, and small vesicles. The basal aspect of these cells also contains microtubules. Their apical surface contains 50 to 60 stereocilia arranged in a "V" shape. The core of the stereocilia contains microfilaments, cross-linked with fimbrin, as in the type I hair cells of the vestibular labyrinth. The microfilaments of the stereocilia merge with those of the terminal web. Although a kinocilium is not present in inner hair cells, a basal body and centriole are both evident in the apical region of these cells. The basal aspects of these cells synapse with afferent fibers of the cochlear division of the vestibulocochlear nerve.

Outer hair cells, supported by outer phalangeal cells, are located near the outer limit of the organ of Corti and are arranged in rows of three (or four) along the entire length of this organ (see Fig. 22-17). The outer hair cells are elongated cylindrical cells whose nuclei are located near their bases. Their cytoplasm contains abundant RER, and their mitochondria are located basally. The cytoplasm of those cells just beneath the lateral walls contains a **cortical lattice,** composed of 5- to 7-nm filaments cross-linked by thinner filaments, that appears to support the cell and resist deformation. Afferent and efferent fibers synapse on the basilar portion of the hair cells. Extending from the apical surface of the outer hair cells are as many as 100 stereocilia organized in the shape of the letter "W." These stereocilia vary in length and are arranged in ordered gradation. Like inner hair cells, outer hair cells do not have a kinocilium but do have a basal body.

Vestibular Function

The vestibular function is the sense of position in space and during movement.

The sense of position in space and during movement is essential to activate and deactivate certain muscles that function in accommodating the body for balance. The sensory mechanism for this function is the **vestibular apparatus,** which is located in the inner ear. This apparatus comprises the utricle, saccule, and semicircular ducts.

Stereocilia of neuroepithelial hair cells located in the ampullae of the utricle and saccule are embedded in the otolithic membrane. **Linear movements** of the head cause displacement of the endolymph, which disturbs the positioning of the otoliths within the otolithic membrane and, consequently, the membrane itself, thereby bending the stereocilia of the hair cells. Movements of the stereocilia are transduced into action potentials, which are conducted by synapses to the vestibular division of the vestibulocochlear nerve for transmittal to the brain.

Circular movements of the head are sensed by receptor sites in the semicircular ducts housed within the semicircular canals. Stereocilia of the neuroepithelial hair cells of the cristae ampullares are embedded in the cupula. Movements of the endolymph within the semicircular ducts disturb the orientation of the cupula, which subsequently distorts the stereocilia of the hair cells. This mechanical stimulus is transduced to an electrical impulse, which is transferred by synapse to branches of the vestibular division of the vestibulocochlear nerve for transmission to the brain.

Information concerning the linear and circular movements of the head, recognized by receptors of the inner ear, is transmitted to the brain via the vestibular division of the vestibulocochlear nerve. There, it is interpreted, and adjustments to the balance are initiated by activation of specific muscle masses responsible for posture.

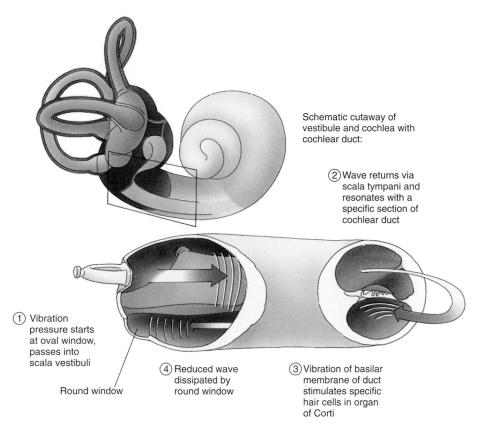

Schematic cutaway of vestibule and cochlea with cochlear duct:

② Wave returns via scala tympani and resonates with a specific section of cochlear duct

① Vibration pressure starts at oval window, passes into scala vestibuli

Round window

④ Reduced wave dissipated by round window

③ Vibration of basilar membrane of duct stimulates specific hair cells in organ of Corti

Figure 22–19 Schematic diagram showing how vibrations of the footplate of the stapes move the membrane on the oval window. This action produces a pressure in the perilymph, located in the scala vestibuli. At the helicotrema, where the scala vestibuli and scala tympani communicate, the pressure wave within the perilymph of the scala tympani sets the basilar membrane and the organ of Corti, sitting on it, into motion. This causes a shearing motion on the hair cells of the basilar membrane, which is transduced into an electric current and in turn is transmitted by a synapse to the cochlear division of the vestibulocochlear nerve for conduction to the brain for processing.

CLINICAL CORRELATIONS

Meniere's Disease is a disorder characterized by hearing loss resulting from excess fluid accumulation in the endolymphatic duct. Other symptoms include vertigo, tinnitus, nausea, and vomiting. Some drugs can relieve vertigo and nausea. However, in severe cases the vestibular division nerve may have to be severed, and the semicircular canals and cochlea may have to be surgically removed.

Cochlear Functions

The cochlea functions in the perception of sound.

Sound waves collected by the external ear pass into the external auditory meatus and are received by the tympanic membrane, which is set into motion. The tympanic membrane converts sound waves into mechanical energy. Vibrations of the tympanic membrane set the malleus, and consequently the remaining two ossicles, into motion.

Because of a mechanical advantage rendered by the articulations of the three bony ossicles, the mechanical energy is amplified about 20 times when it reaches the footplate of the stapes, where it impinges on the membrane of the fenestra vestibuli (oval window). Movements of the oval window membrane initiate pressure waves in the perilymph within the scala vestibuli. Because fluid (in this instance, perilymph) is incompressible, the wave is passed through the scala vestibuli, through the helicotrema, and into the scala tympani. The pressure wave in the perilymph of the scala tympani causes the basilar membrane to vibrate.

Because the organ of Corti is firmly attached to the basilar membrane, a rocking motion within the basilar membrane is translated into a shearing motion on the stereocilia of the hair cells that are embedded in the overlying rigid tectorial membrane. When the shearing force produces a deflection of the stereocilia toward the taller stereocilia, the cell becomes depolarized, thus generating an impulse that is transmitted via the afferent nerve fibers of the cochear division of the vestibulocochear nerve (Fig. 22-19).

How differences in sound frequency or pitch are distinguished is not understood. It has long been thought that the basilar membrane, which becomes longer with each turn of the cochlea, vibrates at different frequencies relative to its width. Therefore, low-frequency sounds would be detected near the apex of the cochlea, whereas high-frequency sounds would be detected near the base of the cochlea. Evidence suggests that outer hair cells contain the necessary machinery to react rapidly to efferent input, causing them to vary the length of their stereocilia and consequently altering the shear force between the tectorial membrane and the basilar membrane, thus "tuning" the basilar membrane. This action then alters the response of the sound-detecting inner hair cells, affecting their reaction to different frequencies.

CLINICAL CORRELATIONS

Conductive deafness may be caused by any condition that impedes the conduction of the sound waves from the external ear through the middle ear and into the organ of Corti of the inner ear. Conditions that can lead to conductive deafness include the presence of foreign bodies, **otitis media,** and **otosclerosis** (fixation of the footplate of the stapes in the oval window).

Otitis media is a common infection of the middle ear cavity in young children. It usually develops from a respiratory infection that involves the auditory tube. Fluid buildup in the middle ear cavity dampens the tympanic membrane, thus constricting the movements of the bony ossicles. Antibiotics are the usual treatment.

Nerve deafness usually results from a disease process that interrupts transmission of the nerve impulse. The interruption may be located anywhere in the cochlear division of the acoustic nerve, from the organ of Corti to the brain. Disease processes that can lead to nerve deafness include rubella, tumors of the nerve, and nerve degeneration.

Index

Note: Page numbers followed by the letter b refer to boxed material; those followed by the letter f refer to figures, and those followed by t refer to tables.

A

α-actin, 43, 45f
α-actinin
  in cytoskeleton, 44t, 45f
  in epithelium, 99
  in skeletal muscle, 164, 165t
  in smooth muscle, 182
A antigens, 224, 224t
A bands
  in cardiac muscle, 178f
  in skeletal muscle, 160, 161f, 162, 162f
α cells, 420, 421, 421t
α-chains
  in tropocollagen, 73, 75, 76t
  synthesis of, 75, 77f
α-globulins, 221t
α-granules, of platelets, 233, 233f, 236t
A-kinase, 22
α-melanocyte-stimulating hormone (α-
  MSH), 310
α-motor neurons, 169, 173, 174f
A-site, ribosomal, 22
α-tubulin, 43f
Abluminal plasmalemma, of capillaries,
  263, 264
ABO blood group system, 224, 224t
Absorption
  by colon, 409
  by small intestine, 405–406, 407f
Absorption cavities, of bone, 152
Accessional teeth (molars), 368, 373
Accessory genital glands, 490f, 504–507
Accessory structures, of eye, 515f,
  525–526
Accommodation, 517, 519b
Acellular cementum, 370
Acetyl coenzyme A (acetyl CoA), 36, 40,
  173b
Acetylcholine
  as neurotransmitter, 203, 204t
  in autonomic nervous system, 208
  in gallbladder, 436
  in HCl secretion, 396
  in lacrimal gland, 184
  in signaling, 20
  in skeletal muscle contraction, 170–171
  in smooth muscle synapses, 182

Acetylcholine (Continued)
  receptors for, 171
    pancreatic, 419
  suprarenal release of, 324
Acetylcholinesterase, 171
Acid hydrolases, 35
Acidophil(s), in pituitary gland, 308, 308f,
  309f
Acidophilic components, 2
Acidosis, 432b
Acinar cells
  mammary, 487f
  pancreatic, 418–419, 418f, 419f
Acinar glands, 107, 107f
Acinus(i)
  hepatic (liver, portal), 426
  in sebaceous glands, 339
  of mixed glands, 104, 104f
  of multicellular exocrine glands, 107, 109f
  of Rappaport, 426
  of salivary gland, 104f, 107, 109f,
    413–414, 414f
  pancreatic, 418, 418f, 419f
Acne, 339b
Acoustic (vestibulocochlear) nerve, 527f,
  528, 529, 531f, 535, 535f
Acquired immunodeficiency syndrome
  (AIDS), 196b, 287b
Acromegaly, 154b
Acrosin, 480, 496
Acrosomal cap, 495, 496f
Acrosomal granule, 495, 497f
Acrosomal phase, of spermiogenesis, 496,
  497f
Acrosomal reaction, 480, 497
Acrosomal vesicle, 495, 497f
Acrosome, 495, 496f
Actin-binding proteins, 43, 44t
Actin filaments
  as vesicle pathway, 31
  bundles of, 43–44
  in cytokinesis, 65
  in cytoplasm, 42, 43, 43f, 44, 44t, 45f
  in eccrine sweat glands, 338
  in epithelial microvilli, 90–91, 93f, 94f
  in erythrocyte cell membrane, 224, 224f
  in skeletal muscle, 161, 164f, 166–167
  in zonulae adherentes, 99

Actin monomer, 43f
Actin ring, of osteoclast, 141
Action potential
  cycle of, 200
  mechanism of, 198–200, 200f
  of cardiac muscle, 178–179
  of skeletal muscle, 171, 178
Activated cells, in immune response,
  276
Activated macrophages, 123
Activation
  of B cells, 280
  of lymphoid cells, 285
Activation gate, 199
Active catalytic subunits, of A-kinase, 22
Active sites
  of synapse, 201
  on axon terminal, 170
  on G-actin, 166
Active transport, 17, 18f, 19
  primary, by Na^+-K^+ pump, 19
  secondary, by coupled carrier proteins,
    20
Activin, ovarian, 466, 468, 472, 473t
Acute myeloblastic leukemia, 246b
Acute myelogenous leukemia, 66b
Adaptin, 31
Adaptive immune system, 273, 276
Addison's disease, 322b, 332b
Adducin, 224
Adenocarcinoma, 102b
  of prostate, 507b
Adenohypophysis, 304, 306–310
Adenoid, 299
Adenoma(s)
  benign pleomorphic, 417b
  pituitary, 311b
Adenosine diphosphate (ADP)
  and clot formation, 233
  in active transport, 19
  in muscle contraction, 168, 168f
Adenosine triphosphate (ATP)
  binding to heavy merosin, 165
  in active transport, 19
  in chromaffin cells, 323
  in mitochondria, 39f, 40
  in muscle contraction, 167, 168, 168f
  in signaling, 20